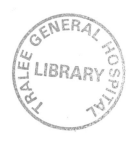

615.5/LAW

y's
plementary &
ative Medicine
CH-BASED APPROACH

Mosby's
Complementary &
Alternative Medicine
A RESEARCH-BASED APPROACH

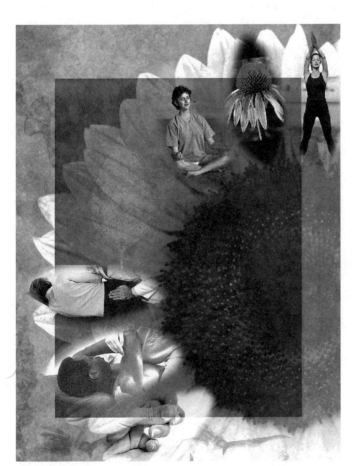

Lyn W. Freeman, PhD
G. Frank Lawlis, PhD

Mosby

A Harcourt Health Sciences Company

St. Louis   London   Philadelphia   Sydney   Toronto

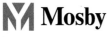

A Harcourt Health Sciences Company

Editor-in-Chief: John Schrefer
Editors: Kellie White
Associate Developmental Editor: Leslie Mosby
Project Manager: Gayle Morris
Internal Design: Dana Peick
Cover Design: Amy Buxton

Mosby, Inc.
A Harcourt Health Sciences Company
11830 Westline Industrial Drive
St. Louis, Missouri 63146

Printed in the United States of America

ISBN 0-323-00697-3

00 01 02 03 04 GC/KPT 9 8 7 6 5 4 3 2 1

Contributors

We gratefully acknowledge the following individuals for the interviews they provided for this text:

Jeanne Achterberg, PhD
Saybrook Institute
San Francisco, California

Robert Ader, PhD
University of Rochester Medical Center
New York, New York

Steven Blair, PhD
Cooper Institute of Aerobics Research
Dallas, Texas

Larry Dossey, MD
Journal of Alternative Therapies in Health and Medicine
Aliso Viejo, California

Helen Erickson, PhD
University of Texas
Austin, Texas

Tiffany Field, PhD
University of Miami School of Medicine
Miami, Florida

Skya Gardner-Abbate, DOM, DiplAc
Southwest Acupuncture College
Santa Fe, New Mexico

Arthur Hastings, PhD
Institute for Transpersonal Psychology
Palo Alto, California

Janice Kiecolt-Glaser, PhD
Ohio State College of Medicine
Columbus, Ohio

G. Frank Lawlis, PhD
Santa Fe Institute of Medicine and Prayer
Santa Fe, New Mexico

Dana Lawrence, DC, FICC
National College of Chiropractic
Lombard, Illinois

Penelope Montgomery, PhD
Health and Rehabilitation Psychology
Kansas City, Missouri

Candace Pert, PhD
Georgetown University Medical Center
Georgetown, Washington, DC

Janet Quinn, PhD
University of Colorado School of Nursing
Denver, Colorado

David Reilly, MD
Glasgow Homeopathic Hospital
Glasgow, Scotland

Beverly Rubik, PhD
Institute for Frontier Science
Oakland, California

Robert H. Schneider, MD
College of Maharishi Medicine, Maharishi University
Fairfield, Iowa

Sandra Sylvester, PhD
Gestalt Institute of Cleveland
Cleveland, Ohio

Andrew Weil, MD
University of Arizona, Program in Integrative Medicine
Tucson, Arizona

Reviewers

Jeanne Achterberg, PhD
Saybrook Institute
San Francisco, California

Larry Dossey, MD
Journal of Alternative Therapies in Health and Medicine
Aliso Viejo, California

Helen Erickson, PhD
University of Texas
Austin, Texas

Skya Gardner-Abbate, DOM, DiplAc
Southwest Acupuncture College
Santa Fe, New Mexico

Harley Goldberg, DO
Kaiser-Permanente Health Systems
San Jose, California

Arthur Hastings, PhD
Institute for Transpersonal Psychology
Palo Alto, California

Joseph Kleinkort, PhD
WorkSTEPS, Inc.
Irving, Texas

Lucille Lawlis-Bennett
BEAR Rehabilitation Center
Anchorage, Alaska

William C. Meeker, DC, MPH
Palmer Center for Chiropractic Research
Davenport, Iowa

Penelope Montgomery, PhD
Health and Rehabilitation Psychology
Kansas City, Missouri

Kathy Murtiashaw, MEd
University of Alaska, Community and Technical College
Anchorage, Alaska

Janet Quinn, PhD
University of Colorado School of Nursing
Denver, Colorado

Beverly Rubik, PhD
Institute for Frontier Science
Oakland, California

Sandra Sylvester, PhD
Gestalt Institute of Cleveland
Cleveland, Ohio

Ruth Townsend, MS
Alaska Regional Hospital Health Management Center
Anchorage, Alaska

Dana Ullman, MPH
University of California
San Francisco, California

Rebecca White, MD
Iliuliuk Family and Health Services
Unalaska, Alaska

To my professor, mentor, and dear friend, Susan Hales, PhD, who always believed in me and who taught me how to think.

To Derek Welton, my husband, companion, and champion. Without your unwavering support and willingness to sacrifice, this book would never have come into being.

Lyn Freeman

Foreword

Education in Alternative Medicine and the Fall of the Bamboo Curtain

In late November 1997, a reporter from *USA Today* interviewed George Lundberg, MD, who was then editor of the *Journal of the American Medical Association (JAMA)*. He was asked to comment on the burgeoning consumer use of complementary and alternative medicines (CAM).

The interview took place only weeks before Lundberg's watershed, December 17, 1997, article in *JAMA* that announced within the year an entire volume of the American Medical Association's (AMA's) flagship journal, together with the AMA's extended family of peer-reviewed publications, would be devoted to scientific studies and editorial content on CAM. Henceforward, the AMA journals would be more open to CAM articles.

The AMA's historic announcement was evidence-based. Consecutive year surveys of editors and advisors to AMA publications discovered a remarkable transformation in attitudes. In a period of only 12 months, the relative rating of CAM as a subject matter for publication in the journals rose from an obscure, bit player (68 of 73 topics) to star billing (in the top 3 among 86 topics).

Lundberg, who would have known these as yet unannounced outcomes and of *JAMA*'s editorial shift at the time of his *USA Today* interview, summed up the moment with a telling metaphor. He spoke of a "bamboo curtain" between alternative and conventional medicine, which he said was "beginning to splinter."

The cold war image is rich in evoking the historic debate over the role of CAM in medicine in the United States. The phrase conjures restrictions on speech, barriers to the free flow of ideas, and fears of reprisal. Consider the need of mainstream providers with a personal interest in or use of CAM keeping this information to themselves or covertly delivering services.

We know that behind such barriers—whether between couples, nations, or health care approaches—ignorance quickly fills with polarizing stories. Each party justifies his or her own place by building up one's positive characteristics and downplaying negative attributes. The party on the other side of the barrier receives the opposite treatment. In a polarized alternative versus conventional medical context, CAM providers are likely to focus on the adverse effects of pharmaceuticals and the over-performance of surgeries. They are less likely to honor the lifesaving qualities of these agents and procedures when appropriately applied. From conventional medicine's perspective, CAM is likely to be painted as "unscientific" without any reference to the limited evidence-based support for many mainstream practices.

The "bamboo curtain" is indeed splintering.

- Numerous studies of physicians find a majority supports the use of one or more CAM treatments.
- Ten years ago, no more than a handful of medical schools offered any education in CAM; by 1997, 75 were doing so.
- Currently, approximately two thirds of health maintenance organizations (HMOs) offer their membership some CAM.
- Of employers offering nonchiropractic CAM in 1999, 50% began doing so in 1995.
- In August 1999 the editorial board of a leading employee benefits periodical published its opinion that employers should "expect to see huge increases in both the credibility and the use of alternative medicine."
- In August 1999 the American Hospital Association (AHA) kicked off a program to help educate the organization's member institutions on how to better offer CAM to AHA members.
- Integrative clinics, in which CAM and conventional providers work side by side, are springing up inside health care systems across the United States.
- At the federal level, direct research into CAM through the National Institutes of Health Center for Complementary and Alternative Medicine swelled to $50 million annually in 1999.

■ Since 1996, numerous other agencies, including the Agency for Health Care Policy and Research, Bureau of Primary Health Care, Centers for Disease Control and Prevention, Health Care Financing Administration, Veterans Administration, and Department of Defense, have each engaged explorations of CAM's role in their service delivery systems.

Today's activity can only be viewed—to extend the cold war metaphor—as a release of pent-up demand and excitement that comes with increased freedom of expression and action. From significant polarization, we have moved in the short space of a half decade toward a discussion of optimal integration. Forward thinkers among all of health care's leading stakeholders are working to discover the appropriate role for CAM products and services for their constituencies. In what ways will CAM help create more effective and cost-effective care?

Resources like Dr. Freeman's text represent free speech moving into a formerly forbidden zone, the leading edge of the system-wide integration process, which will unfold over the next two decades. Newcomers will be pleasantly surprised, upon review of Dr. Freeman's extensive references, to discover what CAM participants have already known: A central problem with CAM science in the United States has not been its existence but its accessibility. Dr. Freeman's book will help make this knowledge available to academics and professionals who choose to integrate this important literature into health care practice.

Given the myriad stresses on mainstream medical payment and delivery at the close of the twentieth century, such integration should be heartily welcomed.

John Weeks
Publisher-Editor, *The Integrator* for the
Business of Alternative Medicine
(<u>onemedicine.com</u>)
Principal, Integration Strategies
for Natural Healthcare
Seattle, Washington

Preface to the Instructor

As an instructor, I know that teaching is more complicated than simply presenting information. A teacher should teach within a framework that is easy to understand, that is readily accessible and enticing to each student, and that challenges the thinking processes. An effective teacher wants to inspire the student to go beyond what is taught and to explore the literature in greater detail. If what is learned by the student is transferred from comprehension to real-life application, the teacher has performed his or her job in a superior manner.

It is my goal to make the process of learning about complementary medicine as intelligible and enjoyable as possible. This does not mean that the information will lack complexity. The information that is covered in this text will be research-dense and application-driven. Printed matter, presented in story format with informative examples, will enhance the learning process. Comments by persons well known in each field, descriptions of timely topics and recent medical advances, case studies, and profiles of the history and philosophy of each discipline will be interwoven into each topic area. Research will be critically reviewed, students will be presented with examples of exceptional and fatally flawed studies, and suggested designs for continuing research will be delineated.

Intended Audience
The domain of complementary medicine cuts across many professional disciplines. This text is written to provide support to as many of those disciplines as possible. The text, in its entirety, provides a comprehensive review of complementary medicine and alternative therapies for health professionals at both the undergraduate and the graduate levels. Graduate students may want to perform research in alternative fields. Detailed descriptions of study designs will provide potential models for replication.

The text is an excellent supplement for continuing education courses. I currently teach much of the information provided in this text as CEU and CME credits for practicing health professionals.

The business sector will also benefit from the information provided in this book. HMOs, hospitals, insurance companies, and health professionals currently struggle with the need to meet client demand for complementary therapies. A review of this text will help these organizations and individuals determine which interventions are safe and appropriate. Physicians, nurses, psychologists, and social workers can determine how to refer patients for alternative care. Health care professionals can teach themselves about the alternative therapies their patients are using, thereby improving their ability to communicate accurately and openly with the patients they serve. Indications and contraindications for therapies are also included, assisting health practitioners in avoiding unexpected complications.

The text can be used in full or in part. For example, psychiatrists, psychologists, and social workers will find Units One and Two (Mind-Body Integration and Mind-Body Interventions) most beneficial. Those individuals interested in learning about the most popular complementary practices will be enlightened by Unit Three (Alternative Professionals). Pharmacists, physical therapists, and fitness trainers will turn their attention to Unit Four (Complementary Self-Help Strategies). Unit Five (Energetics and Spirituality), will appeal to critical care and hospice nurses, environmental health practitioners, and individuals interested in spiritual healing.

Intended Outcome: The Application of Critical Thinking
Critical thinking is disciplined, self-directed, in-depth, rational thinking that leads to clear, relevant, and fair thinking. It is the art of constructive skepticism and of identifying and removing bias, prejudice, and one-sided thought. Critical thinking verifies what we know, and it clarifies and informs when we are ignorant (Paul, 1993, p. 47).

Perhaps no discipline demands critical thinking more than the study of complementary and alternative medicine. Why is this so? All thinking occurs within a domain of thought. That domain is molded by the world view, training, and experiences in the areas being explored. For example, the domain of thought of the medical researcher often resides within the experimental model. The experimental model is the domain most readily accepted as scientifically and medically valid in Western culture. Other cultures problem solve, conceptualize, and reason within different domains of thinking. That which is not measurable by the experimental model is often the foundation of medical systems in other cultures. For example, the chakra system is a frame of reference and the energy called prana, a basic concept of the domain of thinking known as Ayurvedic medicine. The meridian system is a frame of reference and the energy called Qi, a concept underlying the practice of acupuncture. These frames of reference fall within a larger domain of thinking called Chinese medicine. One who studies complementary and alternative medicine must learn to comprehend and effectively evaluate these different systems by thinking critically in the strong sense. There are biologic, mathematical, economic, and psychologic domains of thinking. There are also Ayurvedic, Chinese, and allopathic medicine domains of thinking. One must learn to reason effectively within all of these domains.

Richard Paul, the current leader of the critical thinker movement, points out that critical thinking depends on the ability to adjust one's thinking to differing domains of thought—to conceptualize different questions from various analytical points of view. A critical thinker is capable of effective, accurate, and concise navigation within these differing domains, supporting or disagreeing with various points of view with an unbiased and open mind. Paul goes further. In those instances in which multiple domains of thought must be crossed or are integrated, even more is required. The thinker must perform "higher order" critical thinking. Higher order critical thinking involves:

1. Complexity (the total path is not "visible" from a single vantage point);
2. Multiple solutions, each yielding costs and benefits;
3. Nuanced judgment and interpretation;
4. Application of multiple criteria, which sometimes conflict with one another;
5. Certain amount of uncertainty;
6. Self-regulation of the thinking process;
7. Imposition of meaning (finding structure in apparent disorder); and
8. Effort and considerable mental work (Paul, 1993, p. 282).

For an excellent foundation in critical thinking, I refer the instructor to Paul's (1993) book. For present purposes, I describe the critical thinking strategies that are suggested for this text. I encourage instructors to emphasize these strategies in the classroom to benefit student critical thinking in the strong sense.

Elements of Reasoning

The first strategy refers to using the elements of reasoning, which allow the thinker to avoid trivial, vague, illogical, or superficial thinking. The more important the decision, the more important it is to think systematically and deeply. Therefore before selecting an alternative or, for that matter, a conventional medical treatment, one should formulate, analyze, and assess the following elements:

1. Problem or question at issue (Should this patient be referred, and, if so, for what treatment?)
2. Purpose or goal of thinking (What should be expected from a practitioner? What health goal should be accomplished?)
3. Frame of reference (domain) or point of view involved (e.g., pharmacologic, biochemical, medical, psychologic, Ayurvedic, Chinese medicine)
4. Assumptions (e.g., made by the referring physician, the patient, a practitioner)
5. Central concepts and ideas involved (e.g., healing versus curing, changes in biochemistry versus balancing the prana)
6. Principles or theories underlying the issue (e.g., meridian system versus central nervous system; Qi energy versus stress factors)
7. Evidence, data, or reasons advanced (What research is available?)
8. Interpretations and claims (i.e., those made for treatments, herbs, medications)
9. Inferences, reasoning, and lines of formulated thought (Is the line of reasoning narrow or limited? Is it biased?)
10. Implications and consequences of action or failure to act (Paul, 1993, pp. 422-424)

Perfections of Reasoning

The second strategy refers to the perfections of reasoning (Paul, 1993, pp. 420-421). These perfections refer to thinking, speaking, and writing with clarity, precision, specificity, accuracy, relevance, consistency, logicalness, depth, completeness, significance, fairness, and adequacy (for the purpose). Therefore to apply the strategies of critical thinking to student learning, the instructor should ask students to discuss, in class, questions from the critical thinking section at the end of each chapter. Examples of critical thinking exercises include the following: State precisely (perfection) what evidence or data (element) Ader provided to support his claim (element) that stress can impair immunity. What implications (element) does this have for health care management? Identify, specifically (perfection), the central concepts (element) underpinning acupuncture, and describe the frame of reference (element) on which it was built. What larger domain (element) includes acupuncture, herbology, and Qi Gong?

This book provides the instructor with a ready-made set of critical thinking exercises that will challenge the student and lead to lively dialogue in the classroom. These are intended as only a beginning. It is my hope that instructors will create their own critical thinking exercises to challenge student thinking. The more critical thinking that occurs, the greater the likelihood that learning will be transferred to clinical and problem-solving applications.

Organization and Content

This text is made up of five units encompassing eighteen chapters. Each unit is complete, and individual units can be mastered without compromising subject-matter integrity. The following overview of the text's organization is provided:

Unit One: Mind-Body Integration. Chapter 1 clarifies the pathways of mind-body communications including, the hypothalamic-pituitary-adrenal pathway. Methods for alleviating stress are described, and the work of Candace Pert is emphasized. In Chapter 2, the lines of evidence for the mind's influence on the body are explored, including observational, physiologic, epidemiologic, and clinical research. The immune system is summarized and encapsulated. The history and evolution of the field of psychoneuroimmunology are discussed in Chapter 3. The works of Robert Ader and Nicholas Cohen are synopsized. How physiology and immune cells become conditioned by experience and environment is described. In Chapter 4, the effects of relationships and stressful life events on health are elucidated. The work of Janice Kiecolt-Glaser is summarized.

Unit Two: Mind-Body Interventions. Chapters 5 through 9 present the definitions, history, philosophy, mechanisms, and clinical trials of five mind-body interventions. In Chapter 5, the relaxation response is elucidated, and clinical studies of relaxation as intervention are evaluated.

Theoretical models of relaxation and pain control are discussed, and indications and contraindications for relaxation therapies are defined. In Chapter 6, meditation forms are differentiated and meditation as therapy is considered. Chapter 7 evaluates biofeedback for the treatment of acute and chronic disease. In Chapter 8, hypnosis is described, and hypnosis methods are contrasted with those of relaxation, imagery, and meditation. Imagery for treatment of disease is critiqued in Chapter 9. The differences among imagery, relaxation, and meditation are explored.

Unit Three: Alternative Professionals. In Unit Three, the disciplines of chiropractic, acupuncture, homeopathy, and massage therapy are examined including their definitions, terminologies, history, philosophy, mechanisms, pathways, clinical trials, and indications and contraindications. Methodologic strengths and weaknesses for each discipline are defined.

Chiropractic is examined in Chapter 10. Care is taken to clarify mechanisms and to define traditional and current practices. Systemic effects of chiropractic are considered. Demonstrated effects on beta-endorphin levels, neutrophils, monocytes, and substance P are elucidated.

Chapter 11 explores the philosophic underpinnings of acupuncture, including Tao, yin and yang, the five elements, the eight principles, and the three treasures. The meridian system is reviewed, and acupoints and their electrical conductivity are considered. Physiologic changes induced by acupuncture (e.g., electroencephalographic readings, galvanic skin responses, blood flow, breathing rates) are examined. Effects of acupuncture on the enkephalin, serotonin, and endorphin pathways are investigated. Clinical trials on chronic and acute pain for addiction are emphasized.

Chapter 12 explores the basic concepts and outcomes of homeopathy. The theories of electromagnetic energy and memory of water are described. Homeopathic theories as they relate to Avogadro's law are contemplated.

Chapter 13 summarizes the methodologies of massage therapy; structural, functional, and movement integration methods; and body work interventions. Clinical trials of massage for premature and at-risk infants and for the treatment of anxiety, swelling, and pain are analyzed.

Unit Four: Complementary Self-Help Strategies. Unit Four discusses research outcomes on health-supporting methods used by patients, often without medical supervision. The information presented is valuable because it can be employed by health professionals to maintain their own well-being, as well to advise patients on their self-care.

Chapter 14 explores the history, pharmacology, research, and clinical applications of 10 top-selling herbs in the United States. Special attention is given to contraindications and drug cross reactions. Adverse effects of herbs and health effects of herbs are also discussed.

Chapter 15 reviews the clinical trials on the benefits of exercise interventions as related to longevity, heart disease, cancer, diabetes, stroke, depression, aging, menopause, incontinence, impotence, and HIV and AIDS.

Unit Five: Energetics and Spirituality. Unit Five discusses the most controversial and least researched areas of alternative methods of healing: electromagnetic medicine, spiritual healing (e.g., prayer, distant and intentionality healing), and therapeutic touch.

Chapter 16 discusses electromagnetic spectrum, frequency range, classification, and biologic effects of electromagnetic medicine. Medical applications and clinical outcomes for bioelectromagnetic mechanisms of bone repair, nerve stimulation, wound healing, electroacupuncture, tissue regeneration, immune system stimulation, and neuroendocrine modulations are discussed.

Chapter 17 reviews the spiritual belief systems and clinical outcomes of intercessory prayer and distant intentionality healing. Effects of these interventions and their influences on fungi, bacteria, animals, and human subjects are presented.

Chapter 18 describes the mechanisms and clinical trials of therapeutic touch, a method of healing refined and practiced by nurses. Research on therapeutic touch for anxiety, wound healing, and pain is surveyed.

Special Features

Artwork, Photography, and Figures. Art, photography, and figures play an important role in learning because they allow the student to conceptualize and therefore integrate volumes of information. As will be discussed in Unit Two, imagery is the mind-stuff by which information is experienced, interpreted, stored, and recalled. The use of imagery as a learning tool supports automatic learning and reinforces memory. For example, the artful rendering of the meridian system allows the student to conceptualize acupuncture as an integrated energy system. The meridian system as a frame of reference allows the student to draw connections between the detailed information that follows. Photographs or figures depicting different massage techniques help students conceptualize distinctions among massage methodologies. Art, photography, and figures are liberally sprinkled throughout the text to support learning.

Tables. Tables are used to summarize outcomes from important clinical trials. Thus most chapters will have at least one table that summarizes research on a particular topic in that field.

"A Closer Look." Chapters cover specialized topics. For example, case study reviews, clinical application examples, and medical dilemmas reported in the literature may be summarized. Expanded discussions of important topics may also be discussed. A magnifying glass icon identifies this feature.

"An Expert Speaks." Interviews and comments from well-known researchers and practitioners in each discipline are accentuated. Views on current and future research, descriptions of research contributions, and historical context of research work are expounded. This feature is identified by background color.

In-Chapter Learning Guides

"Why Read this Chapter?" For in-depth learning to occur, the instructor must "hook" the student's curiosity and interest before plowing into the material at hand. This section is intended to provide the reader with a reason for pursuing the chapter. Setting an engaging tone at the beginning of each chapter will encourage students to become committed to the learning process.

"Chapter at a Glance." An opening summary is provided at the beginning of each chapter. It allows the reader to create a clear framework for the more detailed information that is to come. This feature allows the more casual readers to determine whether the chapter is applicable to them and makes the book user-friendly as a reference manual.

"Chapter Objectives." On the second page of each chapter, specific chapter objectives are delineated.

Clinical Terminology and Text Emphasis

When clinical terms relevant to each chapter are first mentioned, a short definition is provided within the body of the text.

Within the text, some headings, words, numbers, or study outcomes are bulleted or typeset in bold to draw attention to critical information. This presentation is beneficial to the reader because some studies are lengthy with multiple outcomes. Bullets are used to break up major points or emphasize different experimental groups. The use of bullets and bold type draws the reader's eye to critical pieces of information, allowing him or her to retain or review data without searching the text.

Review Questions. Multiple choice and matching questions are provided at the end of chapters to encourage thinking. Answers to the questions are located in Appendix B. I want to emphasize that these questions are "knowledge" questions; in other words, accurately answering these questions means only that the reader can essentially repeat what has been presented in the text. To understand the material in the strong sense (i.e., to integrate successfully what is learned for application in complex life scenarios), students must be taught to think critically about what is presented. The critical thinking section that follows will help with the development of these higher order thinking skills.

Critical Thinking and Clinical Application Questions. Critical thinking questions are provided at the end of each chapter. These questions will take more time and effort for students and teachers than knowledge-based questions, because complex, broad, deep, and time-consuming thinking will be elicited. This and only this type of skill practice transforms rote learning into creative and innovative problem-solving processes. Critical thinking exercises will also infuse a lively sense of debate and the sharing of information into the classroom process.

I suggest that students be divided into small groups of three to five persons and assigned one or more questions. Approximately 15 minutes should be allowed for group work, and 3 to 5 minutes are needed for each group to present their findings. The other groups should be asked to offer feedback. Constructive criticism and the strengths of the presentation should be emphasized. Critical thinking comes only with a great deal of practice and is stifled by fear of unbridled and targeted criticism. Each instructor should consider this: Do you want the future physicians, nurses, psychologists, social workers, or manual therapists to be creative problem solvers or mere mechanics? These persons may be offering services to you or your family members some day.

Appendixes. Appendixes offer helpful references for students. They include an overview of research methods and statistics (Appendix A), answers to multiple choice and matching questions (Appendix B), a list of web sites for each topic area (Appendix C), and organizations and associations available for additional information (Appendix D).

Concluding Remarks

It is my hope that the format and content of this text will transform the instructor's experience into a positive and productive one. I would like to hear about your experiences, your suggestions, and any ideas you have for change after using these materials in the classroom. Feel free to write me.

Lyn Freeman, PhD
c/o Mosby, Inc.
Allied Health Editorial
11830 Westline Industrial Drive
St. Louis, Missouri 63146

Paul R: *Critical thinking: what every person needs to survive in a rapidly changing world,* Santa Rosa, CA, 1992, Foundations for Critical Thinking.

Preface to the Student

This text is written to make complex topics unintimidating and enjoyable to learn. The alternative and complementary therapies covered in this book are exciting, dynamic, and evolving disciplines. Learning about them should impart a feeling of interest rather than one of frustration. The text intends to make the research on these topics available to you in one accessible format. To this end, the text is written in such a way as to tell the "story" of each discipline—its history, philosophy, concepts, major players, benefits, failings, and possible future. You will learn to speak the conceptual "language" of each discipline, understand the mind-set of those who helped each discipline evolve, and determine where and how each intervention will fit in the larger scheme of Western medicine.

This information will serve you in a variety of situations. It will help you consider how these alternative therapies may be of value to you, the individual. It will improve your ability to discuss the pros and cons of each method with the patients you will serve. It will allow you to determine if or when cross reactions or contraindications are of concern. This text is created to serve as your guide through what can otherwise be treacherous waters.

The illustrations and tables are designed to assist you in conceptualizing bodies of information at a glance. Tables provide summaries of the most important studies and their outcomes. Illustrations and photographs are included to help you relate to intervention methods. Each "A Closer Look" discusses a case study or clinical applications and medical dilemmas reported in the literature. In each "An Expert Speaks" feature, an interview and comments from well-known researcher and/or practitioner in each discipline are presented. Views on current and future research, descriptions of research contributions, and historical context of research work are expounded.

Learning guides are included to help you structure your learning. At the beginning of each chapter, there are stated objectives. You will also find a chapter review. At the end of the chapters, there are lists of multiple choice, matching, and short essay review question exercises. Most importantly, you will find critical thinking questions that invite you to make many-sided connections between the concepts and information offered. I suggest you first read the objectives and the chapter review, "Chapter At a Glance," and then cruise the major headings of each chapter. This will assist you in structuring a frame of reference for the information to come. Then, and only then, read the entire chapter from scratch. Next, answer all the questions at the end of the chapter. Finally, review the areas where you have questions or need additional time to synthesize the material. Most of all, enjoy what you are learning.

I welcome your comments, suggestions, and ideas for improvement to future editions. Feel free to write to me.

Lyn Freeman, PhD
c/o Mosby, Inc.
Allied Health Editorial
11830 Westline Industrial Drive
St. Louis, Missouri 63146

Table of Contents

Simplified Table of Contents

Mosby's
Complementary &
Alternative Medicine
A RESEARCH-BASED APPROACH

Mind-Body Integration

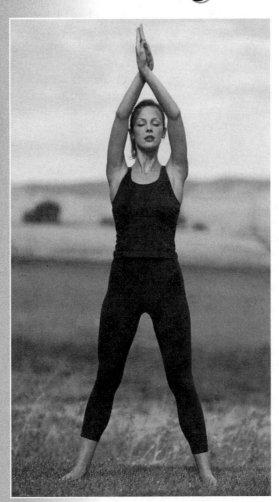

1

Physiologic Pathways of Mind-Body Communication

Lynda W. Freeman

WHY READ THIS CHAPTER?

Chapter 1, "Physiologic Pathways of Mind-Body Communication," explores how what we think and perceive and how we interpret events can alter physiology and biochemistry, affecting health outcomes. In this chapter we answer the question, "By what pathways do these effects occur?"

To understand how stress and emotion can affect health outcomes, it is important to have a clear and complete understanding of the mind-body bi-directional pathways. There are clearly delineated lines of evidence for mind-body communication. These lines of evidence provide information that explains how individuals can take action to modulate the effects of stress on their health. Health management requires an understanding of the potential negative effects of stress and conditioning on health outcomes. It also requires an understanding of what can be done to alleviate some of these negative effects. Chapter 1 defines a simple model of stress management, based on the research explored in this chapter. Sharing the outcomes of this model with patients who must cope with stress may prove beneficial to their health. Application of this model for your own stress management may also be of value.

CHAPTER AT A GLANCE

The mind and body communicate via interactions that occur among the nervous system, the endocrine system, and the immune system. These systems communicate by using two distinctive pathways: the sympathetic-adrenal-medullary axis and the hypothalamic-pituitary-adrenal cortex axis. These pathways use informational substances as messengers. These substances consist of neurotransmitters, neuropeptides, hormones, and immunomodulators. Our interpretation of events and our emotional reactions can affect which informational substances are produced and released at any given moment. These chemical messengers are capable of modulating immune-cell behavior and physiology and thus can affect health outcomes.

Research outcomes have clearly identified a link between emotion and physiologic reactivity and immune competence. Our interpretation of events and our emotional responses to those events are the mechanisms by which the mind affects physiology and biochemistry and, consequently, health outcomes.

Some relatively simple interventions or activities can support or improve immune function, mood state, and health in general. These activities include music and laughter and interventions in the form of group support, counseling, and writing or speaking about traumatic events. Personality style can also have a potential effect on health, with optimistic and pessimistic personality styles becoming topics of study.

> *It is more important to know what sort of a person has a disease than to know what sort of disease a person has.*
>
> HIPPOCRATES

CHAPTER OBJECTIVES

After completing this chapter, you should be able to:

1. Identify the three systems that interact to bring about mind-body effects.
2. Describe the three systems, including the definition and components of each.
3. Define the two brain pathways by which the three systems communicate.
4. Trace the components of the central nervous system through the two divisions of the autonomic nervous system.
5. Define the autonomic nervous system and its two divisions.
6. Name the informational substances used by the sympathetic-adrenal-medullary pathway.
7. Name the informational substances used by the hypothalamic-pituitary-adrenal cortex pathway.
8. Explain the importance of the hypothalamus in mind-body effects.
9. Explain the importance of the limbic system in mind-body effects.
10. Define the stress response.
11. Describe what occurs physiologically and biochemically when the stress response is evoked.
12. Outline the pathways of the stress response.
13. Name and define the four informational substances or chemical messengers used by the three systems in mind-body communication.
14. Describe the characteristics shared by the central nervous and immune systems.
15. List the 11 lines of evidence for mind-body communication.
16. Compare and contrast the research on depression in functional subjects responding to a traumatic life event with the research on depression in hospitalized and clinically depressed subjects.
17. Summarize the findings and limitations of the benefits of music to alleviate pain.
18. Define eustress.
19. Describe the biochemical response during laughter.
20. Summarize the biochemical findings on the effects of writing about traumatic events.
21. Summarize the biochemical findings on the effects of talking about traumatic events.
22. Compare and contrast the potential health benefits of writing, as opposed to talking, about traumatic events.
23. Summarize the findings concerning group support and cancer.
24. Explain how personality style may affect health outcomes.
25. Explain how you will apply the simple interventions discussed in this chapter to your own life experiences.

■ How the Mind and Body Communicate

In the United States the existing medical model strongly suggests it is an absence of organic disease that determines length and quality of life. *Disease* refers to a pathologic condition identified as such by accepted medical procedures and protocols. *Health*, then, is defined as an absence of disease.

Medical models in other parts of the world stress the importance of *illness*, defined to mean the malaise or symptoms experienced by the patient. It is sometimes said that illness is what a patient has on the way to the physician's office. ("I feel achy and sick.") Disease is what the patient has after the physician visit. ("I have the flu.")

The World Health Organization (WHO) defines *health* as "a state of complete physical, mental and social well-being and not simply the absence of disease or infirmity."[67] This is the model of health used most often by practitioners of complementary medicine.

The intent of complementary medicine is to support and encourage a state of physical, mental, and social well being, as well as an absence of disease. To accomplish this objective, we must determine what tools are at our disposal. The mind is the most potent tool available to attain this goal of health because it allows us to determine how to manage our health. Further, it is our most potent weapon in the battle for health because of what is known as mind-body dialog. The mind has been referred to as both "healer" and "slayer" because what we think, feel, and perceive have profound implications for health and longevity. We can assist our bodies in the healing process, or we can exacerbate or create illness with what we express through the minds. This is not an exaggeration. The power of genetics cannot be underestimated, nor can we ignore the fact that exposure to certain viral or bacterial elements is a necessary requirement for certain infectious illness. Nonetheless, disease flowers most profoundly in soil prepared to its liking. The mind—what we think and feel—can modulate whether the body, as "soil," is more likely to support health or disease. Most family members with genetic predispositions to certain disease states do not experience these diseases. We are exposed to viruses and bacteria constantly. Indeed, we carry many types of viruses in our bodies for life. Yet, most of them only reproduce sufficiently to be bothersome when we become physically compromised in some way. Genetics and aging can certainly prepare the "soil" (body) so that it is more likely to nurture disease. Mental and emotional stress is also a factor that can contribute to the likelihood that viruses and bacteria will take hold. Stress can produce biochemical outcomes that contribute to chronic disease states, such as cardiovascular disease. We cannot alter our age or our genetics. We *can,* however, take action to tip the health-disease scales in our favor by using the potent tools of the mind.

The mind and body communicate messages to each other, and these messages result in biochemical and physiologic changes that affect, indeed that drive, both health and disease. In this chapter we explore the pathways by which mind and body communicate. We further describe how perceived stress can have long-term implications for health and longevity, and short-term implications can affect minor illnesses such as viral infections. Of course, if health is already severely compromised (e.g., older adults with compromised immune systems or patients with acquired immunodeficiency syndrome [AIDS]), "minor" illnesses can produce life-threatening consequences.

The opposite of stress is *eustress,* or positive emotion. We discuss how eustress can counteract some of the more negative effects of stress. We begin by describing an event that influences the body via mind-body communication. Then, we investigate the body systems involved in mind-body dialog and the pathways that allow the mind and body to communicate.

A closer look: *The Fear Response*

A rock climber described a situation that resulted in a powerful fear response. Theresa was rock climbing in an area that was indigenous to rattlesnakes. She was careful to wear protective leg gear so she would be safe while she climbed to the top of the bluff. She reached a particularly precarious part of the climb with only one good handhold left, and she was very tired. With as much force as possible, Theresa jammed her fingers into the rock crevice and prepared to swing herself up to the top. At that moment, she heard a rattling sound. In an instant, she was gripped with fear.

In a split second, the thought of being bitten several times, the fear of pain, a picture of her hand swelling, and the fear of an agonizing death all raced through Theresa's mind and body. Her heart began to pound; she began to pant and sweat profusely. Her body stiffened as her gaze froze on a shadow in the crevice. Her thoughts focused, like a laser, on her predicament.

"Don't let go!" a voice screamed in her head. She thought she might survive a snakebite, but never a 2000-foot fall. With all her will, Theresa strengthened her finger grip on the crevice and with tremendous effort swung herself to the top of the bluff. She ripped off her climbing glove and checked for signs of a bite. Her hand was unblemished. Safe, her bodily responses slowly began to return to a more normal state.

A few minutes later, the climber just behind Theresa pulled himself onto the bluff. "Did you encounter the rattler?" Theresa asked. "Oh, do you mean this?" the climber responded. He reached into his shirt and pulled out a chain with snake rattles attached to the end. Shaking the rattles, he said, "This is my good-luck charm."

This real-life event is an example of how the mind communicates with the body, altering physiologic responses in the process. The physiologic responses to fear are obvious to all of us—a pounding heart, an increased breathing rate, a stiff body, sweating, and laserlike attention. The biochemical responses are less obvious. We will review this story again, in greater detail, after we have investigated the mind-body pathways and their informational substances.

───────────── ■ ─────────────

Pathways: An Overview

The mind and body communicate by interactions of the body that occur among (1) the nervous system, (2) the endocrine system, and (3) the immune system.

The *nervous system* is made up of the *central nervous system* (CNS) (i.e., brain and spinal cord) and the *peripheral nervous system* (PNS) (i.e., 31 pairs of spinal nerves and 12 pairs of cranial nerves that branch off from the brain and spinal cord) (Figure 1-1). The PNS also includes the *autonomic nervous system* (ANS) (i.e., neurons that innervate muscles and glands that function to automatically maintain bodily homeostasis) (Figure 1-2). Essentially, the nervous system is how you take in information from the outside world and translate that information to the mind and body. The nervous system also monitors bodily function, relaying this information back to the brain (mind).

The *endocrine system* is made up of glands (i.e., pituitary, thyroid, parathyroid, adrenal, pineal, and thymus) and other hormone-releasing organs (i.e., pancreas, ovaries, testes, hypothalamus) and tissues (i.e., pockets of cells in the small intestines, stomach, kidneys, and heart) (Figure

1-3). The endocrine glands produce substances called *hormones,* which are informational substances. These substances act on the body as needed to monitor or alter bodily processes.

The *immune system* is made up of the thymus and spleen, as well as the lymphocytes and other white blood cells that reside in the lymph nodes, lymph vessels, intestinal lining, appendix, tonsils, and humoral fluids[36] (Figure 1-4 on page 8). These systems interact via two distinctive mind (brain) mediated pathways that can be activated by stress reactions or by conditioning (Figure 1-5 on page 9). The immune system acts to protect the body from foreign invaders (i.e., bacteria, viruses, foreign proteins).

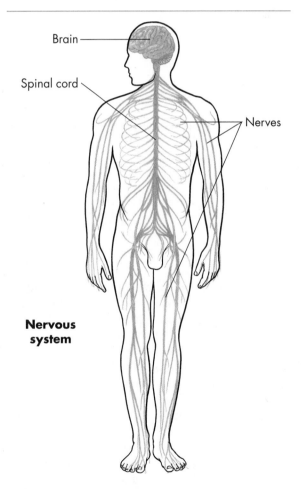

Brain

Spinal cord

Nerves

Nervous system

■ *Figure* **1-1.** Central nervous system. The nervous system includes the brain, spinal cord, and individual nerves. The brain and spinal cord make up the central nervous system and all the nerves, and their branches make up the peripheral nervous system. Nerves originating from the brain are classified as cranial nerves, and nerves originating from the spinal cord are called spinal nerves. *Modified from Thibodeau GA, Patton KT:* Anatomy and physiology, *ed 4, St Louis, 1999, Mosby.*

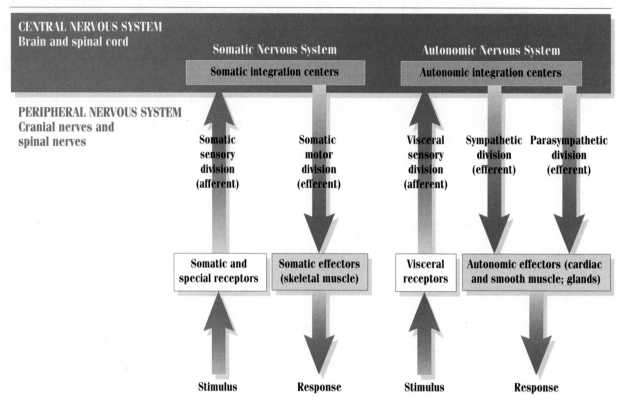

■ *Figure* 1-2. Organizational plan of the nervous system. Diagram summarizes the scheme used by most neurobiologists in studying the nervous system. Both the somatic and autonomic nervous systems include components in the central and peripheral nervous systems. Somatic sensory pathways conduce information toward integrators in the central nervous system, and somatic motor pathways conduct information toward somatic effectors. In the autonomic nervous system, visceral sensory pathways conduct information toward the central nervous system integrators, whereas the sympathetic and parasympathetic pathways conduct information toward autonomic effectors.
Modified from Thibodeau GA, Patton KT: Anatomy and physiology, ed 4, St Louis, 1999, Mosby.

The first and most direct brain pathway is the sympathetic-adrenal-medullary (SAM) axis. The SAM pathway functions by activating the ANS. Motor neurons of the ANS innervate lymphoid tissues and cardiac and smooth muscles, using *neurotransmitters* and *neuropeptides* as their informational substances (Table 1-1). These informational substances can communicate directly with immune cells and tissues and alter immune reactivity.[22,23]

The second and indirect brain pathway is the hypothalamic-pituitary-adrenal (HPA) axis. It alters both the physiology and immune functions by signaling the endocrine system to release informational substances called *hormones*.[13] This pathway is more indirect in how it affects the body and health outcomes because the brain must trigger hormones to be released that then, secondarily, modulate both physiology and immunity.

In essence, changes in the CNS, brought on by internal or external environmental stressors or conditioned stimuli, result in the production of these informational substances. Our interpretation of events, perceived by the body as *messages* for action, determines which *informational substances* are produced and released. Let us examine mind-body communication in greater detail, beginning with the ANS that is activated by the SAM pathway.

Autonomic Nervous System
The ANS refers to the *motor* or *efferent neurons* that are embedded in smooth and cardiac muscles and glands (Figure 1-6 on page 10). Motor or efferent neurons are cells of the nervous system that carry signals *away* from the brain and spinal cord (i.e., CNS) and back to the organs or glands, whereas sensory or afferent neurons carry signals *from* the organs or glands *back* to the spinal cord

TABLE 1-1	Examples of Neurotransmitters

NEUROTRANSMITTER	LOCATION*	FUNCTION
ACETYLCHOLINE	Junctions with motor effectors (muscles, glands); many parts of brain	Excitatory or inhibitory; involved in memory
AMINES		
Serotonin	Several regions of the CNS	Mostly inhibitory; involved in moods and emotions, sleep
Histamine	Brain	Mostly excitatory; involved in emotions and regulation of body temperature and water balance
Dopamine	Brain; ANS	Mostly inhibitory; involved in emotions, moods, and regulation of motor control
Epinephrine	Several areas of the CNS and in the sympathetic division of the ANS	Excitatory or inhibitory; acts as a hormone when secreted by sympathetic neurosecretory cells of the adrenal gland
Norepinephrine	Several areas of the CNS and in the sympathetic division of the ANS	Excitatory or inhibitory; regulates sympathetic effectors; in brain, involves emotional responses
NEUROPEPTIDES		
VIP	Brain, ANS and sensory fibers; retina; GI tract	Function in nervous system uncertain
CCK	Brain; retina	Function in nervous system uncertain
Substance P	Brain; spinal cord, sensory pain pathways; GI tract	Mostly excitatory; transmits pain information
Enkephalins	Several regions of CNS; retina; GI tract	Excitatory or inhibitory; act like opiates to block pain
Endorphins	Several regions of CNS; retina; GI tract	Excitatory or inhibitory; act like opiates to block pain

*These are examples only; most of these neurotransmitters are also found in other locations, and many have additional functions.
ANS, Autonomic nervous system; *CCK,* cholecystokinin; *CNS,* central nervous system; *GI,* gastrointestinal; *VIP,* vasoactive intestinal peptide.
Modified from Thibodeau GA, Patton KT: *Anatomy and physiology,* ed 4, St Louis, 1999, Mosby.

and brain. The ANS receives a constant flood of signals from our visceral (i.e., internal) organs. This glut of information is constantly being processed, and the body must adapt to these signals to maintain homeostasis and support changing bodily activities and needs. In this capacity the ANS performs impressively.

In response to these changes, the ANS shunts blood to needed areas, increases or decreases respiration and heart rates, and modulates blood pressure (BP), body temperature, and stomach secretions. The ANS determines when we need to adapt to "fight-or-flight" or "rest-and-digest" scenarios— or to a condition in-between. Theresa's experience is an example of a "fight-or-flight" experience; sleep is a "rest-and-digest" scenario. The ANS is often referred to as the involuntary or *automatic* nervous system, because much of what it does is not in our consciousness. We are not typically aware, for example, when our pupils dilate or contract or when our BP goes up. For a long time, scientists believed we could do little to alter the functions of the ANS (Figure 1-7 on page 10).

The activities of the ANS are regulated by the spinal cord, brainstem, hypothalamus, and cerebral cortex (Figure 1-8 on page 11). The *brainstem* controls our heartbeat, BP, respiration, and swallowing—unconscious functions vital to basic

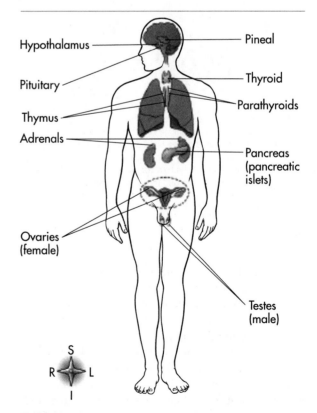

■ **Figure 1-3.** Principle organs of the lymphatic system. *Modified from Thibodeau GA, Patton KT:* Anatomy and physiology, *ed 4, St Louis, 1999, Mosby.*

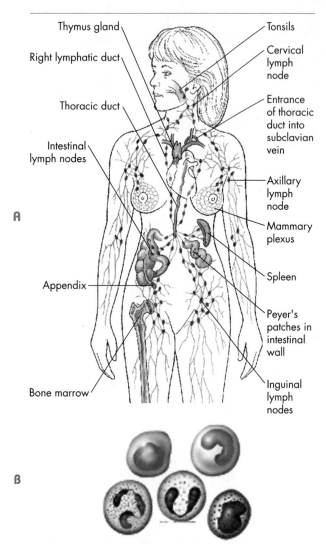

Thymus gland

Right lymphatic duct

Thoracic duct

Intestinal lymph nodes

Tonsils

Cervical lymph node

Entrance of thoracic duct into subclavian vein

Axillary lymph node

Mammary plexus

A

Appendix

Spleen

Peyer's patches in intestinal wall

Bone marrow

Inguinal lymph nodes

B

■ *Figure 1-4.* **A,** Principle organs of the lymphatic system. **B,** Immune cells. Some immune cells have outer membranes that engulf other cells, some have systems that manufacture antibodies, and some are able to destroy other cells. The function of immune cells is to recognize and destroy "nonself" cells, such as cancer cells and invading bacteria. *Modified from Thibodeau GA, Patton KT: Anatomy and physiology, ed 4, St Louis, 1999, Mosby.*

matic and preconscious functions of the ANS.

The ANS has two divisions that affect the same internal organs, but they have opposite effects. The two divisions are called *sympathetic* and *parasympathetic* (see Figure 1-7). The sympathetic division generally *stimulates* certain smooth muscles to contract or glands to secrete, whereas the parasympathetic division typically *inhibits* this action. The sympathetic division mobilizes the body during emergency or stressful situations (e.g., fear, exercise, rage), whereas the parasympathetic division acts to unwind and relax us and to conserve bodily energy. The two divisions serve to counterbalance each other's activities.

Sympathetic-Adrenal-Medullary Axis: Our First and Most Direct Pathway. The ANS controls SAM, the first pathway. The ANS's tissues and organs are heavily laced with nerve fibers, which provide support for immune-cell populations, many of which are mobile cells. The motor neurons in these nerve fibers have receptors for neurotransmitters, the brain chemicals we use to send messages throughout the body. Cell traffic into these organs takes place in areas that are supplied with a large variety of nerves using several different neurotransmitters. These neurotransmitters include, but are not limited to, norepinephrine (NEP), epinephrine (EPI), substance P (SP), and vasoactive intestinal peptide (VIP). When these chemical messengers are released from the nerves, they initiate or alter actions of the lymphocytes, macrophages, and granulocytes (i.e., immune cells). This action is possible because, although the nervous and immune systems function in different ways, they share common receptors for neurotransmitters and neuropeptides. Receptors can be thought of as "docking sites" for neurotransmitters and neuropeptides. When they "dock," cellular responses are activated or altered.

Immune cells are like neurons, in that they have receptors to which neurotransmitters and neuropeptides can attach. Once neurotransmitters have attached to immune cells, they can affect the immune cells' ability to multiply, travel, or kill invaders. Since these chemicals are released during times of strong emotion, it follows that emotions may modify our susceptibility to disease.

Hypothalamic-Pituitary-Adrenal Axis: Our Indirect, Second Communication Pathway. The hypothalamus is the integration center of the ANS—the telephone switchboard that combines visceral,

survival. The *spinal cord* is our conduction pathway, which passes messages to and from the brain; it is also our major reflex center. The *cerebral cortex* is the "executive" of the brain, allowing us to remember, perceive, communicate, comprehend, and initiate voluntary action.[37] These qualities are associated with conscious behavior. The ANS is activated via the *hypothalamus.* Later in this chapter we explore a variety of methods that do, indeed, allow us to alter how the ANS behaves. For now, we begin by discussing the auto-

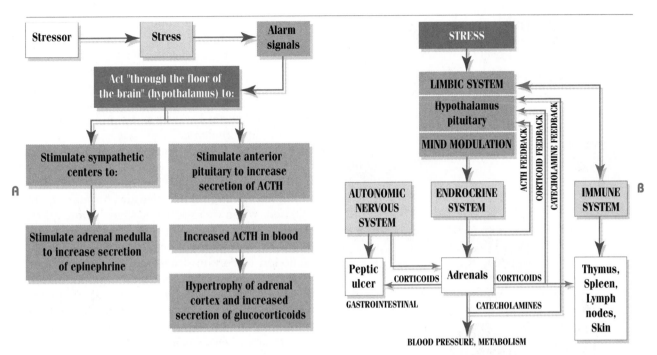

■ **Figure 1-5. A,** Stressors produce a state of stress, which, in turn, inaugurates a series of responses that Selye called the "General Adaptation Syndrome." A state of stress, Selye hypothesized, turns on the stress response mechanism, which activates the organs that produce the syndrome. Selye stated that "alarm signals" produced by stress acted "through the floor of the brain" (presumably the hypothalamus) to stimulate the sympathetic nervous system and pituitary gland. This figure represents Selye's original hypothesis in diagram form. **B,** An updated version of Selye's General Adaptation Syndrome, this figure portrays the mind-modulating role of the limbic-hypothalamic system on the autonomic, endocrine and immune systems, emphasizing how what we think, feel, and believe interacts to create a mind-body effect. *Modified from Thibodeau GA, Patton KT:* Anatomy and physiology, *ed 4, St Louis, 1999, Mosby.*

emotional, and interpretive responses (Figure 1-9). The hypothalamus contains the centers that modulate our heart activity, body temperature, BP, and endocrine activity according to our need. At the same time, it contains centers that modulate our emotional condition (e.g., rage, pleasure) and our most basic biological drives (i.e., sex, thirst, and hunger).

Emotional Brain. The emotional part of the brain (the limbic system) contains a structure called the *amygdala* that links our emotional responses to our memories and to the situation we are currently facing. Not surprisingly, the limbic system also has strong connections to the hypothalamus. When the amygdala in the limbic system responds to danger or stress, it "signals" the hypothalamus to invoke a "fight-or-flight" response from the sympathetic nervous system (SNS). It is the hypothalamus, consequently, that serves as the connection between emotion and visceral responses, and it is the hypothalamic center that frequently directs our behaviors.[3,21] It

is this secondary pathway that gives us some conscious control over ANS activities. This control, in turn, allows us to modulate hormonal reactions that affect physiology, biochemistry, immune function, and stress-related health outcomes.

The emotional brain works something like this. Stressors, such as fear and anxiety, cause nerve impulses to be transmitted from the periphery of the body through unknown higher centers of the brain to the hypothalamus. When the hypothalamus receives a stress or fear reaction from the limbic system, the hypothalamus responds by secreting a *corticotropin-releasing hormone* (CRH) that then incites the pituitary gland to release an *adrenocorticotropic hormone* (ACTH). The ACTH, in turn, stimulates the adrenal cortex to release *cortisol,* a major stress hormone. This process of cascading stimulation with its related hormones is accomplished by the HPA axis.[8]

The known effects of cortisol include the mobilization of energy stores for immediate energy needs, the enhancement of tissue sensitivity to

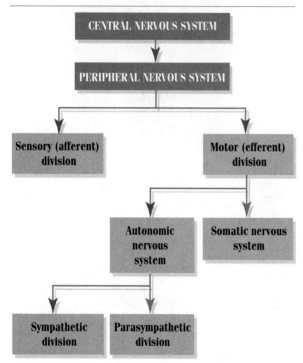

■ **Figure 1-6.** Overview of the organization of the central nervous system. This figure emphasizes the role of the autonomic nervous system in the central nervous system and the flow of information between the central and autonomic systems, as these relate to mind-body effects.

other stress-related neurohormones, and the inhibition of immune and inflammatory responses. These effects provide the organism with the capacity to respond quickly to acute stressors. After the acute stressor is removed, negative feedback mechanisms turn off the heightened secretion of cortisol and cortisol returns to its prior level.

The hypothalamus also releases hormones that regulate emotion and behavior in a more pleasant way. If messages of pleasure are received by the hypothalamus, the *enkephalins* or *endorphins,* our "feel good" or pleasure hormones, are released. When we experience sexual stimulation, the hypothalamus via the anterior pituitary gland can elicit an increase in sex hormones. Even addiction to certain drugs can be related to the hypothalamic pleasure centers.

An interesting piece of research was conducted whereby immune cells (i.e., natural killer [NK] cells) were conditioned or "trained" to respond in a unique way when the subject was exposed to camphor odor. These researchers identified that when the conditioned stimulus (i.e., camphor odor) was presented, a direct input occurred into the hypothalamus, resulting in a redirection of the activity of NK cells by the release of certain mediator chemicals.[30] This suggested that a hypothalamic "inter-

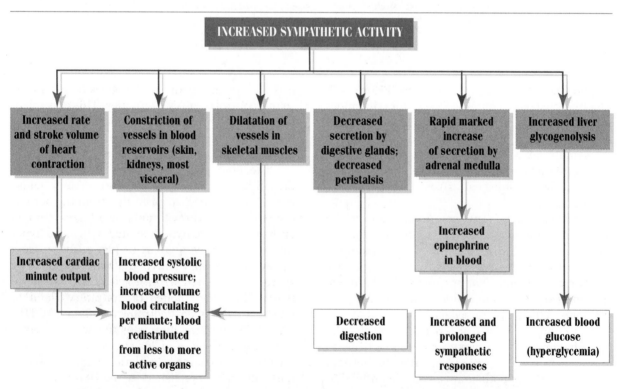

■ **Figure 1-7.** The "fight-or-flight" response activated by the sympathetic-adrenal-medullary pathway. This alarm reaction results from increased sympathetic activity. *Modified from Thibodeau GA, Patton KT: Anatomy and physiology, ed 4, St Louis, 1999, Mosby.*

pretation" of events affects how the body responds to life events. How we interpret these events can determine what informational substances are released, thereby affecting our response to those events and, indirectly, our biochemical reactions. It also appears that the hypothalamus is involved in the *learning* of conditioned immunologic responses. This finding has implications related to susceptibility to both acute and chronic illnesses. Let us take a look at the stress response itself, how it activates the mind-body communication pathways and their informational substances, and how the stress response affects the body.

Stress Response

Anxiety, fear, and other strong emotions can activate the sympathetic nervous division of the ANS, evoking the stress response. This response increases blood flow to skeletal muscles and modulates endocrine gland responsivity[57] (Figure 1-10).

The two pathways of the stress response (i.e., the two-alarm reaction pathways) are the HPA axis and SAM axis, as previously mentioned. When these pathways are activated, numerous neuroendocrine changes are triggered including elevations in the levels of hormones and proteins (e.g., EPI, NEP, renin, calcitonin, cortisol, thyroxine, parathyroid hormone, gastrin, insulin, erythopoietin). The outcomes of a stress response include elevations or increases in BP, heart rate, galvanic skin response (e.g., sweating), blood glucose levels, coagulation time, and muscle tension.[14,38] Although the capacity for these responses are critical for survival, if prolonged unnecessarily, these changes can lead to heightened physiologic and emotional reactivity and immunosuppression. Persons experiencing chronic stress and therefore chronic physiologic hyperreactivity demonstrate an increased risk of illness and premature death (Table 1-2).

Chronically stressed persons frequently exhibit increased muscle tension, decreased peripheral skin temperatures, and a hyperreactive response to an acute stressor. They have difficulty returning to a hypoactive or relaxation state. The expression of a stress response is typically assessed by measurements of SNS responses, such as BP, heart rate, sweat rate, peripheral skin temperature.[63]

Stress can be induced both physiologically and psychologically. For example, psychologic stress can lead to immune impairment and to illness. On the other hand, a disease state can

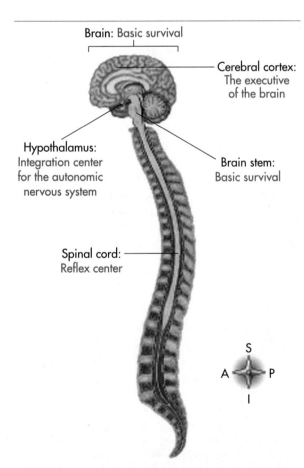

■ **Figure 1-8.** The activities of the autonomic nervous system are regulated by the spinal cord, brain stem, hypothalamus, and cerebral cortex. *From Thibodeau GA, Patton KT: Anatomy and physiology, ed 4, St Louis, 1999, Mosby.*

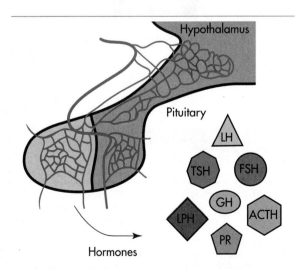

■ **Figure 1-9.** The hypothalamus-pituitary-adrenal axis—the indirect communications pathway. The hypothalamus is the integration center of the autonomic nervous system—the telephone switchboard that combines visceral, emotional, and interpretative responses.

induce a psychologic stressor (e.g., fear, anxiety) that further impairs the body's ability to recover. The two effects are intertwined (Figure 1-11). We will now revisit our mountain climber and review her fear response in greater detail.

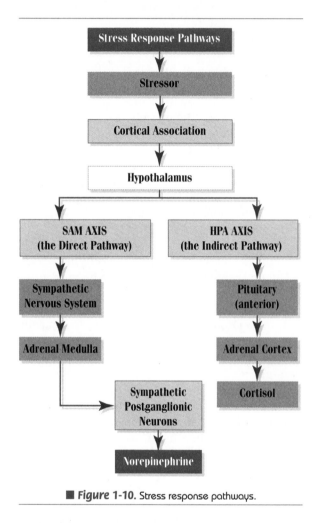

■ **Figure 1-10.** Stress response pathways.

A closer look: *The Fear Response*

A rock climber described a situation that resulted in a powerful fear response. Theresa was rock climbing in an area that was indigenous to rattlesnakes. She was careful to wear protective leg gear so she would be safe while climbing to the top of the bluff. She reached a particularly precarious part of the climb with only one good hand-hold left, and she was very tired. With as much force as possible, Theresa jammed her fingers into the rock crevice and prepared to swing herself up to the top. At that moment, she heard a rattling sound. In an instant, she was gripped with fear.

What was going on, literally, inside her head and body at that moment? The limbic system and the ever-active amygdala quickly made a connection between her responsive fear reaction to snakes and her current situation. In a split second, the thought of being bitten several times, the fear of pain, a picture of her hand swelling, and the fear of an agonizing death were all integrated, and these powerful "signals" were accepted by the hypothalamus.

The hypothalamus responded. It secreted CRH via the HPA axis, which signaled the pituitary gland to release ACTH, which stimulated the adrenal glands to pour cortisol into her body. Simultaneously, the SNS via the SAM pathway triggered the release of EPI, NEP, and other neurotransmitters and neuropeptides, preparing Theresa for the struggle of her life. Her heart raced, her breathing became rapid, her BP jumped, and she began to sweat profusely. Her pupils dilated and her body stiffened as her gaze froze on a shadow in the crevice. Her thoughts focused, like a laser, on her predicament.

TABLE 1-2	Effects of Stress, Leading to Exhaustion	
ALARM	**RESISTANCE**	**EXHAUSTION**
Increased secretion of glucocorticoids and resultant changes	Glucocorticoid secretion returns to normal	Increased glucocorticoid secretion but eventually marked decreased secretion
Increased activity of sympathetic nervous system	Sympathetic activity returns to normal	Stress triad (hypertrophied adrenal glands, atrophied thymus and lymph nodes, bleeding ulcers stomach and duodenum)
Increased norepinephrine secretion by adrenal medulla	Norepinephrine secretion returns to normal	
"Fight-or-flight" syndrome of changes	"Fight-or-flight" syndrome disappears	
Low resistance to stressors	High resistance (adaptation) to stressor	Loss of resistance to stressor; may lead to death

The prefrontal cortex had been simultaneously stimulated, assessing the danger and preparing for a decision. "Don't let go!" is the message she heard screaming in her head. She may survive the snakebite, but she would never survive a 2000-foot fall. With all her will, Theresa strengthened her finger grip on the crevice and with tremendous force swung herself to the top of the bluff. She ripped off her climbing glove and checked for signs of a bite. Her hand was unblemished. She was safe and her bodily responses slowly returned to a more normal state.

A few minutes later, the climber just behind Theresa pulled himself onto the bluff. "Did you encounter the rattler?" Theresa asked. "Oh, do you mean this?" the climber responded. He reached into his shirt and pulled out a chain with snake rattles attached to the end. "This is my good-luck charm."

Did this experience have an immediate effect on Theresa's physiology and biochemistry? Of course. Will this experience have a permanent effect on her health? Probably not. However, long-term stress of considerably less intensity can affect health and longevity. A one-time acute stressor event of short duration is potentially harmful only for individuals with severely compromised immune systems or severely degraded health. The pathways are, nonetheless, the same.

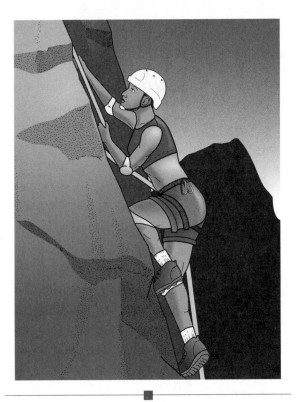

Chemical Messengers

So, in essence, we have chemical messengers in the body that the brain and the nervous and immune systems use to communicate with each other.[10] These chemical couriers travel throughout the lymphatic system and bloodstream to deliver their messages. These chemical messengers are known as:

- Neurotransmitters
- Neuropeptides
- Hormones
- Immune modulators

Chemical signals (e.g., neurotransmitters, neuropeptides, hormones) traveling from the brain and ANS to the immune cells can modify migration, killing ability, and reproduction of immune cells. Simultaneously, chemical messengers (e.g., lymphokines, neurotransmitters, neuropeptides, and hormones) from the immune cells travel to the brain, keeping the brain informed as to the effective workings of the immune system and influencing mood state and physiologic responses in the body.

Neurotransmitters

Neurotransmitters are the "language" of the nervous system—the means by which neurons communicate with each other and with the rest of the body. Neurotransmitters are released in the brain, upon excitation by a presynaptic cell. They then cross the synapse to stimulate or inhibit a postsynaptic cell. In this way, neurotransmitters (e.g., acetylcholine, EPI, NEP, dopamine, Gaba, serotonin) dispatch their messages. Receptors for neurotransmitters are found on immune cells; further, immune cells produce neurotransmitters.[29,55,61]

Neuropeptides

Neuropeptides typically affect their target neurons at lower concentrations than the "classical" neurotransmitters. Neuropeptides are essentially short strings of amino acids that produce very diverse effects (Box 1-1). Neuropeptides can act as hormones, neurotransmitters, and neuromodulators. Some neuropeptides act as neurotransmitters at some synapses and as neuromodulators at other synapses.

Although a neurotransmitter changes the conductance of the target cell, thereby changing membrane potential, a neuromodulator modulates synaptic transmission. A neuromodulator may act presynaptically to change the amount of transmitter released, or it may act on a postsynaptic cell to modify its response to the neurotransmitter.

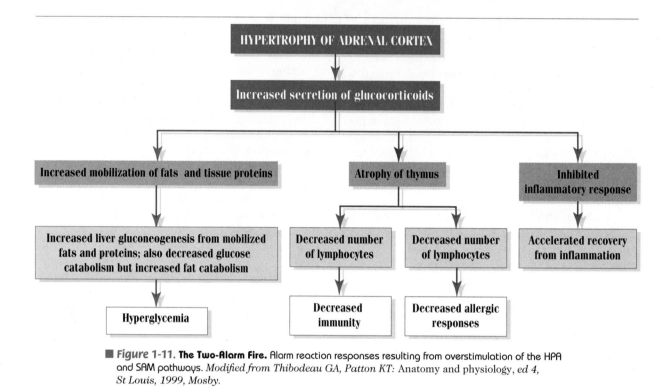

■ **Figure 1-11. The Two-Alarm Fire.** Alarm reaction responses resulting from overstimulation of the HPA and SAM pathways. *Modified from Thibodeau GA, Patton KT:* Anatomy and physiology, *ed 4, St Louis, 1999, Mosby.*

BOX 1-1 Some Neuroactive Peptides

Gut-brain peptides
Vasoactive intestinal polypeptide (VIP)
Cholecystokinin octapeptide (CCK-8)
Substance P
Neurotensin
Methionine enkephalin
Leucine enkephalin
Motilin
Insulin
Glucagon

Hypothalamic-releasing hormones
Thyrotropin-releasing hormone (TRH)
Luteinizing hormone-releasing hormone (LHRH)
Somatostatin (growth hormone releasing-inhibiting factor [SRIF])

Pituitary peptides
Adrenocorticotropin (ACTH)
β-Endorphin
α-Melanocyte-stimulating hormone (a-MSH)

Others
Dynorphin
Angiotensin II
Bradykinin
Vasopressin
Oxytocin
Carnosine
Bombesin

Modified from Synder SH: *Science* 209:976,1980. Copyright ©1980 by American Association for the Advancement of Science.

The SP neuropeptide is a mediator of pain signals. The endorphin and enkephalin neuropeptides are our natural opiates, elevating mood and reducing our perception of pain in stressful situations. Enkephalins increase dramatically during labor, whereas endorphins are enhanced with exercise. It has been suggested that neuropeptides are responsible for the placebo effect because they have a kind of morphine or opiate effect on the body. Other neuropeptides, like somatostatin, VIP, and cholecystokinin are produced by body tissues and are widespread in the gastrointestinal tract. These peptides are referred to as "gut-brain" peptides. The saying, "I know this in my gut..." may be a more accurate statement than we think.

Neuropeptides are secreted by the brain, immune system, and nerve cells in other organs. The areas of the brain (i.e., limbic system) that regulate our emotional responses are particularly rich in receptor sites for neuropeptides. At the same time, the brain contains receptor sites for protein molecules produced by immune cells (e.g., lymphokines, interleukins), allowing a two-way communication link between the brain and immune system.[15,27]

The research on neuropeptides has provided some of the most revealing factors behind the effects of the mind on immunity. Much of this

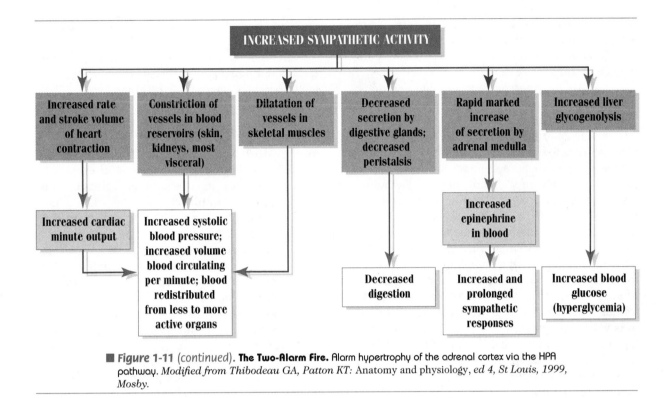

INCREASED SYMPATHETIC ACTIVITY

Increased rate and stroke volume of heart contraction	Constriction of vessels in blood reservoirs (skin, kidneys, most visceral)	Dilatation of vessels in skeletal muscles	Decreased secretion by digestive glands; decreased peristalsis	Rapid marked increase of secretion by adrenal medulla	Increased liver glycogenolysis

Increased cardiac minute output

Increased systolic blood pressure; increased volume blood circulating per minute; blood redistributed from less to more active organs

Increased epinephrine in blood

Decreased digestion

Increased and prolonged sympathetic responses

Increased blood glucose (hyperglycemia)

■ **Figure 1-11** (continued). **The Two-Alarm Fire.** Alarm hypertrophy of the adrenal cortex via the HPA pathway. *Modified from Thibodeau GA, Patton KT:* Anatomy and physiology, *ed 4, St Louis, 1999, Mosby.*

groundbreaking work has come about through the efforts of Dr. Candace Pert. Dr. Pert was chief of brain chemistry in the clinical neuroscience branch at National Institute of Health in the 1980s. Her major interest was the research on brain receptors, particularly their biochemistry. It was her work as a graduate student that led to the discovery of neuropeptides and their critical role in mind-body interactions.[49]

According to Pert, the very essence of communication between the immune system and the mind occurs via the neuropeptides. Through the research, much of it from her own laboratory, she discovered that immune cells carry receptors for ALL the neuropeptides. She believes that mind and body are bound by the communication among these neuropeptides. Dr. Pert shares some of her ideas and experiences.

An Expert Speaks: Dr. Candace Pert

Question. When did you realize your peptide receptor research was linked to health and healing?

Answer. In the early 80s, two shocking discoveries were made by two key scientists, Ed Blalock and Michael Ruff. The discovery was that the same neuropeptides found in the brain could also be found in immune cells. Now, everyone believes that the immune system is not only responsible for fighting against infections, but it does the actual healing; so, if you cut your finger, certain immune cells rush in and secrete peptides and make everything work. Blalock discovered that immune cells have peptides in them, endorphins being the first one. Then Ruff discovered that [the immune cells] have receptors, too, not just biochemical receptors, but functional receptors that affect which way the immune cells work.

In 1985, Ruff and I and several other scientists published a pivotal paper in the *Journal of Immunology* called "Neuropeptides and their Receptors: A Psychosomatic Network." In the paper we talked about the psychoimmunoendocrine network. We said, "Look, there's this common language. It's got to be a network. It's sending information through peptides that are being released by cells all over and they are receiving information." Based on the distribution patterns of these receptors that I had been studying for 10 years, we said, "Look, they're in the amygdala, they're in the hypothalamus, they're in the parts of the brain thought to be important in emotions. This is obviously the biochemical foundation of emotions." And that's where we started to bridge into the spiritual, if you will. There were a lot of jokes, because, let's just say that emotions, ironically, are not dealt with in Western science.

Question. Isn't that odd, since we all experience emotions every day?

Answer. We not only experience emotions, but as it turns out, they run every system of your body. These neuropeptides (receptors) run your physiology, your health, or your tendency toward disease. And we have a culture that's in complete denial, not just about their importance, but almost their very existence. Certainly in medicine, there's not time for it. Psychiatry theoretically deals with emotional pathology, but there's not much emotion, is there, in mainstream medicine?

There's a key difference [between mainstream and alternative medicine]. Alternative practitioners are almost going in the other direction. They explain, "Well, I was trying to get rid of her virus, and I was using energy medicine. It was working, but she had unresolved issues with her mother." I'm not making fun of that because I can see how there could be a connection. I think that's the void that alternative medicine is filling because it has an emotional approach.

Question. So, when I get mad, my brain releases neuropeptides?

Answer. Angry ones.

Question. And these neuropeptides find their receptors through my body, and they trigger physiologic actions within my body?

Answer. Wrong. It's not a brain-centered system where everything—thoughts, mind, emotions—comes from the brain and then peters down to the poor second-rate body, which is just this dangling appendage. The truth is so weird that I've only recently come to believe in it and experience it. Emotions are not in the head. There's a cellular consciousness. There's a wisdom in every cell. Every single cell has receptors on it. The emotional energy comes first and then peptides are released all over. It's not that they're just coming out of the pituitary gland and diffusing down and hitting cells.

For example, there is a peptide that when dropped into the brain of a rat, the rat will start drinking water and act like it's thirsty. Drop [this peptide] into the receptors of the lung, the lung will conserve water. Drop it onto the angiotensin receptors of the kidney, the kidney will conserve water. So it's happening everywhere. Everywhere simultaneously the molecules are manifesting. This gets almost into—I don't want to call it the metaphysical—but it goes beyond reductionist Western thought. Somehow the feeling is there first, and then the molecules manifest themselves.

Question. So consciousness has the feeling first?

Answer. Yes. Consciousness precedes matter. It's not like a peptide creates the feeling. The feeling creates the peptide on some level.

Question. How can we use this knowledge?

Answer. To heal ourselves and to heal each other. I think that it gets used all the time except in classical Western medicine. Stanley Krippner studied cross-cultural healing, and in every single culture they have emotional release, emotional catharsis. In our culture, there is a denial of it. So the first thing is just to recognize that emotional changes or releases can be part of a culture. But I have a whole rationale for embracing many aspects of alternative medicine, based on the fact that they would be expected to perturb peptides and do things to them.

Question. In your published work, you use peptides to explain mind-body healing, but you also used it to explain acupuncture, didn't you?

Answer. Yes. As we published in 1980, there is clear scientific evidence that acupuncture and analgesia are mediated by the release of endorphins. However, acupuncture does a lot more than analgesia and we suspect that it also releases some of the other 60 or 70 active peptides.

But everyone is into biochemistry. It's reductionist, and that's okay. But emotions are in two realms. They're in the realm of the physical, the molecular, the material; and they're also in the realm of the spiritual. It's almost like the transition element. It slides back and forth. That's why emotions are so critically important.

Take breathing. Breathing is used in almost every alternative modality I've been exposed to. People talk about breathing through or projecting your consciousness and breathing into an injury, exhaling through it. Now, hundreds of scientists have mapped the location of the neuropeptides and any one can be found in the floor of the fourth ventricle, which is where breathing is controlled. Peptides are released into the ventricular fluid, and they affect how fast the breaths are, how shallow, how deep.

Question. Can you talk about your AIDS work?

Answer. In 1986, my lab at NIH discovered that the brain and immune system have the same receptors. Every time we would take any receptor found in the brain and look for it in the immune system, it would be there. We'd take any immune system receptor, look for it in the brain, and find it there. Then we heard that the AIDS virus used a molecule called CD-4, which is a receptor, to get into cells. We said, "Well, let's look." And sure enough, we tested it and found it in the brain. So we started to study it.

We hypothesized that if you could find the peptide that usually uses this receptor.... This was the thinking: Here's the opiate receptor. God didn't put the opiate receptor there so we could all get high from opium, and so we found the endorphins. The marijuana receptor has recently been found and there's a substance that binds to it. It's actually not a peptide, but it appears to be a very important cellular communication molecule. So I said, "Hey, if we could figure out what peptide [uses this receptor], this would be a great drug, because it would block the AIDS virus from getting in." That was the rationale. We used a computer-assisted database search, and we looked for peptides that were shared in common between the known database and the AIDS viral envelope, which is the part of the virus that encircles it and holds the nucleic acid. This is the part of the cell that sees. So we figured out this structure, and we had great faith and hope and optimism on this.

The peptides came back in the very first experiments. It not only blocked the binding of GP-120, the virus envelope, but it blocked the binding of GP-120 to the CD-4 receptor in both brain and immune cells. And it also blocked the virus from growing, just as we had predicted. The easy part was discovering the AIDS [peptide]. The hard part was convincing people I had discovered it. AZT had been invented 3 months before peptide T. All the research money went to AZT.

Early on, I sent a sample of the drug to Dr. Wetterberg, the head of the Karolinska Institute's psychiatry department. They have a rule that in a fatal disease, the chairman at his prerogative can give [a new drug]. He gave it to four terminally ill men, and they all had surprising rebounds. Well, that was enough for me to dedicate my life to it after that. We began doing trials of peptide T.

Let me say that peptide T isn't a cure. A cure in my mind would be: You give the drug and the virus is gone. I think peptide T may be part of a cure, but it's going to be in conjunction with a second drug.

Question. Do you have any final words for the readers?

Answer. My intuition is there's something wonderful and exciting and promising about alternative medicine. It's sorely needed. And I think it's really frustrating for alternative practitioners right now. It's important to seek scientific validation for what you do, but I have the feeling sometimes that maybe we are holding alternative practitioners to a higher standard. So I think alternative practitioners are too humble. They should be more proud of what they do and more assertive, because I believe that they have something very valuable that helps people.

Other researchers support many of Dr. Pert's assertions. Morley and associates refer to the neuropeptides as the "conductors of the immune orchestra."[42] Carr and Blalock suggest that psychosocial factors alter our response to infections and neoplasms (i.e., tumors).[15] Goetzl and colleagues identified the cell source of production of neuropeptides and described how cells in the immune system recognize neuropeptides.[26] Through Pert's research and the research of others, neuropeptides may become the clear pathway by which mind affects body, health, and many life-threatening illnesses such as AIDS.*

Hormones

In essence, hormones released via the HPA axis control the activity and release of hormones from all the other glands (Figure 1-12). The endocrine system produces hormones (e.g., gonadal steroids, thyroid hormones, adrenal hormones), and these have a direct effect on immune responses through their dialog with immune cells.[7] Hormones affect target cells by altering (i.e., increasing or decreasing) rates of cellular processes. Further, immune cells can produce hormones themselves, leading again to bi-directional dialog.[52] It is interesting to note that cancer cells synthesize hormones identical to the endocrine glands, but in an excessive and uncontrollable fashion.

Immune Modulators

The immune modulators (cytokines) are the chemical messengers of the immune cells (e.g., cytokines). Cytokines include the hormonelike *lymphokines,* soluble proteins released by activated T-cells, and monokines that are secreted by macrophages (Figure 1-13). The names of some individual cytokines include *chemotactic factor, migration inhibition factor, macrophage activating factor, and lymphotoxin.* Chemotactic factors attract macrophages, causing them to migrate to sensitized T-cells. Migration inhibition factors stop the migration of macrophages. Macrophage activating factors enhance and speed up the ability of the macrophages to destroy antigens by

---

*Modified with permission from *Alternative Therapies in Health and Medicine* 1(3):70, July 1995.

phagocytosis (i.e., engulfing and digesting it). Lymphotoxin is a potent poison that directly kills any cell it attacks.[65]

These immune modulators communicate and direct the type of immune defense that is necessary. Macrophages and T-cells in the immune system release cytokines, which influence other immune cells.[33] These immunomodulators can also communicate directly with nonimmune cells in the brain via lymphokines. For example, Besedovski and colleagues and Blalock reported that activated lymphocytes, containing lymphokines, induced the release of CRF in the hypothalamus and the subsequent rise of blood cortisol levels.[9,11] This chemical language between the brain and immune system, and its subsequent effects on stress hormones, is one pathway by which conditioning and stress affect immunity.[44]

Chemical Messengers: A Summary

Neurotransmitters, neuropeptides, hormones, and immune modulators have been reported to modulate immune-cell behavior. For example, macrophages become sluggish when we are depressed, high levels of endorphins suppress NK cell activity, and hormones that are released in large amounts during stress (e.g., cortisol, epinephrine) depress T-cell activity.[23]

The CNS and PNS and the immune system share certain characteristics:
■ Ability to communicate at a distance
■ Ability to develop memory
■ Ability to use many of the same chemical messengers,[3] which essentially allows them to communicate with each other

Neurotransmitters from the brain alter immune reaction. For example, NEP, also called

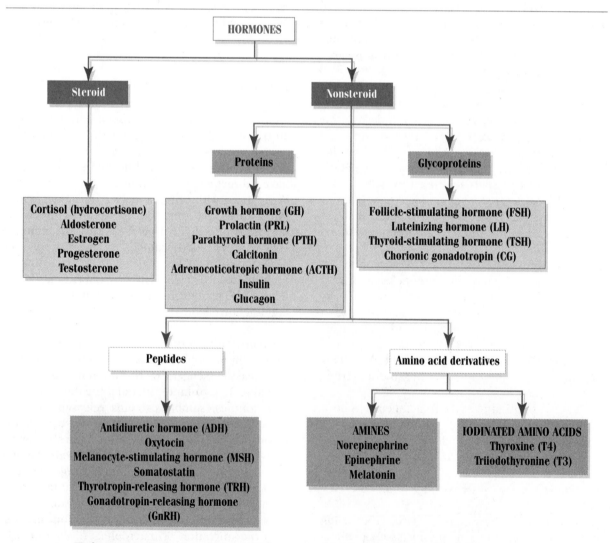

■ **Figure 1-12.** Chemical classification of hormones. *Modified from Thibodeau GA, Patton KT: Anatomy and physiology, ed 4, St Louis, 1999, Mosby.*

noradrenaline, is released by ANS neurons. Receptors for NEP and other neurotransmitters have been identified on immune cells, specifically, lymphocytes.

Bi-directional communication allows the brain to keep track of immune function, and it allows the immune system to affect the brain, specifically the emotions. This ability of the brain and immune system to communicate seems to depend on lymphokines and hormones released by immune cells.

Immune cells can receive chemical messages from other bodily sources (e.g., endocrine system, nervous system) because they have receptor sites that allow hormones, neurotransmitters, and neuropeptides to "dock" on their membranes.[55] Further, immune cells can directly synthesize neuropeptides (e.g., endorphins) and hormones, including ACTH, growth hormone (GH), thyroid-stimulating hormone (TSH), and reproductive hormone, allowing immune cells to communicate in return. Immune cells can behave almost as if they are a secondary pituitary gland. This ability to produce and receive chemical messengers, as well as the mobility of immune cells, is one of the reasons why the immune system is sometimes referred to as the "floating brain."

So, these chemical messengers (i.e., neurotransmitters, neuropeptides, hormones, immunomodulators) are attracted to the receptor sites on cells where they communicate their messages, not unlike a key turning in a lock. Our combined chemical messengers are like the codes that make up the body's software program. As functional changes occur in these chemicals, we temporarily rewrite our software, altering the body's functioning in subtle, but meaningful, ways. This informational substance-driven dialog between the brain and the systems of the body (e.g., nervous, endocrine, immune) is the circuitry by which our interpretation of life events can influence our immunity and physiologic condition.

■ Lines of Evidence for Mind-Body Communication

Ader and others have clearly delineated the lines of evidence that demonstrate that communication pathways exist between the CNS and immune systems.[1] These studies are reviewed individually in coming chapters. A summary of their findings is listed below.

1. **Nerve endings are embedded in the tissues of the immune system.** Bone marrow, thymus gland, spleen, and lymph nodes are innervated (i.e., embedded with nerve endings) by the CNS. All lymphocytes originate in bone marrow, and B-cells develop immunocompetence in the bone marrow. Immature lymphocytes migrate

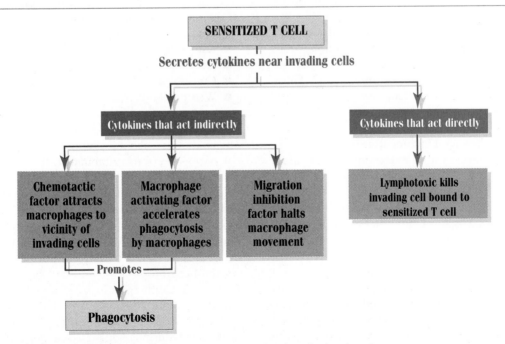

■ *Figure* 1-13. Illustration shows how cytokines act directly and indirectly on immune response.
Modified from Thibodeau GA, Patton KT: Anatomy and physiology, *ed 4, St Louis, 1999, Mosby.*

from bone marrow to the thymus gland where, under the influence of thymic hormones, they develop immunocompetence. After acquiring immunocompetence, lymphocytes seed the lymph nodes, spleen, and other lymphoid tissues where antigen challenge occurs. The CNS therefore has direct contact with immune tissues and access to immune cells.

2. **Changes in the CNS (i.e., brain and spinal cord) alter immune responses. When an immune response is triggered, CNS activity is also altered.** Animal experiments dating back to the 1960s demonstrate that damage to the hypothalamus suppresses or enhances immune response. Further, when an immune response is triggered, nerve cells in the hypothalamus become more active, and this brain cell activity peaks at the same time antibody levels are at their highest. It appears that the brain monitors immunologic changes very closely.

3. **Changes in hormone and neurotransmitter levels alter immune activity and vice versa.** Stress hormones typically suppress immune response; other hormones, such as GH, also affect immunity. In experiments when animals are immunized, they alter their hormone levels.

4. **Lymphocytes can produce both hormones and neurotransmitters.** Lymphocytes can act like mini–pituitary glands. For example, when an animal is infected with a virus, lymphocytes produce infinitesimal amounts of many of the same chemicals produced by the pituitary gland.

5. **Activated lymphocytes produce substances recognized by the CNS.** Immune cells "talk" to each other by using chemical messengers, such as interleukins and interferons. These same chemicals trigger receptors on cells in the brain, confirming that the immune and nervous system speak the same language.

6. **Psychosocial factors alter the susceptibility to or progression of autoimmune and infectious diseases.** (This research is discussed in Chapters 3 and 4.)

7. **Immunologic reactivity can be influenced by stress.** Chronic or intense stress generally makes immune cells less responsive to a challenge.

8. **Immunologic reactivity can be influenced by relaxation techniques, hypnosis, and biologically targeted imagery.** Allergic reactions have been both produced and reduced by the use of hypnosis or imagery. Relaxation techniques have been demonstrated to down regulate some allergic responses. (These studies are discussed in detail in later chapters.)

9. **Immunologic reactivity can be modulated by classical conditioning.** Ader's animal experiments, which are reviewed in Chapter 3, demonstrated that the immune system can "learn" to react a particular way as a conditioned response.

10. **Psychoactive drugs and drug abuse influence immune function.** Drugs that affect the CNS include alcohol, marijuana, cocaine, heroin, and nicotine. They also suppress the immune response. Some psychotropic medications, such as lithium, also modulate immunity.

11. **Stress can interfere with the effectiveness of an immunization program.** In one research study, stressed medical students receiving hepatitis B vaccinations required one or two booster immunizations before they formed antibodies; unstressed students formed antibodies with the first injection. This effect of stress has implications for public health practices.

In the next two chapters, the studies that define these lines of evidence are reviewed in detail. We now turn our attention to what we can do to support immune function.

■ Suggestions for Supporting Immune Function

Are there some relatively simple things we can do to support healthy immune function, positive mood state, and health in general? The literature suggests that there are. Actions or interactions that have been demonstrated to counteract some of the effects of stress include:

- Music
- Laughter
- Group support
- Counseling
- Writing about traumatic events

Music Therapy

Music therapy can be defined as the controlled use of music and its influence on the human being to aid in physiologic, psychologic, and emotional integration of the individual during the treatment of an illness or disease (Figure 1-14). A 1929 study found that the volume, pitch, melody, rhythm, and type of music all affect BP. The greatest effects on BP were related to the listener's interest and comprehension.[66] Other studies have suggested that music can help reduce pain, even the pain of cancer patients.[32]

In more recent years, music has been used as an entrainment mechanism to reduce pain or alter the mood state in a variety of settings. The term *entrainment* refers to any stimuli (e.g., music, imagery, hypnosis), which matches or models the current mood state of an individual and then moves that person in the direction of a more positive or pleasant mood state. For example, an erratic, fast, off-pitch musical selection might be a match for a highly agitated, anxious person. Beginning with this music and moving slowly into a mellow, slower-paced, more melodic musical piece could possibly reduce the subject's anxiety level. Music and imagery, alone and in combination, have been used to entrain mood states, reduce acute or chronic pain, and alter certain biochemical properties, such as plasma B-endorphin levels.[39,60] The following is one of the better studies that assesses the use of entrainment music for pain reduction.

Rider Study of Entrainment Music and Pain Reduction

Rider chose to study the effects of different types of music on (1) the vividness and activity level of suggested imagery, (2) the ability to reduce pain, and (3) the ability to reduce electromyographic (EMG)–assessed muscle tension.[53] He hypothesized that there would be significant pain reduction for each music-imagery intervention, that there would be significant EMG-assessed muscle relaxation for each music-imagery intervention, that music would significantly increase the vividness of the imagery produced, and that music would significantly increase the activity level of the imagery produced.

Method. Twenty-three patients with spinal cord injury were admitted to a spinal pain clinic. In this randomized, counter-balanced, double-blind

designed study, the patients received one of seven taped musical conditions each day for a 7-day period. The following five dependent variables were measured before and after intervention: (1) pain, (2) EMG-assessed muscle tension, (3) imagery vividness, (4) imagery activity, and (5) musical preference. All but EMG outputs were measured on self-report questionnaires.

The musical conditions were 20 minutes in duration and consisted of 9 minutes of muscle relaxation, 1 minute of imagery instruction, and 10 minutes of music. During the imagery instructions, the patients were taught to imagine their pain being subdued by their endorphin system. The seven types of music were described as follows:

1. Trancelike or habituating music (e.g., Steve Reich's "Music for Mallets, Voices and Organ" and synthesized music simulating crystal goblets on a guitar synthesizer) that was highly repetitive with no mood shift or ending climax.
2. Impressionistic music (e.g., Debussy's "Prelude to the Afternoon of a Faun" [classical], and Pat Metheny's "If I Could" [jazz]) that also contained no mood shift.
3. Entrainment musical condition, containing both synthesized and acoustic guitar music that exhibited a definite and strong mood shift from an unpleasant mood to a pleasant mood state, with a climax in the pleasant mood occurring after 3 minutes. (Mood state shifts were accomplished by moving from an accelerating 7/8 meter to a more pleasant and melodic 4/4 meter.)
4. Twenty minutes of muscle relaxation and pain relief imagery with no music. (This tape preceded the musical and imagery conditions.)
5. One taped condition of the patient's preferred music with no imagery induction or suggestions. (The music was brought to the clinic by the patient, or it was selected by the patient from "new age" tapes housed in the clinic.)

Outcome. Analysis of variance (ANOVA) found that there were significant effects of music intervention treatment for pain ($p=0.006$) with the *entrainment condition demonstrating the most effective method for pain reduction* ($p<0.05$). *Patient-preferred music produced the least significant effects.* Posttreatment EMG levels of stress were significantly reduced for music interventions ($p<0.0001$). Entrainment music was again the most effective intervention for EMG reduction ($p<0.05$). Neither imagery vividness nor activity were significantly affected by music condi-

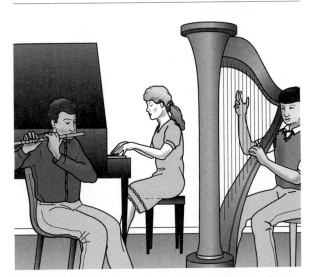

■ *Figure 1-14.* Music has the capacity to modulate mood state.

tion, although the highest imagery scores were obtained in the entrainment condition. The order of music effectiveness was found to be: (1) entrainment, (2) Reich, (3) Metheny, and (4) crystal simulation. *Of most interest was the finding that the two most effective conditions for pain reduction (entrainment and Reich) were the least preferred types of music and that the preferred type of music was the least effective intervention. Music preference may reflect the current mood rather than the music most effective in shifting mood state and affecting endorphin activation.*

Points to Ponder   Entrainment music was the most effective method for pain reduction. Preferred music produced the least significant effects.   ■

Conclusions and comments. The authors concluded that entrainment music, where the prevalent mood is shifted from tension to relaxation and negative to positive, was the most effective condition for reducing pain and EMG tension levels. Further, entrainment-mediated imagery invoked psychologic and possibly physiologic pain relief mechanisms.

Other Music Outcomes

A controlled study of 50 surgeons who reported that they listened to music during surgery evaluated the effects of music on physiologic response and task performance. Skin conductance, diastolic and systolic BP, pulse rate, and task speed and accuracy were assessed while performing a serial subtraction stressor task. In three treatment conditions, surgeons listened to (1) self-selected music, (2) experimenter-selected music, and (3) no music. All physiologic measures of stress were significantly lower for the surgeon-selected music condition, and the speed and accuracy at task were significantly higher, as opposed with the experimenter-selected music condition.[2]

A review of 21 studies on the use of music and relaxation to control postoperative pain found that the combination was consistently effective in reducing affective and observed pain, but less effective in reducing sensory pain or opioid intake.[28] The author found that benefits fluctuated with the type of relaxation and music used, the type of surgery, the amount of preoperative practice, and the period of ambulation (i.e., time until walking).

A metaanalysis of 30 studies using music in medical and dental treatments evaluated the *effect size* (ES) of 55 variables assessed in music research studies.[60] The ES was defined as +1.00, meaning the experimental group was one standard deviation above the control group. The authors of this study found that music enhanced medical objectives, whether measured by physiologic (mean ES=0.97), psychologic self report (mean ES=0.85), or behavioral observation (mean ES=1.10). Estimated ES sizes by population were greatest for dental procedures (2.26), cardiac patients (1.15), and surgical patients (1.13); they were the lowest for neonates (0.21), cancer patients (0.55), and obstetric patients (0.65). ES for psychologic or physiologic outcomes ranged from +3.28 for pain relief, +3.00 for reduction of pulse rate and +2.49 for reduced need of analgesia to +0.06 for neonate crying and −0.17 for stress hormone levels.

Not all studies found beneficial results. In a randomized controlled study, 75 patients in a coronary unit were assigned to one of three groups. Those who (1) listened to music, (2) listened to white noise, or (3) were part of a silent control group. There were no significant differences between the groups for state anxiety scores or physiologic parameters (i.e., BP, heart rate, digital skin temperature). Silence and white noise were as effective in lowering BP, heart rate, skin temperature, and anxiety as was music selected by the patients. Authors concluded that the therapeutic intervention was actually 30 minutes of uninterrupted relaxation.[68]

The research suggests that music can affect mood state, decrease pain, and increase cognitive function. To be effective, music selection must be appropriate for the intended outcome. Music selection based on personal preference may represent the subject's current mood state, which can potentially reinforce the problem (e.g., depression, anxiety, fear) rather than provide relief. Music selection may be most beneficial when initially "entrained" to current mood state, but then designed to move the individual from the current mental state of mind into one more conducive to inducing relaxation, producing endorphins, promoting alertness, or some other intended outcome.

Laughter and Its Effects on Stress Hormones

It has been reported that healthy children laugh as many as 400 times per day and adults only

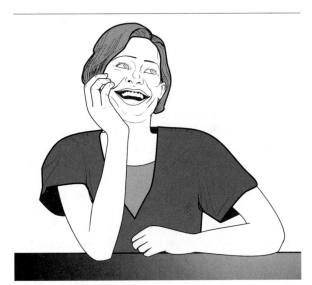

■ **Figure 1-15.** Laughter is considered a positive form of stress or "eustress," which can have positive health benefits.

about 15 times a day (Figure 1-15).[19] Some persons believe that this reduction in expressed joy is a result of repressed emotion and life stress. Stress has been demonstrated to impair immune function.

The classical stress response consists of psychologic, neural, and endocrine components involving the CNS and HPA axis.[17,62] In response to stress, the body increases ACTH, cortisol, catecholamines, beta-endorphin, GH, and prolactin. These are collectively referred to as stress hormones. In an amusing study, Berk and others hypothesized that although laughter invokes a form of stress, it is qualitatively different in effect from the classical increases in stress hormones observed in the types of stress known to downregulate immunity.

In Berk's study, the authors sought to assess the effects of laughter on the neuroendocrine hormones involved in the classical stress response. They hypothesized that laughter would invoke qualitatively different neuroendocrine responses from those invoked by a classical stress response.

Method. In a controlled trial, the blood hormones of healthy men were compared when experimental subjects (N=5) were shown a humorous video and control subjects (N=5) sat quietly for the same period of time.[4] The video was "Gallagher-Over Your Head", the comedian Gallagher's personal view of politicians, ancient history, and child rearing, including his famous "Sledge-O-Matic" finale.

Outcomes. Although both groups decreased the stress hormone cortisol (0.0005), the experimental group decreased the hormone significantly more rapidly (0.016). EPI (i.e., adrenaline) remained lower for the experimental group, but it increased for the control group (0.0003). There were no changes in GH for control subjects, whereas GH levels in the experimental group decreased over intervention (0.0005). ACTH, beta-endorphin, prolactin, and NEP levels did not significantly increase.

Conclusions and comments. In summary, video watchers significantly reduced the stress hormones of cortisol, GH, and EPI and as compared with resting controls. Because laughter has been reported to reduce certain stress hormones, it may be considered a health-generating behavioral habit. The authors therefore described the effects of laughter as "eustress" or a healthy, positive form of stress. In previous studies the authors found that laughter also increased spontaneous lymphocyte reproduction and NK cell activity.[5,6] Since increased cortisol and EPI levels during stress suppress immune function, decreasing these levels may improve immune competency.

Writing or Talking about Traumatic Events

Accumulating evidence suggests that if an extremely upsetting life event or experience is not expressed, over time this failure to express feelings may be related to disease processes and an increased susceptibility to illness.[47,64] Research was designed to determine whether expression of feelings in written form would benefit subjects. This was of interest because some subjects may not be able or willing to verbally express feelings about a traumatic event to others and because, if effective, this method would be potentially beneficial to an unlimited number of subjects.

Effects of Writing on Illness Susceptibility

The authors of the Pennebaker study examined the effects of divulging traumatic events independent of social feedback (i.e., written form). The questions at issue were the following: (1) What aspects of expressing a traumatic event reduce physiologic levels and disease rates? (2) Is the discharge of emotion alone sufficient to help heal?

Method. In a randomized, double-blind, placebo-controlled study, 46 subjects, divided into four groups, were required to write an essay on 4 nights.[46] Group 1, the trauma-fact group, narratively described a traumatic event without referring to their feelings about it. Group 2, the trauma-emotion group, described their feelings about the event without writing about the event itself. Group 3, the trauma-combination group, wrote about the traumatic event and their feelings about it. Group 4, the control group, wrote about a trivial event like describing the appearance of their shoes.

Outcomes

1. The subjects in groups 1, 2, and 3 had short-term significant increases in physiologic stress responses (i.e., increased BP and negative mood states prewriting to postwriting sessions) with these effects, then, consistently decreasing with each writing session. Only BP reached a significant decline ($p<0.001$) with separate ANOVAs on heart rate and diastolic BP yielding no significant condition of main effect or interaction (i.e., no significant differences between groups). Subjects in group 4 had the least response of the four groups.

2. There was a long-term (6 months) reduction in health center visits for illness among the subjects in Groups 2 and 3 ($p=0.055$), but those in Group 1 and 4 both experienced similar nonsignificant changes in health status.

3. Subjects in groups 2 and 3 reported thinking a great deal about their topic for months after the study ($p=0.05$).

4. Subjects who never discussed the trauma with others experienced greater short-term stress and long-term health benefits than those who shared the experience.

Conclusions and comments. The authors concluded that the need to express emotion, as well as cognitively organize the event, is necessary if health outcomes are to be optimal. Subjects described developing a new "coping strategy" for dealing with trauma. This is an important point to consider. The concept that one should practice only "positive thinking," which is interpreted to mean evading or denying negative emotions, may not be the best strategy for health maintenance.

Effects of Writing on Mitogen Responses

In a randomized, placebo-controlled study of the same design, but with only two groups (N=50), half of the undergraduate subjects were assigned to write about traumatic experiences (experimental group) and half were instructed to write about superficial topics (control group) for 20 minutes a day for 4 days. The experimental group was instructed to write about their deepest feelings about a topic they had not shared with others. Blood samples from the subjects of both groups were taken on three occasions: (1) the day before the writing, (2) the last day of the writing, and (3) 6 weeks after the writing. The experimental group had a significantly higher response to cellular stimulation (i.e., the ability to reproduce when needed) when compared with their baseline than did the control subjects ($p=0.04$). The experimental group required less health center visits than they did before the writing and as compared with the control subjects ($p<0.05$)[48] (Figure 1-16).

Is writing the most effective method for releasing repressed feelings? Other studies have suggested that orally expressing feelings is a more effective method than writing for strengthening immunity and improving health outcomes.

Writing Versus Speaking: A Modulator of Epstein-Barr Virus Antibody Titers

The authors of the Esterling study sought to replicate an earlier study, which reported that subjects who were classified as "repressors" of emotion (i.e., those who abstained from disclosing an emotional event on a writing task) had a higher rate of reactivation of Epstein-Barr virus (EBV) than subjects who were classified as nonrepressors.[18] Most have been exposed to EBV and carry the virus in their bodies for life. When an individual's immune

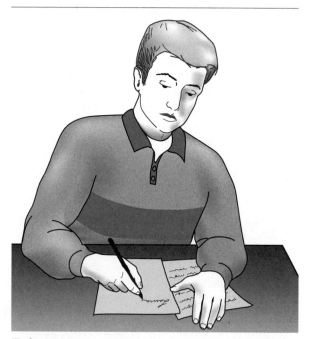

■ *Figure 1-16.* Research suggests that writing about negative life events may help improve health outcomes.

system is strong, these viruses are kept in check; when the immune system becomes weakened, these viruses can multiply. If they multiply, the human body produces more antibodies to fight them. Changes in the amount of antibody are measured in titers. Thus when antibody titers increase, it suggests we have compromised our immune system to some degree and our bodies are attempting to beat back the invaders. The authors of the Esterling study asked the following questions: (1) Will experimentally manipulating emotional expression modulate EBV antibody titers? (2) Will oral or written disclosure of stressful events elicit different EBV reactivation levels? (3) Will the seriousness of the event disclosed alter the health outcomes?

Method. Seventy-two volunteer subjects were assessed for seropositive status to EBV; 57 were determined to be EBV seropositive (i.e., they had been previously exposed to EBV). Data from only these 57 subjects were used in the study. Subjects completed the Millon Behavioral Health Inventory, which assesses individual differences in interpersonal coping styles. Based on the scores on the inventory, subjects were placed into one of three classifications: (1) emotional repressors, (2) emotional sensitizers, or (3) neither personality style. Subjects classified as repressors are said to have an inner need to deny negative feelings to self and to others; they may appear content when facing problems and they may attempt to please others with self-sacrificing behaviors. Those classified as sensitizers may present themselves as overbearing, aggressive, rivalrous, and confident. They may have a low frustration tolerance level and express negative feelings quickly.[40]

The 57 undergraduates were randomly assigned to one of three groups: (1) writing about a stressful event; (2) talking about a stressful event; or (3) writing about a trivial event (control group). In Groups 1 and 2, the subjects were asked to disclose a traumatic event about which they felt very guilty and had not shared with many people. They were then asked to either write an essay (N=21) or speak into a tape recorder (N=17) about the event, as if they were writing or speaking to someone they trusted. Each trial lasted 20 minutes. The subjects in the trivial event group were asked to write about the contents of their bedroom closets, bedrooms, or cars. All subjects participated in three weekly sessions in which they received the same instructions.

Blood was collected between 1:00 PM and 4:00 PM 1 week before the first session and at the same time of day, and 1 week after the last session. Oral sessions were transcribed into a written format. Then, both written and oral comments were assessed for content and the number of emotional words. They were also assessed for positive cognitive appraisal change, self-esteem improvements, and adaptive coping strategies.

Outcomes. The subjects uniformly disclosed highly personal and upsetting experiences in their essays, and the frequency of these themes did not differ between the written and oral stressful disclosure groups. The oral stressful group had significantly greater evidence of cognitive change, as compared with the written stressful group, and both groups demonstrated more cognitive change than the control group ($p<0.0001$). The oral group had a higher self-esteem rating than the written group, which scored similarly to the control group ($p<0.001$). The oral group displayed significantly more adaptive coping strategies than the written or control groups, which did not differ from each other ($p<0.0001$). Randomly assigned groups had equivalent EBV antibody levels at baseline. No significant changes occurred in the control group, from preintervention to postintervention. This finding was in contrast to the antibody levels of the written stressful group ($p<0.01$) and oral stressful group ($p<0.001$), the latter of which demonstrated significant decreases in EBV antibody titer levels after intervention. Thus the subjects in classification 1 (repressors) had the highest levels of EBV antibody titers; subjects in classification 3 (neither personality style) had the second highest levels of titers; and classification 2 (sensitizers) had the lowest levels, although differences between classification 2 and 3 were not significant. Further, personality style significantly predicted changes in EBV antibody titer levels. Sensitizers demonstrated greater decreases in antibody titers than repressors. The number of expressed negative emotional words also predicted greater decreases. Greater cognitive change, enhanced self-esteem, and seriousness of the event, but not the adaptive coping strategies, predicted greater decreases in EBV antibody titers.

Conclusions and comments. Participation in three written or oral emotional disclosure interventions significantly decreased EBV antibody titers over a 4-week period, with oral expression producing significantly lower antibody titer levels than written expression, an indicator of a more efficient immune system. Subjects in the writing group expressed significantly more total emotional words and more negative and positive emotional words than subjects in the oral group. Subjects classified as emotional repressors had significantly higher EBV antibody titers than those classified as emotional sensitizers, who expressed their feelings readily and strongly.

Other Studies on Oral and Written Expression of Emotion

Other authors have also found speaking about traumatic events healing. Pennebaker, Barger, and Tiebout found that Holocaust survivors, who expressed the most emotional words when disclosing particularly traumatic war-related experiences, had lower skin conductance levels and demonstrated the greatest health improvements (i.e., fewer physical symptoms and physician visits) in the year after an interview.[45] These authors concluded that disclosing an extremely traumatic event, even 40 years after its occurrence, can have positive health benefits.

Murray and others contrasted brief psychotherapy with written expression in a study similar to the one reviewed in the previous text. They found written expression effective in temporarily releasing negative effect, but it did not change the feelings about the traumatic events. Oral expression aroused less negative effect, but it provided more cognitive reappraisal and a strong shift to a positive effect and a change in attitude about stressful events.[43] These findings were replicated in the previously mentioned study.

Earlier, Pennebaker and Beall demonstrated that emotional written expression about a stressful event decreased health center visits in the 6 months after the study.[46] The current authors suggested that one immunologic pathway by which this occurs may be in the body's ability to control viral replication.

Petrie and others assessed 40 medical students who tested negative for hepatitis B antibodies. These subjects were then given their first hepatitis B vaccination, with booster injections at 1 and 4 months after writing. Compared with control group subjects, treatment subjects who wrote about their emotions demonstrated significantly higher antibody levels against hepatitis B at the 4- and 6-month follow-up periods.[50]

Most importantly, attention should be paid to the difference between an experience of emotion and the expression of emotion. The distinction between emotional experience and expression

may explain the low correlations between measures of negative effect, neuroticism, and anxiety with health outcome measures. Chronically anxious persons (sensitizers) may be at the highest risk for degradation of health, but they may also receive maximal benefit from expressive therapies. On the other hand, persons who appear to be less anxious, but who are not in touch with their emotional feelings and do not therefore express them (repressors), are at greatest risk. It has been suggested that verbalizing an event produces a deeper awareness of the emotional issues around a stressor. The person essentially "rehearses" the experience when they express it orally. Several researchers have suggested that the ideal approach to emotional expression for health purposes should include written homework combined with orally expressive psychotherapy. Others have suggested that even the homework should be completed orally, perhaps with a tape recorder.[35,51] In any case, the importance of emotional expression is worthy of consideration in maintaining emotional and physical well being.

Group Support and Cancer Outcomes

In the mid-1970s, David Spiegel, a psychiatrist, never anticipated his work would show that the mind had an effect on physical health (Figure 1-17). He led support groups for women in treatment for advanced breast cancer that had spread throughout their bodies. This condition provided the grimmest of prognoses. He began his study with the belief that positive psychologic and symptom effects could occur without affecting the course of the disease. He expected a potential improvement in the quality of life, but not an

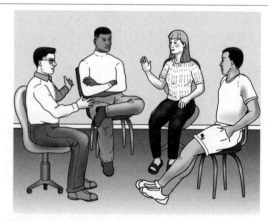

■ **Figure 1-17.** Group support may benefit health outcomes in those facing chronic or potentially fatal diseases such as cancer.

increase in survival time. His original intention was to assess improvement level in the quality of the emotional life for patients during their survival time. An additional original intent, he recalled, was to disprove the superficial notion that emotions affected the actual course of cancer. Unexpectedly, the women in the support group survived an average of 18 months longer, almost twice as long as controls who did not participate in the support group. At this phase of their disease, the added months of life exceeded the time expected from cancer medication. Ten years later, the only three survivors were all patients in Spiegel's support group. We examine this and other studies and the effects of emotional support on mortality.

Group Support for Terminal Cancer Patients.
In the Spiegel study, the authors wanted to determine whether group therapy for in-patients with metastatic breast cancer had any effect on survival time.

Method. The survival outcomes of patients with metastatic breast cancer (N=86), who were assigned to either a weekly 1-year support group (Group 1) or a control group (Group 2), were assessed in a randomized, controlled, 10-year follow-up study.[59] Intervention groups met weekly for 90 minutes and were led by a psychiatrist and a social worker. At no time were the patients told that participation would affect the course of their disease. The patients expressed feelings and shared physical problems, including discussions of side effects. They also discussed and learned a self-hypnosis strategy for pain control.

Chemotherapy and radiation treatments between the groups and the severity of the illnesses were not significantly different.

Outcomes. The length of survival for patients in Group 1 doubled, with this group obtaining a survival mean of 37 months, compared with the survival mean of 19 months for Group 2. Survival divergence began 8 months after treatment. Psychologic assessments did not significantly predict survival; the only variable that affected survival time was the complex psychosocial intervention itself.

Conclusions and comments. This study, performed at Stanford University, was considered to be profoundly compelling. The authors believed that social support may have been an important factor in patient survival. They suggested that neuroendocrine and immune systems may also be linked with the emotional process, affecting the course of cancer. They also noted that treated patients learned about hypnosis for pain control and therefore may have been more able to maintain exercise and routine activities, both conducive to health.

Other Group Support Studies
A well-designed study evaluated the health effects of a 6-week structured group intervention that provided health education, enhancement of problem-solving skills, relaxation training, and psychologic support.[20] The subjects had Stage I or II malignant melanoma and received no treatment other than surgical removal of the malignant cells. The subjects met in groups of seven to ten for 90 minutes, once a week for 6 weeks. Compared with patients assigned to a control group (N=26), patients in the intervention group (N=35) demonstrated significant increases in percentages of NK cells, an increase in NK cytotoxicity (i.e., ability to kill invaders), and a decrease in the percentage of helper-inducer T-cells. Psychologic distress was also reduced for those in the intervention group. Results began to emerge 6 months after group intervention. The magnitude of change in immunologic measurements was frequently greater than 25% for the intervention group, and the majority of intervention subjects demonstrated these changes. On the other hand, less than one third of controls demonstrated these changes.

In an earlier controlled study, Spiegel and others reported on 54 women with metastatic breast cancer who attended weekly group therapy sessions with or without self-hypnosis training.[58] Both groups had suffered less intense pain, but there was no difference in duration or frequency of pain. The hypnosis-trained group controlled pain intensity more effectively. These combined studies may indicate the efficacy of psychosocial interventions.

Other studies have failed to replicate Spiegel's positive findings. For example, Gellert and colleagues conducted a 10-year, retrospective, matched survey. In this study, 34 patients with breast cancer who attended weekly cancer support groups, family therapy, and individual counseling and who practiced positive imagery were compared with 102 patients with breast cancer who did not.[26] Although the program may have had a beneficial effect on the quality of life, no significant difference in survival rates was found nor did the program serve as a social locus for exceptional survivors. These findings differed sharply from Spiegel's outcomes. This difference may be accounted for in part by the fact that Gellert's study used group support, meditation, and imagery for pain control, whereas Spiegel's intervention emphasized personal relationships and hypnosis. Spiegel noted that it was quite possible that the subjects in his original study were more compliant with treatment, had better exercise and diet habits, and differed on other health-related behaviors. These differences could contribute to his original findings. Nonetheless, the overall findings can only be considered suggestive as program designs and outcomes differ and the number of studies is low.

Personality Style and Illness

Previous studies have suggested that personality styles may be related to what has been termed a *disease-prone personality.* As we have discussed earlier in this chapter, depression can suppress immune function and play a role in chronic disease states. Repression of feelings may also produce unnatural psychophysiologic arousal, leaving persons more susceptible to a variety of illnesses.[25] Hostility has been found to influence the course of life-threatening illnesses, such as coronary heart disease. For example, in a retrospective study, 1877 men between the ages of 40 and 55 with high levels of hostility demonstrated higher death rates from both cardiovascular disease and other causes. When those with the highest scores were compared with those with the lowest, risk of death was 42% higher.[56] Several reports have linked coronary heart disease and cardiac death with anxiety, depression, worry, and mental stress.[12,24,31,34,41]

The question is: Are these individual emotional states predictive factors or are combined states of negative emotion more predictive (Figure 1-18)?

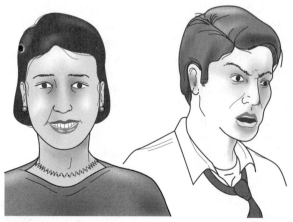

■ **Figure 1-18.** Research has suggested that personality style can potentially affect health outcomes.

In a more comprehensive approach, Denollet and Brutsaert followed 87 patients who suffered myocardial infarctions, a study that lasted 6 to 10 years. They hypothesized that emotional stress in these patients (1) was unrelated to the severity of the cardiac disorder, (2) may predict future cardiac events, and (3) was a function of a basic personality trait (e.g., Type D). Type D refers to a personality with a negative affectation, consisting of the combined states of anxiety, pessimism, despair, and anger. The Type D personality experiences a great many of these negative emotions and simultaneously inhibits the self-expression of these emotions.

During follow-up, Type D personalities were more likely to experience a cardiac event, including cardiac death, than their non–Type D counterparts ($p=0.00005$). The authors concluded that although emotional distress was unrelated to the severity of disease, personality type definitely influenced the clinical course of cardiac disease in patients with a decreased left ventricular ejection fraction (i.e., patient with a poor prognosis).[16]

The literature has attempted to describe both the disease-prone personality and another style known as the *self-healing personality. Self-healing personalities* are described as enthusiastic, spontaneous, creative, playful, humorous, and philosophic rather than hostile, as well as concerned with issues of beauty, justice, ethics, and understanding.

Another way these personalities are often labeled is *pessimistic* versus *optimistic.* A recent study found this "either-or" approach unconvincing, as related to sickness versus health. Robinson-Whelen and others found that pessimism, not optimism, was the unique predictor of subsequent psychologic and physical health in samples of both stressed and nonstressed individuals.[54] The authors suggested that optimism and pessimism should be explored separately to determine how one can specifically benefit from optimism. Do these benefits come from thinking optimistically, avoiding pessimistic thinking, or a combination of both? Being optimistic may not be as important as simply avoiding undue negative thinking. In this context, optimism should not be interpreted as denying or evading negative feelings; rather, it should be considered as avoiding the reinforcement of negative thought patterns. Forced optimism could serve to repress emotions that need to be experienced and released.

It would appear that cognitive organization and the expression and release of negative emotional experiences in written and oral form may be beneficial to health. Repression of feelings in the form of forced optimism is not. In later chapters, we explore more formalized intervention methods of health intervention.

■ Implications for Stress Management and Optimal Wellness

The combined research suggests that the following factors contribute to health:

1. Written and oral expression
2. Group support
3. Entrainment music that modifies the mood state from a negative to a more positive condition
4. Reasonable amount of entertainment with generous doses of laughter

A sense of purpose and belief in one's ability to affect and have control over one's life and one's health is also critical for well-being. How can you apply these approaches to your life? What can you recommend to your patients who need stress management strategies?

To determine the formula that supports health, the patient can begin by taking stock—taking control and determining which of these approaches can contribute to the management of his or her stress. Most importantly, the patient must decide which approaches are appealing enough to put into practice.

Written Expression

Keeping a journal is a creative, fulfilling, insightful, and therapeutic exercise. It can provide a sense of constancy in an otherwise chaotic world. Writing in a journal takes as little as 5 minutes a day and is a permanent record of life's events, the feelings about these events, and one's goals, dreams, and frustrations. It is an acknowledgement of, and an ongoing conversation with, one's self.

How the patient wants to keep a journal is a very personal matter:

- Some patients feel it is absolutely essential to handwrite their feelings and thoughts in an empty book or notepad purchased for this specific purpose.
- Other patients use their computer, because they find it easier and faster to use to express their thoughts.
- Some patients use predefined, structured formats. For example, there may be categories entitled, "What I did today," "How I felt today," and "What I learned and experienced today."
- Others simply pour their thoughts and feelings for the day into the journal—in a stream-of-consciousness fashion.
- Some patients include prayers as part of their journals.
- Some persons include artwork in their journals.

The critical point is that patients write in the journal every day, for a minimum of 5 minutes. Then once a month, the patients can review the entries and write their thoughts about what they have learned from their experiences and what they will do with what they have learned. Many persons perform a more thorough review of their journals at the 1-year anniversary.

Oral Expression

There are several ways that oral expression can be implemented as part of a self-awareness and stress reduction program. The patient could, as described in one study, keep a tape-recorded account of his or her day—the equivalent of keeping an oral journal. Then once a month, he or she could listen to the recordings and write down thoughts about what was experienced, what was learned, and what will be done with the new insights.

Some patients who keep journals perform their monthly review by reading their entries aloud to a family member, therapist, or friend and then discuss their feelings about the experiences of the month and their feelings about them.

One patient spends 5 minutes each night, right after dinner, talking to her spouse about her day and her feelings; her spouse then does the same to her. These oral expressions serve to keep them in touch with each other and provide a consistent format for expression.

Again, the important issue is to have a committed process for oral expression with which the patient is comfortable and consistent.

Support Groups

Support groups are used for a wide variety of purposes, including psychological therapy, weight loss, grief work, and personal development. The patient can decide if a support group would be helpful and if he or she is committed to attending and working with a group. If so, the patient can seek a group that is facilitated by a licensed, well-trained professional. Support groups allow oral expression with other persons living through similar challenges.

Support groups that are not structured as therapy sessions can also be beneficial. For example, in one community a local support group was created for widows and widowers with children. The format is one of entertainment and social interaction. Picnics, camping trips, movie outings, or dinner parties were held once a week.

Entrainment Music

To be effective, entrainment music must, in the first few minutes, match the prevalent mood (e.g., depression, anxiety, anger) and then shift from this mood to a more positive one. When used effectively, entrainment music can significantly reduce pain, tension, depression, and anxiety and significantly improve general mood state, energy levels, and cognitive functioning. Care must be taken to select music that does not reinforce the patient's current undesired mood state. The following steps should be taken to use entrainment music effectively:

1. Determine which mood state is most problematic (e.g., anxiety is a typical problem for patients).
2. Spend time previewing music that is representative of both the undesired mood state and the mood state the patient wants to entrain.
3. Combine music selections so that the first few minutes of music matches the current mood state and then shifts to music that represents the desired mood state.

Another, simpler method for accomplishing entrainment is to identify records or radio stations (the ones with music only formats) and select music from those that match the mood state. Then, the patient moves from the matched music to a station with music that matches a mood between the undesired and the desired mood state. Finally, he or she moves to a station matching the desired state of consciousness. For example, if the patient is in an anxious mood and wants to move to a deeply relaxed state, he or she could start with a frenetic rock tune that matches the anxious mood state, move to jazz music, and then to alternative music, which is repetitive, soothing, and slow-paced.

It is important that the mood of the music successfully drift from the undesired to the desired state of consciousness. For suggested music, the previous music studies can be reviewed, with consideration given to the types of music used by these researchers.

Laughter

Many patients with anger problems attend movies that contain a great deal of violence in them. They claim this gives them a sense of release. "I can imagine," said one patient, "that I am throttling my boss while Bruce Willis throttles the bad guy." Research has consistently demonstrated that images entrain and reinforce our moods, just as mood music entrains mood state. There may be a temporary sense of release of tension, but the anger is, in fact, reinforced by exposure to aggressive images. Patients should select television programming and movie entertainment carefully and actively seek out and participate in forms of entertainment that are fun, light hearted, and matched to the mood state they wish to cultivate.

■ Chapter Review

There are many things in life that we are exposed to that we cannot control. We can, however, make choices about how we cultivate our inner thoughts and where we focus our attention. We can decide how to interact with our world and ourselves. The strategies discussed in this chapter are but a few ideas for taking control of the inner self and of health.

In later chapters, we learn how to incorporate meditation and relaxation practices, exercise, and herbs into a wellness program. The services, benefits, and limitations of alternative practices are reviewed, and beneficial effects of spirituality on health are described. How these practices complement conventional medicine is delineated. The suggestions in this chapter are a beginning point—simple interventions that can be helpful for health professionals and patients alike.

Matching Terms and Definitions

Match each numbered definition with the correct term. Place the corresponding letter in the space provided.

_____ 1. Brain and spinal cord

_____ 2. Nerves branching from the brain and spinal cord

_____ 3. Thymus, spleen, lymph nodes, appendix, tonsils, and white blood cells

_____ 4. Pituitary, thyroid, parathyroid, adrenal, pineal, and thymus glands; pancreas, ovaries, testes, and hypothalamus; and other specialized cells

_____ 5. Neurons innervating muscles and glands

_____ 6. Most direct mind-body pathway that uses neurotransmitters and neuropeptides

_____ 7. Second mind-body pathway that uses hormones as messengers

_____ 8. Chemicals that communicate between nervous, endocrine, and immune systems

_____ 9. Carry messages away from brain and spinal cord and back to organs and glands

_____ 10. Carry signals from organs and glands back to spinal cord and brain

_____ 11. Controls heart beat, BP, respiration, and swallowing

_____ 12. Conduction to and from brain and major reflex center

_____ 13. Executive of the brain, allowing us to remember, perceive, communicate, comprehend, and initiate voluntary action

_____ 14. Two divisions of the ANS

_____ 15. NEP, acetylcholine, EPI, dopamine, Gaba, serotonin

_____ 16. Integration center of the ANS that modulates heart activity, body temperature, BP, and endocrine activity

_____ 17. Emotional part of brain

_____ 18. CRH, ACTH, cortisol, TSH, and GH

_____ 19. Activation of the SNS division of the ANS in response to anxiety, fear, or strong emotion

_____ 20. Neurotransmitters, neuropeptides, hormones, and immune modulators

_____ 21. VIP, somatostatin, cholecystokinin, endorphins, and enkephalins

_____ 22. Cytokines, including lymphokines and monokines

a. Sympathetic and parasympathetic
b. Spinal cord
c. Limbic system
d. Sympathetic-adrenal-medullary axis
e. Endocrine system
f. Neurotransmitters
g. Informational substances
h. Peripheral nervous system
i. Brainstem
j. Hormones
k. Immune modulators
l. Chemical messengers, information substances
m. Motor or efferent neurons
n. ANS
o. Neuropeptides
p. Central nervous system
q. Hypothalamus
r. Hypothalamic/pituitary/adrenal cortex axis
s. Sensory or afferent neurons
t. Stress response
u. Immune system
v. Cerebral cortex

CRITICAL THINKING AND CLINICAL APPLICATION EXERCISES

1. Design a "laughter therapy program" for a professional workaholic.
2. Evaluate the research in this chapter concerning group support and cancer. What are the limitations of the research? What do you consider to be the best combination of components for a group support intervention?
3. Compare and contrast the research in the chapter on writing as opposed to talking about traumatic events. Under what circumstances is one preferred over the other? Suggest populations for which one might be more beneficial than another.
4. Think deeply about your own mood states and lifestyles. How can you use the research in this chapter to optimize your own emotional and physical well being?
5. Do you think personality style influences health outcomes? How? If it does, suggest one way to use knowledge about personality style to work with a patient's health outcomes.
6. Review the research on music provided in this chapter. Design a model music intervention for lifting a depressive mood state.

References

1. Ader R: *Commentary: on the teaching of psycho-neuroimmunology.* Proceedings of the 1996 Meeting of the Psychoneuroimmunology Research Society, Center for Psychoneuroimmunology Research and Department of Psychiatry, Rochester, NY, 1996, University of Rochester, School of Medicine and Dentistry.
2. Allen K, Blascovich J: Effects of music on cardiovascular reactivity among surgeons, *JAMA* 272(11):882, 1994.
3. Ballieux RE, Heijnen CJ: Brain and immune system: a one-way conversation or a genuine dialogue? *Prog Brain Res* 72:71, 1987.
4. Berk LS, Tan SA, Fry WF, et al: Neuroendocrine and stress hormone changes during mirthful laughter, *Am J Med Sci* 298(6):390, 1989.
5. Berk LA, Tan SA, Napier BJ, Eby WC: Eustress of mirthful laughter modifies natural killer cell activity, *Clin Res* 37:115A, 1989.
6. Berk LS, Tan SA, Nehlsen-Cannarella S, Napier BJ, Lewis JE, Lee JW, Eby WC: Humor associated laughter decreases cortisol and increases spontaneous lymphocyte blastogenesis, *Clin Res* 36:435A, 1988.
7. Besedovsky HO, del Rey A: Physiological implications of the immune-neuro-endocrine network. In Ader R, Felten DL, Cohen N, editors: *Psychoneuroimmunology,* New York, 1991, Academic Press.
8. Besedovsky HO, del Rey A, Sorkin E: Antigenic competition between horse and sheep red blood cells as a hormone-dependent phenomenon, *Clin Exp Immunol* 37:106, 1979.
9. Besedovsky HO, del Rey A, Sorkin E, Lortz W, Schwulera W: Lymphoid cells produce an immunoregulatory glucocorticoid increasing factor (GIF) acting through the pituitary gland, *Clin Exp Immunol* 59:622, 1985.
10. Besedovsky HO, Sorkin E: Immunologic-neuroendocrine circuits: physiological approaches. In Ader R, editor: *Psychoneuroimmunology,* New York, 1981, Academic Press.
11. Blalock JE: Production and action of lymphocyte-derived neuroendocrine peptide hormones—summary, *Prog Immunol* 6:27, 1986.
12. Blumenthal JA, Jiang W, Waugh RA, Frid DJ, Morris IJ, Coleman RE, Hanson M, Babyak M, Thyrum ET, Krantz DS, O'Connor C: Mental stress-induced ischemia in the laboratory and ambulatory ischemia during daily life: association and hemodynamic features, *Circulation* 92:2102, 1995.
13. Bulloch K, Pomerantz W: Autonomic nervous system innervation of thymic-related lymphoid tissue in wild-type and nude mice, *J Comp Neurol* 228:57, 1984.
14. Calabrese JR, Wilde C: Alterations in immunocompetence during stress: a medical perspective. In Plotnikoff N, Murgo A, Faith R, Wybran J, editors: *Stress and immunity,* Boca Raton, FL, 1991, CRC Press.
15. Carr DJJ, Blalock JE: Neuropeptide hormones and receptors common to the immune and neuroendocrine systems: bidirectional pathway of intersystem communication. In Ader R, Felton DL, Cohen N, editors: *Psychoneuroimmunology,* New York, 1991, Academic Press.
16. Denollet J, Brutsaert DL: Personality, disease severity, and the risk of long-term cardiac events in patients with a decreased ejection fraction after myocardial infarction, *Circulation* 97:16, 1998.
17. Dunn AJ, Kamarcy NR: Neurochemical responses in stress: relationship between the hypothalamic-pituitary-adrenal and catecholamine systems. In Iversen LL, Iversen SD, Snyder SH, editors: *Handbook of psychopharmacology,* vol 18, New York, 1984, Plenum Press.
18. Esterling BA, Antoni MH, Kumar M, Schneiderman N: Emotional repression, stress disclosure responses and Epstein-Barr viral capsid antigen titers, *Psychosom Med* 52:397, 1990.
19. *Family Practice News:* Research is showing healthful effects of laughter, May 15:52a, 1992.
20. Fawzy FI, Kemeny ME, Fawzy NW, Elashoff R, Morton D, Cousins M, Fahey JL: A structured psychiatric intervention for cancer patients, *Arch Gen Psychiatry* 47:729, 1990.
21. Felten, DL, Cohen N, Ader R, Felten SY, Carlson SL, Roszman TL: Central neural circuits involved in neural-immune interactions. In Ader R, Felten DL, Cohen N, editors: *Psychoneuroimmunology,* New York, 1991, Academic Press.
22. Felten DL, Felten SY, Carlson SL, Olschowka JA, Livnat S: Noradrenergic and peptidergic innervation of lymphoid tissue, *J Immunol* 135:755S, 1985.
23. Felten SY, Felten DL: Innervation of lymphoid tissues. In Ader R, Felton DL, Cohen N, editors: *Psychoneuroimmunology,* New York, 1991, Academic Press.
24. Frasure-Smith N, Lesperance F, Talajic M: Depression and 18-month prognosis after myocardial infarction, *Circulation* 91:999, 1995.
25. Friedman HS, Vandenvos GR: Disease-prone and self-healing personalities, *Hosp Com Psychiatry* 43(12):1177, 1992.
26. Gellert GA, Maxwell RM, Siegal BS: Survival of breast cancer patients receiving adjunctive psychosocial support therapy: a 10-year follow-up study, *J Clin Oncol* 11(1):66, 1993.
27. Goetzl EJ, Turck CW, Sreedharan SP: Production and recognition of neuropeptides by cells of the immune system. In Ader R, Felten DL, Cohen N, editors: *Psychoneuroimmunology,* New York, 1991, Academic Press.
28. Good M: Effects of relaxation and music on postoperative pain: a review, *J Adv Nurs* 24:905, 1996.
29. Hall NR, Goldstein AL: Neurotransmitters and the immune system. In Ader R, editor: *Psychoneuroimmunology,* New York, 1981, Academic Press.
30. Hiramoto R, Ghanta V, Solvason B, Lorden J, Hsueh C, Rogers C, Demissie S, Hiramoto N: Identification of specific pathways of communication between the CNS and NK cell system, *Life Sci* 53:527, 1993.
31. Kawachi I, Colditz GA, Ascherio A, Rimm E, Giovannucci E, Stempfer MJ, Willet WC: Prospective study of phobic anxiety, and risk of coronary heart disease in men, *Circulation* 89:1992, 1994.
32. Kerkvliet GJ: Music therapy may help control cancer pain, *J Natl Cancer Inst* 82(5):350, 1990.
33. Krippner S: Psychoneuroimmunology. In Raymond J, Corsini N, editors: *Encyclopedia of psychology,* ed 2, New York, 1994, Wiley.
34. Kubzansky LD, Kawachi I, Spiro A, Weiss ST, Vokonas PS, Sparrow D: Is worrying bad for your heart? A prospective study of worry and coronary heart disease in the Normative Aging Study, *Circulation* 95:818, 1997.
35. L'Abate L: The use of writing in psychotherapy, *Am J Psychother* 45:87, 1991.
36. Lyon ML: Psychoneuroimmunology: the problem of the situatedness of illness and the conceptualization of healing, *Cult Med Psychiatry* 17:77, 1993.
37. Marieb EN: *Human anatomy and physiology,* ed 3, New York, 1995, Benjamin/Cummings.
38. McGuinan FJ: Progressive relaxation: origins, principles, and clinical applications. In Lehrer P, Woolfolk RL, editors: *Principles and practice of stress management,* ed 2, New York, 1993, The Guilford Press.
39. McKinney CH, Tims FC, Kumar AM, Kumar M: The effect of selected classical music and spontaneous imagery on plasma B-endorphin, *J Behav Med* 20(1):85, 1997.
40. Millon T, Green CJ, Meagher RB: *Millon Behavioral Health Inventory,* Minneapolis, Minn, 1982, Interpretive Scoring Systems.

41. Mittleman MA, Maclure M, Sherwood JB, Mulry RP, Tofler GH, Jacobs SC, Friedman R, Benson H, Muller JE: Triggering of acute myocardial infarction onset by episodes of anger, *Circulation* 92:1720, 1995.

42. Morley JE, Key NE, Solomon GF, Plotnikoff NP: Neuropeptides: conductors of the immune orchestra, *Science* 42:527, 1987.

43. Murray EJ, Lamnin AD, Carver CS: Emotional expression in written essays and psychotherapy, *J Soc Clin Psychol* 7:414, 1989.

44. O'Grady MP, Hall NRS: Long-term effects of neuro-endocrine-immune interactions during early development. In Ader R, Felten DL, Cohen N, editors: *Psychoneuroimmunology,* New York, 1991, Academic Press.

45. Pennebaker JW, Barger SD, Tiebout J: Disclosure of traumas and health among Holocaust survivors, *Psychosom Med* 51:577, 1989.

46. Pennebaker JW, Beall S: Confronting a traumatic event: toward an understanding of inhibition and disease, *J Abnorm Psychol* 95:274, 1986.

47. Pennebaker JW, Hoover CW: Inhibition and cognition: toward an understanding of trauma and disease. In Davidson RJ, Schwartz GE, Shapiro D, editors: *Consciousness and self-regulation,* vol 4, New York, 1986, Plenum Press.

48. Pennebaker JW, Kiecolt-Glaser JK, Glaser R: Disclosure of traumas and immune function: health implications for psychotherapy, *J Consult Clin Psychol* 56:239, 1988.

49. Pert CB: *Molecules of emotion: why we feel the way we feel,* New York, 1997, Scribner.

50. Petrie JK, Booth RJ, Pennebaker JW, Davison KP, Thomas MG: Disclosure of trauma and immune response to a hepatitis B vaccination program, *J Consult Clin Psychol* 63(5):787, 1995.

51. Phillips EL, Weiner DN: *Short term psychotherapy and structured behavior change,* New York, 1966, McGraw-Hill.

52. Renoux G, Biziere K: Neurocortex lateralization of immune function and of the activities of imuthiol, a T-cell specific immunopotentiator. In Ader R, Felten DL, Cohen N, editors: *Psychoneuroimmunology,* New York, 1991, Academic Press.

53. Rider MS: Entrainment mechanisms are involved in pain reduction, muscle relaxation, and music-mediated imagery, *J Music Ther* 22(4):183, 1985.

54. Robinson-Whelemn S, Kim C, MacCallum RC, Kiecolt-Glaser JK: Distinguishing optimism from pessimism in older adults: is it more important to be optimistic, or not to be pessimistic? *J Pers Soc Psychol* 73(6):1345, 1997.

55. Roszman TL, Carlson SL: Neurotransmitters and molecular signaling in the immune system. In Ader R, Felten DL, Cohen N, editors: *Psychoneuroimmunology,* New York, 1991, Academic Press.

56. Shekelle RB, Gale M, Ostfeld AM, Oglesby P: Hostility, risk of coronary heart disease and mortality, *Psychosom Med* 45(2):109, 1983.

57. Siegman AW: Paraverbal correlates of stress: implications for stress identification and management. In Goldberger L, Breznitz S, editors: *Handbook of stress. Theoretical and clinical aspects,* ed 2, New York, 1993, The Free Press.

58. Spiegel D, Bloom JR: Group therapy and hypnosis reduce metastatic breast carcinoma pain, *Psychosom Med* 45(4):333, 1983.

59. Spiegel D, Kraemer HC, Bloom JR, Gottheil E: Effect of psychosocial treatment on survival of patients with metastatic breast cancer, *Lancet* 2(8668):888, 1989.

60. Standley JM: Music research in medical/dental treatment: meta-analysis and clinical applications, *J Music Ther* 23(2):56, 1986.

61. Stead RH, Tomioka M, Pezzati P, Marshall J, Croitoru K, Perdue M, Stanisz A, Bienenstock J: Interaction of the mucosal immune and peripheral nervous system. In. Ader R, Felten DL, Cohen N, editors: *Psychoneuroimmunology,* New York, 1991, Academic Press.

62. Stone EA: Stress and catecholamines. In Friedhoff AJ, editor: *Catecholamines and behavior: neuropsychopharmacology,* vol 2, New York, 1975, Plenum Press.

63. Stoyva JM, Budzynski TH: Biofeedback methods in the treatment of anxiety and stress disorders. In Lehrer P, Woolfolk RL, editors: *Principles and practice of stress management,* ed 2, New York, 1993, Guilford Press.

64. Susman JR: *The relationship of expressiveness styles and elements of traumatic experience to self-reported illness,* Unpublished master's thesis, University Park, Tex, 1986, Southern Methodist University.

65. Thibodeau GA, Patton KT: *Anatomy and physiology,* St Louis, 1998, Mosby.

66. Vincent S, Thompson JH: The effects of music upon the human blood pressure, *Lancet* 534, 1929.

67. World Health Organization: *The first ten years of the World Health Organization,* Geneva, 1958, WHO.

68. Zimmerman LM, Pierson MA, Marker J: Effects of music on patient anxiety in coronary care units, *Heart Lung,* 17:560, 1988.

2

Research on Mind-Body Effects

Lynda W. Freeman

WHY READ THIS CHAPTER?

To comprehend the information concerning how life events modulate health, you must have a foundation in the "basics." This chapter covers these "basics," including (1) an overview of the lines of research that demonstrate the effects of stress on health; (2) an explanation of how immune cells are conditioned to respond in particular ways; (3) the delineation of how immune cells interact and communicate; and (4) a summary of how researchers assess immune competency in human subjects. Without some knowledge of these topics, you will be unable to understand, evaluate, and synthesize the outcomes of mind-body research. This chapter also serves as a mini–reference manual to which you can repeatedly refer as you study this text.

CHAPTER AT A GLANCE

Physiologic and immunologic responses can become conditioned by exposure to certain stimuli, such as taste, touch, or heat; by certain chemicals, such as immunosuppressive drugs; and by events that are emotionally meaningful or traumatic. The pathways by which these events occur are most clearly defined by an emerging interdisciplinary field called psychoneuroimmunology. Psychoneuroimmunology describes the interactions among behavior, neural and endocrine function, and immune processes.

There are four lines of evidence for the mind's influence on the body: observational, physiologic, epidemiologic, and clinical. Observational evidence includes individual case studies of responses to otherwise neutral substances, such as patients who are allergic to flowers and become symptomatic at the sight of an artificial rose. Walter B. Cannon performed the original physiologic research. Cannon discovered the "fight-or-flight" response, defined as a physiologic response that occurs when the emotions of anger, fear, or rage are expressed. These emotions include increased adrenaline, elevated blood pressure and blood sugar, and accelerated heart rate. Epidemiologic research, dating from the 1960s, describes how psychosocial factors and patterns of illness are correlated. Clinical trials refer to the testing of immediate and ongoing health effects of stressful situations. Serious life changes such as divorce or job loss, distressing life events such as role conflicts and family stress, unhappiness or clinical depression, and social isolation were all found to be major risk factors for mortality from a wide variety of causes.

Most outcomes of mind-body research are evaluated by measuring the changes in values of immune cells and their by-products with the use of immune assays.

The immune system protects the body through its ability to recognize and respond to invaders. It uses specific and nonspecific defense systems. One way the immune system protects the body is with white blood cells and their by-products. White blood cells include neutrophils, lymphocytes, monocytes, eosinophils, and basophils. Neutrophils, eosinophils, and basophils are called granulocytes because they have granules that contain hydrogen peroxide–reducing agents, compound-splitting enzymes, and digestive enzyme–containing cells. Lymphocytes and monocytes are agranulocytes, because they contain no granules; however, they perform their work with molecular substances created as by-products. These by-products include antibodies and cytokines.

Primary immune deficiencies include antibody, cellular, combined cellular and antibody, and complement deficiencies. Phagocytic disorders are another primary immune deficiency. Methods that determine whether primary immune deficiencies exist include the delayed skin hypersensitivity T-cell assays; lymphocyte classification assays that use flow cytometry and monoclonal antibodies; radial immunodiffusion and enzyme-linked immunosorbent assays; quantification of serum proteins; in vitro–stimulation of T-cells; cytotoxic assessments; adhesion, and phagocytic and intracellular killing assays; and chemotaxis or migration assays. External factors that affect immunologic competence include aging, nutrition, starvation, obesity, drugs, alcohol, circadian rhythms, and endocrine factors.

CHAPTER OBJECTIVES

After completing this chapter, you should be able to:

1. Define the four lines of evidence for the mind's influence on the body.
2. Describe a research study from the text for each line of evidence.
3. Define and describe the nonspecific and specific defense systems.
4. Define the five leukocyte cell types.
5. Compare and contrast the functions of the three granulocytes with the two agranulocytes.
6. Explain the "Clonal-Selection Theory."
7. Distinguish between antibody and cytokine function and the cells that produce them.
8. Categorize the five types of primary immune deficiencies and state the prevalence of each.
9. Define and describe two immunodeficiency assays for T-cell function.
10. Define and describe one lymphocyte classification assay.
11. Explain why cellular proliferation tests are performed.
12. Describe one antibody assay.
13. Describe one test each for cellular adhesion, cytotoxicity, and chemotaxis.
14. Define in vivo, in vitro, cytotoxicity, and monoclonal antibodies.
15. Name three external factors that can affect immunologic competence.

■ Research on Mind-Body Effects: An Overview

Scientific research strongly suggests that what we think and believe and how we behave can improve or exacerbate a variety of illnesses, including asthma, heart disease, gastrointestinal disorders, musculoskeletal diseases, endocrine disorders, and obesity.[6] Studies have demonstrated that animal and human physiologic and immune responses can be altered and even conditioned to respond in a particular way by environment, experience, or interpretation of an event.[2,3] It has been well documented that highly stressful events suppress immunity. Certain chemicals, such as cyclophosphamide (CY) are immunosuppressant agents. When these agents or stressful events occur simultaneously with certain conditions (e.g., novel tastes, type of touch, heat, certain sights or images), the result can be the "learning" of a conditioned immune response.

The evidence that supports stress as an immune suppressor and the "learning" of a conditioned immune response has been clearly delineated by an emerging and interdisciplinary field called *psychoneuroimmunology* (PNI). PNI can be defined as the study of interactions among behavior, neural and endocrine function, and immune processes.[4] In human studies, interactions are explored between mind and its variables, because these interactions relate to the neural, endocrine, and immune processes. The variables of the mind include our thoughts and their accompanying images and emotions, stress, conditioning stimuli (cues), and interpretations of life events.

■ Mind-Body Dilemma

Philosophers and scientists have grappled with the mind-body problem for centuries. Is there a distinct separation between the mind and body? If the answer is "yes," mental events may be entirely explained by physical events in the brain. However, if mind and body communicate, their bidirectional dialogue may have powerful implications for physical and psychologic well being. In Chapter 1, we traced the pathways that allow the mind and body to communicate. In this chapter, we explore the lines of research that seek to demonstrate specific outcomes related to the mind's influence on the body.

■ History of Research: Mind-Body Influence on Health

Lines of Research for the Mind's Influence on the Body

Four lines of research explore the mind's influence on the body. They are: (1) observational, (2) physiologic, (3) epidemiologic, and (4) clinical.

1. *Observational research* is made up of documented case studies. For example, a patient who is allergic to flowers sneezes uncontrollably at the sight of an artificial rose in a physician's office. The physician records the observations in detail and submits them for publication as a case study of mental stimulation of an allergic response. However, dust in the office or other factors could be the actual trigger for the sneezing, since these observations take place in an uncontrolled environment. An observational finding is considered to be a weak line of evidence because unlimited variables may contribute to the observed outcomes. Nonetheless, observational evidence is invariably our first indication that a cause-effect relationship may exist.

2. *Physiologic research* investigates specific biological or biochemical connections between the mind and other body systems and defines the pathways that allow for physiologic modulations. For example, while delivering a public speech, the presenter typically experiences a rise in blood pressure (BP) and an increase in cortisol and other stress hormones. The mouth becomes dry and the heart races. These are physiologic and biochemical responses elicited by the mind's interpretation of the event of public speaking and the brain's messages to the rest of the body in response to that interpretation. In the case of public speaking, hormones and biochemicals are released by the brain, which then elicits a stress response. These pathways are delineated in Chapter 1.

3. *Epidemiologic research* of the mind-body arena pursues *retrospective* (i.e., past events) or *prospective* (i.e., future events) correlations between physical and psychologic stress factors and the development of certain illnesses. It also explores the relationship among factors that determine the frequency and distribution of disease in human beings. Epidemiologic research uses survey data, as well as physiologic, biochemical, and psychologic assessments, which are gathered historically over time. Common subjects

of epidemiologic research are the correlations among isolation, depression, and stress and the development or exacerbation of chronic or acute disease states. For example, epidemiologic studies have found that persons experiencing *marital disruption* (e.g., divorce, separation) experience more *morbidity* (i.e., illness) and live shorter lives than their happily married counterparts. Epidemiologists can identify correlations between events and health outcomes, but they do not describe precisely what occurs in the body that leads to these outcomes.

4. *Clinical research* tests the effects of stress and conditioning on physiology and the immune function. Clinical interventions may be tested for their ability to induce, alleviate, or treat disease. Randomized controlled trials are often designed and delivered to a specified audience (e.g., hospitalized patients with pain or with a psychologic condition and medical students under stress during examination time). The exact stress-related physical reactions leading to illness can be delineated with clinical research. For example, we know students produce more stress-related hormones and demonstrate immune impairment just before an examination. Conversely, their immune systems seem to be strongest when they are just returning from summer vacation. With this type of research data, scientists can design intervention models intended to improve health. Stress management strategies and methods for preventing negative conditioning outcomes (e.g., conditioned nausea to hospital settings in the case of the patient taking chemotherapy) are examples of intervention models created from the findings of clinical research.

Observational Research

Observations of the mind's effects on the body have been documented for centuries. In 1557, Amatus Lusitanus wrote about a Dominican monk who was seized with fainting and fell to the ground unconscious when he observed a rose from a great distance. In 1896, Mackenzie described an experiment in which he intentionally evoked the so-called "rose cold" in a patient who was allergic to flowers by presenting an artificial rose.[20] This experiment was replicated by Osler who, with an artificial rose, induced an asthma attack in a patient.[28] In 1930, Hill found that the picture of a hay field was sufficient to elicit hay fever attacks in sensitive subjects.[13] These early observational studies were the first indicators that physiologic and immunologic responses could be conditioned and then elicited by otherwise neutral stimuli.

While performing research with adult asthmatic patients in Anchorage, Alaska, this author unintentionally induced asthmatic symptoms in more than 30 subjects by displaying graphic pictures of allergens (i.e., dust particles, dust mites) that would most likely induce an attack.[9] The intent was to educate these patients on what allergic triggers to avoid. The results were an immediate need for bronchodilator (inhaler) treatments for the patients, a perturbed class, and an apologetic researcher.

Physiologic Research

The original research on the physiology of emotion dates to Walter B. Cannon, a Harvard physiologist who discovered the *"fight-or-flight"* response. Cannon's interest in emotion centered on its bodily associations. He documented striking physical responses to the individual experiences of anger, fear, and rage. Human expression of these emotions led to a cessation of stomach digestive movement, an increase in BP, an accelerated heart rate, and elevated epinephrine (adrenaline) into the bloodstream. Epinephrine was responsible for the rise in BP and for increased blood sugar. Blood clotting time was accelerated as well. All of these responses served to prepare the person for emergency action and was believed to be an adaptive, evolutionary response. Most of these functions were mediated by the *sympathetic nervous system* (SNS).[12] Further research found the ability of the SNS to evoke dilation of the pupils, clammy skin, galvanic skin resistance, dilation of bronchioles, and increased oxygen uptake. In short, if the person was required to run from a mugger, both lunch and siesta time—the *rest-and-digest* response—could wait! These studies were important because, unlike the observational studies that answered "what" happened, these studies began to explain "how" emotional and perceptual responses elicit physiologic and biochemical changes in the body.

Epidemiologic Research

Epidemiologic research (dating back to the 1960s) studied the relationships among psychosocial factors and patterns of illness. Specific events or mood states were found to be associated with an increased risk of illness. The following are some of the landmark epidemiologic studies that span the last 45 years.

- Research performed in the U.S. Navy found that men who experienced *serious life changes* (e.g., divorce, move, job loss) had an increased risk of becoming seriously ill within months after these upsets.[7,11,25,26,27]

- Meyer and Haggerty systematically investigated 100 lower middle-class families to determine the factors responsible for the variability π individual susceptibility to streptococcal acquisition and illness.[23] Acquisition was defined as the detection of a new streptococcus or the reappearance of the same type after 8 weeks of negative cultures. Illness was defined as the appearance, in association with a positive culture, of infectious symptoms (e.g., red throat, cough, rash). Throat cultures were taken from all participants every 3 weeks for 1 year. Approximately 52% of the persons who colonized the virus did not become ill, although 24% of all family illnesses were associated with streptococci. The streptococcal group, type, and number of colonies did not correlate with the illnesses or with the severity of the illnesses. However, the *assessed level of chronic family stress was associated with the number of acquisitions, the prolonged periods of carriers, and the number of illnesses.*

- Jacobs, Spilken, and Norman hypothesized that the *development of serious upper respiratory infections are predated by distressing life conflicts.*[15] These authors compared 29 ill male college students with 29 symptom-free, randomly selected male students. A battery of assessments revealed those who were ill had significantly more disappointments, failures, and role crises than did the healthy subjects. Defiant coping patterns and heightened unpleasant effects also characterized the ill group. The authors performed another study of respiratory illness using a larger population base (N=179 male college students). The increased number of life stressors occurring in the preceding year was directly associated with the more incapacitating illnesses.[16]

- Luborsky and colleagues evaluated the effects of mood state on symptom activation in subjects carrying the herpes simplex virus. In 1976, one third of the population carried antibodies for herpes simplex, making it a relatively convenient illness to study. A battery of psychologic and immunologic assessments with a retrospective design indicated that the *factor labeled "unhappy" was associated with more herpes-related cold sores, more illnesses in general, and more psychologic complaints.* The authors then decided to perform a prospective study. They reasoned that since mood, especially the "unhappy" factor, had predicted the number of later episodes of cold sores and ulcers in colds, then daily self-ratings may show a buildup of this factor on the days just before the actual episodes. That expectation was not confirmed, leading the authors to question retrospective epidemiologic studies as a predictor of future illnesses.[19]

- In 1988, House, Landis, and Umberson reviewed the literature on social relationships and health.[14] These authors determined the retrospective studies of the 60s and 70s were more suggestive than conclusive. However, the completion of *prospective studies controlled for baseline health status consistently demonstrated an increased risk of death among persons with a low quantity or quality of social relationships.* Further, experimental and quasiexperimental *studies of human beings and animals implicated social isolation as a major risk factor for premature death from a wide variety of causes.*

In summary, the epidemiologic studies found that serious life changes, chronic family stresses, distressing life conflicts, unhappiness or depression, and social isolation were correlated with increased health risks. These results were only suggestive because a causal relationship could not be determined by epidemiologic data. It would take experimental trials to determine whether psychologic and conditioning factors were the causes of immunologic modulation and increased *morbidity* (i.e., a diseased state) and *mortality* (i.e., a fatal outcome).

Early Clinical and Experimental Findings

In past decades, it has been argued that all events of the mind can be explained by the physical and chemical workings of the brain. Neuroscientific findings of the past 50 years restructured this limited perspective and reported that direct communication between the mind and body has been repeatedly demonstrated in animal and human studies.[5]

Experimental research on mind-body effects essentially evolved into two different but overlapping approaches.

Testing the immediate and ongoing health effects of stressful or emotional situations. In clinical trials, physiologic, biochemical, and immunologic changes were evaluated in persons (1) before, during, and after stressful examinations; (2) experiencing separation or divorce; (3) during marital conflict; (4) during the bereavement period; (5) during a 7- to 10-year period of intense care giving; and (6) during stressful work times.

Testing the conditioned immune response. In research studies, animals were injected with CY, an immunosuppressive agent, at the same time that heating pads were applied to a particular part of their bodies (e.g., feet, underbelly). The "event" of the heating pad was paired with the CY injections on several occasions. After a period of time, applying the heating pad without giving the injection resulted in a suppression of specific immune cells, as had occurred naturally in response to the CY. The immune cells of the rats "learned" to respond to the heating pad as if it were an immunosuppressing chemical.

In upcoming chapters, we review in detail the epidemiologic and clinical and experimental studies of the effects of consciousness on morbidity and mortality. In Chapter 1, we review the stress pathways and the chemical messengers (e.g., hormones, neurotransmitters, neuropeptides, immunomodulators) that drive these pathways. To fully understand how the mind affects morbidity and mortality outcomes, it is necessary to investigate the effects of stress and conditioning on immune function. To understand this information, you must possess a basic understanding of the immune system, its cells and its cellular by-products. You must also possess some basic knowledge of how immune competence is assessed by the researchers in the mind-body community.

■ Immune System: Its Cells and Assessment of Immune Competence

At this point, it may be beneficial to review the basics of (1) how the immune system is structured, (2) how immune cells function, and (3) how researchers use immune cell assays to demonstrate immune competence or incompetence. If you are a physician, an immunologist, or a health researcher and use this kind of information on a regular basis, you may wish to skip the next three sections. However, it is strongly advised that most readers carefully review the following sections.

Table 2-1 provides a schematic of the structure of the immune system, and the textual overview describes the structural processes in detail.
- The table and overview offer a "picture" of how the components of immunity interact.
- In-depth definitions and information about the immune cell types are delineated. These definitions flesh out the various functions of the cellular components of the immune system.
- The types of assays that researchers use to evaluate immune response are discussed.

The overview of the immune system should be committed to memory. A description of immunologic assays is included to provide a general explanation of how immune competence is measured in a laboratory setting. It is included only to offer a sense of how this type of work is performed and is intended for individuals interested in pursuing mind-body research. Those who are not may choose to skip this section.

Once the remainder of this chapter is reviewed, you will be prepared to evaluate the animal and human trials that are discussed throughout this text.

Immune Defense System: An Overview

We live in a hostile environment. Our skin is exposed to microorganisms minute by minute. Airborne bacteria and environmental pollutants invade our lungs. Viruses attack our cells, sometimes turning them into reproductive "factories" that manufacture more viruses. To protect itself, the body must learn to recognize that which is "self"—the body's own cells and by-products—and that which is "not self"—foreign cells and by-products. To accomplish this, bodily defenses must be well organized and maintain an excellent communication system. There are two bodily defense systems that act independently, but cooperatively, to protect the body. The first system is our nonspecific defense system; the second system is our specific defense system. (It should be noted that the organizational structure of the immune defense system [e.g., our nonspecific or innate immunity and our specific or adaptive immunity] is presented in Table 2-1. In the bottom half of this table, the separate components of the specific and nonspecific systems are further categorized, with arrows pointing to subcomponents. Readers should frequently refer to this table as they read the next few pages.)

The term *nonspecific immunity* refers to those mechanisms that do not act against one or two types of invaders; rather, they act to destroy

TABLE 2-1	Organizational Structure of the Immune Defense System

NONSPECIFIC (INNATE IMMUNITY)	SPECIFIC (ADAPTIVE IMMUNITY)
FIRST DEFENSE BARRIER: IMMEDIATE, NO MEMORY	THIRD DEFENSE BARRIER: ANTIGEN SPECIFIC, TAKES SEVERAL DAYS, HAS MEMORY FOR ANTIGEN

Intact skin epidermis
Acidic skin secretions
Intact mucous membranes
    Mucus, nasal hairs
    Cilia
    Gastric juices
    Tears, saliva
    Urine
	Cellular
	    Recognizes intracellular pathogens (viruses, bacteria, fungi)
	    First effectors: T-lymphocytes, macrophages, NKC
	Humoral
	    Attacks extracellular pathogens, including encapsulated bacteria
	    First effectors:
	        B-lymphocytes
	        Phagocytic cells
	        Antibodies
	        Complement cascades

SECOND DEFENSE BARRIER	

Inflammation mediated
Phagocytes
Neutrophil—in blood, contains lysosome, defensin
Monocyte—in blood, presents to T-cells via Il1
            —produces complement proteins
Macrophage—in fixed tissue
NKC—attacks invader membranes
Eosinophil—kills parasitic worms
Basophil—in blood, releases inflammatory mediators
Mast cell—in tissues
Fever—kills microbes, boosts immune response
Slow-wave sleep—releases growth hormone
Antimicrobial proteins
    Interferon—molecules released by virus infected cells
            that "interfere" with viral replication;
            complement-cascading series of enzymes
            and proteins	

SPECIFIC OR ADAPTIVE IMMUNITY	
CELLULAR IMMUNITY	HUMORAL IMMUNITY

Proliferation/differentiation regulated by cytokines
Cytotoxic T—kills tumors with chemicals
T-helper—facilitates antibody production, activates phagocytes
T-suppressor—calls off the battle
T-cell
First effectors of cell-mediated immunity
First regulatory cells of T/B lymphocytes
Monocyte function by lymphokine production and
    direct cell contact
Regulates cell maturation in bone marrow
	Classic pathway: Fast
	    Activated by immune complexes; B-cell to
	        plasma cell to immunoglobulins (IgG, IgM)
	Alternate pathway: Slow
	    Activated by microbial components
	    Antigen independent
	    Endotoxin or IgA

ACTIVATION OF COMPLEMENT	
CLASSICAL PATHWAY	ALTERNATE PATHWAY
Antigen-antibody complex plus 1 C1, C4, C2	Microorganisms' cell wall polysaccharide 1 Factors B, D, P

C3b
    Opsonization (to make tasty) by coating with
        antibody increases blood vessel permeability;
        chemotactic
	C3a
	    Causes inflammation, stimulates histamine release,
	        and complement proteins; enhances

C3
C4
C5
C6
C7
C8

NKC, Natural killer cells.

anything recognized as "not self." By contrast, *specific immunity* involves mechanisms that recognize and act against specific threatening agents that are *assigned* to them and to no other. Because of this specialization, the specific defense system takes longer to "gear up" a response than it takes the nonspecific system to do the same.

Nonspecific and Innate Defense System

First Defensive Barrier

The nonspecific defense system erects two barriers to protect the body from foreign invaders. The *first defensive barrier* consists of our intact skin with its acid mantle and keratinized membrane and the intact mucous membranes and their components (e.g., mucus, nasal hairs, cilia, gastric juice, urine, and secretions [i.e., tears, saliva]).

The skin prevents pathogens from entering the body. Skin secretions of perspiration and sebum make the epidermis acidic. This acidic mantle inhibits bacterial growth, and sebum contains bactericidal chemicals. The skin protein, keratin, protects the skin from acids (Figure 2-1).

Mucous membranes line all body cavities that open to the exterior environment. In the mucous membranes, mucus traps organisms in respiratory and digestive tracts; nasal hairs serve as filters in the nasal passages; and cilia catapult mucous-trapped debris away from lower respiratory passages. Gastric juices containing hydrochloric acid and digestive enzymes destroy microorganisms in the stomach. Tears lubricate and cleanse the eyes, and saliva lubricates the oral cavity and teeth. Tears and saliva contain lysozyme, an enzyme that destroys microorganisms. Finally, the acid pH in urine inhibits bacterial growth in the urinary tract.

Second Defensive Barrier

If our first defensive barrier is penetrated, which occurs when we cut ourselves, the first barrier is compromised. The second defensive barrier is then recruited into action by chemical messengers that send out an "alarm" to the body. The inflammation process is triggered whenever bodily tissues are injured and the "alarm" is sounded. The inflammation process recruits macrophages, mast cells, and white blood cells (WBCs), as well as other chemical substances (e.g., antimicrobial proteins) to kill microorganisms and assist in tissue repair, rebuilding the first defensive barrier (Figure 2-2). Antimicrobial proteins (e.g., complement and interferon [IFN]) and the recruited cells respond to the battle site and prevent the foreign invader's advance into other bodily tissues.

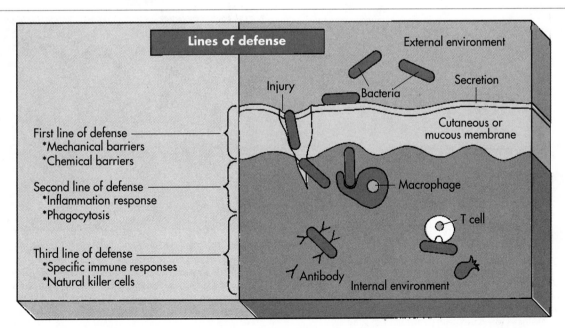

■ **Figure 2-1.** Nonspecific and specific defensive barriers. *Modified from Thibodeau GA, Patton KT: Anatomy and physiology, ed 4, St Louis, 1999, Mosby.*

Invaders advancing to the second defensive barrier are engaged by *phagocytes,* or cell eaters, the main ones of which are macrophages—voracious destroyers that are derived from circulating monocytes (Figure 2-3). Neutrophils, the most abundant WBCs, also turn phagocytic when they engage pathogens, which are any microorganisms that cause disease. *Eosinophils* become weakly phagocytic by depositing their enzymatic and digestive chemicals onto invading parasitic worms. Natural killer (NK) cells act as the border police, spontaneously targeting invading cells. NK cells recognize changes in cell surface membranes that occur in tumor cells or in virus-infected cells and then destroy them. NK cells are not phagocytic, but they kill by attacking the cell's membrane and releasing chemicals into the infected cell. Antimicrobial proteins—complement and IFNs—also enter the fray by directly attacking microorganisms or inhibiting their ability to reproduce.

Complement refers to twenty or more plasma proteins that circulate in the blood in an inactive state. Proteins include *C1* through *C9, factors B, D,* and *P,* as well as other regulatory proteins. When activated, complement mediators amplify all aspects of the inflammatory process, killing bacteria and other foreign types of cells. Our own cells are equipped with proteins to inactivate complement mediators. This is a self-protective

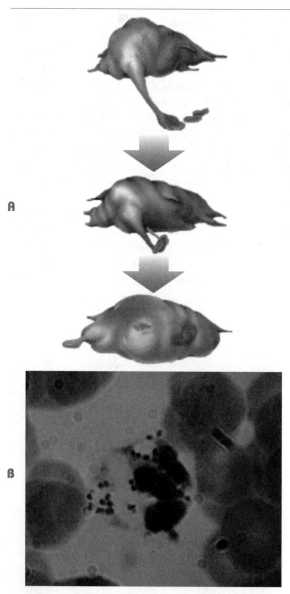

■ **Figure 2-3. Macrophage with pseudopod engulfing its prey. A,** Series of steps in phagocytosis of bacteria. The plasma membrane extends (as a pseudopod) toward the bacterial cells and then envelops them. Once trapped, they are engulfed by the cell and destroyed by lysosomes. **B,** Micrograph showing phagocytized streptococcus pheunmonia bacterial being destroyed in a neutrophil. *Modified from Thibodeau GA, Patton KT:* Anatomy and physiology, *ed 4, St Louis, 1999, Mosby.*

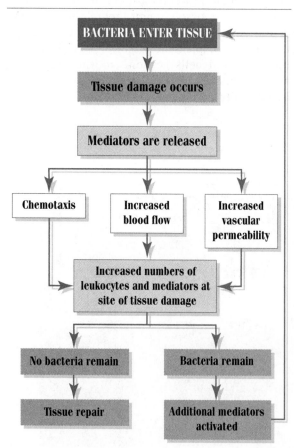

■ **Figure 2-2. Inflammatory response.** Tissue damage caused by bacteria triggers a series of events that produces the inflammatory response and promotes phagocytosis at the site of injury. These responses tend to inhibit or destroy the bacteria. *Modified from Thibodeau GA, Patton KT:* Anatomy and physiology, *ed 4, St Louis, 1999, Mosby.*

mechanism that keeps the complement from harming "self" (i.e., so we do not harm our own healthy tissues or cells).

Complement enhances the effectiveness of both nonspecific and specific defense systems and *can be activated by either the classical pathway or the alternate pathway.* The classical pathway depends on the binding of antibodies to the pathogen and the subsequent binding of C1 to antigen-antibody complexes, a process called complement fixation (Figures 2-4 and 2-5). The alternate pathway is triggered by factors B, D, and P and molecules present on the surface of microorganisms. Both pathways involve a cascade effect in which complement proteins are activated in an orderly sequence, thereby activating subsequent steps. Both pathways converge on C3, cleaving it into two pieces (C3a and C3b).

Opsonization is a process whereby C3b binds to the surface of a target cell, inserting groups of complement proteins that stabilize an open hole in the membrane of the target cell. This process leads to cell *lysis,* or destruction. The C3b coating on the target cell acts like a handle to which macrophages and neutrophils can adhere, making engulfment and destruction of the pathogen an easy process.

Once body cells are infected with viruses, they can do little to save themselves. However, they can act to warn and protect other cells from viral infection. IFNs are small proteins secreted by virus-infected cells that travel to nearby healthy cells and stimulate them to synthesize molecules that inhibit or interfere with viral replication. This is a nonspecific interaction, in that an IFN produced against a particular virus also helps protect the cells from many other viruses. In addition to the antiviral function, IFNs activate macrophages and mobilize NK cells. They play a role in protecting the body from cancer.

Fever occurs in response to infection and is regulated by the *hypothalamus,* sometimes referred to as the body's thermostat. When exposed to bacteria or foreign substances, leukocytes and macrophages secrete chemicals called *pyrogens,* which turn up the body's temperature. Moderate fevers help the body fight bacteria by inhibiting the available amounts of iron and zinc, requirements for bacteria proliferation and reproduction. Fever also increases the metabolic rate, accelerating defensive action and tissue repair.

Specific or Adaptive Defense System: An Overview

The specific or adaptive defense system maintains divisions of specialists—highly complex cellular and molecular troops—that individually recognize and inactivate one specific *antigen,* or enemy. Technically, antigen refers to any substance that induces a resistance response to infection after a latent period, typically 8 to 14 days. Less technically, antigen refers to what the body perceives as a threat. For example, in one cellular division referred to as B-lymphocytes, each individual cell

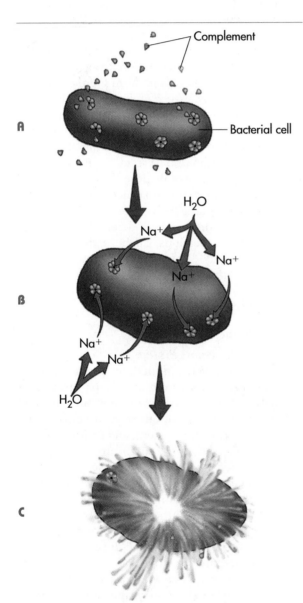

■ *Figure 2-4.* **Complement fixation. A,** Complement molecules activated by antibodies form doughnut-shaped complexes in a bacterium's plasma membrane. **B,** Holes in the complement complex allow sodium (Na^+) and then water (H_2O) to diffuse into the bacterium. **C,** After enough water has entered, the swollen bacterium bursts. *Modified from Thibodeau GA, Patton KT: Anatomy and physiology, ed 4, St Louis, 1999, Mosby.*

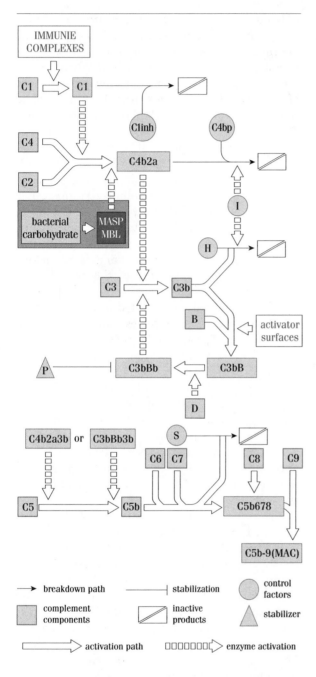

■ **Figure 2-5.** Complement pathways: classical and alternative. *Modified from Male D:* Immunology: an illustrated outline, *ed 3, St Louis, 1998, Mosby.*

ping it cold in its tracks. Antibodies function somewhat like a stun gun. They must first actually make contact with the antigen. To accomplish this, the antibody and the receptor on the antigen fit together just like a key into a lock (Figure 2-6). Once the key is engaged, the stunning effect occurs. Antibodies both stop the enemy and visibly mark it for destruction by other "less specialized troops" that bring up the rear. These "troops" can "spear" the pathogen or inject a chemical agent, thereby dissolving or bursting the invader.

The specific defense system contains a great many cellular commanders that can order the immune system to provide more troops. *Helper T-cells* help existing troops perform more efficiently, whereas *suppressor T-cells* tell the defense system when the war is over and when to stop the attack.

The individual types of cells in the body are reviewed in detail, with emphasis on those that make up the immune system. It is helpful to review Table 2-2, which describes the types of WBCs in the bloodstream (which can be thought of as our "white knights"). Their numbers will be discussed, and their unique defensive duties will be described. Questions, such as the following, will be answered: "How long does it take to train and prepare these cells for duty (their maturing time)?" "How long they can function 'in the field' (their life span)?"

Makeup of the Bloodstream

Blood: Our Transport System

The blood, in a sense, functions like a transport unit, hauling various immune troops throughout the body. It transports *erythrocytes,* our red blood cells (RBCs), which are our oxygen delivery and carbon dioxide refuse system, and *leukocytes,* our WBCs (leuko=white), which are our "white knight" defense divisions. These leukocytes include neutrophils, lymphocytes, monocytes, eosinophils, and basophils (see Table 2-2).

Erythrocytes. Erythrocytes, or RBCs, are our most abundant cells (Figure 2-7). We have 4 to 6 million RBCs per mm³ of blood. It takes them 5 to 7 days to prepare for duty and they survive for 100 to 200 days. Their purpose is to transport oxygen throughout the body and remove carbon dioxide from the body by transporting it to the lungs.

Leukocytes. Leukocytes, or WBCs, are complete cells that account for less than 1% of the total blood volume. We average 4,000 to 11,000 WBCs per mm³ of blood. The various divisions of leukocytes serve as our bodily defense systems against disease, protecting us from bacteria, virus-

is taught to recognize a different enemy by its shape or appearance. When an individual B-lymphocyte recognizes the foe it is trained to detect, it launches "magic bullets" called *antibodies* (also called *immunoglobulins*) at the enemy. These antibodies are created to attack only this one type of adversary. The antibodies lock onto the receptors on the surface of the enemy, stop-

TABLE 2-2	White Blood Cells

Cell Type	Number of Cells per mm³ (μL) of Blood	Developmental Time (DT) and Lifespan (LS)	Function
Erythrocytes (RBCs) 	4-6 million	DT: 5-7 days LS: 100-200 days	Oxygen and carbon dioxide transport
Leukocytes (WBCs) 	4-11 thousand		
Granulocytes Neutrophils 	3-7 thousand	DT: 6-9 days LS: 6 hours to a few days	Phagocytosis of bacteria
Eosinophils 	100-400	DT: 6-9 days LS: 8-12 days	Kills invasive parasitic worms; destroys antigen-antibody complexes; inactivates inflammatory chemicals of allergy functions in hypersensitivity states
Basophils 	20-50	DT: 3-7 days LS: a few hours to a few days	Releases histamine and other inflammatory mediators; contains the anticoagulant heparin; active in delayed hypersensitivity
Agranulocytes Lymphocytes 	1½-3 thousand	DT: days to work LS: hours to years	Immune response by antibody or direct cell attack
Monocytes 	100-700	DT: 2-3 days LS: months	Phagocytosis; develops into macrophages in tissue

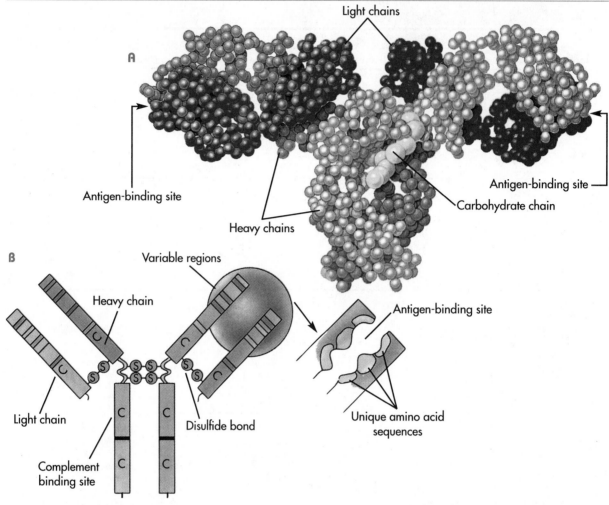

■ *Figure 2-6.* **Structure of the antibody molecule. A,** In this molecular model of a typical antibody molecule, the light chains are represented by strands of green spheres (each represents an individual amino acid). Heavy chains are represented by strands of gray spheres. Notice that the heavy chains can complex with a carbohydrate chain. **B,** This simplified diagram shows the variable regions, highlighted by colored bars that represent amino acid sequences unique to that molecule. Constant regions of the heavy and light chains are marked "C." The inset shows that the variable regions at the end of each arm of the molecule form a cleft that serves as an antigen-binding site.

es, parasites, toxins, and tumor cells.[22] Although RBCs are confined to the bloodstream, our WBCs (leukocytes) are more mobile, moving out of capillary blood vessels by a process called *diapedesis,* which means "leaping across." The circulatory system is simply a transportation medium, allowing the leukocytes access to other areas of the body—mostly to connective and lymphoid tissues—where they are needed to initiate inflammatory or immune responses. Once leukocytes leave the bloodstream, they move through tissue spaces by what is known as *amoeboid* motion. They form *cytoplasmic pseudopods* or footlike extensions that allow them to flow or slither along. Leukocytes leave chemical trails of molecules released from damaged cells or other leukocytes, similar to the scent that bloodhounds sniff as they track their prey. This process, known as *chemotaxis,* allows leukocytes to converge in large numbers at the location of tissue damage or infection. Once leukocytes are recruited into action, their production is accelerated. Within a few hours, the number of leukocytes in the blood may double. A WBC count of more than 11,000 is a medical indicator of a bacterial or viral assault and is referred to as *leukocytosis.*

Leukocytes are divided into two categories: *granulocytes* and *agranulocytes.* Granulocytes are so named because they contain specialized cytoplasmic granules. The cells known as granu-

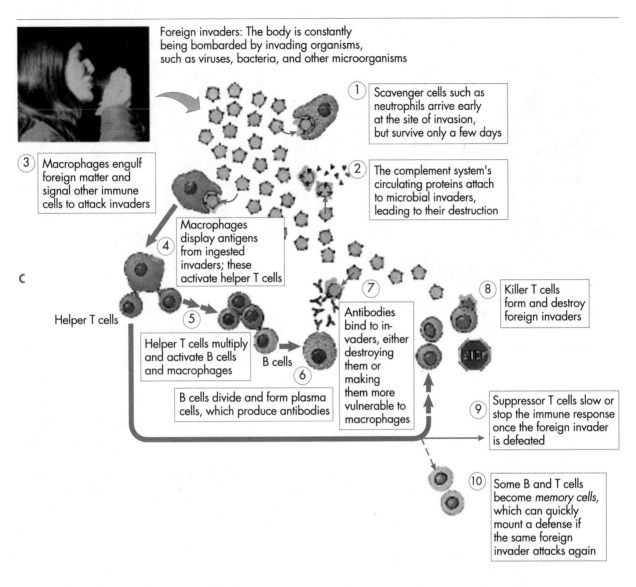

Foreign invaders: The body is constantly being bombarded by invading organisms, such as viruses, bacteria, and other microorganisms

① Scavenger cells such as neutrophils arrive early at the site of invasion, but survive only a few days

② The complement system's circulating proteins attach to microbial invaders, leading to their destruction

③ Macrophages engulf foreign matter and signal other immune cells to attack invaders

④ Macrophages display antigens from ingested invaders; these activate helper T cells

C

Helper T cells

⑤ Helper T cells multiply and activate B cells and macrophages

B cells

⑥ B cells divide and form plasma cells, which produce antibodies

⑦ Antibodies bind to invaders, either destroying them or making them more vulnerable to macrophages

⑧ Killer T cells form and destroy foreign invaders

⑨ Suppressor T cells slow or stop the immune response once the foreign invader is defeated

⑩ Some B and T cells become *memory cells,* which can quickly mount a defense if the same foreign invader attacks again

■ **Figure 2-6. C, Biological warfare.** A brief summary of the immune response. *Parts A-C modified from Thibodeau GA, Patton KT:* Anatomy and physiology, *ed 4, St Louis, 1999, Mosby.*

locytes are part of our nonspecific defense system. Agranulocytes lack these granules.

Students are often taught to remember leukocytes in the order of their abundance. The phrase, "Never let monkeys eat bananas," or neutrophils, lymphocytes, monocytes, eosinophils, basophils, may help jog one's memory. The second and third of the leukocytes—lymphocytes and monocytes—are agranulocytes; the remaining three—neutrophils, eosinophils, and basophils—are granulocytes (refer to Table 2-1).

Granulocytes

Granulocytes, or neutrophils, eosinophils, and basophils, are part of our nonspecific defense system.

Neutrophils—Marine battalion. *Neutrophils,* the most abundant leukocytes, account for more than one half of the WBCs (Figure 2-8). Neutrophils, like the Marines, perform hand-to-hand combat with invading enemies (e.g., bacteria, fungi). They use peptides, or protein molecules, that function like "spears." They also carry the internal equivalent of chemical weapons (e.g., lysosomes, defensins) that are stored in their granular sacs. Neutrophils trek to the sites of greatest action (i.e., locations of inflammation), engulf their enemy, and quite literally "eat them for breakfast."

Some of the granules in neutrophils contain both *peroxidases,* which are hydrogen peroxide-

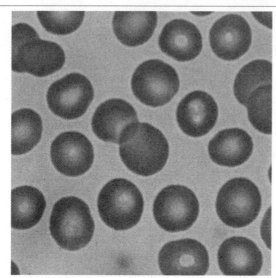

■ **Figure 2-7.** Erythrocytes. Color-enhanced scanning electron micrograph shows normal erythrocytes. *From Thibodeau GA, Patton KT:* Anatomy and physiology, *ed 4, St Louis, 1999, Mosby.*

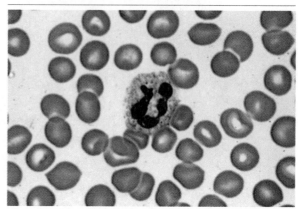

■ **Figure 2-8.** Neutrophils. *From Thibodeau GA, Patton KT:* Anatomy and physiology, *ed 4, St Louis, 1999, Mosby.*

reducing agents, and other hydrolytic or compound-splitting enzymes. They are therefore considered as *lysosomes,* or digestive enzyme-containing cells. Other small granules contain antibiotic-like proteins called *defensins.*

Neutrophils are chemically attracted to regions of inflammation and are active *phagocytes,* or cell eaters, their diet consisting mostly of bacteria and some fungi. Bacterial killing is actively promoted by neutrophils through a process called respiratory burst. A *respiratory burst* occurs when oxygen is actively metabolized to produce potent germ-killing substances, such as bleach and hydrogen peroxide. *Defensin-mediated lysis,* or cellular bursting, is a potent bodily process for destroying bacteria. The granules containing defensins merge with a *phagosome*—a vesicle formed during phagocytosis—that has engulfed a microbe. The defensins then form long peptide "spears" that literally pierce holes in the membrane of the foe ingested by the phagocyte. During acute bacterial infections (e.g., meningitis, appendicitis) neutrophil numbers increase tremendously, aiding the body in fighting off these invaders.

Neutrophils are easily recognizable and countable in assays because neutrophil cytoplasm, when stained, is a pale lilac color (refer to Table 2-2).

Eosinophils—tank destroyers. Eosinophils make up 1% to 4% of all leukocytes. They can be thought of as the equivalent of tank destroyers, because they eliminate "armored" invaders too large to be engulfed. These adversaries are invasive parasitic worms. Eosinophils also serve to eliminate some allergic responses by inactivating inflammatory responses (Figure 2-9).

When stained, the eosinophil nucleus turns blue-red and is shaped somewhat like a telephone receiver. Its granules appear brick red to crimson when stained with an eosin dye. These granules are packed with a variety of digestive enzymes, but they lack the enzymes necessary to digest bacteria. The main function of eosinophils is to attack parasitic worms such as tapeworms, flukes, pinworms, and hookworms, which are too large to be engulfed for digestion (i.e., phagocytized). Eosinophils reside in the loose connective tissue where these worms thrive (e.g., in the intestinal and respiratory mucosae). The eosinophils release enzymes from their granules directly onto the parasite's surface, like pouring a potent acid on a tank until it disintegrates, which kills and partially digests the parasite. *Major basic protein* (MBP) is the enzyme responsible for this digestion process.

Eosinophils also reduce allergic reactions by destroying the *antigen-antibody complexes* and by inactivating some of the inflammatory mediators produced during an allergic attack. Antigen-antibody complexes are formed when antibodies bind to the surface of the antigen.

One of the defensive mechanisms used by antibodies during complex formation is called *complement fixation* and *activation.* When antibodies bind to cellular targets and form complexes, they change their shape and expose complement-binding sites on the segments that remain constant. This process triggers complement fixation

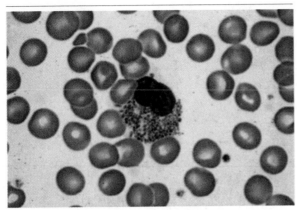

Figure 2-9. Eosinophils. *From Thibodeau GA, Patton KT: Anatomy and physiology, ed 4, St Louis, 1999, Mosby.*

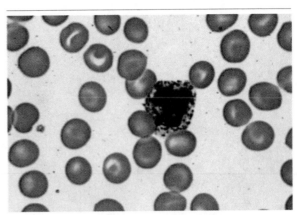

Figure 2-10. Basophils. *From Thibodeau GA, Patton KT: Anatomy and physiology, ed 4, St Louis, 1999, Mosby.*

and activation in the surface of the antigen cell and leads to lysis (refer to Table 2-1). As a side effect, molecules released during complement activation amplify the inflammatory response and promote phagocytosis. Therefore the neutrophilic eating of antigen-antibody complexes degrades both the inflammation and phagocytosis processes.

Basophils—trail markers. *Basophils* average less than 0.5% of the leukocyte population and contain coarse granules with histamine (Figure 2-10). Basophils act as trail markers, laying down a "scent" for other WBCs to follow, using histamine as the chemical attractant. Histamine acts as a vasodilator by making blood vessels leaky and attracts WBCs to the site of inflammation.

Mast cells are microscopically similar to basophils, are found in connective tissues, and are sometimes referred to as tissue basophils, although they are a unique type of cell (Figure 2-11). Both basophils and mast cells bind to the antibody immunoglobulin E (IgE), which causes the granules to release histamine. Basophils and mast cells are also responsible for the release of the major mediators of immediate hypersensitivity (e.g., leukotrienes, prostaglandins, platelet-activating factors). Basophils are present in the circulation, whereas mast cells are found only in tissue.

The nuclei of basophils form a U or S shape, and when stained, the nuclei are purple. The basophilic granules are readily recognizable because they have an affinity for basic dyes and stain purple-black.

Agranulocytes

Agranulocytes, or lymphocytes and monocytes, are part of our specific defense system. They are recognizable because they lack visible cytoplasmic granules. The nuclei of both are spherical or shaped like a kidney. Although they resemble each other, they are distinctively different cell types with different functions.

Lymphocytes—military specialists. *Lymphocytes,* when stained, have a large, dark purple nucleus that occupies almost all of the cell volume. The nucleus is spherical and surrounded by a thin border of pale blue cytoplasm. They are smaller than monocytes. Although a great many lymphocytes exist in the body, only a small number of them—typically the smallest lymphocytes—are found in the bloodstream. Most are embedded in lymphoid tissues (e.g., lymphoid nodes, spleen) where they lead a critical role in immune protection.

Lymphocytes are "trained" to become either *T-lymphocytes* or *B-lymphocytes*. Between 70% and 80% become T-cells and 10% to 15% become B-cells, depending on (1) where they migrate and (2) where they mature or get trained (Figure 2-12). If they migrate to the thymus and mature there, thymic hormones determine their maturation and they become T-cells. Lymphocytes that mature in bone marrow become B-lymphocytes. During maturation, both T- and B-lymphocytes develop the ability to identify foreign antigens.

The remaining lymphocytes that become neither T- nor B-cells are called null. Null cells probably become a number of different types of cells, including NK cells.

When B- and T-cells become mature, they display a special type of receptor on their surfaces. These receptors enable the lymphocyte to recognize and bind to specific antigens, which are substances that induce a state of sensitivity or resist-

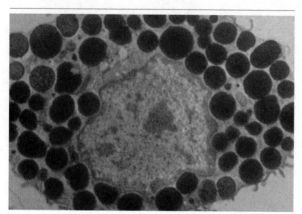

■ *Figure 2-11.* Mast cells. *From Thibodeau GA, Patton KT: Anatomy and physiology,* ed 4, St Louis, 1999, Mosby.

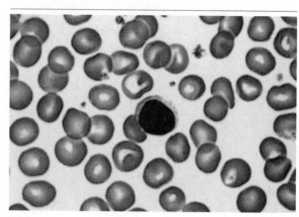

■ *Figure 2-12.* Lymphocytes. *From Thibodeau GA, Patton KT: Anatomy and physiology,* ed 4, St Louis, 1999, Mosby.

ance. Once these receptors appear, a lymphocyte can react to one—and only one—distinct antigen. For example, receptors on one lymphocyte may recognize only a single antigenic determinant of hepatitis A virus; another may recognize only pneumococcus bacteria.

Our lymphocytes become immunocompetent before ever meeting the antigens they attack. Thus it is our genes—our heredity—not antigens that determine the specific foreign substance our immune system can both recognize and resist. Only the antigens to which we are exposed in our lifetime will activate the related lymphocytes. Therefore many of our lymphocytes will not be conscripted into battle, but they will remain idle for life.

After becoming immunocompetent, both T- and B-cells disperse to the lymph nodes, spleen, and other lymphoid organs where they may encounter antigens (Figures 2-13 and 2-14). Only when lymphocytes bind with the antigen they recognize do they complete their differentiation into fully functional T- and B-cells. They obtain the "rank" to undertake their assigned missions.

T-lymphocytes attack virus-infected cells and tumor cells directly. B-lymphocytes, on the other hand, create plasma cells that produce antibodies (i.e., the magic bullets—immunoglobulins, such as IgA, IgD, IgE, IgM) that are released into the blood cells (Figures 2-15 and 2-16 on page 54).

This process begins when antigens that are binding to the surface receptors of the B-cells activate the B-lymphocytes. At that point, B-cells are stimulated to grow, multiply, and form an army of cells exactly like themselves, bearing the same antigen-specific receptors. Most of these clone cells become plasma cells—anti-

body-secreting cells of humoral (i.e., bodily fluid) immunity. Each plasma cell can produce antibodies at a remarkable pace for 4 to 5 days, but then they burn out and die. The antibodies secreted by these plasma cells circulate in the blood or lymph systems, binding to free antigens. This binding not only inactivates the antigen, but it also marks it for destruction by other specific and nonspecific mechanisms. The clone cells that do not differentiate into plasma cells become long-lived memory cells, which can elicit an immediate humoral response if they encounter more of the same antigen. As depicted in Table 2-3, immunity can be viewed as an activation of immune cells and of molecules, both of which are involved in the immune response.

A closer look: "Clonal-Selection Theory" versus "Side-Chain Theory"

How do B-cells make such an incredible variety of antibodies? One antibody can neutralize only one specific type of antigen, yet antigens come in unlimited shapes, sizes, and chemical compositions. Bacteria, viruses, pollens, incompatible blood cells, and man-made molecules all qualify as antigens.

Historically, there have been two schools of thought concerning how this occurs. One group of scientists believes that antigens serve as templates, directing the creation of matching antibodies. A second group of scientists believes lymphocytes maintain a pool of predesigned antibodies from which the antigen picks its approximate match. In time, and with research, the second theory proved to be correct.

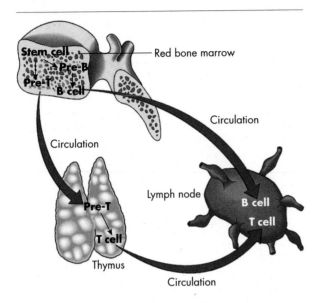

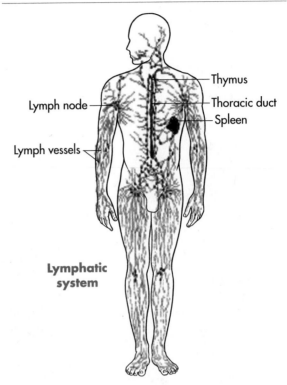

■ **Figure 2-13. Development of B cells and T cells.** Both types of lymphocytes originate from stem cells in the red bone marrow. Pre-B cells that are formed by dividing stem cells develop in the "bursa-equivalent" tissues in the yolk sac, fetal liver, and bone marrow. Likewise, pre-T cells migrate to the thymus, where they continue developing. Once they are formed, B cells and T cells circulate to the lymph nodes and spleen. *From Thibodeau GA, Patton KT:* Anatomy and physiology, *ed 4, St Louis, 1999, Mosby.*

■ **Figure 2-14.** Lymphatic system. *From Thibodeau GA, Patton KT:* Anatomy and physiology, *ed 4, St Louis, 1999, Mosby.*

Reactions between antibodies and antigens have been observed in test tubes for a long time, because the reactants form aggregates visible to the naked eye. At the turn of the century, Paul Erhlich devised a technique for quantifying antibody production. This new method disclosed an explosive generation of antibodies following B-cell contact with an infectious agent. Ehrlich explained these phenomena with his "Side-Chain Theory."

This theory postulated that the surface of a WBC contains receptors with side chains. Foreign substances can link chemically with these chains. When this chemical binding occurs, the cell is prompted to produce numerous copies of the bound receptor. The excess receptors, or antibodies, are then shed into the blood. Ehrlich assumed that cells naturally make side chains that are capable of binding all foreign substances.

There are some flaws with this theory, however. The theory does not explain the exponential rise in antibody production in the early stages of an immune response. If a template is required to make each antibody, it is hard to comprehend how antibodies can outnumber their templates so quickly. Also, the theory does not account for the quickened pace of antibody production that

occurs when a person or animal encounters the same antigen for a second time.

F. Macfarlane Burnet, an Australian scientist, accepted a different hypothesis formulated by other researchers. This hypothesis states the body is endowed with preexisting (i.e., genetically inherited) antibodies that can recognize all antigens. He proposed, as had others, that the binding of an antigen with an antibody receptor triggers the cell to multiply and manufacture more of the same receptor. Then he went a step further and made the daring assertion that each individual cell and its clones can produce only one specific kind of receptor. He named this genetic process the "Clonal-Selection Theory."

This theory resolved a variety of problems associated with the "Side-Chain Theory." The incredible rise in antibody production after contact with an antigen is the result of the explosive rise in the number of antibody-producing cells. Therefore a second reaction to the antigen is more rapid, because there are more cells that respond to stimulation. The binding ability of antibodies improves with time because the antigen "selects" for replication cells that carry genetic mutations that promote this match between

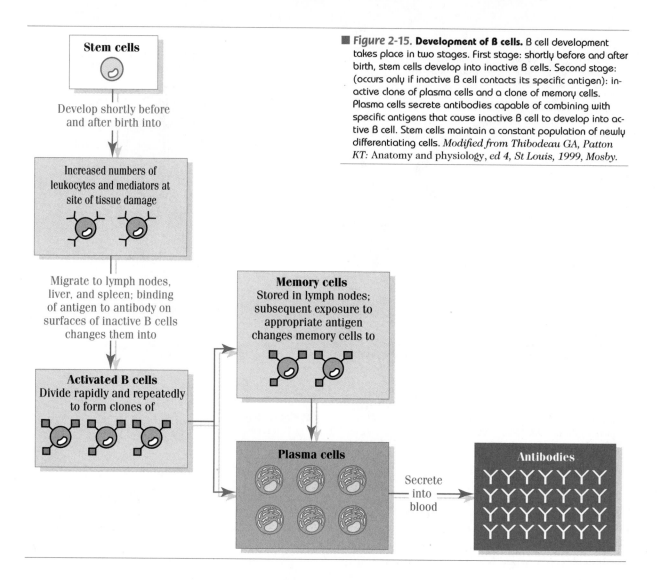

Stem cells

Develop shortly before
and after birth into

Increased numbers of
leukocytes and mediators at
site of tissue damage

Migrate to lymph nodes,
liver, and spleen; binding
of antigen to antibody on
surfaces of inactive B cells
changes them into

Activated B cells
Divide rapidly and repeatedly
to form clones of

Memory cells
Stored in lymph nodes;
subsequent exposure to
appropriate antigen
changes memory cells to

Plasma cells

Antibodies

Secrete
into
blood

■ *Figure 2-15.* **Development of B cells.** B cell development takes place in two stages. First stage: shortly before and after birth, stem cells develop into inactive B cells. Second stage: (occurs only if inactive B cell contacts its specific antigen): inactive clone of plasma cells and a clone of memory cells. Plasma cells secrete antibodies capable of combining with specific antigens that cause inactive B cell to develop into active B cell. Stem cells maintain a constant population of newly differentiating cells. *Modified from Thibodeau GA, Patton KT:* Anatomy and physiology, *ed 4, St Louis, 1999, Mosby.*

antibody and antigen. The "Clonal-Selection Theory" also explains immunologic tolerance, or the ability not to attack "self." The deletion of an entire clone of cells could occur before or soon after birth if an antigen overwhelmed the metabolic abilities of the cell.

Burnet conceived of the immune response as a kind of Darwinian selection of the fittest. The antibody-producing cells are subject to mutation and selection. In this case, the "fittest" cell is the one that "fits" best between a cell's antibody and antigen. Along with Medawar, Burnet was awarded the Nobel Prize in 1960 for his understanding and conceptualization of acquired immunologic tolerance. Burnet, himself, believed articulating the "Clonal-Selection Theory" was his most significant achievement.[1]

Natural killer cells—trained assassins. NK cells make up a distinct group of large granular lymphocytes. Unlike other lymphocytes that only react against specific virus-infected or tumor cells, NK cells recognize, lyse, and kill any cancer cells or virus-infected cells, even before the immune system is activated. This capability is possible because they recognize changes in the cell's surface, which occur on tumor or virus-infected cells. NK cells are not phagocytic or cell eaters, however. They attack the membrane of the target cell and release toxic chemicals into the cell. Soon after this attack, the cell's membrane and its nucleus disintegrates.

NK cells are also capable of binding IgG because they have a receptor for this antibody on their cell surface. When a cell is coated with antibody and then destroyed by an NK cell, this attack

TABLE 2-3	Cells and Molecules Involved in Specific Immunity

CELLS

B-CELLS	Lymphocytes residing in lymph nodes, spleen, or other lymphoid tissue; stimulated to replicate by antigen-binding and helper T-cell interactions; clones form memory and plasma cells.
PLASMA CELL	The antibody-producing cell, producing immunoglobulins with the same antigen specificity.
HELPER T-CELL	This regulatory cell binds with the antigen presented by a macrophage; it then circulates into the spleen and lymph nodes, stimulating production of other cells (killer and B-cells) to fight invaders; acts by releasing lymphokines.
KILLER T-CELL	Also called killer cells; activated by antigen presented by any cell; recruited by helper T-cells; it kills virus-invaded body cells and cancer cells; it is involved in the rejection of foreign tissue grafts.
SUPPRESSOR T-CELL	Activated by antigen presented by macrophages; slows or prevents activity of B- and T-cells once infection is overcome.
MEMORY CELL	Descends from activated B- or T-cells; produced during primary immune response; can live in body for years, enabling a quicker response if the same antigen is presented.
MACROPHAGE	Engulfs and eats antigens; presents part of it on its plasma membrane for T-cells with same antigen to recognize; releases chemicals that activate T-cells and prevent viral multiplication.

MOLECULES

ANTIBODY (IMMUNOGLOBULIN)	Protein produced by B- or plasma cells; antibodies produced by plasma cells are released into body fluids (e.g., blood, saliva, mucus, lymph) where they attach to antigens, marking them for destruction by complement or phagocytes; antibodies include IgA, IgD, IgE, IgG, and IgM.
CYTOKINES	**Lymphokines:** Chemicals released by sensitized T-cells. Includes *inhibitory factor, interleukin 2*, which stimulated proliferation of T- and B-cells and activates natural killer cells; *interleukin 4*, which causes plasma cells to secrete IgE antibodies; *interleukin 5*, which causes plasma cells to secrete IgM and IgA; *gamma interferon*, which stimulates macrophages to become killers and renders tissue cells resistant to viral infection, *lymphotoxin*, which causes DNA fragmentation; *perforin*, which causes cell lysis; *tumor necrosis factor* produced by macrophages. **Monokines:** Chemicals released by activated macrophages. Includes *interleukin 1*, which stimulates T- and B-cells to proliferate and causes fever; *tumor necrosis factor*, like perforin, causes cell killing; *interleukin 6* causes differentiation of B-cells into plasma cells and enhances proliferation of T-cells; triggers complement binding to bacteria.
COMPLEMENT	Group of proteins activated after binding to antibody-covered antigens; causes lysis of microorganisms and enhances inflammatory responses.
ANTIGEN	Provokes immune responses; large complex protein molecules not normally present in the body.

is called *antibody-dependent, cell-mediated cytotoxicity* (ADCC).

Monocytes—Paul Revere of the immune system. *Monocytes* are the largest leukocytes with gray-blue staining cytoplasm and a dark blue-purple, distinctively U or kidney-shaped nucleus (Figure 2-17). Once in tissue, monocytes differentiate into macrophages, which are highly mobile and have enormous appetites. The main job of macrophages is to engulf foreign particles and "present" fragments of these antigens on their own surfaces—like signal flags—so that the foreign particles will be easily recognized by T-cells. Then, like Paul Revere, they "ride" throughout the body announcing which "foe" has invaded. This is called *antigen presentation* (Figure 2-18).

Macrophages also secrete proteins that activate T-cells, and T-cells release chemicals that

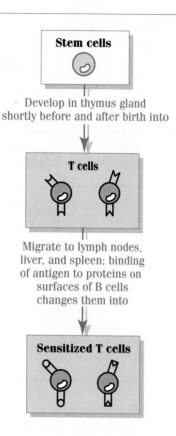

■ *Figure 2-16.* **Development of T cells.** The first stage occurs in the thymus gland shortly before and after birth. Stem cells maintain a constant population of newly differentiating cells as they are needed. The second stage occurs only if a T cell is presented an antigen, which combines with certain proteins on the T cell's surface. *Modified from Thibodeau GA, Patton KT: Anatomy and physiology, ed 4, St Louis, 1999, Mosby.*

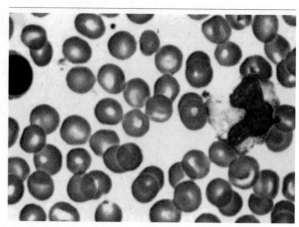

■ *Figure 2-17.* Monocyte. *Modified from Thibodeau GA, Patton KT: Anatomy and physiology, ed 4, St Louis, 1999, Mosby.*

direct macrophages to turn into true killers that will phagocytize the enemy and secrete bactericidal chemicals. In chronic infections, such as tuberculosis, macrophages increase their numbers and become actively phagocytic. They are vital in the body's defense against viruses and intracellular bacterial parasites.

It is apparent that interactions among different categories of lymphocytes and between lymphocytes and macrophages are the foundation of virtually all immune responses.

■ How Researchers Assess Immune Competence

This section discusses the types of assays, or measurements, commonly used in PNI research, how they are performed, and how their results are interpreted. Essentially, PNI researchers want to determine whether stress or conditioning mod-

ulates immunologic competence, which is the ability of the body to identify and reject foreign or unhealthy substances while not rejecting or attacking one's own healthy body tissues and fluids. This differentiation is accomplished by a complex system that includes both cellular and humoral (i.e., fluid) factors[24] (see Table 2-3). This definition suggests that infections and tumors are the result of a failure to recognize and mobilize appropriate bodily defenses against an invader. Autoimmune diseases, on the other hand, are the result of a failure of these defenses to recognize markers of self, leading to an attack on one's tissues or fluids.

Mind-body researchers hypothesize that stressors alter immune function and that immune responses can be conditioned. To support or refute those hypotheses, immunologic activity must be assessed, which involves performing a variety of tests on immune cells and their byproducts.

The ultimate goal of mind-body research is to determine under what conditions and to what degree stressors and conditioning factors alter immunity. Once this information is elucidated, new methods for the management of immune dysfunction can be developed.

Prevalence of Immunodeficiency Disorders

Primary immune deficiencies can be classified into one of the following five categories:
1. Antibody deficiencies
2. Cellular deficiencies
3. Combined cellular and antibody deficiencies
4. Phagocytic disorders
5. Complement deficiencies

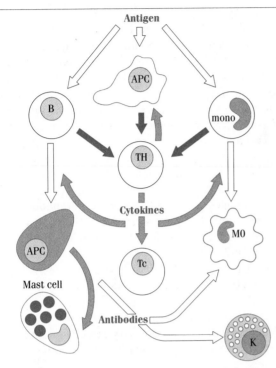

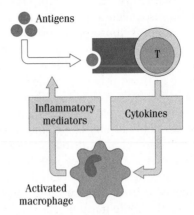

Figure 2-19. Delayed hypersensitivity response. *Modified from Male D:* Immunology: an illustrated outline, *ed 3, St Louis, 1997, Mosby.*

■ **Figure 2-18.** Antigen presentation. *Modified from Male D:* Immunology: an illustrated outline, *ed 3, St Louis, 1997, Mosby.*

Antibody (B-cell) deficiencies make up 50% to 60% of all primary immunodeficiencies, and cellular (T-cell) deficiencies comprise 5% to 10% of all immune failures. Most B-cell disorders are associated with some difficulty in the ability to form antibodies.[17] Combined cellular and antibody deficiencies account for another 20% to 25%, and phagocytic disorders (e.g., granulocytes, monocytes) account for 10% to 15% of immunodeficiencies. Complement deficiencies make up less than 2% of immune dysfunction.

Assessing or measuring the competence of various immune cells and their by-products identifies these immune disorders. The measurements, or assays, used in the research are described and discussed later in this text. In no way does this overview represent all immune assessments currently available. For a more detailed review of immune assessment, the reader is referred to Lawlor and colleagues and Male.[18,21]

Commonly Used Immunodeficiency Assays

Delayed Skin Hypersensitivity: T-Cell Assay
An often-used clinical measurement of immunologic competence is the induction of delayed skin

hypersensitivity (DSH).[17] A DSH response is one that occurs 12 to 24 hours after encountering an antigen and is mediated by CD4+cells. These cells release *cytokines,* or chemical messengers, that attract macrophages to the site and activate them (Figure 2-19).[21] Essentially, the DSH immunocompetence test assesses the ability of T-cells to initiate an inflammatory response. For this assessment, an *intradermal* (i.e., in the dermis) injection of a recall antigen is administered. A *recall antigen* is a protein derivative or bacterial product to which the patient has been previously exposed. Unless a severe cellular deficiency exists, the patient will develop resistance to this product and a positive response. A significant skin *induration,* or skin hardening, will occur 48 to 72 hours after the injection. This induration is composed of macrophages and lymphocytes. Failure to respond can be the result of an immune dysfunction or a lack of previous exposure to test antigens. Therefore a panel of antigens is typically used and can include *Candida,* tetanus toxoid, mumps, and *Trichophyton.*

DSH usefulness is limited in human research because persons who are repeatedly tested for DSH can develop tolerance and diminished skin responsiveness or they can develop immunization that will enhance the size of induration.[8] Corticosteroid and immunosuppressive agents can also cause false negative results.

Flow Cytometry and Monoclonal Antibodies: Lymphocyte Classification Assay
Lymphocytes can be classified using flow cytometry and monoclonal antibodies to identify different surface antigens.

The *flow cytometry* is a technique that measures cell characteristics, including size, granularity, and fluorescence. Cells can be stained with up to three different fluorescent antibodies to quantify the density of three different molecules. Populations are then identified based on the expression of these three molecules.

Obviously, if fluorescent antibodies are to be used during flow cytometry, the "right" antibodies must be available in sufficient quantities. This is the reason monoclonal antibodies are so important. *Monoclonal antibodies* are antibodies produced by a single clone, created by fusing an immortal cell line with normal plasma cells (Figure 2-20). Unlike normal cells that have a limited lifespan, these cells virtually live and reproduce forever. Immortal cells can be selected for a specific antibody before cell expansion, providing an unlimited supply of antigen-specific antibodies. These monoclonal antibodies, specific to each lymphocyte cell surface antigen, are categorized according to a *cluster of differentiation* (CD) number.

In lymphocyte identification, monoclonal antibodies are used to evaluate cell lineage, differentiation, activation, and functional capacity. They determine the presence of particular cells and their potential function by identifying cell surface proteins that are unique to specific lymphocyte populations (e.g., T-cells, B-cells, subpopulations of T-cells, such as helper and suppressor cells, NK cells, and macrophages).[8]

It is easy to understand why flow cytometry with its use of monoclonal antibodies and CD antigens is so convenient. NK cells, B-cells, and macrophages can be identified simultaneously by their CD antigens. For example, CD11 and CD18 are markers for monocytes, whereas CD16, CD56, and CD57 are markers for NK cells. Identifying CD1 through CD8 often assesses T-cells. Researchers in human immunodeficiency viral (HIV) infection and acquired immunodeficiency syndrome (AIDS), for example, identify a CD4:CD8 ratio imbalance related to HIV infection and AIDS (i.e., a helper to suppressor T-cell imbalance).

Electrophoresis: Separation of Serum Proteins

Electrophoresis separates proteins based on electric charge by subjecting a solution (e.g., serum, cerebral spinal fluid, urine) to an electropotential gradient. Zone electrophoresis is a semiquantitative technique that is useful for assessing total protein status and for identifying immunoglobulins.[8] Serum electrophoresis typically yields five bands, consisting of albumin, alphas 1 and 2, beta, and gamma globulin fractions (Figure 2-21). A densitometer generates a tracing representative of fraction percentages. Immunoglobulins normally fall within the gamma globulin band.

Nephelometry Method: Measurement of Serum Proteins

Nephelometry is a method that quantifies different proteins in a solution by scattering the light from soluble immune complexes generated by the addition of specific antibodies to the sample. This method enables accurate measurement of IgG and IgG subclasses—IgA, IgM, IgE, C3, C4, C-reactive protein (CRP)—and a number of other serum proteins. It is the standard clinical laboratory method for quantifying immunoglobulins (Figure 2-22).[8]

Radial Immunodiffusion and Enzyme-Linked Immunosorbent Assays: Quantification of Immunoglobulins and Other Serum Proteins

Radial immunodiffusion can be used to quantify immunoglobulins, complement components, and other proteins. This method quantifies a protein

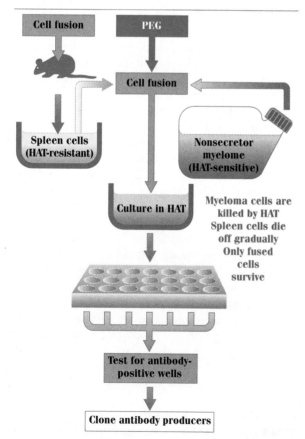

■ **Figure 2-20.** Monoclonal antibody production. *Modified from Male D:* Immunology: an illustrated outline, *ed 3, St Louis, 1997, Mosby.*

by adding serum to wells (i.e., a deep impression) cut into agarose, a solidifying agent, containing specific antiserum. The diameter of the precipitant ring formed by this interaction is proportional to the concentration of the protein being evaluated (Figure 2-23).[8]

Enzyme-linked immunosorbent assays (ELISA) use polystyrine plates, tubes, or beads to provide a binding site for specific antigens under study. ELISA can be used to quantify a number of specific antibodies or antigens, is simpler to perform than immunodiffusion, and requires no radioactive isotopes, using enzymes as a substitute. Antigen is absorbed to a solid phase, and test antibody is added. Antibody is detected using enzyme-labeled

protein G, which binds IgG. Enzymes such as peroxidase and phosphatase are often used. A chromogenic substrate is later added, which generates a colored end-product. The optical density of this solution is then measured and is proportional to the amount of the enzyme, which is related to the amount of antibody.[2] ELISA is the standard laboratory assay for antiviral antibody testing, including HIV (Figure 2-24).

In Vitro Stimulation of T-Cells

In severe T-cell immune deficiencies, the maturation or differentiation of T-cells or T-cell percentages and numbers may be impaired. This impairment can be evaluated by assessing the ability of

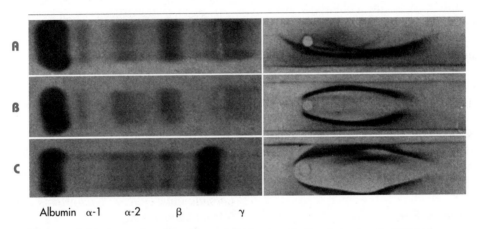

Albumin   α-1   α-2   β   γ

∎ *Figure 2-21.* **Electrophoresis and immunoelectrophoresis.** The electrophoretic (left) and immunoelectrophoretic (right) patterns of a normal individual (A), a patient with hypogammaglobulinemia (B), and a patient with a monoclonal IgG (C). *From Rich RR, editor:* Clinical immunology: principles and practice, *vol 2, St Louis, 1995, Mosby.)*

Nephelometry

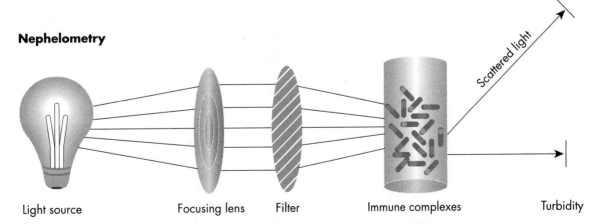

Light source   Focusing lens   Filter   Immune complexes   Turbidity

Scattered light

∎ *Figure 2-22.* Principle of nephelometry. Light rays from a high-intensity source are collected in focusing lens and pass through a sample tube containing antigen-antibody complexes. Light emerging at 70-degree angle is collected and focused into an electronic detector. The signal is converted to a digital recording of the amount of turbidity that is proportional to the antigen concentration in the sample. *From Rich RR, editor:* Clinical immunology: principles and practice, *vol 2, St Louis, 1995, Mosby.)*

Antigen-containing gel

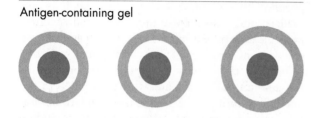

■ **Figure 2-23.** Single radioimmunodiffusion. *Modified from Male D:* Immunology: an illustrated outline, *ed 3, St Louis, 1997, Mosby.*

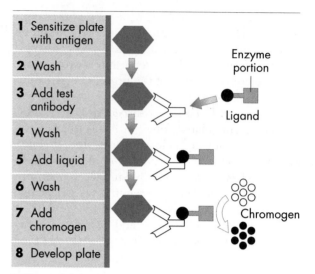

■ **Figure 2-24.** Enzyme-linked immunosorbent assay (ELISA). *Modified from Male D:* Immunology: an illustrated outline, *ed 3, St Louis, 1997, Mosby.*

T-cells to proliferate, or reproduce, when challenged. T-cells are stimulated to reproduce by specific antigens, antibodies to T-cell surface antigens, and *mitogens,* such as concanavalin A (con A), phytohemagglutinin (PHA), and pokeweed. Mitogens nonspecifically stimulate T-cells, whereas antigens stimulate only the T-cells, seeking the antigen-specific receptor. Lymphocytes are cultured with one or more of these stimuli. At the end of the response period, proliferation is evaluated by quantifying the incorporation of a radioactively labeled nucleoside (e.g., titiated thymidine) into newly synthesized deoxyribonucleic acid (DNA). The cells are then harvested and counted by their radioactivity. Mitogens require 3 days of culturing, whereas antigens require 6 to 7 days.[8]

Nitroblue Tetrazolium Test: Phagocytic Assessment

The *nitroblue tetrazolium* (NTB) test is a dye reduction assay that assesses the increased metabolic activity of normal granulocytes (e.g., neutrophils, eosinophils, basophils) during phagocytosis. Most specifically, it is used to assess phagocytosis, or engulfment, rates. Basically, the phagocytic cell absorbs the dye during a set timeframe. How much is engulfed determines the rate of phagocytosis.[17]

Bacterial Phagocytosis and Killing Tests

In bacterial phagocytosis and killing tests, peripheral blood leukocytes are incubated and agitated with fresh bacteria (usually Staphylococcus aureus or Escherichia coli) for 2 hours. The mixture is then centrifuged so that leukocytes, with their phagocytized bacteria, and the unphagocytized bacteria are separated. Normally, leukocytes can be expected to phagocytize and kill 95% of the bacteria within 120 minutes. Sometimes, phagocytized but still living bacteria are found in the leukocyte mixture, indicating that intracellular killing, but not phagocytosis, is deficient.[17]

Cytotoxicity Assessments

Cytotoxicity testing determines the ability of T-cells to kill target cells. In standard assays the target cells are labeled with a radioactive probe Cr (creatinine). Destruction of the target cell is measured by the radioactivity released in the solution.

Chemiluminescence, Phagocytosis, and Intracellular Killing

Chemiluminescence is an alternative method for evaluating phagocytosis and intracellular killing. During phagocytosis, healthy neutrophils and monocytes generate oxygen radicals that react with microbes to form unstable intermediates. When these elements revert to their normal ground state, light energy is released. This light can be measured by chemiluminescence. The amount of light released is a measurement of the killing capacity.

Adhesion Tests

Leukocyte adhesion ability is determined using flow cytometry and analyzing CD11 or CD18 antigens on neutrophils, monocytes, and lymphocytes. In leukocyte adhesion defects, adhesive proteins are significantly decreased and in some cases absent. This deficiency can lead to an impaired ability to fight infection. Neutrophil adhesion can also be quantified by assessing their adherence to single layers of endothelial cells.

Chemotaxis or Migration Assays

The migration, or chemotaxis, of cells (usually granulocytes or monocytes) to sites of infection or inflammation result in the rapid destruction of foreign invaders. If chemotaxis does not readily occur, the patient becomes susceptible to infections. Several tests are used to assess the migration rates of effector cells. These are the in vivo Rebuck skin window assessment and the in vitro chemotaxis tests (Boyden chamber method) and agarose test.[17]

Rebuck skin window assessment. In the Rebuck skin window test, patient skin is abraded, or scraped, with a scalpel blade, producing fine capillary bleeding. Coverslips are placed on the site and changed at intervals of 1/2 to 2 hours. The coverslips with adhering leukocytes are stained and analyzed. In healthy subjects there is an influx of polymorphonuclear granulocytes within 2 hours. Mononuclear cells then replace the polymorphonuclear granulocytes within 12 hours.

In vitro chemotaxis tests. Granulocytes or monocytes are separated from peripheral blood and exposed to chemotaxis factors. The number of cells moving toward the factor can be quantified by using the Boyden chamber method, which uses a Millipore filter, or by using agarose in a plastic Petri dish. Agarose is a seaweed derivative used as a solidifying agent. The rate at which cells move through the agarose can be evaluated.

■ How Researchers Assess Individual Leukocyte Competence

Now that descriptions of the basic assays have been provided, more detail is given about when and how these assays are selected and used for assessing individual leukocyte competence.

Assaying Neutrophils

When assessing neutrophil competence, scientists need to determine the following:
- Adherence of neutrophils to endothelial cells, which occurs when neutrophils leave the bloodstream and enter tissue
- Rate and direction of migration, or chemotaxis, into tissues in response to chemical attractants
- Rate of neutrophilic engulfment of bacteria and foreign particles
- Quantitative analysis of microbe killing by neutrophils

Neutrophil Adhesion

Neutrophils mature in bone marrow and are released into the bloodstream where they spend approximately 6 hours. They then reach the tissues where they are needed by adhering to or migrating among endothelial cells of the blood vessels. One measurement of neutrophil reaction to infection or stress would be to assess the rate at which they adhere to endothelial tissues in preparation for transport to infected tissue sites. In some of the studies that are discussed in this text, researchers produce adherence to endothelial cells *in vitro* (i.e., in a dish) by assessing the *adherence* of neutrophils in *heparinized* (i.e., an anticoagulant that prevents clotting) blood to nylon fibers or to glass beads. Nylon fibers are the best choice for this test because they most accurately reflect the ability of neutrophils to adhere to endothelial cells *in vivo* (i.e., in the body). Therefore this assay is an extremely valuable measurement of neutrophil competence.

Today, researchers are more likely to assess the presence of surface adhesion molecules by seeking three specific cell surface receptors on neutrophils. These molecules are LFA-1, Mac-1, and p150,95. These receptors are identified by flow cytometry using monoclonal antibodies. Patients with leukocyte adhesion defects will demonstrate depressed or absent expression of these surface antigens in resting and in activated neutrophils. The degree to which an individual's neutrophils fail to adhere correlates with (1) a decrease of neutrophil accumulation at infected tissue sites, (2) an increase in the severity of infections, (3) a delay in wound healing, and (4) an absence of pus at infected sites.[8]

Neutrophil Chemotaxis or Migration

Neutrophil migration into tissues can be studied by isolating peripheral blood neutrophils and using an apparatus called a *Boyden chamber*. This chamber has a filter that separates the neutrophils from their chemical attractants or control material. After a set time period, the filters are removed to determine the presence of neutrophil migration. Impaired migration, or chemotaxis, toward the appropriate chemical attractants coexists with slowed or decreased neutrophil accumulation at the infected site. This impairment leads to increased frequency of the infection and contributes to its severity.[10] An alternative approach involves a soft-agar system in response to chemical attractants. In vivo chemotaxis can be assessed by the Rebuck skin window method. In this method, the skin is abraded with a scalpel to produce fine capillary bleeding. Coverslips are placed on the site and changed at various intervals over a 24-hour period. Coverslips, along with the adhering leukocytes, are stained and analyzed[8] (Table 2-4).

TABLE 2-4	Assessing Bodily Defense Systems

DEFENSE SYSTEMS	ASSAY
CELLULAR DEFENSES **Phagocytes**	**White Blood Cell Count and Morphology**

• Neutrophils
  adherence
  engulfment
  bactericidal response
  chemotaxis
	Adherence in vitro
	Migration/chemotaxis by skin window or Boyden chamber or under agarose or in gel
	Rate of engulfment
	• Counting the number of ingested particles or neutrophils engaged in engulfment
	• Can be radioactively labeled
	Killing calculated by quantitative bacterial culturing
	  IgE level
	  Chemiluminescence
	  CD11/CD18

• Monocytes—macrophages	*Phagocytic rate*—disappearance of radioactive
• Phagocytosis	Albumin in peripheral blood; white blood cell count and morphology; nitroblue tetrazolium reduction; chemiluminescence
• Antigen presentation	*Mitogens* to affect lymphocytic stimulation
• Cytotoxic action	Release of creatinine from tagged erythrocytes incubated with monocytes *Delayed skin hypersensitivity*—induration
Lymphocytes	

• T-cells	Absolute lymphocyte count; delayed skin hypersensitivity, proliferation of DNA
	  synthesis. (PHA/Con A stimulation)
	  T-cell and subpopulations numbers
	  Acquisition of activation molecules
	  Cytokine synthesis

• Cytotoxic action	Creatinine release from target cells (in tumor research)

• Subpopulations include:
  T-helper cells
  T-suppressor cells
  Natural killer cells
	No immunoglobulin receptors; no rosettes to sheep erythrocytes

• B-cells (antibody production)	Attaching fluorescent antibodies to human immunoglobulins Preexisting antibodies before immunizations: tetanus, diphtheria, rubella, *H. influenzae,* and poliomyelitis Isohemagglutinins Quantitative immunoglobulin: immunoglobulins G, A, and M *Mitogen*—pokeweed and lipopolysaccharides
HUMORAL DEFENSES • Humoral immunity (immunoglobulins G, M, A)	Immunochemical methods Radial diffusion Complement binding/hemagglutinating capacity
MISCELLANEOUS • Serum complement factors	Serum opsonic and chemotactic assays; individual complement levels

Neutrophil Engulfment

After a microorganism becomes attached to the surface of the neutrophil, the cell engulfs it. The *rate of engulfment* can also be measured. Bacteria or artificial particles can be labeled radioactively to make the counting procedure more accurate. Chemiluminescence can also assess phagocytosis, because the result of chemiluminescence is the release of light energy.[8]

Neutrophil Microbe Killing

Killing microbes is calculated by a quantitative bacterial culturing technique, wherein neutrophils, opsonins (i.e., a substance that enhances phagocytosis), and bacteria are mixed in vitro. Patients with chronic granulomatous disease will show diminished killing of *S. aureus* in this assay. Killing is also dependent on the *respiratory burst,* a process that follows neutrophil activation and phagocytosis and causes an increase in oxygen consumption, hydrogen peroxide production, and superoxide radical formation. In one process the NBT test, neutrophil activation, and phagocytosis reduce the dye into insoluble crystals of formazan, which are detected with microscopic examination. An absence of dye is an indication of chronic granulomatous disease. The alternative test is evaluation of *chemiluminescence.* When respiratory bursts occur, light is generated by activated neutrophils. In this test, neutrophils may be stimulated to action by adding ingestible particles such as zymosan. The chemiluminescence that is then obtained from the patient is compared with the chemiluminescence obtained from cells of healthy patients.

The effectiveness of these uptake and killing steps are critical measurements because a large number of congenital and acquired pathologic conditions are related to the failure of uptake or killing. Therefore these assessments can accurately predict the immunologic competence before, during, and after conditioning or stress events. Persons with uptake and killing disorders typically exhibit an increased susceptibility to bacteria and fungi, but not to viruses.[8]

In summary, all these tests demonstrate high methodologically accurate results with low variability, which means these tests can be used effectively and repeatedly in the same individual. They are effective assessments of bodily defense against stress events.

Assaying Monocytes

To determine the immunologic competence of monocytes, researchers often perform the following:

- Assess effective monocyte surveillance by the rate at which radioactive albumin disappears from peripheral blood
- Quantify monocyte stimulation of lymphocytes by assessing their response to mitogen challenge (e.g., lymphocyte cell proliferation)
- Measure skin *induration* (i.e., when skin becomes hard or firm) 48 to 72 hours after a bacterial injection
- Determine cytotoxic activation of lymphocytes by macrophages as measured by the release of Cr from tagged erythrocytes incubated with monocytes

The monocytes found in peripheral blood eventually become macrophages. Monocytes migrate in response to chemotactic stimulation (i.e., the sniffing phenomenon) so they can phago-

cytize invaders. The greatest value of monocytes lies in their surveillance of the circulating blood entering the connective tissue between the liver and spleen. One way to evaluate the ability of monocytes to phagocytize is to assess the rate of disappearance of radioactive *albumin,* which is a simple protein, from peripheral blood.

Monocytes also play an important role in specific immunity through their interactions with lymphocytes. Monocytes display antigens to lymphocytes, stimulating lymphocytic action. Many mitogens and bacterial products in assays are used to assess how stimulated these lymphocytes become. They measure the degree of response by assessing the incorporation of new DNA as occurs when cells proliferate. This process, previously described, is dependent on the interaction between monocytes and lymphocytes.

Macrophages can also be activated by lymphocytes to become cytotoxic. Cytotoxicity makes macrophages more effective at killing adjacent cells. The cytotoxic effect can be assessed as the release of Cr from tagged erythrocytes incubated with isolated monocytes. These tests are all extremely simple to administer and reflect clinically important aspects of host defense.[8]

Assaying Lymphocytes

Lymphocytes fall into one of two basic categories: B-lymphocytes and T-lymphocytes. B-lymphocytes make antibodies, whereas T-cells engage in surveillance in peripheral blood. There are additional subclasses of lymphocytes. NK cells look like traditional lymphocytes, but they lack some of their basic characteristics. T-cells, called helper cells, and suppressor cells affect lymphocyte DNA synthesis and antibody production.

T-Cell Assays

In vitro stimulation of T-lymphocytes can determine their ability to become activated. T-lymphocytes can be stimulated by the presence of the following:

- Mitogens (PHA, con A, and pokeweed)
- Soluble antigens (*Candida albicans* and tetanus toxoid, which stimulate memory T-cells)
- Allogeneic cells (mixed lymphocyte culture)
- Antibodies specific to T-cell surface antigens (CD2, CD3, CD43)

The potency of the activation in T-cells is then determined by the following:

- Amount of lymphocyte proliferation that occurs

- Secretion of specific cytokines (interleukins 2, 4, and 5; tumor necrosis factor [TNF]; and IFNs)
- Expression of activation molecules (CD25, major histocompatibility complex [MHC] class II)
- T-cell cytotoxicity

When unstimulated T-lymphocytes are exposed to mitogens, antigens, or allenogeneic cells, they react by synthesizing DNA and multiply. Lymphocyte activation can then be measured by the uptake of a radio-labeled nucleotide and thymidine, which quantifies the amount of DNA produced.[17]

B-Cell Assays

Monoclonal antibodies and flow cytometry (as previously described) are also used to identify B-cells. B-lymphocytes in peripheral blood are identified by their surface-bound immunoglobulins and by the monoclonal antibodies specific to B-cell surface proteins (e.g., CD19, CD20). Assessment of antibody responses to mitogens, proteins, and polysaccharide antigens are valuable measurements of B-cell function.

When incubated in vitro with mitogens or bacterial products, B-lymphocytes will proliferate. Their ability to proliferate is measured by the incorporation of the amino acid, thymidine, which is required for DNA replication. The mitogens—pokeweed and certain lipopolysaccharides—selectively stimulate B-cells to divide.

If B-lymphocytes are challenged, they or their plasmic cells will produce antibodies. Levels of antibodies are typically measured by the *nephelometry method* or by radial *immunodiffusion.* Antibody levels in response to childhood immunizations or infections are another alternative measurement. For example, IgG antibody competence is determined by the response of antibody titers to diphtheria and tetanus toxoids. Antibody responses to poliomyelitis and hepatitis B vaccines after vaccination are other methods used to evaluate antibody effectiveness. To assess antibody response to polysaccharide antigens, pneumococcal and meningococcal vaccines are used.[17]

Plasma levels of immunoglobulins are typically stable in response to what is regarded as a severe challenge (i.e., total starvation for 10 days). Therefore commonly encountered everyday stressors do not affect immunoglobulin levels in such a way that the risk of infection is increased. Less is known about the changes of local production of antibodies in the mucous membranes in airways.

Natural Killer Cell Assays

As previously prescribed, labeling target cells with the radioactive probe Cr assesses NK cell cytotoxicity. Cytokine-enhanced cytotoxicity is also assayed by introducing a preincubation step with specific cytokines, including IFN and interleukin-2. NK cells are responsive in viral infections, graft rejection, and tumor rejection. NK activity is sometimes diminished in cancer patients.[8]

Complement Assays

A total hemolytic complement, CH50, value is used to assess functional complement activity for C1 through C9, although abnormalities can exist even with a normal value. C3 and C4 are assayed by radioimmunodiffusion using a precipitating antibody to measure the amount of each protein in serum. These assays do not measure functional activity, however, only the amount. By comparing the values of CH50 values with those of C3 and C4, a variety of immune deficiencies can be identified including active viral hepatitis, malaria, and systemic lupus erythematosus.[17]

■ Researcher Practices

It is normal practice for researchers to use a battery of assays to gain a more in-depth view of the effects of a stressor. A drawback of many immune tests in human beings is that these tests may have a high degree of assay variability. The day-to-day variation in a single subject can be high. Therefore comparison of several assays provides a more accurate picture of immune reaction.

■ Chapter Review

Physiologic and pharmacologic factors can alter immunologic functioning. They are therefore considered stressors in their own right. When performing research, pertinent variables must be taken into consideration and these extraneous factors must be controlled. These factors include aging, nutrition (including starvation or obesity), drugs (e.g., analgesics, tranquilizers), and alcohol. Researchers are concerned with the variables of circadian rhythms (i.e., daily physiologic cycles) and endocrine factors (e.g., hormonal cyclical changes).

The next chapters provide a detailed profile of the events that launched PNI and mind-body medicine in the United States. You will want to refer back for details related to research methods, since this chapter discusses some of the landmark studies in detail.

Matching Terms and Definitions

Match each numbered definition with the correct term. Place the corresponding letter in the space provided.

_____ 1. "Rose cold," pictures of hay fields, asthma attacks

_____ 2. Increased blood sugar, elevated epinephrine, accelerated heart rate, clammy skin, dilated pupils

_____ 3. Serious life changes, chronic family stress, distressing
life conflicts, unhappiness, depression, social isolation

_____ 4. Observational, physiologic, epidemiologic, clinical

a. Epidemiologic research findings of
factors that affect mortality

b. Four lines of evidence for mind-
body communication

c. Examples of observational
research of conditioned responses

d. Examples of the "fight-or-flight"
response mediated by the SNS

Multiple Choice

Select the correct answer or answers.

_____ 1. Which of the following are granulocyte
cells?
 a. Neutrophils
 b. Lymphocytes
 c. Monocytes
 d. Eosinophils
 e. Basophils

_____ 2. Which of the following are agranulocyte
cells?
 a. Neutrophils
 b. Lymphocytes
 c. Monocytes
 d. Eosinophils
 e. Basophils

_____ 3. Which of the following are called WBCs?
 a. Leukocytes
 b. Erythrocytes
 c. Lymphocytes

_____ 4. Which of the following are found in
neutrophils?
 a. Peptidelike spears
 b. Chemical weapons called lysosomes
 c. Lysosomes in their granular sacs
 d. Defensins in their granular sacs
 e. All the above
 f. a, b and d

_____ 5. Which of the following are performed by
eosinophils?
 a. Destroying parasitic worms
 b. Releasing histamine
 c. None of these
 d. Both a and b

_____ 6. Lymphocytes mature into which of the
following?
 a. T-cells
 b. B-cells
 c. NK cells
 d. a, b, and c
 e. only a and b

_____ 7. Which of the following perform antigen
presentation?
 a. Eosinophils
 b. Neutrophils
 c. Macrophages
 d. Basophils
 e. Lymphocytes

Continued

Multiple Choice—cont'd

Select the correct answer or answers.

_____ 8. Which of the following include chemical by-products activated by immune cell activity?
   a. Antibodies
   b. Lymphokines
   c. Complement
   d. Monokines
   e. Antigen
   f. All the above
   g. a, b, c, and d

_____ 9. Assays of protein serum proteins include which of the following?
   a. Electrophoresis
   b. Nephelometry
   c. Radial immunodiffusion
   d. ELIZA
   e. All the above
   f. a, b, and c

_____10. Which of the following are common mitogens that are used to stimulate T-cells?
   a. Con A
   b. PHA
   c. Alloantigens
   d. Antigens
   e. a and b
   f. c and d

CRITICAL THINKING AND CLINICAL APPLICATION EXERCISES

1. Explain how the Rebuck skin window test is performed. What does it determine?
2. Provide a definition for antigen.
3. Define phagosome.
4. Graph specific and nonspecific immunities, including first, second, and third defense systems, the related cell types, and the complement pathways.
5. Define PNI.
6. Define antibodies. Which types of cells produce them?
7. Explain the "Clonal-Selection Theory."
8. Name the five primary immune deficiencies. List them in the order of their prevalence.
9. Explain how the DSH test is used.
10. Explain what respiratory burst is. How does it occur?
11. Define chemotaxis. Why is it important to assess chemotaxis in immune cells? How does chemotaxis relate to immune competence?
12. Explain the term adherence as it relates to immunity. How does adherence relate to immune competence?
13. What is rate of engulfment? How does rate of engulfment relate to immune competence?
14. What is the difference between engulfment and killing by phagocytic cells? Why are both important?
15. What is mitogen challenge? What are the common mitogens used to stimulate T-cells?

References

1. Ade GL, Nossal Sir G: The clonal-selection theory. In Epaul W, editor: *Immunology: recognition and response,* New York, 1990, WH Freeman.
2. Ader R: A historical account of conditioned immunological responses. In Ader R, editor, *Psychoneuroimmunology,* New York, 1981, Academic Press.
3. Ader R: *Psychoneuroimmunology,* New York, 1981, Academic Press.
4. Ader R, Cohen N: Psychoneuroimmunology: conditioning and stress, *Annu Rev Psychol* 44:53, 1993.
5. Ader R, Felten DL, Cohen N, editors: *Psychoneuroimmunology,* New York, 1991, Academic Press.
6. Cheren S: *Psychosomatic medicine: theory, physiology and practice,* Monograph 2, Madison, Conn, 1989, International Universities Press.
7. Doll RE, Rubin RT, Gunderson EK: Life stress and illness patterns in the US Navy. II. Demographic variables and illness onset in an attack carrier's crew, *Arch Environ Health* 19(5):748, 1969.
8. Fleischer TA, Gracy DG: Diagnostic immunology. In Lawlor GJ, Fischer TJ, Adelman DC, editors: *Manual of allergy and immunology,* Boston, 1995, Little Brown.
9. Freeman LW: *Outcome evaluation of two psychoneuroimmunological intervention programs on asthma symptoms and mood state in adult asthmatic patients,* 1997, Manuscript submitted for publication.
10. Gallin JI, Quie PG: *Neutrophil chemotaxis,* New York, 1977, Raven.
11. Gunderson EK, Rahe RH, Arthur RJ: The epidemiology of illness in naval environments. II. Demographic, social background, and occupational factors, *Mil Med* 135(6):453, 1970.
12. Hilgard ER: *Psychology in America: a historical perspective,* New York, 1987, Harcourt Brace Jovanovich.
13. Hill LE: Philosophy of a biologist, London, 1930, Arnold.
14. House JS, Landis KR, Umberson D: Social relationships and health, *Science* 241:540, 1988.
15. Jacobs MA, Spilken AZ, Norman MM: Relationship of life change, maladaptive aggression, and upper respiratory infection in male college students, *Psychosom Med* 31(1):31, 1969.
16. Jacobs MA, Spilken AZ, Normal MM, Anderson LS: Life stress and respiratory illness, *Psychosom Med* 32(3):233, 1970.
17. Knutsen AP, Fischer TJ: Primary immunodeficiency diseases. In Lawlor GJ, Fischer TJ, Adelman DC, editors: *Manual of allergy and immunology,* Boston, 1995, Little Brown.
18. Lawlor GJ, Fischer TJ, Adelman DC, editors: *Manual of allergy and immunology,* ed 3, New York, 1995, Little Brown.
19. Luborsky L, Mintz J, Brightman JV, Katcher AH: Herpes simplex virus and moods: a longitudinal study, *J Psychosom Res* 20:543, 1976.
20. Mackenzie JN: The production of the so-called "rose-cold" by means of an artificial rose, *Am J Med Sci* 91:45, 1896.
21. Male D: *Immunology: an illustrated outline,* London, 1998, Mosby.
22. Marieb EN: *Human anatomy and physiology,* New York, 1995, Benjamin/Cummings.
23. Meyer RJ, Haggerty RJ: Streptococcal infections in families: factors altering individual susceptibility, *Pediatrics* 539, 1962.
24. Palmblad J: Stress and immunologic competence: studies in man. In Ader R, editor: *Psychoneuroimmunology,* New York, 1981, Academic Press.
25. Pugh WM, Gunderson EK, Rahe RH, Rubin RT: Variations of illness incidence in the Navy population, *Mil Med* 37(6):224, 1972.
26. Rahe RH, Pugh WM, Erickson J, Gunderson EK, Rubin RT: Cluster analyses of life changes. I. Consistency of clusters across large Navy samples, *Arch Gen Psychiatry* 25(4):30, 1971.
27. Rubin RT, Gunderson EK, Arthur RJ: Life stress and illness patterns in the US Navy. III. Prior life change and illness onset in an attack carrier's crew, *Arch Environ Health* 19(5):753, 1969.
28. Smith GH, Salinger R: Hypersensitiveness and the conditioned reflex, *Yale J Biol Med* 5:387, 1933.

3

Psychoneuroimmunology and Conditioning of Immune Function

Lynda W. Freeman

WHY READ THIS CHAPTER?

The challenge for health care professionals and for those in the field of medicine is no longer the treatment of acute diseases or traumatic injuries. Medicine has excelled in the treatment of these conditions. Rather, the future challenges for health care professionals reside with the effective treatment of chronic diseases, many of which are autoimmune diseases, such as systemic lupus erythematosus and multiple sclerosis, or diseases where the immune system fails to perform its surveillance duties adequately, as occurs with cancer.

In the past 25 years, we have learned a great deal about how both physiologic and immunologic responses become conditioned in animals and in human beings. This information has great potential for the development of new and less invasive ways to treat some of our most debilitating diseases. It also has implications for how, in some cases, medical intervention should be provided today.

In this chapter, you will learn in specific detail how conditioning occurs. You will also learn how undesirable immunologic and physiologic responses become conditioned in the patients you treat. The health care environment, itself, may reinforce some of these undesirable responses. An example of this conditioning occurs in chemotherapy-induced anticipatory-nausea. You will learn how to limit some of this undesirable reinforcement. Finally, you will learn how psychoneuroimmunology, as an applied field, offers promise for the development of less debilitating forms of treatment for autoimmune and dysfunctional immune disorders.

Psychoneuroimmunology is literally in its infancy. However, it is important that the health professional knows about research in this area because methods developed in psychoneuroimmunology are likely to become a part of our future health care practices. The reader is cautioned: No other chapter in this text is as complex or will require as much concentration as this chapter. Simultaneously, no chapter provides information as likely to mold the future of complementary medicine.

CHAPTER AT A GLANCE

Physiologic and immunologic responses can become conditioned by exposure to certain conditions, such as taste, touch, or heat; by certain chemicals, such as immunosuppressive drugs; and by events that are emotionally meaningful or traumatic. The pathways by which these events occur are most clearly defined by the emerging interdisciplinary field of psychoneuroimmunology, which describes the interactions among behavior, neural and endocrine function, and immune processes.

The clinical works of Ivan Pavlov, a Russian researcher, demonstrated the ability to condition a salivary response in dogs by pairing a neutral stimulus (a light) with the presentation of food. Later, the presentation of the light alone elicited salivation in dogs. Other Russian researchers believed that immune responses could be conditioned in the same manner as physiologic responses. Two Russian researchers, Metal'nikov and Chorine, succeeded in eliciting a change in cellular response in animals by pairing the scratching of a single area of the skin with the injection of antigenic material. After many pairings, the scratching of the skin alone elicited a conditioned cellular response. Similar studies were replicated by these two researchers and by other Russian scientists.

Years later, two important events heralded a renewed interest in the mind-body domain in the United States. Solomon and Moos published their theoretical integration of emotion, immunity, and disease, and Robert Ader published his serendipitous findings demonstrating classical conditioning of immune function. Solomon and Moos' theoretical assumption was that autoimmunity may be related to immunologic incompetence and that this incompetence might be related to emotional stress associated with elevated adrenal cortical steroid hormones.

Robert Ader was performing an experiment with rats, which induced a conditioned taste aversion. He paired the drug, cyclophosphamide, which unconditionally induces stomach upset and nausea, with a novel tasting solution. Although cyclophosphamide is also an immunosuppressive drug, the amount injected into the rats was insufficient to induce long-term immune suppression. As expected, the animals developed an aversion to the taste of the novel solution. Unexpectedly, because the animals continued to receive the solution, they began to sicken and die. It appeared they had become conditioned to respond to the novel solution as if it were the immunosuppressive drug.

Ader and immunologist Nicholas Cohen designed an elaborate experiment to test the hypothesis that immune responses can become conditioned. The outcomes supported Ader's original observations. By the 1990s, more than thirty well-designed replication studies supported Ader and Cohen's findings. Studies of conditioned modulation using odors, environment, and other drugs demonstrated similar findings. The effects of conditioning on autoimmune diseases and on cancer were also evaluated.

Later, case studies and clinical trials were designed to test similar hypotheses with human subjects. The areas of exploration included (1) the means by which chemotherapy induces anticipatory physiologic and immunologic conditioning; (2) the ability of placebo pills to act as stimuli; (3) the use of taste and imagery as stimuli in the treatment of lupus erythematosus; (4) and the effects of conditioning on multiple sclerosis.

CHAPTER OBJECTIVES

After completing this chapter, you should be able to:

1. Define conditioned stimulus, unconditioned stimulus, conditioned response, and unconditioned response.
2. Describe Ivan Pavlov's experiment with salivary reflexes in dogs.
3. Explain why Russian researchers hypothesized that the immune system could be conditioned in the same manner as physiologic responses.
4. Explain how Solomon and Moos deduced their theoretical integration of emotion, immunity, and disease.
5. Describe Robert Ader's serendipitous discovery concerning stress and immunity.
6. Describe the treatment and control groups used in Ader and Cohen's groundbreaking study.
7. Explain the major conclusions reached by Ader and Cohen from their study.
8. Discuss why the study of the interactions between mind, body, and immune system may have value for the medical community.
9. Describe the findings from one animal study related to autoimmune disease progression.
10. Describe three neutral substances used as conditioning stimuli in animal studies.
11. Define chemotherapy-induced anticipatory nausea, and explain what can be done in the health care setting to discourage its development.
12. Describe one human study of conditioning and explain the outcomes.
13. Discuss how conditioning may be used in the future to treat chronic disease states.

■ Birth of the Field of Psychoneuroimmunology

Psychoneuroimmunology describes the interactions between behavior, neural and endocrine function, and immune processes. The beginning scientific research leading to the development of this field originated with the works of Ivan Pavlov (1928), a Russian physiologist. Pavlov developed a new method for studying animal learning while exploring the conditioned salivary reflexes of dogs.[37] Dogs were trained to stand quietly in a harness while the flow of saliva was meticulously recorded in time sequences and in relation to the presentation of a stimulus. A light, the *conditioned stimulus* (CS), was displayed in a window at the same time that meat, the *unconditioned stimulus* (UCS), was placed in a food bowl, just beneath the dog's nose. The *unconditioned response* (UCR) was salivation, which occurred naturally when the food was presented. After simultaneous pairings of meat with light, the dog would salivate in response to the light alone, a physiologically *conditioned response* (CR) (Figure 3-1).

In other trials, sounds, tastes, smells, and touch stimuli have also been used successfully to evoke CRs, although not all of these responses were identical to the UCRs.

Pavlov found that repeated presentations of a CS that was not reinforced by a UCS eventually resulted in the disappearance of the CR. This disappearance of response is an outcome referred to as *extinction*. For example, if a light had been repeatedly presented to the dog in the previous study without occasionally pairing it with meat, eventually the dog would no longer salivate at the sight of the light in the window.

Russian Studies on Conditioning of Immunity

Pavlov's early trials were the first recorded experiments of *physiologic conditioning.* Russian investigators also conducted the first experiments of *immune conditioning.* These investigators maintained controversial beliefs regarding the mechanisms of antibody formation. *Antibodies* are by-products created by B-cells in the immune system. Early Soviet investigators believed that immunologic phenomena, including B-cell activity, were essentially the same as physiologic phenomena and therefore regulated by the *central nervous system* (CNS). Because of this belief, Soviet researchers decided to study the possibility of direct antigenic stimulation of the nervous system. *Antigens* are substances that stimulate B-cells to produce antibodies.

From a behavioral point of view, they began studying the differences in immunologic reactivity between animals characterized as having different types of nervous systems (e.g., calm versus fearful; sluggish versus overactive). The following is a description of one of the earliest recorded studies of immunologic conditioning.

Metal'nikov and Chorine Study

Modeling their study on the Pavlovian paradigm, Metal'nikov and Chorine injected antigenic bacterial elements (e.g., tapioca, *Bacillus anthracis,* or staphylococcus filtrate), the UCS, into guinea pigs *intraperitoneally* (i.e., into the body cavity), while associating these injections with an external CS (e.g., scratching a single area of the skin).[28,29] These UCS-CS pairings were administered once daily for 18 to 25 days. After a 12- to 15-day rest period to allow the *exudates,* or tissue fluid, in the peritoneum to return to normal, the CS (skin scratching) was delivered several times without the UCS (the injection of antigenic material).

Undisturbed peritoneal exudates normally contain mostly mononuclear white blood cells (WBCs) (i.e., lymphocytes and monocytes). However, in response to the USC (antigenic injection), polynucleated cells or neutrophils, in one of the guinea pigs, made up as much as 90% of the exudate within 5 hours of the injection of a tapioca emulsion. (You may recall from Chapter 2 that neutrophils respond to and engulf bacteria and other foreign particles.) After the 13-day rest period, presenting the CS (scratching the skin) alone increased polynucleated cells in the guinea pig from 0.6% to 62% within 5 hours of presenting the

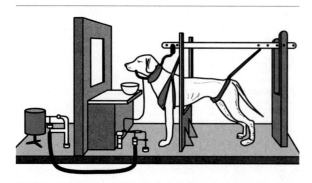

■ *Figure 3-1.* Classical conditioning apparatus used by Pavlov in his experiments with classical conditioning of salivation. Mechanical arrangements (not shown) permitted the light, the conditioned stimulus, to appear in the window, and the meat, the unconditioned stimulus, to appear in the bowl. *Modified from Hilgard E: Psychology in America: a historical survey, New York, 1997, Harcourt Brace College Publishers.*

CS. When results were replicated, two other animals demonstrated similar outcomes. Although the reaction to the CS (skin scratching) alone was somewhat weaker than the response to the USC (injection), the reaction was still clearly evident. This study demonstrated that the immune systems of the guinea pigs had "learned" to respond to the skin scratching phenomena as if the bacterial antigen had been presented. As previously noted, the response was not identical to the actual presentation of antigen; it was somewhat weaker.

Other Studies

In further studies, animals were exposed to multiple pairings of heat or tactile stimulation—scratching the flank and applying a heat plate to the stomach or heat behind the ear, the CS—along with injections of a foreign protein, the UCS.[34,36,38] Foreign proteins are known to elicit an immune response. With time, the CS alone elicited conditioned increases in various defense responses and, in some cases, in antibody responses. The *nonspecific cellular responses* included changes in leukocyte (WBC) numbers, *phagocytosis* (e.g., cell eating, such as macrophages ingesting bacteria or foreign tissue), and inflammatory responses (e.g., swelling, redness, fever). Conditioning could also induce a reversed response—a weakening of immune reactivity. **In summary, when immune-suppressive or immune-enhancing substances were paired with a neutral stimulus, subsequent exposure to the neutral stimulus alone successfully depressed or enhanced immunologic reactivity.**

Limitations of Russian Studies

Early Russian trials were poorly designed and produced questionable outcomes by today's rigorous scientific standards. They often failed to describe important procedural details, results were inadequately portrayed, and outcomes were poorly analyzed. For example, studies would only describe the outcomes for one animal and then state that all other animals in the study demonstrated similar outcomes. Nonetheless, the findings were impressive enough to suggest that just as behavioral and physiologic responses can become conditioned, so can immune responses. An excellent review of these early studies can be found in the Ader's first edition of *Psychoneuroimmunology* (1981), including the use of conditioning stimuli to combat infection and increase antibody titers.[7]

Interestingly, in some of the early antibody conditioning experiments, thermal and tactile stimulation, the CS, was successful in increasing antibody *titers* (i.e., strength of solution), whereas auditory stimuli, also the CS, were not. It was also observed that variables affecting outcomes included (1) the strength of dose of the antigen, the UCS; (2) the intervals between and frequency of the UCS presentation; and similarly, (3) the nature and strength of the CS.

Psychoneuroimmunology in the United States

Two important events heralded a renewed interest in the mind-body domain in the United States. In 1964, Solomon and Moos published their bold paper on the theoretical integration of emotion, immunity, and disease.[40] In 1975, Robert Ader published his serendipitous findings demonstrating classical conditioning of immune function.[4]

Solomon and Moos: Integration of Emotion, Immunity, and Disease

Solomon and Moos based their theoretical integration of emotion, immunity, and disease on two bodies of work: (1) their own work with personality factors in rheumatoid arthritis, an autoimmune disease, and (2) Jeffrey Fessel's extensive work on serum protein abnormalities and autoimmunity in mental illness.[15-17,30-32]

They first analyzed evidence supporting the theory that emotion plays an important role in disease pathogenesis, especially rheumatoid arthritis, a condition where autoantibody to γ-globulin rheumatoid factor is usually present. They then compared data on the emotional aspects of other diseases in which autoimmune factors are found, most specifically, the *dysproteinemias,* an abnormality in plasma proteins, usually immunoglobulins, associated with mental illness. Their major theoretical assumption was that autoimmunity may be related to immunologic incompetence and that this incompetence might, in turn, be related to specific emotional stress (e.g., anxiety, depression) associated with stress elevated cortical steroid hormones. The poor antibody response of patients with schizophrenia was also cited as literature supporting the susceptibility of illness during stress. Their theoretical work was bold, daring, and the first serious attempt to integrate these factors into one theory of disease progression or remission.

Robert Ader and Psychoneuroimmunology

As often happens, breakthrough discoveries are the result of scientific accidents, not rational theories. Such was the case with Robert Ader's experiment with the illness-induced, taste-aversion paradigm. In fact, at the time Ader performed his experiments, he was totally unaware that attempts to condition immune responses had been initiated by Russian investigators almost 50 years before (Figure 3-2).

Illness-induced taste-aversion paradigm. An effective technique known as the *illness-induced taste-aversion paradigm* is often used for establishing CRs. In this paradigm, consumption of a distinctively flavored drinking solution is paired with an injection of a pharmacologic agent known to induce gastrointestinal upset (e.g., nausea, diarrhea). The behavior-elicited CR is the aversion to drinking the flavored liquid. In most studies, the distinctive flavor has been a saccharine solution, although coffee, tea, sucrose, almond, and even garlic-flavored water have been used. Because these substances alone do not induce symptoms, they are neutral stimuli and are effective choices for CS.

In earlier studies, UCS included substances such as lithium chloride (LiCl) or cyclophosphamide (CY), both of which induced nausea and diarrhea. This paradigm was often used because it rapidly induced conditioning (in one trial as opposed to numerous trials required with other models) and because the CR (aversion to the liquid that caused upset) was retained, without reinforcement, for as long as 3 months. Another feature of this paradigm was that several hours could intervene between the presentation of the CS and

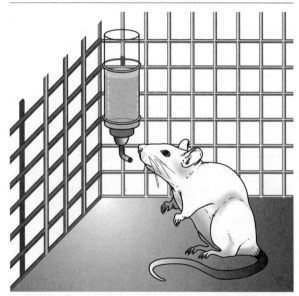

■ **Figure 3-2.** In the illness-induced taste-aversion paradigm, the consumption of a distinctively flavored drinking solution is paired with an injection of a pharmacologic agent known to induce gastrointestinal upset.

the presentation of the UCS with conditioning still occurring. The phenomenon elicited with this paradigm was **highly reproducible** (i.e., outcomes were the same when the experiment was repeated many times).

Ader's serendipitous discovery. Ader was conducting an experiment in which a saccharine-flavored solution was paired with the drug CY.[1] The purpose of the study was to determine whether varying the volume of saccharin would affect the acquisition or extinction of a conditioned taste aversion. What Ader accidentally discovered would launch a new field of mind-body research.

Experimental animals received intraperitoneal (IP) injections of 50 mg CY 30 minutes after the animals drank one of the following volumes: (1) 1 ml, (2) 5 ml, or (3) 10 ml of a 0.1% saccharine solution. Control animals received IP injections of a neutral alcohol solution.

For 2 days after the injections, all rats were allowed plain water during their drinking periods. On day 3, a saccharine solution was provided instead of plain water. The 2-day water, 1-day saccharine solution intervals were repeated twenty times.

As expected, the extent of the demonstrated aversion to saccharin and the resistance to extinction measured in 3-day intervals was directly related to the dosage (1, 5, or 10 ml) of the saccharine solution, the CS, received on the day of conditioning. Extinction did not occur in most animals until 50 days after the one-time pairing of CY with the solution.

Beginning 45 days after conditioning, **some animals from the experimental, but not the control, group began to die.** The first animals to die were from the group given the strongest (10 ml) saccharine solution on day 1. This suggested that the volume of the strength of the saccharine solution, the CS, received was directly related to the death rate. The experiment was concluded at day 60.

Ader's conclusions. While analyzing why the experimental animals died, Ader discovered that CY was an immunosuppressive drug. However, the single dose given during the experiment was insufficient to cause long-term illness.

In conditioning experiments, one can expect the magnitude of conditioning and increased resistance of extinction to be related to the volume of the CS administered, in this case, saccharine solution. Ader hypothesized that perhaps the rats had not only become behaviorally conditioned (i.e., the taste aversion), but their immune cells had become conditioned as well (i.e., immunosuppression). The conditioned immunosuppression, he hypothesized, left the most strongly conditioned animals—those who received the 10 ml of solution—highly susceptible to latent *pathogens* (i.e., any virus or substance causing disease) in the environment.

Ader and Cohen's conditioning of immunity experiment. Ader's findings sent shock waves through the scientific community. The wisdom of the day was that the immune system could not "learn" anything; only the brain or CNS could adapt in such a manner. Based on these initial findings, Ader teamed with Nicholas Cohen, an immunologist, and tested his hypothesis.

The following study is thoughtfully designed and demonstrates the complexity required to eliminate confounding variables in a research study. It will require intense concentration to follow the purposes and outcomes for each group, but it will be worth the effort. (Referring to the color-coded Table 3-1 will simplify the design. Groups are

coded and the colors or shadings will be referenced as each group is identified in the text.)

Ader designed a new study to test the hypothesis that conditioning can alter immune responses. He wanted to determine whether a neutral substance such as a saccharine solution, the CS, when paired with the immunosuppressive CY, the UCS, would later enable the saccharine solution alone, the CS, to influence antibody responses after an immunization with sheep red blood cells (RBCs).[4] Foreign proteins like sheep RBCs will automatically elicit an immune reaction in healthy animals and can therefore be an effective agent for assessing immune suppression or enhancement.

During a 5-day *adaptation period*, rats were provided with and consumed their total daily allotment of water during a single 15-minute period between 9 AM and 10 AM. This regimen was maintained throughout the experiment. The adaptation period provided baseline data for fluid consumption. The experiment that followed lasted for 9 days.

TABLE 3-1 | **Ader and Cohen's Protocol of Conditioned Immune Response**

				DAYS AFTER CONDITIONING			
				0	3	6	9
						DAYS AFTER ANTIGEN	
Group	Conditioning Day	Subgroup		Antigen 0	1-2	3	4-5	6
Conditioned (N=67)	Saccharin+CY	CG$_1$ (11) (9)	Saccharin+saline H$_2$O	H$_2$O H$_2$O	H$_2$O Saccharin+saline	H$_2$O H$_2$O	Sample Sample
		CG$_2$ (9)	Saccharin+saline	H$_2$O	Saccharin+saline	H$_2$O	Sample
		CG$_3$ (10) (9)	H$_2$O+CY H$_2$O	H$_2$O H$_2$O	H$_2$O H$_2$O+CY	H$_2$O H$_2$O	Sample Sample
Specialized controls		CG$_4$ (10) (9)	H$_2$O+saline H$_2$O	H$_2$O H$_2$O	H$_2$O H$_2$O+saline	H$_2$O H$_2$O	Sample Sample
Unconditioned (N=19)	H$_2$O+CY	UCG (10) (9)	Saccharin+saline H$_2$O	H$_2$O H$_2$O	H$_2$O Saccharin+saline	H$_2$O H$_2$O	Sample Sample
Placebo (N=10)	H$_2$O+placebo	P (10)	H$_2$O	H$_2$O	H$_2$O	H$_2$O	Sample

CONDITIONED ANIMALS:

CG$_1$ Green group: Conditioned subgroup 1 received one exposure to saccharin

CG$_2$ Black-on-white group: Conditioned subgroup 2 received two exposures to saccharin

CG$_3$ White-on-black group: Conditioned subgroup 3 received one additional CY injection

CG$_4$ Black-on-green group: Conditioned subgroup 4 received one additional injection

On the day of conditioning, (Day 0) rats were randomly assigned to one of three groups referred to as the conditioned group (CG) (N=67), the unconditioned group (UCG) (N=19); and the placebo group (P) (N=10) (see Table 3-1).

On Day 0, all 67 conditioned animals (subgroups CG_1 [green], CG_2 [black on white], CG_3 [white on black], and CG_4 [gray on black]) received a 0.1% solution of saccharin in tap water and 30 minutes later received an injection of CY. It was expected that the novel taste of saccharin paired with CY would later induce, in all these animals, a conditioned immunosuppressive response to saccharin.

UCG (black on color) were given plain water, and 30 minutes later they also received an injection of the immunosuppressive CY. Because water is not a novel-tasting substance, no conditioning of immunity was expected. In other words, receiving plain water at a later time should have had no effect on immune function. Also, no behaviorally conditioned aversion to the taste of water was expected, since water is not a novel substance. The purpose of this group was to allow the authors to evaluate any residual effects of immunosuppression from the injection of CY. This had to be determined so that any effect could be eliminated as a confounding variable.

P animals (black on striped background) received plain water and an injection of neutral saline. Because handling animals can be stressful to them and since stress can alter immunity, the identical treatment of this group *without* the CY injection would assess any changes in immunity caused by the stress of handling.

For the next 2 days, all rats in all groups were simply given tap water during the 15-minute drinking periods. Three days after conditioning, all rats were injected with sheep RBCs. Thirty minutes after the injections, randomly selected subgroups of both the conditioned (CG) and unconditioned (UCG) animals received either saccharine solution **or** plain water, and then they received an injection of either saline **or** CY (see Table 3-1).

CG_1 animals (green) were divided into two groups. On day 3, half of the animals in this subgroup received saccharin on the day that sheep RBCs—the antigen—was normally given. On day 6, 3 days after the antigen was delivered, the other half received saccharin. This schedule was set up to determine if delaying the exposure of saccharin, the CS, would affect the strength of the immunosuppressive response.

CG_2 animals (black on white) received saccharin on both day 3 and 6, the antigen day and 3 days later. It should be noted that **the animals in subgroup CG_2 received twice the exposure to saccharin, as did the animals in CG_1.**

The remaining two subgroups of the CG animals—CG_3 (white on black) and CG_4 (black on gray)—served as specialized control groups.

The CG_3 animals (white on black) received additional CY injections, either on the day the sheep RBC injection was given or 3 days later. This schedule determined the immunosuppressive effects of CY in the CG animals without providing the saccharin. The CG_4 animals (black on gray) received plain water and an injection of saline on the day the sheep RBCs were administered, or 3 days later, to determine the prior effects of conditioning without additional CY or saccharine exposure.

The UCG animals (color background), which received only plain water with the injection of CY on conditioning day (day 3), were subdivided into groups and received saccharin and saline on the same schedule as the CG_1 animals.

Finally, the P animals (black on striped background) received no injections or saccharine solution, but they were given water during the same 15-minute period each day. On day 9 (6 days after receiving the sheep RBC injections), all animals were killed and their blood collected for antibody assays.

The information about drinking solutions and injections of CY or saline were maintained on coded data sheets, and all laboratory procedures were conducted without knowledge of the group to which the animals belonged. This satisfied double-blind procedures.

Outcomes. As expected, pairing the CS (saccharin) and CY resulted in a conditioned aversion to the taste of saccharin. All of the animals in subgroup CG_1—those that received saccharin on day 3 or day 6—did not differ in their outcomes. This group was therefore collapsed into one, CG_1 (green). This subgroup, as a whole, was defined as receiving one as opposed to two exposures to the CS (saccharin). The special control groups, CG_3 and CG_4 (white on black and black on gray) also did not differ in outcomes from their subgroups. Therefore all CG_3 animals became one group defined as animals receiving an additional CY injection. All CG_4 animals were collapsed into one group and defined as animals exposed to an additional saline injection.

As expected, P animals (black on striped background) that never received CY injections produced the highest antibody titers (i.e., maintained the strongest immune response). No difference in outcomes was found between the UCG animals (color background) and the animals in the CG_4 subgroup, which were not reexposed to the CS (saccharin). Both CG_1 and CG_2 had lower antibody titers than the P group, however. This result was judged to be a residual effect of receiving the initial injection of CY. Therefore the CG_4 and UCG groups were the two that were used for comparison to determine whether any additional immunosuppression had or had not occurred because of conditioning alone.

- CG animals that received either one or two exposures of saccharin after the antigen injection (CG_1 and CG_2) showed a diminished antibody response significantly different from the UCG and CG_4 groups.
- Subgroup CG_2, which received two exposures of CS, demonstrated greater attenuated immunity than CG_1, which received only one exposure.
- ***These results demonstrate that saccharin paired with CY, an immunosuppressive drug, enabled saccharin alone to later elicit a conditioned immunosuppressive response. Further, the effect was heightened with multiple exposures.*** (Figure 3-3).

Conclusions and comments. This experiment, pairing saccharin and CY, has been highly reproducible and has demonstrated successful outcomes in more than 30 animal studies (Table 3-2). Immunosuppressive conditioning has now been verified in numerous animal studies and under a variety of experimental conditions.[8] Similar experiments using other pharmacologic agents (LiCl, Poly I:C, methotrexate) and various forms of conditioning stimuli (e.g., taste, odor, touch, even electric shock) have produced a similar type of conditioning (Table 3-3).

Because of the concerns that water deprivation may have affected antibody titers, this model has also been replicated with a two-bottle model—one bottle with saccharine water and the other with plain water. With this model, outcomes were assessed by preference rather than avoidance.

Findings from these studies suggest that **conditioned immunosuppression may affect T-cells more readily than B-cells**. Of particular note is the finding that **when cells are transferred from conditioned animals to unconditioned animals,** the cells elicit immune responses in the unconditioned animals.

Antibody response has been demonstrated to be highly specific. For example, the antibody IgM stimulated in vitro with pokeweed can be suppressed with no apparent suppression of the antibodies IgG or IgA. Proliferation response to concanavalin A (con A) and phytohemagglutinin (PHA) and two T-cell mitogens were successfully suppressed in other studies. Not surprisingly, previous exposure to the CS *before* conditioning trials can delay the creation of a CR, whereas continued, unreinforced exposure to the CS will eventually extinguish the CR. (For an extremely thorough review of these trials, see Ader and Cohen, 1993.)[9]

The early Ader and Cohen trials (1974) fueled the development of the field of PNI. The question at issue was, "Could conditioning be applied as a treatment for specific disease states?" A series of studies suggested that it could.

> **Points to Ponder**   The early Ader and Cohen trials (1974) fueled the development of the field of PNI. The question at issue was, "Could conditioning be applied as a treatment for specific disease states?" A series of studies suggested that it could.

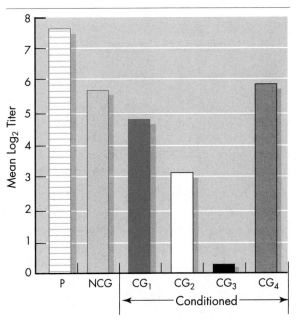

■ *Figure 3-3.* Elicitation of a conditioned immune suppression response in Ader & Cohen's groundbreaking experiment.

TABLE 3-2	**Replication Studies of Conditioned Modulation of Immunity**

CONDITIONED STIMULUS	MEASURE	SPECIES	REFERENCE
Saccharin	Ab (SRBC)	Rat	Ader R, Cohen N: Behaviorally conditioned immunosuppression, *Psychosom Med* 37:33, 1975.
Saccharin	Ab (SRBC)	Rat	Ader R, Cohen N: Conditioned immunopharmacologic responses. In Ader R, editor: *Psychoneuroimmunology*, New York, 1981, Academic Press.
Saccharin	Ab (SRBC)	Rat	Ader R, Cohen N, Grota LJ: Adrenal involvement in conditioned immuno-suppression, *Int J Immunopharmacol* 1:141, 1979.
Saccharin	Ab (SRBC)	Rat	Ader R, Cohen N, Bovbjerg D: Conditioned suppression of humoral immunity in the rat, *J Comp Physiol Psychol* 96:517, 1982.
Saccharin	Ab (SRBC)	Rat	Rogers MP, Reich P, Strom TB, Carpenter CB: Behaviorally conditioned immunosuppression: replication of a recent study, *Psychosom Med* 38:447, 1976.
Saccharin	Ab (SRBC)	Rat	Wayner EA, Flannery GR, Singer G: The effects of taste aversion conditioning on the primary antibody response to sheep red blood cells and *Brucella abortus* in the albino rat, *Physiol Behav* 21:995, 1978.
Saccharin	Ab (SRBC)	Rat	MacQueen GM, Siegel S: Conditioned immunomodulation following training with cyclophosphamide, *Behav Neurosci* 103:638, 1989.
Saccharin	Ab (SRBC)	Mouse	Schulze GE, Benso, RW, Paule MG, Roberts DW: Behaviorally conditioned suppression of murine T-cell dependent but not T-cell independent antibody responses, *Pharmacol Biochem Behav* 30:859, 1988.
Sucrose	Ab (SRBC)	Rat	Ader R, Cohen N: Conditioned immunopharmacologic responses. In Ader R, editor: *Psychoneuroimmunology*, New York, 1981, Academic Press.
HCL	Ab (SRBC)	Rat	Wayner EA, Flannery GR, Singer G: The effects of taste aversion conditioning on the primary antibody response to sheep red blood cells and *Brucella abortus* in the albino rat, *Physiol Behav* 21:995, 1978.
Saccharin/Environment	Ab (SRBC)	Mouse	Krank MD, MacQueen GM: Conditioned compensatory responses elicited by environmental signals for cyclophosphamide-induced suppression of antibody production in mice, *Psychobiol* 16:229, 1988.
Saccharin/Environment	Ab (SRBC)	Rat	MacQueen GM, Siegel S: Conditioned immunomodulation following training with cyclophosphamide, *Behav Neurosci* 103:638, 1989.
Saccharin	PFC (SRBC)	Mouse	Gorczynski RM, Macrae S, Kennedy M: Factors involved in the classical conditioning of antibody responses in mice. In Ballieux RE, Fielding JF, L'Abbate A, editors: *Breakdown in human adaptation to "stress": towards a multidisciplinary approach*, Hingham, MA, 1984, Martinus Nijhof.
Saccharin	PFC (SRBC)	Mouse	McCoy DF, Roxman TL, Miller JS, Kelly KS, Titus MJ: Some parameters of conditioned immunosuppression: species differences and CS-US delay, *Physiol Behav* 36:731, 1986.
Saccharin	PFC (SRBC)	Mouse	Bovbjerg D, Cohen N, Ader R: Behaviorally conditioned enhancement of delayed type hypersensitivity in the mouse, *Brain Behav Immun* 1:64, 1987.
Saccharin	IgM	Rat	Kusnecov AV, Husband AJ, King MG: Behaviorally conditioned suppression of mitogen-induced proliferation and immunoglobulin production: effect of time span between conditioning and reexposure to the conditioned stimulus, *Brain Behav Immun* 2:198, 1988.

Ab, Antibody; *CR (−)*, conditioned immunosuppression; *CR (0)*, no conditioned immunosuppression; *DTH*, delayed type hypersensitivity; *GcH*, graft vs host response; *HCL*, hydrochloric acid; *IgM*, immunoglobulin M; *LiCl*, lithium chloride; *LPS*, lipopolysaccharide; *NK*, natural killer; *PFC*, plaque-forming cells; *SRBC*, sheep red blood cells; *WBCs*, white blood cells.

TABLE 3-2	Replication Studies of Conditioned Modulation of Immunity—cont'd

CONDITIONED STIMULUS	MEASURE	SPECIES	REFERENCE
Saccharin	PFC (TNP-LPS)	Mouse	Cohen N, Ader R, Green N, Bovbjerg D: Conditioned suppression of a thymus independent antibody response, *Psychosom Med* 41:487, 1979.
Saccharin	Ab (Brucella ab.)	Rat	Wayner EA, Glannery GR, Singer G: The effects of taste aversion conditioning on the primary antibody response to sheep red blood cells and Brucella abortus in the albino rat, *Physiol Behav* 21:995, 1978.
Saccharin	*Pneumococcal P.*	Mouse	Schulze GE, Benson RW, Paule MG, Roberts DW: Behaviorally conditioned suppression of murine T-cell dependent but not T-cell independent antibody responses, *Pharmacol Biochem Behav* 30:859, 1988.
Saccharin	GvH Response	Rat	Bovbjerg D, Ader R, Cohen N: Behaviorally conditioned suppression of a graft-vs-host response, *Proceedings of the National Academy of Sciences of the United States of America* 79:583, 1982.
Saccharin	GvH Response	Rat	Bovbjerg D, Ader R, Cohen N: Acquisition and extinction of conditioned suppression of a graft-vs-host response in the rat, *J Immunol* 132:111, 1984.
Saccharin	DTH Response	Mouse	Bovbjerg D, Cohen N, Ader R: Behaviorally conditioned enhancement of delayed-type hypersensitivity in the mouse, *Brain Behav Immun* 1:64, 1987.
Saccharin	DTH Response	Mouse	Bovbjerg D, Cohen N, Ader R: Behaviorally conditioned enhancement of delayed-type hypersensitivity in the mouse, *Brain Behav Immun* 1:64, 1987.
Saccharin	Lymphocyte Prolif.	Mouse	Neveu PJ, Dantzer R, Le Moal M: Behaviorally conditioned suppression of mitogen-induced lymphoproliferation and antibody production in mice, *Neurosci Lett* 65:293, 1986.
Saccharin	Lymphocyte Prolif.	Rat	Kusnecov AV, Sivyer M, King MG, Husband AJ, Cripps AW, Clancy RL: Behaviorally conditioned suppression of the immune response by anti-lymphocyte serum, *J Immunol* 130:2117, 1983.
Saccharin	NK cell activity	Rat	O'Reilly CA, Exon JH: Cyclophosphamide-conditioned suppression of the natural killer cell response in rats, *Physiol Behav* 37:759, 1986.
Saccharin/LiCl	NK cell activity	Mouse	Hiramoto RN, Hiramoto NS, Solvason HB, Ghanta VK: Regulation of natural immunity (NK activity) by conditioning, *Ann N Y Acad Sci* 496:545, 1987.
Saccharin/vanilla	Total WBC	Rat	Klosterhalfen S, Klosterhalfen W: Classically conditioned effects of cyclophosphamide of white blood cell counts in rats, *Ann N Y Acad Sci* 496:569, 1987.
Saccharin/vanilla	Inflammation	Rat	Klosterhalfen W, Klosterhalfen S: Pavlovian conditioning of immunosuppression modifies adjuvant arthritis in rats, *Behav Neurosci* 4:663, 1983.
			Klosterhalfen W, Klosterhalfen S: Conditioned immunopharmacologic effects and adjuvant arthritis: further results. In Spector NH, editor: *Neuroimmunomodulation: proceedings of the first international workshop on neuroimmunomodulation*, Bethesda, MD, 1985, IWGN.
Saccharin	Lupus	Mouse	Ader R, Cohen N: Behaviorally conditioned immunosuppression and murine systemic lupus erythematosus, *Science* 214:1534, 1982.
Saccharin	Plasmacytoma	Mouse	Gorcyznski RM, Kennedy M, Ciampi A: Cimetidine reverses tumor growth enhancement of plasmacytoma tumors in mice demonstrating conditioned immunosuppression, *J Immunol* 134:4261, 1985.

TABLE 3-3	Conditioned Modulation of Immunity Studies Using Different Unconditioned Stimuli

UNCONDITIONED STIMULI	CONDITIONED STIMULI	MEASURE	SPECIES	REFERENCE
Methotrexate	Saccharin/LiCl	Ab (SRBC)	Rat	Ader R, Cohen N: Conditioned immunopharmacologic responses. In Ader R, editor: *Psychoneuroimmunology*, New York, 1981, Academic Press.
Levamisole	Saccharin	T-helper/suppressor	Rat	Husband AJ, King MG, Brown R: Behaviorally conditioned modification of T cell subset ratios in rats, *Immunol Lett* 14:91, 1986, 1987.
Antilymphocyte serum	Saccharin	Mixed lymphocyte	Rat	Kusnecov AV, Sivyer M, King MG, Husband AJ, Cripps AW, Clancy RL: Behaviorally conditioned suppression of the immune response by antilymphocyte serum, *J Immunol* 130:2117, 1983.
Same	Saccharin	Same	Rat	King MG, Husband A, Kusnecov AW: Behaviorally conditioned immunosuppression using anti-lymphatic serum: duration of effect and role of corticosteroids, *Med Sci Res* 15:407, 1987.
Allogeneic cells	Environment	CTL	Mouse	Gorczynski RM, Macrae S, Kennedy M: Conditioned immune response associated with allogeneic skin grafts in mice, *J Immunol* 129:704, 1982.
Bovine serum albumin	Odors	Histamine	Guinea pig	Russell M, Dark KA, Cummins RW, Ellman G, Callaway E, Peeke HVS: Learned histamine release, *Science* 225:733, 1984.
Same	Same	Same	Same	Dark K, Peeke HVS, Ellman G, Salfi M: Behaviorally conditioned histamine release, *Ann N Y Acad Sci* 496:578, 1987.
Same	Same	Same	Same	Peeke HVS, Ellman G, Dark L, Salfi M, Reus VI: Cortisol and behaviorally conditioned histamine release, *Ann N Y Acad Sci* 496:583, 1987.
Egg albumin	Environment	Mast cell protease II	Rat	MacQueen GM, Marshall J, Perdue M, Siegel S, Bienenstock J: Pavlovian conditioning of rat mucosal mast cells to secrete rat mast cell protease II, *Science*, 243:83, 1989.
Poly I:C	Saccharin/LiCl	NK activity	Mouse	Hiramoto RN, Hiramoto NS, Solvason HB, Ghanta VK: Regulation of natural immunity (NK activity) by conditioning, *Ann N Y Acad Sci* 496:545, 1987.
Poly I:C	Saccharin/LiCl	NK activity	Mouse	Solvason HB, Ghanta VK, Hiramoto RN: Conditioned augmentation of natural killer cell activity. Independence from nociceptive effects and dependence on interferon-B, *J Immunol* 140:661, 1988.
Poly I:C	Saccharin	NK activity	Mouse	Gorczynski RM, Kennedy M: Associative learning and regulation of immune responses, *Prog Neuropsychopharmacol Biol Psychiatry* 8:593, 1984.

Modified from Ader R, Cohen N: The influence of conditioning on immune responses. In Ader R, Felten DL, Cohen N, editors: *Psychoneuroimmunology*, New York, 1991, Academic Press.

Ab, Antibody; *CR (−)*, conditioned immunosuppression; *CTL*, cytotoxic T lymphocytes; *CY*, cyclophosphamide; *DTH*, delayed type hypersensitivity; *HCL*, hydrochloric acid, *LiCl*, lithium chloride; *LPS*, lipopolysaccharides; *NK*, natural killer; *PFC*, plaque-forming cells; *Poly I:C*, polycytidylic acid; *CR (+)*, conditioned immunoenhancement; *SRBC*, sheep red blood cells; *WBC*, white blood cells.

Conditioning of Immunity and Autoimmune Disease Progression

Several animal studies have found that, indeed, autoimmune disease progression can be postponed by conditioning. The following text examines two of these studies.

Systemic Lupus Erythematosus and Conditioned Immunosuppression

A 1982 study by Ader and Cohen sought to determine if suppression of an immune response could be conditioned in such a way as to slow the progression of the autoimmune disease, *systemic lupus erythematosus* (SLE).[5] SLE is an inflammatory connective tissue disease with symptoms that include fever, weakness, fatigue, joint pain, and skin lesions on the face, neck, or upper extremities.

Groups of rats bred to have a genetic predisposition to SLE were divided into four groups and were treated for 8 weeks. Group 1 received CY injections and saccharin once weekly on the same

TABLE 3-3	Conditioned Modulation of Immunity Studies Using Different Unconditioned Stimuli—cont'd

UNCONDITIONED STIMULI	CONDITIONED STIMULI	MEASURE	SPECIES	REFERENCE
Poly I:C	Odors	NK activity	Mouse	Ghanta V, Hiramoto RN, Solvason B, Spector NH: Neural and environmental influences on neoplasia and conditioning of NK activity, *J Immunol* 135:848S, 1985.
Poly I:C	Odors	NK activity	Mouse	Solvason HB, Ghanta VK, Hiramoto RN: Conditioned augmentation of natural killer cell activity. Independence from nociceptive effects and dependence on interferon-B, *J Immunol* 140:661, 1988.
LiCl	Saccharin	Ab (SRBC)	Rat	Ader R, Cohen N: Behaviorally conditioned immunosuppression, *Psychosom Med* 37:333, 1975.
LiCl	Saccharin	Ab (SRBC)	Rat	MacQueen GM, Siegel S: Conditioned immunomodulation following training with cyclophosphamide, *Behav Neurosci* 103:638, 1989.
LiCl	Saccharin	DTH-Response	Mouse	Kelley KW, Dantzer R, Mormede P, Salmon H, Aynaud J: Conditioned taste aversion suppresses induction of delayed-type hypersensitivity immune reactions, *Physiol Behav* 34:198, 1985.
Rotation/acute/CY	Environment	Ab (SRBC)	Mouse	Gorczynski RM, Kennedy M: Associative learning and regulation of immune responses, *Progr Neuropsychopharmacol Biol Psychiatry* 8:593, 1984.
Rotation/ chronic/CY	Environment	Ab (SRBC)	Mouse	Gorczynski RM, Kennedy M: Associative learning and regulation of immune responses, *Progr Neuropsychopharmacol Biol Psychiatry* 8:593, 1984.
Electric shock	Environment	PFC (SRBC)	Mouse	Sato K, Flood JF, Makinodan T: Influence on conditioned psychological stress on immunological recovery in mice exposed to low-dose X-irradiation, *Radiat Res* 98:381, 1984.
Electric shock	Environment	Lymphocyte prolif.	Mouse	Drugan RC, Mandler R, Crawley JN, Skoolnick P, Barker JL, Novotny B, Paul SM, Weber RJ: Conditioned fear-induced rapid immunosuppression in the rat, *Neurosci* (abstract) 12:337, 1986.
Electric shock	Environment	Same	Rat	Lysle DT, Cunnick JE, Fowler H, Rabin B: Pavlovian conditioning of shock-induced suppression of lymphocyte reactivity: acquisition, extinction, and preexposure effects, *Life Sci* 42:2185, 1988.

day of the week. Group 2 received saccharin and a CY injection on the same schedule. However, on four occasions, two times for each of 4 weeks in random sequence, saline, not CY, was administered to this group. Group 2 therefore received **only one half the amount of CY as did Group 1.** Group 3, like Group 2, received **one half of the dose of Group 1,** but additionally the injections were administered on different days of the same week (i.e., noncontiguously). Group 4 **received no immunosuppressive therapy,** but it received

saccharin followed by intermittent injections of saline. Since Groups 2 and 3 received one half the dose of CY of Group 1, it was expected that Group 1 would live significantly longer than the other two groups. Since Group 2 received a *consistent* pairing of CY and saccharin on the same day and time of the week, but Group 3 did not, it was anticipated that no conditioning would occur for Group 3. Group 3 therefore should die more readily than Group 2, even though the doses of CY were the same.

Proteinuria is a severe, prolonged loss of protein in the urine and is an indicator that SLE is progressing. As anticipated, animals in Group 1 developed proteinuria later than any of the other groups ($p<0.001$ in each instance). Animals in Group 2 developed proteinuria significantly more slowly than Group 3 ($p<0.05$) and Group 4 ($p<0.01$). Group 3 did not differ in disease development from Group 4. By contrast, Group 2, the conditioned group that received one half the dose of CY, survived significantly longer than Groups 3 and 4 ($p<0.001$). Further, Groups 3 and 4 did not differ in death rates.

Most importantly, Group 2, which received one half the dose of CY, did not differ in death rate from Group 1. This finding is particularly important because even though CY was administered to Group 2 in quantities that would normally have little affect on disease course, Group 2, but not Groups 3 or 4, still demonstrated significant delays in disease onset and death ($p<0.05$).

The author hypothesized that **prescribing chemotherapy and pharmacologic treatments on a conditioned, noncontiguous but consistent schedule versus a continuous drug regimen may have application in the pharmacotherapeutic control and regulation of a variety of physiologic systems.** It appears that **autoimmune diseases may be possibly postponed by conditioning, as occurred in the previous study.**

> **Points to Ponder**   Outcomes demonstrated that the pairing of saccharin and CY enabled the CS, saccharine solution, to delay the onset of and death rate from the autoimmune disease SLE. ■

Conditioning and Immune Enhancement

If conditioning can decrease hyperreactive immune responses, researchers began to wonder if it could also be used to accomplish the opposite effect. Could it be used to enhance immunity? More animal studies were undertaken and their results suggested that this, too, might be a possibility.

Conditioned Enhancement of Immune Response as Demonstrated by Skin Grafting

In 1982, Gorczynski, Macrae, and Kennedy wanted to determine whether an enhanced, rather than suppressed, immune response could be conditioned by a consistent environmental event.[21] They undertook an unusual method for demonstrating immune response, a method that involved skin grafting, not unlike the procedure used when patients are severely burned.

For this experiment, the authors used two different inbred strains of mice. They grafted the skin from one strain onto the mice of a different strain. Because the strains were different, an *alloantigen,* (i.e., an antigen occurring in some members of the same species, but not others) was produced. If a foreign alloantigen is introduced into an animal by skin grafting tissue from a different strain of mouse, a natural-occurring immune response is elicited. This natural immune response in this case was an increase in cytotoxic T-lymphocytes in the blood. (The reader should recall that cytotoxic refers to the ability of T-cells to kill foreign or invading cells or microorganisms.) In this instance, the T-lymphocytes would attempt to destroy the foreign tissue applied to the open wound of the animal.

In addition to the usual skin grafting procedure, *sham grafts* were also used in this experiment. Sham grafts refer to the removal and reapplication of the rodent's own skin tissue. Since this tissue is not foreign, there is no natural-occurring cytotoxic T-cell activation.

In this experiment, the behaviorally consistent actions, or *cues,* associated with the technique of skin grafting in small rodents (e.g., handling for injections of anesthetic, shaving the grafted area, cutting the skin, encasement of the area in gauze and plaster of Paris for 10 days) served as the CS. This point is extremely important; if behavioral cues in the environment can lead to a CR, then potentially any consistent combination of behavioral cues paired with an immune response can lead to conditioning. The alloantigen introduced into the different strain of mice by the skin graft was the UCS.

If the authors were correct in their hypothesis, a CR would be elicited, that is, an increase in blood cytotoxic T-lymphocytes, when sham grafts were applied to the animals. This response would occur only if several skin grafts and their accompanying environmental cues had successfully produced a CR.

Grafting procedures occurred at 40-day intervals, the minimum time needed for the wounds to heal and for peripheral blood precursors to return to normal levels. After three completed trials, sham grafts were applied to all animals in all groups.

Outcome. Only 50% to 60% of the allografted animals developed an increased frequency of antigen-specific cytotoxic T-lymphocyte precursors in the peripheral blood in response to the sham graft. Therefore these mice were named, "responders," that is, they were capable of demonstrating conditioning. This is a very important point. Some animals (and human beings, for that matter) are more resistant to conditioning than others.

Additional experimentation with these "responders" demonstrated the following:

1. Regrafting with allogeneic skin could reinforce the CR (e.g., the increased frequency of precursor cells in blood in response to sham grafting).
2. Repeated application of sham grafts in the absence of a reinforcing UCS (e.g., allograft) could extinguish the CR.

Conclusions and comments. The authors concluded that in this animal study, a consistent environmental event could successfully condition an enhanced immune response in susceptible animals ("responders"). This conclusion has potent implications. For example, life events may serve as CS, resulting in altered immune responses.

> **Points to Ponder**   The authors concluded that in this animal study, a consistent environmental event could successfully condition an enhanced immune response in susceptible animals ("responders"). This conclusion has potent implications. For example, life events may serve as CS, resulting in altered immune responses. ■

Conditioning Effects of Stress on Natural Killer Cells and Cancer

The ability of environmental events to serve as conditioning cues has led to more studies that examine the potential conditioning effects of stress.

Ghanta and others created an experiment to assess the effects of being forcefully restrained, a behavioral stressor, on cancer development. They also sought to determine whether conditioning of natural killer (NK) cells—the immune cells that destroy cancer cells—occurred in response to restraint stress.[20] They believed that the stress produced by physical restraint would speed tumor growth and decrease survival time in mice inoculated with tumor cells. They further hypothesized that the administration of poly I:C, which increases interferon (IFN) titers and NK cell activity, would decrease the growth rates of tumors and increase survival time.

Two groups of mice with induced myeloma or osteosarcoma tumors were assessed. *Myeloma* is a tumor derived from malignant proliferation of plasma cells, whereas *osteosarcoma* arises from bone-forming cells, affecting chiefly the ends of long bones.

Both types of tumor were divided into the following identical groups: Group 1 mice were handled only and injected with saline three times a week; Group 2 mice received 7 consecutive hours of forced physical restraint, three times a week; Group 3 mice received injections of poly I:C three times a week; and Group 4 received the restraint combined with the poly I:C injections.

The effects of **physical restraint alone were detrimental to the myeloma group, leading to early death of the mice** (100% mortality rate at 85 days for the restrained group versus 99 days for control groups). **When combined with the group that received injections of poly I:C during the early course of the disease, restraint stress neutralized the beneficial effects of the poly I:C treatment.**

Conversely, **restraint stress delayed tumor growth and increased the median survival time in mice with osteosarcoma** (median survival 19 days for the control groups, 27 for the restrained group). When restraint stress was combined with poly I:C, tumor size decreased and survival time substantially increased over those in the control groups (nearly twice that of those with no treatment alone).

A second trial was then undertaken. Because poly I:C therapy delayed tumor growth, the authors attempted to strengthen this response by conditioning. For example, they paired poly I:C, the UCS, and camphor odor, the CS, in groups of rats. They believed this pairing could induce an increase in NK cell activity, a CR, when the camphor odor was later introduced alone.

Outcomes demonstrated that **response to poly I:C treatment as measured by the elevation of the NK cell activity could be conditioned with camphor odor.** The CR group demonstrated enhanced NK cell activity, greater than 50% of the poly I:C–injected groups.

Thoughts on Animal Studies of Stress and Immunity

Animal studies on stress and immunity are important because they explore the connection between stress and resistance to disease, and because conditioning of a host to increase immune activity may have potential for altering disease outcome in human subjects.

Outcomes were surprising because one type of cancer, osteosarcoma, was helped, not hindered, by stress. The authors believe this phenomenon is true because osteosarcoma is not regulated by T-cell function, whereas myeloma is. This study suggests that diseases driven by T-cell dysfunction may worsened with stress (e.g., grief, anxiety, depression) to a greater extent than diseases driven by other forms of cellular dysfunction. More research is needed on these different mechanisms and the effects of stress on outcomes for different forms of cancer. This study implicates stress as a helper or a hindrance to immune function, depending on the type of disease, the pathways involved in the disease, and whether the stressor is chronic or acute.

Could these findings from animal studies have relevance for human subjects? Could similar forms of conditioning or the management of stress be applied to the management of disease in human subjects? If so, could interventions work for both immune deficiency and autoimmune diseases? The possibilities seemed promising. Next, we explore the human trials of the effects of stress on the conditioning of physiologic and immune responses in humans.

> **Points to Ponder**   The outcomes of the Ghanta study were surprising because one type of cancer, osteosarcoma, was helped, not hindered, by stress. ■

■ Conditioned Immune Suppression in Response to Chemotherapy Treatment: Human Trials

We now turn our attention to how specific conditioning of biochemical responses occurs in human subjects. We know that biochemical responses can become conditioned, just as behaviors can become conditioned. In fact, stress-related environmental cues may themselves become CS. Since stress can degrade health, the concept that stress-related cues may continue to reinforce biochemical responses has implications for health and for health care interventions. Let us explore how conditioning actually occurs in human subjects.

When we speak about CRs in human subjects, we are speaking about both physiologic responses (e.g., nausea, increased adrenaline when speaking in public) and immune responses (e.g., immune cell or mediator suppression or enhancement). For ethical reasons, much less research is available on the conditioning of immunologic responses in human subjects. However, natural-occurring conditioned phenomena are observable every day in hospitals around the country. The classic example of human conditioning is the response of patients with cancer to chemotherapy treatments.[39] We therefore review in detail this living laboratory of a learned CR.

Many patients receiving chemotherapy become nauseated as they approach the hospital for treatment, when they see the oncology nurse, or as they wait for an infusion. Some patients state that even talking about the treatments can induce nausea. Other patients report being nauseated for the entire day before treatment. This condition is not only stressful, but it is also humiliating. Susceptible patients often begin vomiting as they enter the treatment hospital or while in the waiting room.

> **Points to Ponder**   Many patients receiving chemotherapy become nauseated as they approach the hospital for treatment, when they see the oncology nurse, or as they wait for an infusion. Some patients state that even talking about the treatments can induce nausea. ■

An associate, Jacob, who was an oncology nurse, told the following story. Jacob had administered infusion treatments to a particularly ill patient over a period of months. By the third treatment, the patient was suffering terribly from nausea and vomiting both before and after treatment. Treatment with antiemetic drugs failed to alleviate her sickness. Fortunately, with time, her cancer went into remission and she recovered. Jacob soon lost contact with his former patient. A year later, Jacob saw this woman at a New Year's party and approached her to ask how she was doing. He tapped her on the shoulder, she turned around, looked him squarely in the eye, and immediately vomited all over his tuxedo.

"It's hard not to take it personally," Jacob commented. "It's bad enough that former patients cross the street to avoid me after treatment. Now, I guess the very sight of me makes them ill." Jacob and his former patient were victims of a CR called *anticipatory nausea*. Research continues to shed light on this conditioned phenomenon.

Conditioning of Immunity and Nausea

Between 25% and 75% of patients develop anticipatory nausea and vomit during the course of repeated chemotherapy.[10,13,33] This effect is believed to be the result of classical conditioning. Nausea, the CR, is induced by reexposure to hospital or infusion cues. These cues become CS because they are paired with the infusion of cytotoxic drugs, the UCS, which invoke nausea and vomiting, the UCR. This type of conditioning is amazingly robust, with patients reporting nausea in response to hospital cues years after chemotherapy has ended. The problems of nausea and vomiting can lead to complications, such as anorexia, metabolite imbalance, and general psychologic deterioration. Patients may insist on reduced chemotherapy doses or even prematurely terminate treatment rather than endure the distress and humiliation of nausea and vomiting.[23,24] In the studies that follow, we explore this phenomenon in detail.

Anticipatory Nausea in Response to Chemotherapy: Conditioned Immunosuppression

In an uncontrolled study, Bovbjerg and colleagues wanted to determine whether patients with cancer (N=20) who displayed anticipatory nausea and vomiting during a course of chemotherapy would also demonstrate *anticipatory immunosuppression* of immune function.[12] No control group was possible because ethical considerations prevented administering immunosuppressive drugs to healthy subjects.

Based on earlier animal studies that demonstrated behavioral conditioning of immune function, the authors hypothesized that measures of immune function would be lower in blood samples taken while in the hospital setting just before chemotherapy infusion, as compared with blood samples taken while in the patients' homes 3 to 8 days before treatment. Specifically, they hypothesized that a proliferative response to mitogen stimulation and NK cell activity would be impaired, as had occurred in Ader's previous animal studies.

Patients in this study were being treated for ovarian cancer and had no history of chemotherapy treatments for any disease. Psychosocial adjustment to illness, as assessed by the "Global Adjustment to Illness Scale," indicated normal adjustment for group members.

Patients received intravenous chemotherapy treatments of CY and other drugs every 4 weeks. The intravenous infusions were administered between 11:00 AM and 1:00 PM to control circadian rhythm effects. Patients were admitted to the program after they had completed no less than three chemotherapy sessions. After admission, patients were scheduled for home assessments between 3 and 8 days *before* their next infusion.

During home assessment, blood was drawn and psychologic and behavioral questionnaires were administered. Patients were reassessed and blood redrawn in the hospital each morning before beginning infusion. Functional measures included proliferative responses to mitogens (PHA, con A, and *Staphylococcus aureus)* Protein A, and NK cell activity.

As hypothesized, proliferative responses to the three mitogens, PHA, con A, and *Staphylococcus aureus,* were significantly lower when the patients were in the hospital than when they were in their homes (p<0.001).

NK cell activity, contrary to hypothesis, was not significantly lower when the patients were in the hospital. There were also no significant differences in other quantitative assays. Visual analog scales (VAS) demonstrated that nausea was significantly higher when the patients were in the hospital than when they were in their homes. Also, patients reported significantly higher anxiety when in the hospital.

Patients were then divided post hoc into subjects who had low PHA responses when in the hospital before infusion and subjects who did not—the anticipatory immunosuppressive group versus no anticipatory immune suppression. The authors discovered that patients with the greatest differences of immune suppression between hospital and home also had the highest levels of nausea when in the hospital.

In conclusion, the authors noted that some patients suppressed immune function more strongly than others (i.e., some were more susceptible to conditioning). One patient demonstrated a 50% reduction in PHA response when comparing measures taken at home with those taken in the hospital. Methods to minimize the affect of such potent conditioning in highly susceptible patients warranted additional research. The following study conducted by Andrykowski addressed the issue of the antecedents of anticipatory nausea.

Points to Ponder The authors noted that some patients suppressed immune function more strongly than others (i.e., some were more susceptible to conditioning).

Antecedents to the Development of Anticipatory Nausea

In a prospective research study, Andrykowski sought to identify factors associated with the subsequent development of anticipatory nausea.[11] This study asked, "What factors make patients more susceptible to the development of anticipatory nausea?"

Patients in chemotherapy treatment (N=71) were interviewed before and after each infusion during the first 6 months of treatment. These subjects had not previously received intravenous cytotoxic chemotherapy.

Results of these interviews were consistent with earlier research on anticipatory nausea. **Posttreatment nausea and state anxiety are elevated in patients who then develop anticipatory nausea.** *Trait anxiety* is a personality trait, whereas state anxiety is a temporary, event-induced condition. **In this study the primary factor contributing to the development of anticipatory nausea was, quite clearly, the strength of posttreatment nausea experienced early in treatment.** Since state anxiety was a contributing factor to conditioned nausea, the authors suggested that patient education, hypnosis, desensitization, or relaxation training and the reduction of hospital waiting times might contribute to less pretreatment nausea. (The effectiveness of these types of intervention for anticipatory nausea is reviewed in the chapter on hypnosis.)

More than thirty studies have now been conducted on the CR of nausea and vomiting in patients with cancer receiving chemotherapy treatments. Some of those studies are listed in Table 3-4.

Classical Conditioning and the Placebo Effect in Relation to Drug Action

The *placebo effect* is a phenomenon whereby an inactive substance (e.g., a sugar pill) or treatment is used to determine the effects of suggestion on the psychology, physiology, or biochemistry of experimental subjects. Historically, researchers regard the placebo effect as an annoyance that has obstructed the accurate assessment of therapeutic effects. A more recent hypothesis contends that the placebo effect is actually a CR that genuinely alters physiology and biochemistry and therefore

TABLE 3-4	**Frequency of Conditioned Anticipatory Nausea and Vomiting in Patients Taking Chemotherapy**		
STUDY		**SUBJECTS**	**PERCENT***
Scogna DM, Smalley RV: Chemotherapy-induced nausea and vomiting, *Am J Nurs* 79:1562, 1979.		41	78%
Nesse RM, Carli T, Curtis GG, Kleinman PD: Pre-treatment nausea in cancer chemotherapy: a conditioned response? *Psychosom Med* 42:33, 1980.		18	44%
Palmer BV, Walsh G, McKinna JA, Greening WP: Adjuvant chemotherapy for breast cancer: side effects and quality of life, *Br Med J* 281:1594, 1980.		24	22%
Schultz LS: Classical (Pavlovian) conditioning of nausea and vomiting in cancer chemotherapy, Proceedings, *Am Soc Clin Oncol* 21:244, 1980.		68	31%
Morrow GR, Arseneau JC, Asbury RF, Bennett JM, Boros L: Anticipatory nausea and vomiting in chemotherapy patients, *N Engl J Med* 306:431, 1982.		406	24%
Nicholas DR: Prevalence of anticipatory nausea and emesis in cancer chemotherapy patients, *J Behav Med* 5:461, 1982.		71	18.3%
Wilcox PM, Fetting JH, Nettesheim KM, Abeloff MD: Anticipatory vomiting in women receiving cyclophosphamide, methotrexate, and 5-FU (CMF) adjuvant chemotherapy for breast carcinoma, *Cancer Treat Rev* 66(8):1601, 1982.		52	33%
Fetting JH, Wilcox PM, Iwata BA, Criswell EL, Bosmajian LS, Sheidler VR: Anticipatory nausea and vomiting in an ambulatory medical oncology population, *Cancer Treatment Rep* 67(12):1093, 1983.		123	31%
Ingle RJ, Burish TG, Wallston KA: Conditionability of cancer chemotherapy patients, *Oncol Nurs Forum* 11:97, 1984.		60	25%
Weddington WW, Miller NJ, Sweet DL: Anticipatory nausea and vomiting associated with cancer chemotherapy, *J Psychosom Res* 28:73, 1984.		50	38%
Andrykowski MA, Redd WH, Hatfield AK: Development of anticipatory nausea: a prospective analysis, *J Consult Clin Psychol* 53:447, 1985.		71	37%
Dobkin P, Zeichner A, Dickson-Parnell B: Concomitants of anticipatory nausea and emesis in cancer chemotherap, *Psychol Rep* 56:671, 1985.		125	32%
van Komen RW, Redd WH: Personality factors associated with anticipatory nausea/vomiting in patients receiving cancer chemotherapy, *Health Psychol* 4:189, 1985.		100	33%
Dolgan MJ, Katz ER, McGinty K, Siegel SE: Anticipatory nausea and vomiting in pediatric cancer patients, *Pediatrics* 75:547, 1985.		80	29%
Nerenz DR, Leventhal H, Easterling DV, Love DD: Anxiety and drug taste as predictors of anticipatory nausea in cancer chemotherapy, *J Clin Oncol* 4:224, 1986.		192	38.5%
Olafsdottir R, Sjöden P-O, Westling B: Prevalence and prediction of chemotherapy-related anxiety, nausea, and vomiting in cancer patients, *Behav Res Ther* 24:59, 1986.		50	40%
Andrykowski MA: Do infusion-related tastes and odors facilitate the development of anticipatory nausea? A failure to support hypothesis, *Health Psychol* 6:329, 1987.		78	33%

Modified from Ader R, Cohen N: The influence of conditioning on immune responses. In Ader R, Felten DL, Cohen N, editors: *Psychoneuroimmunology,* New York, 1991, Academic Press.

*Percent of anticipatory nausea or vomiting.

serves as a treatment itself. This viewpoint suggests that sight, sensation, and taste are all CS capable of producing a physiologic or immunologic CR. If these stimuli are paired with the delivery of an active drug, a CR that is qualitatively similar to the drug or treatment response can be elicited.

One study used a crossover drug trial to detect potential CRs to a placebo pill.[41] The authors believed that the placebo response would be greater after drug exposure than before, demonstrating a CR.

Twenty-four patients with mild-to-moderate hypertension were randomized to one of three treatment groups. Group 1 received a placebo daily for 1 week. This was followed by a daily dose of 50 mg atenolol (a substance that reduces blood pressure) for 1 week. Finally, no treatment was prescribed for 1 week.

Group 2 received a daily dose of 50 mg atenolol for 1 week, followed by daily doses of placebo for 1 week, and then no treatment for 1 week. Group 3 received atenolol daily for 1 week followed by no treatment for 2 weeks, to assess residual drug effects. The authors noted that any difference between group 3 subjects during the no-treatment period and the patients treated with the placebo where the possibility of prior conditioning existed (group 2) could be attributed to the conditioning effect of the placebo pill.

Twice a day, the patients took blood pressure measurements while in their homes. Once a week, a nurse recorded measurements of blood pressure and heart rate.

Before treatment, there were no differences in the antihypertensive responses of patients taking the placebo and patients with no treatment. Further, all three groups exhibited similar decreases in mean arterial pressure in response to atenolol. However, **after atenolol treatment, the placebo treatment produced a significantly greater antihypertensive response than no treatment in both morning and evening blood pressure readings.** Similar patterns were observed for heart rate, but not for blood pressure readings taken in the office. **The placebo response after atenolol was more than a residual drug effect, which was consistent with a conditioning model and reflected the acquisition of a CR.**

Weekly measurements of blood pressure recorded by a nurse failed to demonstrate a significant difference, which was attributed to the extinction of the CR. Home blood pressure readings reflected measurements made on days 4 through 7 of each treatment period, whereas measurements obtained by the nurse were recorded

only on day 7. More unreinforced presentations of the CS were made before the nurse's recording than during in-home recordings, providing greater opportunity for extinction. This study has powerful implications for medical research. Crossover drug trials are common as a means to assess the efficacy of new drug therapies. If the findings from this study are consistently replicated, it will indicate that outcomes from drug crossover trials are essentially flawed, and conditioned effects are elicited as a result of prior drug exposure. Prior drug exposure will then be a confounding variable of this research design.

Other Findings of Conditioned Responses in Human Subjects

Anticipatory nausea reflects a classically conditioned physiologic and immunologic response. Other studies involving human subjects confirm the clinical suggestion that exposure to symbolic and nonallergic stimuli previously associated with allergens (e.g., artificial roses, pictures of allergens) are capable of inducing asthma symptoms in some patients.[14,26] An uncontrolled Japanese study induced eczema in human subjects by pairing the extract of a lacquer tree—known to unconditionally induce eczema—with methylene blue, a neutral substance. After several pairings, the methylene blue singularly induced eczema in all subjects.[25]

> **Points to Ponder** Studies involving human subjects confirm the clinical suggestion that exposure to symbolic and nonallergic stimuli previously associated with allergens (e.g., artificial roses, pictures of allergens) are capable of inducing asthma symptoms in some patients.

These and other similar findings have implications for health practices. Health professionals may, unknowingly, condition patient mood, physiology, and immune responses by creating conditioning cues in offices and hospitals. The CR to a placebo pill, as occurred in the previous study, is an example of cueing to a behavioral stimulus (i.e., the behavior of ingesting a pill).

Because visual cues reinforce conditioning phenomena, some hospitals have made arrangements for patients to rotate through locations or rooms where they receive chemotherapy, so as to reduce the likelihood of conditioning nausea to the hospital setting. In addition to the visual and behavioral cues, odors and tastes are particularly effective as conditioning agents.

It has even been observed that medication designed to reduce vomiting symptoms produces a CR in some patients. Patients consistently treated with antiemetic (i.e., nausea-reducing medication) while already nauseated may become conditioned to the taste of the medication, which then becomes a cue that causes the patient to be nauseated and to vomit.[13]

The critical question is this: If conditioning can create physiologic symptoms and immunosuppression in human subjects, why is this knowledge not being used in the management of autoimmune diseases? At this point in time, there have been few attempts to use this information as potential intervention, but a few such scenarios do exist. The following case study uses conditioning in the treatment of SLE.

Immune Conditioning of a Patient with Systemic Lupus Erythematosus

SLE is a disease in which tissue damage is caused by pathogenic subsets of *autoantibodies*—antibodies directed against the host's own tissues—and immune complexes. Abnormal immune responses include hyperactivity of antigen-specific T- and B-lymphocytes and the body's inability to regulate this hyperactivity. Clinical manifestations can include a flat or raised rash covering the cheeks and cheekbones, a disk-shaped rash with scaling, photosensitivity, oral ulcers, arthritis, inflammation of the membranous lining of the walls of the lungs or heart, renal disorders, seizures, blood disorders such as anemia or leukopenia (i.e., subnormal leukocyte counts), immunologic disorders, and antinuclear antibodies. Any four of these manifestations result in a diagnosis of SLE.[22]

Symptoms can include fatigue, malaise (i.e., general discomfort, uneasiness), fever, anorexia (e.g., refusal to eat), nausea, weight loss, and pain in the stomach, musculoskeletal system, head, and other areas.

In one case study, an 11-year old female adolescent was diagnosed with severe SLE.[35] She was aggressively treated with pharmaceutical drugs (i.e., phenobarbital, antihypertensives, diuretics, corticosteroids). Between the ages of 11 and 13, her condition deteriorated, resulting in nephritis (i.e., kidney inflammation), severe hypertension, seizures, and bleeding episodes caused by an antibody to factor II. She experienced frequent headaches, anxiety, and pain associated with diagnostic and treatment procedures. At age 13, biofeedback treatment was implemented to manage her hypertension and headaches, from which she received some benefit. Some months later, she was experiencing frequent bleeding and intermittent heart failure. It was decided that intravenous infusions of CY must be implemented to inhibit the out-of-control immune hyperreactivity.

The patient's mother, a psychologist, was familiar with the animal conditioning trials conducted by Robert Ader. She gained the support of her physician and the hospital board to attempt immune conditioning with her daughter. It was her hope that by reducing the amount of the drug required to control the disease, her daughter's side effects would be more controlled, and the child's quality of life would be elevated.

Both a taste and an odor were chosen for the conditioning trials. The taste was cod liver oil, the odor a strong rose scent. During trial 1, 500 mg/M2 of CY was injected over a 5-minute period while the mother instructed her daughter to slowly sip 8 ml of the cod liver oil. Three minutes into the injection, the child commented that the cod liver oil "makes me feel like vomiting." After completion of the treatment, the odor of a rose was administered. The child stated that she clearly imaged a rose during this time, creating an association between the rose and the treatment. The child was nauseous for 3 days after the treatment.

The pairing of the cod liver oil and rose scent with CY continued once monthly for 3 months. After the second pairing, the child was nauseated whenever she sipped the oil. Pairing occurred in three consecutive trials. After the three trial pairings, the cod liver oil and rose scent were presented once a month, but the CY was only administered in conjunction with the scent and oil, once every 3 months. Thus over a 12-month period, the actual infusions of CY were reduced by one half. After 15 months, the child refused the cod liver oil because it immediately triggered nausea, but she continued to imagine the rose, believing she had successfully linked this to the effects of CY.

After treatment, the child maintained clinical stability, with improved factor II and normal blood pressure levels for 13 months. She then developed a pericardial effusion, a leakage of fluid into the heart sac, and was hospitalized for 4 days.

During the subsequent 3 years, her prednisone (corticosteroid) dose was reduced, the enalapril (antihypertensive) was eliminated, and she performed well clinically. She continued to take antiseizure medications—calcitril and sodium bicarbonate—daily. Her condition was maintained for 5 years.

Although the outcome seemed as successful as might be expected from a full-dose regimen, no conclusions can be drawn from a single case study. Because the natural history of SLE is varied, it is possible that the outcomes were a result of the natural disease course as opposed to the conditioning paradigm. Nonetheless, the level of improvement received with one half the normal drug dosage is worthy of consideration.

Based on the suggestive findings of this case study, a classical conditioning study was undertaken involving patients with multiple sclerosis (MS). A therapy of CY infusions is widely used for patients with chronic and progressive MS who are unresponsive to less toxic treatments. The following study was designed around CY treatments for ten patients with MS.

Conditioning of Leukopenia in Patients with Multiple Sclerosis

Nerve fibers inside and outside of the brain are wrapped with many layers of insulation called the *myelin sheath.* The myelin sheath permits electrical impulses to be conducted with speed and accuracy along the nerve fibers. It functions similar to the insulation surrounding an electrical wire. When the myelin sheath is damaged, nerves do not properly conduct impulses. Certain conditions can destroy the myelin sheath in the adult, a process called *demyelination.*

MS is a disorder in which the nerves of the eye, brain, and spinal cord lose patches of myelin. When the disease worsens with time, affected persons usually have periods of relatively good health—remission periods—alternating with debilitating flare-ups. About 400,000 Americans, mostly young adults, have the disease.

It has been suggested that a virus or some unknown antigen that somehow triggers an autoimmune response causes MS. The body, then, for unknown reasons, produces antibodies that attack its own myelin. The antibodies provoke inflammation and damage the myelin sheath.

Symptoms generally appear in people between 20 and 40 years old. Symptoms can include problems with movement, disturbances in sensation, tingling, numbness, and peculiar feelings in the arms, legs, trunk, or face. A person may lose strength or dexterity in a leg or hand. Some persons develop symptoms only in the eyes—double vision, partial blindness, and pain. Early symptoms can include mild emotional or intellectual changes. These changes are an indication of demyelination in the brain.

The purpose of one case study was to determine if a significant decrease in peripheral leukocyte (WBC) count, a condition referred to as *leukopenia,* could be induced by conditioning in human subjects with MS.

Researchers believed that the leukopenia (a CR) produced as a result of conditioning would not be as pronounced as leukopenia produced in response to the UCS alone (i.e., a full dose of CY). They hypothesized that the CR would, nonetheless, produce a significant change from baseline and a similar change to that produced by a full dose of CY.

Ten subjects received first-cycle infusions of 500 ml methylprednisolone for 3 days followed by a single infusion of CY. Five additional cycles of CY infusions, the UCS, ranging in doses from 1100 to 1826 ml, were administered and paired each time with an anise-flavored syrup, the CS. At either cycle five or six, only 10 ml of CY (an insignificant amount, less than 1% of the normal dose) and the CS were administered. Therefore treatment was spread out over 7 months with one treatment consisting of the CS and the insignificant 10 ml CY.

WBC counts were assessed on days 7, 14, and 26 after CY administration. The counts from days 7 and 14 were used to determine the dose (1100 to 1826) necessary to obtain a WBC count between 2000/mm^3 and 4,000/mm^3 in the following cycle. The 10 ml of CY was administered so that the words, "low dose," could be used instead of the word, "placebo," when explaining the protocol to the patients. This explanation prevented the likelihood of placebo conditioning, as occurred in earlier drug trials. All routines, including environmental cues, were maintained as consistently as possible to assist with the conditioning effect. Although no separate control group existed, double-blind procedures were satisfied by assigning a pharmacist to code which day (cycle six or seven) that the anise-flavored syrup and lose-dose CY would be administered.

Because of the administration of methylprednisolone in cycle one, the WBC count increased after this treatment. The next four cycles demonstrated decrements of WBC counts on day 14 after CY dosing. As doses increased between cycles two and five, WBC count depression was more prominent.

Eight of the ten subjects (P=0.044) demonstrated statistically significant declines in WBC counts (i.e., leukopenia) in response to the conditioning agent of anise-flavored syrup and low-dose CY. Side effects were less severe in response to the conditioned day, with six of the ten subjects demonstrating less nausea and vomiting with the anise-flavored syrup and low-dose CY, the CS, as compared with the full-dose CY, the UCS.

In conclusion, outcomes suggest that WBC counts, after infusions of CY, can be conditioned in human subjects, indicating that the CNS can exert an effect on WBC count. It is important to note that one patient whose WBC count increased with the CS and one patient whose WBC declined only slightly had both been previously exposed to CY treatments, potentially attenuating a conditioning effect. Further, one subject experienced conditioned nausea without demonstrating a decrease in WBC count, whereas three subjects experienced no conditioned nausea but produced decreased WBC counts. This outcome suggested that the conditioning of gastrointestinal and immunologic effects of CY may be independent of each other. Perhaps in some patients, immunologic effects can be produced without the physiologic side effects. The authors also suggested that studies in which control groups perform better than expected may actually be a result of CNS modification of the immune system (i.e., classical conditioning).

■ Thoughts on Conditioning Trials

We have reviewed the research that demonstrates how stress regulates downward immunity and degrades health. We have also seen how immune competence is suppressed or enhanced by conditioning. Since stress itself induces immune suppression, a stressful event can become a CS without being paired with an immunosuppressive drug. This is one possible explanation for the reason a chronic stressor can sufficiently impair immune function to degrade long-term health.

Conditioning immune function can, indeed, occur without the use of drugs.[6] Lysle and others conditioned animals by pairing auditory or visual cues, the CS, with electric shock in the foot, a stressor and UCS. Reexposure to the auditory and visual cues without pairing the shock resulted in significant proliferative responses in vitro to con A and PHA as compared with unconditioned controls exposed to the same novel auditory and visual cues.[27]

This and similar trials demonstrated that environmental cues associated with stress, a natural-occurring immunosuppressive agent, can indeed lead to the conditioning of immune function. Although exposure to the stressor itself can be immunosuppressive, reexposure to conditioning cues that "prime" or remind the person of the stressor may also affect immunity through the conditioning pathways.

Why Study Mind, Body, and Immune Interactions?

All of us struggle to understand systems that are complex and interactive, such as our economic, political, and ecologic systems. How much easier and less frustrating it would be to study these issues if they could be readily quantified. Scientific experimental methods seek to provide the cause-and-effect explanations whenever possible and to delineate clearly defined solutions to our problems. Science succeeds quite well at meeting these challenges in certain medical arenas. Cures have been found for many physical ailments for which we have an obvious cause—most noticeably, the infectious diseases and physical deformities or organ failures that are amenable to surgical intervention. However, these arenas are not where current medical challenges lie. Chronic ailments fueled by multiple factors that defeat bodily homeostasis are the present-day enemies. Cancer and cardiovascular and autoimmune diseases are the challenges of the twenty-first century. These problems reside in complex human bodies affected by many factors, all of which interact daily to modulate health and well-being. We are sorely equipped to address this multidimensional puzzle with our current scientific methods and compartmentalized disciplines.

In each body there are three systems—nervous, endocrine, and immune—that are involved in maintaining equilibrium. Each is a highly complex unit unto itself, and each interacts with the other, increasing the complexity of the whole. Add to these internal complexities the external factors of stress, emotion, and perception and you have the reason for studying PNI. PNI is a brave attempt to comprehend at least some of the interactions between these three systems, external modulating factors, our environment, and disease states. To accomplish this task, Western reductionist ideas will be tested. New models of intervention, more adept at integrating these elaborate interactions, will have to be created if those in this field are to succeed.

This dimensional puzzle will only be comprehended by understanding the immune and nervous interactions at the molecular, cellular, tissue, and organ levels, as well as in the context of the whole entity. As Cunningham points out, with multilevel organized entities like the human body, properties emerge at higher levels of organization than could be predicted or conceived by analysis of the lower parts. In other words, the old scientific, compartmentalized rules no longer apply.[2]

Perhaps the most reasonable way to conceptualize this interaction is with a systems-theory approach. As can be seen in Figure 3-4, human beings, as whole organisms, are dynamic open systems interacting with the environment. Any theory attempting to assess health outcomes on such an open and complex system must take into account the social, psychologic, and somatic events affecting the body. The body's two most adaptive systems are the mind-brain and immune systems. Exchanges taking place between the environment and organism involve the transmission of information and the interpretation of that information—memory, emotion, stress, and meaning-making. With this new discipline of PNI, we must comprehend the physiologic, psychologic, social, immunologic, environmental, and hormonal influences acting on the body. This effort must be comprehensive and multidisciplined. As you can see from the research discussed in this chapter, the field of PNI has already begun to bite off huge chunks of these interactive areas.

There is one other point that needs to be emphasized. The greatest number of benefits from PNI research will not be realized by simply determining what psychosocial factors contribute to or cause disease; rather, it will be by determining what multiple factors alter individual susceptibility to disease. You need to think of this concept this way: a pathogenic agent or a psychologic stressor or both may cause any given disease, but the issue is the degree to which the disease can be related to each of these factors. In statistical language, we may want to determine the percentage of the total variance for which each of these factors account.

We know that the presence of germs is insufficient to induce a disease state. Many of us are repeatedly exposed to viruses. My associate may become ill while I may not. Therefore the virus is a necessary but insufficient determinant of illness. There must also exist a susceptibility to illness—a weakness in the immune or in another system. The research presented in this text clearly demonstrates that psychosocial stressors and immunologic conditioning can, in fact, increase the susceptibility to a variety of illness states. As research in PNI expands, medicine will be required to transform its methods for treating patients. No longer will it be sufficient to treat the patient in the context of the body and its systems. Rather, all diseases will be viewed as the result of the

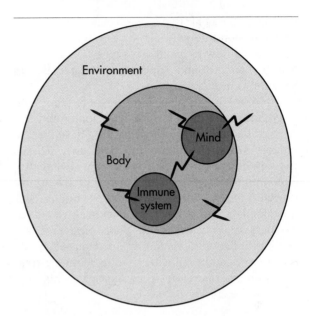

■ **Figure** 3-4. Interaction among the environment, mind, body, and immune system. *Modified from Ader R:* Psychoneuroimmunology, *New York, 1990, Academic Press.*

social context of the individual, as well as the patient's genetic history. In these approaches lie the potential to slow the progression of chronic disease in society at large.

Some researchers suggest that the only method that will allow significant progress is to follow individuals over extended periods, documenting changes in a number of chosen variables. Stress, viral infections, and mucosal immunoglobin levels could be one combination. Hypervigilant work environments, lymphocyte function, and development of chronic disease in the workplace population may be another interesting 25-year study. Research that connects chosen internal emotional environments (e.g., meditation, relaxation, cognitive processes) with immune function and the prevention of disease is another fascinating and promising area for exploration. Such are the challenges for those in the field of PNI. Of course, the greatest challenge of all will not come from solving the mysteries; rather, it will come from convincing humankind to put into practice what is learned. Let us turn our attention back to what we have already discovered and the implications of those findings.

Psychoneuroimmunologic Findings

You may be wondering what implications these findings have for health management in general and how eliciting such outcomes can be beneficial in a disease model. In a general sense, if immunity can be conditionally suppressed, it may benefit us to learn how to avoid the types of events that lead to conditioned suppression, especially in relation to human subjects.

In relation to disease models, there are specific circumstances where immune suppression can extend life and improve its quality. These disease models are the autoimmune diseases, such as rheumatoid arthritis, SLE, and Type I diabetes. Autoimmune diseases stem from overactive or imprecise immune functioning where immune cells mistakenly identify the body's own healthy cells as invaders and attack them. The outcomes are chronic inflammation and organ damage. In the future, will conditioning be used to routinely treat autoimmune diseases? The author of this text believes the answer is "yes."

■ What Should We Do Now?

Implications for Pharmacologic Approaches to Health Care Management

Robert Ader has suggested the potential development of pharmacotherapeutic regimens using a series of conditioning trials. For patients who must be maintained long term on drugs with noxious or debilitating side effects (e.g., adrenal steroids or immunosuppressive agents), prescribing a partial schedule of drug reinforcement may allow a reduction in the drug amount required to treat pathophysiologic conditions successfully. This reduced drug administration could be highly beneficial from the standpoint of patient compliance and health outcomes. Side effects could be reduced, potentially leading to increased patient adherence to the treatment protocol. The fact that a less active drug would be present in the system could have consequences for target organ damage and might potentially address problems related to drug dependence and withdrawal. A less active drug could also result in a considerable reduction in the cost of long-term treatment.[3]

Dr. Ader pointed out that the ideal schedule for patients cannot be known in advance, but it would need to be titrated based on patient response and condition. Several potential approaches were suggested. One method was a slow reduction in reinforcement schedules in stabilized patients or a partial schedule of reinforcement in which the CS-only trials actually consisted of the CS in conjunction with a low, ineffective or minimally effective dose of the active ingredient. Another protocol could be used in which the original dose is held constant, but a placebo is used to decrease the number of occasions per day or week in which the medication is taken. The latter protocol would serve to increase the potency of medication without increasing the medication itself.

If such pharmacotherapeutic regimens are developed and demonstrated to be effective, it could have important implications for the treatment of a variety of autoimmune and chronic diseases. Asthma, for example, would serve as an excellent model for research. Steroidal side effects could possibly be reduced. In Alaska, protocols are currently being developed to assess pharmacotherapeutic conditioning regimens of patients who are poorly maintained by medication alone.[19]

An Expert Speaks: Dr. Robert Ader

Dr. Robert Ader is the George L. Engel Professor of Psychosocial Medicine, Director of the Division of Behavioral and Psychosocial Medicine in the Department of Psychiatry, and Director of the newly created Center for Psychoneuroimmunology Research at the University of Rochester School of Medicine and Dentistry.

Dr. Ader received his B.S. from Tulane University and his Ph.D. in experimental psychology from Cornell University in 1957. He joined the University of Rochester faculty in 1957 as an instructor in psychiatry and psychology. He became a professor of psychiatry and psychology in 1968 and also holds a secondary appointment as professor of medicine.

Since 1969, Dr. Ader has held the continuing Research Scientist Award from the National Institute of Mental Health. In 1992, Dr. Ader was awarded an honorary doctor of medicine degree from the University of Trondheim in Norway. During the 1992 and 1993 academic year, Dr. Ader was a Fellow at the Center for Advanced Study in the Behavioral Sciences at Stanford.

Dr. Ader edited *Psychoneuroimmunology,* the "signature volume of a new field of research," and he co-edited the second edition in 1991. He serves on the Editorial Boards of several journals and is Editor-in-Chief of *Brain, Behavior, and Immunity.* Dr. Ader is a past president of the American Psychosomatic Society, the International Society for Developmental Psychobiology, the Academy of Behavioral Medicine Research, and founding president of the Psychoneuroimmunology Research Society. In this interview, Dr. Ader shares his ideas on the past, present, and future on the field of psychoneuroimmunology.

Question. Dr. Ader, can you provide us with your definition of psychoneuroimmunology?

Answer. Psychoneuroimmunology refers, most simply, to the study of the interactions among behavioral, neural, and endocrine (or neuroendocrine), and immunologic processes of adaptation. Its central premise is that homeostasis is an integrated process involving interactions among the nervous, endocrine, and immune systems. The term was first used in 1980 in my presidential address to the American Psychosomatic Society.

Question. Can you tell us how you, personally, became involved in the study of psychoneuroimmunology?

Answer. When asked how I became involved in psychoneuroimmunology, I can't refer to a logical starting point. I say it was an accident; I was "forced" into it by my data. I was studying taste aversion learning in rats. When a novel, distinctively flavored conditioned stimulus (CS), saccharin, is paired with the unconditioned effects of a drug, cyclophosphamide (CY), which induces a transient stomach upset, the animal learns in one such conditioning trial to avoid saccharine-flavored drinking solutions. We were conducting an experiment on the acquisition and extinction of a conditioned aversive response as a function of the strength of the CS (i.e., the volume of saccharin consumed before the animal was injected with CY). As expected, the magnitude of the conditioned response was directly related to the volume of saccharin consumed on the single conditioning trial. Also, repeated presentation of the CS [saccharin] in the absence of the drug [CY] resulted in extinction of the aversive response, and the rate of extinction was inversely related to the magnitude of the CS. However, in the course of these extinction trials, animals began to die. As more animals died, it became evident that mortality, like the magnitude of the conditioned response, varied directly with the volume of saccharin consumed by the animals on the one drug trial, a troublesome but interesting effect.

As a psychologist, I was unaware [by current day theory] that there was no connection between the brain and immune system. Therefore I was free to make up any story I wanted in an attempt to explain this orderly relationship. My hypothesis was that, in the course of conditioning the avoidance behavior, we were also conditioning the immunosuppressive effects of CY. If every time the conditioned animals were reexposed to the CS previously paired with the drug, the CS induced a conditioned immunosuppressive response, then these animals might be more susceptible to low levels of pathogenic stimulation that may have existed in the laboratory environment. Moreover, if the strength of the conditioned response was a function of the magnitude of the CS, the greater the immunosuppressive response, the greater the likelihood of an increased susceptibility to environmental pathogens. Thus it was the serendipitous observation of mortality in a simple conditioning study—and the need to explain an orderly relationship between mortality and a conditioned aversive response—that gave rise to the hypothesis that immune responses could be modified by conditioning operations.

I did not have much luck in generating any interest in this hypothesis—let alone the help I would need to examine it—until I met Nicholas Cohen. Cohen was the first person with sophistication in immunology who didn't think these notions were too "far out," and we began a collaboration that is as active today as it was in 1974. Still oblivious of the Russian studies of the 1920s, Cohen and I designed a study to examine directly the hypothesis that immune responses could be modified by classical conditioning. For better or worse (sometimes, we're not sure), the first experimental paradigm we adopted was successful and, with some evident trepidation on the part of the reviewers and editor, "Behaviorally conditioned immunosuppression" was published in 1975. This study demonstrated that, like other physiologic processes, the immune system was subject to classical (Pavlovian) conditioning, providing dramatic evidence of an inextricable relationship between the brain and the immune system. The biomedical community, however, was, to be generous, guarded and, to be precise, quite negative. Such a phenomenon simply could not occur because, as everybody knew, there were no connections between the brain and the immune system.

Question. This brings up an important point I would like to understand a little better. There has been and still is great resistance to the idea that our perceptions or thoughts, stresses, or classical conditioning can effect immunity. Why was this resistance so powerful historically, and why, with all we have learned in the past 25 years, is resistance still so ingrained today?

Answer. Traditionally, the immune system had been considered an autonomous agency of defense—a system of bodily defenses regulated by cellular interactions that were independent of neural influences. Besides, there were no known connections between the brain and the immune system. Even when interactions or effects were observed (for example, adrenal hormones influencing immunity; brain lesions influencing immune responses; observations that emotional states were associated with the development of progression of disease related to the immune system), few scientists took these observations seriously. After all, there were no mechanistic explanations for how such things could occur.

Among other contributing factors—scientific disciplinary boundaries tend to keep insiders in and outsiders out. The field of psychoneuroimmunology could only evolve in an interdisciplinary arena. In the past, other hybrid disciplines have emerged and significantly extended our understanding of the functions and the components of interacting systems.

Question. Why, then, does the field of psychoneuroimmunology still engender so much resistance and enmity in scientific circles?

Answer. Certainly, the attention that psychoneuroimmunology has captured in the popular press and its exploitation by those who redefine and use psychoneuroimmunology as the scientific umbrella for their own undisciplined and untested theories and practices cannot have endeared psychoneuroimmunology or investigators who study brain-immune system interactions to the remainder of the scientific community. In my unsubstantiated view, however, the reasons lie as much within as without the biomedical community. Some scientists are willing to say they "don't believe" there's anything of substance in psychoneuroimmunology (although they are not necessarily willing to be quoted). Of course, scientists do not have recourse to "I don't believe it" as grounds for rejecting hypotheses. One can argue "I don't believe it because..." as in "I don't believe it because there are no connections between the brain and the immune system." Such arguments are capable of disproof, and with respect to psychoneuroimmunology, all such arguments have been contradicted by experimental data. There is, too, a sense of unease among some so-called "hard" scientists who seem to view the scientific study of behavior as an oxymoron. In truth, the sophistication in experimental design and analysis of research by the behavioral sciences far exceeds that of the more classical biomedical sciences and is essential for addressing the quantitative questions (e.g., when, how much, under what conditions) that are raised by factoring behavioral, neural, and endocrine variables into the experimental analysis of immunoregulatory processes.

Question. Yet, in spite these issues, psychoneuroimmunology as a viable discipline has come into its own. How did this occur?

Answer. The systematic research initiated during the 1970s seemed to finally be "the right stuff at the right time." No one study can be said to have been (or could have been) responsible for psychoneuroimmunology. There was a convergence of evidence of brain-immune-system interactions being provided by many others at about the same time. Studies of brain-immune system relationships had been appearing in the literature for many, many years. However, it was the coalescence of interdisciplinary research initiated during the 1970s and sustained thereafter—and the identity provided by the label, psychoneuroimmunology, itself—that reawakened long-standing interests and attracted new investigators into this "new" field.

Question. Where do we go from here? How can what has been learned in the field of psychoneuroimmunology be applied to the treatment of human disease and to disease prevention?

Answer. The question of application may be a little premature—except, perhaps, for the adoption of conditioning principles in the design of drug treatment regimens. There is every reason to believe that we could capitalize on conditioned physiologic (e.g., immune) responses and thereby decrease the cumulative amount of active drug required to maintain some physiologic response within homeostatic bounds.

There is, of course, the need to demonstrate in humans—as has been done in animals—that behaviorally induced changes in immune function are, in interaction with other biological factors, sufficient to influence the development, exacerbation, or progression of disease.

To be quite speculative, I would say that the most significant contribution of psychoneuroimmunology thus far has been the demonstration that there are, in fact, interactions between the brain and the immune system. The integrative study of immunoregulatory processes will, I believe, contribute to the dissolution of arbitrary disciplinary boundaries which will, in turn, lead to more research on the relationships among systems in addition to the more typical study of the relationships within systems. This strategy could lead to a better understanding and even a redefinition of the nature of some pathophysiologic processes. It is that knowledge that will lead to the development and application of new intervention or treatment strategies.*

*Modified in part and updated from Ader R: Historical perspectives on psychoneuroimmunology. In Freidman H, Klein TW, Friedman AL, editors. *Psychoneuroimmunology, stress, and infection,* Boco Raton, 1995, CRC Press.

■ Chapter Review

Clearly, if we are to *manage* health care, the issues of stressful life events and the conditioning related to these events must be addressed. Many persons suggest that these events and their related conditioning are both private issues that cannot be addressed by health professionals. However, health programs that provide comprehensive interventions, including skills training, can contribute significantly to the management of stress and its effects on health outcomes.

Health education provides information about how to manage a chronic illness. A comprehensive intervention provides the same information, but with several additional and intensive components. Those components include the following:

- Skills development in critical thinking and problem-solving techniques
- Identification of the unique issues that must be addressed for the patient to successfully manage his or her health outcomes
- Psychosocial evaluation that assesses relationship issues that may sabotage patient care and elicits family support for disease management
- Development of an individualized health management plan based on patient lifestyle, natural coping strategies, and personality profile
- Patient follow-up to fine tune the health management plan as circumstances (e.g., relationships or lifestyle) change

"The Asthma Self-Regulation Intervention," a model asthma intervention program, was developed, tested, and delivered in Anchorage, Alaska. Before asthma training was offered, a battery of assessments were administered that provided data on the patient's medical history, coping style, personality profile, health attributes, lifestyle issues contributing to asthma symptoms, current patient knowledge about asthma, and patient response to asthma treatment. Patients were then educated in the following areas related to asthma management:

1. Cause and course of the disease
2. Common asthma triggers
3. Psychosocial stressors that act as exacerbating contributors
4. Stress reduction techniques
5. Conditioning of immunity as related to asthma
6. Effects of relaxation and imagery on lung function
7. Asthma medications
8. Unique conditions of Alaska that contribute to asthma
9. How to communicate with your physician
10. Systematic methods for managing asthma emergencies

During each step of the education process, patients were taught to apply critical thinking strategies for gleaning information specific to the unique expression of their disease state. (Note: asthma is not a clear-cut disease, but it consists of a cluster of many different disease manifestations.) The information was adapted to become as compatible as possible to patient lifestyles, natural coping strategies, and personality. Family members were also taught about asthma so they could offer support to the asthmatic family member and because a genetic predisposition for asthma is likely to be inherited by other family members. Patients identified issues in the family that served to sabotage asthma management in the past. These issues were addressed and strategies for psychosocial management were implemented. Finally, a comprehensive and long-term asthma management plan was developed including a follow-up plan.

At a 6-month follow-up review, patients receiving the comprehensive intervention improved statistically and clinically, as compared with extended baseline subjects and as compared with an asthma record-keeping control group. Areas of improvement included knowledge, attitude, self-efficacy, mood state, lung function as assessed by peak flows, number of attacks and asthma symptoms, and application of asthma management behaviors.[18] This example of a health intervention applies education, stress management, and conditioning components to the management of a chronic disease.

Health management requires that the complexity of the individual be addressed as in the program previously described. Providing education alone does not translate into health care management, as has been repeatedly demonstrated by education-only approaches. Further, to be successful, persons trained in psychosocial, conditioning, and problem-solving strategies must be the ones to deliver this type of program. If we are to manage health care, the type of intervention just described is required. Individuals with both the knowledge and inclination to provide such interventions are also required. To date, the medical community finds it easier and more cost-effective to offer medication rather than treat the whole mind and body. With emerging medical problems such as the escalation of chronic diseases and the side effects and organ damage caused by many of the medications used to treat them, we may soon find we can no longer afford the luxury of the pill-only approach. The interdisciplinary field of PNI and the conditioning of immunologic and physiologic responses may be one answer to these continuing medical dilemmas.

Matching Terms and Definitions

Match each numbered definition with the correct term. Place the corresponding letter in the space provided.

_____ 1. "Rose cold," pictures of hay fields, asthma attack
_____ 2. Neutral substance paired with a UCS to elicit a CR
_____ 3. Increased blood sugar, elevated epinephrine, accelerated heart rate, clammy skin, dilated pupils
_____ 4. Serious life changes, chronic family stress, distressing life conflicts, unhappiness, depression, social isolation
_____ 5. Salivary reflexes of dogs
_____ 6. Disappearance of a CR when not reinforced by the UCS
_____ 7. Substance that naturally elicits a physiologic or biochemical response
_____ 8. Effect caused by the pairing of a CS with a UCS
_____ 9. Physiologic or biochemical response to the presentation of an UCS
_____10. Observational, physiologic, epidemiologic, experimental

a. Epidemiologic research findings of factors that affect mortality
b. Extinction
c. Four lines of evidence for mind-body communication
d. CR
e. Examples of observational research of CRs
f. UCS
g. Examples of the "fight-or-flight" response mediated by the sympathetic nervous system
h. UCR
i. Experiments of Ivan Pavlov
j. CS

SHORT ANSWER ESSAY QUESTIONS

1. Explain the illness-induced, taste-aversion paradigm.
2. What is the assumption underlying Solomon and Moos' theory of integration of emotion, immunity, and disease? How did they arrive at this theory?

CRITICAL THINKING AND CLINICAL APPLICATION EXERCISES

1. Based on the information in this chapter, precisely state what conclusions can be drawn from the animal research concerning the effects of conditioning on immune function. Clearly describe at least three medical implications this research may have for the management of cancer and autoimmune diseases and for the use of drug therapy.

2. Design a drugless study that assesses the effects of the variable "restraint stress" on cancer progression in mice inoculated with tumor cells. You need not attempt to duplicate the complexities of the studies provided in this text. However, clearly state a purpose for your study and the method you will use. Define your hypotheses and defend why you believe these hypotheses to be correct based on prior research.

3. Asthma is driven by both physiologic, or bronchoconstriction, and immunologic, or inflammation, effects. There are several case studies that suggest a strong conditioning influence in the exacerbation of asthmatic symptoms in some patients. Approximately 20 years ago, some physicians and researchers believed asthma to be a psychosomatic illness, that is, they believed the symptoms were imagined. They thought giving attention to an asthmatic child increased the likelihood of future attacks. Based on what we know today about CRs, delineate the following points:
   ■ The assumptions leading to the belief that asthma was a psychosomatic condition, in this case, imagined
   ■ The consequences this belief may have produced for asthmatic children 20 years ago
   ■ The implications of current conditioning research for the treatment of asthma

4. Chronic, as opposed to acute, diseases have now become the medical challenge for the twenty-first century. Included are autoimmune diseases such as arthritis and SLE, various types of cancer, and immune disorders such as asthma. Select one chronic disease; discuss the research presented in this chapter that may be relevant to the treatment of your chosen disease in human subjects. Explain how the evidence from these studies may provide new insight into the treatment of this disease state.

5. A physician reported a case of a middle-aged woman who, after 9 years of marriage, developed an allergic reaction to her second husband's sperm. This case was particularly interesting because this same patient developed a similar allergic reaction to the sperm of her first husband just before ending the marriage in divorce. Describe the implications this case study may have for conditioned immunologic responses.

6. A child experienced an emotional response to an immunization and vomited profusely. Preparation for the immunization included liberal swabbing with alcohol before and after the injection. Years later, this same person still becomes nauseous at the smell of alcohol. Compare and contrast this situation with the animal study using camphor odor.

7. A medical student experienced a particularly difficult time during her internship; she was constantly on call to handle gruesome cases in the emergency room. The beeper she used during those years had a distinctive tone. Currently, hearing a similar tone on television or the telephone elicits a pounding heart, elevated blood pressure, and clammy palms. When she hears this tone today, the strength of these responses has been observed to be correlated with her physical distance from an emergency room. Describe the pathways by which this CR occurs. How might this CR impair her immune competence?

References

1. Ader R: Behaviorally conditioned immunosuppression, *Psychosom Med* 36(2):183, 1974.
2. Ader R: Mind, body, and immune response. In Ader R, editor: *Psychoneuroimmunology,* New York, 1981, Academic Press.
3. Ader R: The role of conditioning in pharmacotherapy. In Harrington A, editor: *Placebo,* Cambridge, 1997, Harvard University Press.
4. Ader R, Cohen N: Behaviorally conditioned immunosuppression, *Psychosom Med* 37:333, 1975.
5. Ader R, Cohen N: Behaviorally conditioned immunosuppression and murine systemic lupus erythematosus, *Science* 215:1534, 1982.
6. Ader R, Cohen N: Conditioned immunopharmacologic effects on cell-mediated immunity, *Int J Immunopharmacol* 14(3):323, 1992.
7. Ader R, Cohen N: Conditioned immunopharmacologic responses. In Ader R, editor: *Psychoneuroimmunology,* New York, 1981, Academic Press.
8. Ader R, Cohen N: The influence of conditioning on immune response. In Ader R, editor: *Psychoneuroimmunology,* New York, 1991, Academic Press.
9. Ader R, Cohen N: Psychoneuroimmunology: conditioning and stress, *Annu Rev Psychol* 44:53, 1993.
10. Andrykowski MA, Jacobsen PB, Marks E, Gorfinkle K, Hakes TB, Kaufman RJ, Currie VE, Hooland JC, Redd WH: Prevalence, predictors and course of anticipatory measure in workmen receiving adjuvant chemotherapy for breast cancer, *Cancer* 62:2607, 1988.
11. Andrykowski MA, Redd WH, Hatfiel AK: Development of anticipatory nausea: a prospective analysis, *J Consult Clin Psychol* 53(4):447, 1985.
12. Bovbjerg DH, Redd WH, Maier LA et al: Anticipatory immune suppression and nausea in women receiving cyclic chemotherapy for ovarian cancer, *J Consult Clin Psychol* 58(2):153, 1990.
13. Carey MP, Burish TG: Etiology and treatment of the psychological side effects associated with cancer chemotherapy: a critical review and discussion, *Psychol Bull* 104(3):307, 1988.
14. Dekker E, Pelser HE, Groen J: Conditioning as a cause of asthmatic attack, *J Psychosom Res* 2:97, 1957.
15. Fessel WJ: Mental stress, blood proteins, and the hypothalamus: experimental results showing effect of mental stress upon 4S and 19S proteins; speculation that functional behavior disturbances may be expressions of general metabolic disorder, *Arch Gen Psychiatry* 7:427, 1962.
16. Fessel WJ, Forsyth RP: Hypothalamic role in control of gamma globulin levels (abstract), *Arthritis Rheum* 6:770, 1963.
17. Fessel WJ, Grunbaum BW: Electrophoresis and analytical ultracentrifuge studies in sera of psychotic patients: elevation of gamma globulins and macroglobulins and splitting of alpha 2 globulins, *Ann Intern Med* 54:1134, 1961.
18. Freeman LW: *Outcome evaluation of two comprehensive psychoneuroimmunological intervention programs on asthma symptoms and mood states in adult asthmatic patients,* 1997, Dissertation abstracts.
19. Freeman LW, White R: *Personal communication,* June 18, 1997.
20. Ghanta VK et al: Neural and environmental influences on neoplasia and conditioning of NK activity, *J Immunol* 135(2):848s, 1985.
21. Gorczynski RM, Macrae S, Kennedy M: Conditioned immune response associated with allogeneic skin grafts in mice, *J Immunol* 129(2):704, 1982.
22. Hahn BH: Systemic lupus erythematosus. In Fauci AS, Braunwald E, Isselbacher KJ, Wilson JD, Martin JB, Kasper DL, Hauser SL, Longo DL, editors: *Harrison's principles of internal medicine,* ed 14, 1998, New York, McGraw-Hill.
23. Hoagland AC, Morrow GR, Bennett JM, Carnrike CLM: Oncologist's view of cancer patient noncompliance, *Am J Clin Oncol* 6:239, 1983.
24. Holland J: Psychological aspects of oncology, *Med Clin North Am* 61:737, 1977.
25. Ikemi Y, Nakagawa S: A psychosomatic study of contagious dermatitis, *Kyushu J Med Sci* 13:335, 1962.
26. Khan AU: Effectiveness of biofeedback and counterconditioning in the treatment of bronchial asthma, *J Psychosom Res* 21:97, 1977.
27. Lylse DT, Cunnick JE, Fowler H, Rabin B: Pavlovian conditioning of shock-induced suppression of lymphocyte reactivity: acquisition, extinction and pre-exposure effects, *Life Sci* 42:2185, 1988.
28. Metal'nikov S, Chorine V: Role des reflexes conditionels dans l'immunite, *Ann Inst Pasteur (Paris)* 40:893, 1926.
29. Metal'nikov S, Chorine V: Role des reflexes conditionnels dans la formation des anticorps, Comptes Rendus Seances, *Soc Biol Ses Fil* 102:133, 1928.
30. Moos RH, Engel BT: Personality factors associated with rheumatoid arthritis: review, *J Chronic Dis* 17:41, 1964.
31. Moos RH, Solomon GF: Personality correlates of the rapidity of progression of rheumatoid arthritis, *Ann Rheum Dis* 23:145, 1964.
32. Moos RH, Solomon GF: Personality differences among symptom-free relatives of rheumatoid patients (preliminary report [abstract]), *Arthritis Rheum* 6:784, 1963.
33. Morrow GR, Dobkin PL: Anticipatory nausea and vomiting in cancer patients undergoing chemotherapy treatment: prevalence, etiology and behavioral interventions, *Clin Psychol Rev* 8:517, 1988.
34. Nicolau I, Antinescu-Dimitriu O: Role des reflexes conditionnels dans la formation des anticorps, *C R Seances Soc Biol Fil* 102:133, 1929.
35. Olness K, Ader R: Conditioning as an adjunct in the pharmacotherapy of lupus erythematosus, *Dev Behav Pediatrics* 13(2):124, 1992.
36. Ostravskaya OA: Le reflex conditionnel et les reactions de l'immunite, *Annales del' Institute Pasteur* 44:340, 1930.
37. Pavlov IP: *Lectures on conditioned reflexes,* Gantt WH, Volborth G, (translators), New York, 1928, International.
38. Podkopaeff NA, Saatchian RL: Conditioned reflexes for immunity. I. Conditioned reflexes in rabbits for cellular reaction of peritoneal fluid, *Bull Battle Creek Santarium Hosp Clin* 24:375, 1929.
39. Redd WH, Andrykowski MA: Behavioral interventions in cancer treatment: controlling aversive reactions to chemotherapy, *J Consult Clin Psychol* 50:1018, 1982.
40. Solomon GF, Moos RH: Emotions, immunity and disease: a speculative theoretical integration, *Arch Gen Psychiatry* 11:657,1964.
41. Suchman AL, Ader R: Classic conditioning and placebo effects in crossover studies, *Clin Pharmacol Ther* 52:372, 1992.

4

How Relationships and Life Events Affect Health: Human Studies

Lynda W. Freeman

WHY READ THIS CHAPTER?

We all pass through a series of life challenges. These challenges may include learning to cope with social networks or enduring periods of loneliness, depression, or emotional isolation. Challenges are often presented during a series of events called relationship passages. Relationship passages include (1) newlywed and marital adaptation period; (2) disruption of the marital state (e.g., separation, divorce, bereavement); and (3) caregiving when a spouse or family member becomes chronically ill. We can also experience chronic stressors (e.g., job-related stress, fear from a nuclear accident) and acute, short-term stressors (e.g., academic stress) not necessarily related to family or friends. All these events have important health consequences. This chapter provides information on how these challenges affect health on both a short- and long-term basis. It also provides information on what can be done to manage the emotional challenges that affect our health.

Most critical is the realization that if health care dollars are to be managed, the psychosocial aspects of life cannot be overlooked. It is hoped that this literature will serve as a wake-up call to health care professionals and a reminder that psychosocial interventions and support systems are not luxuries; rather, they are necessities in a comprehensive health care program.

CHAPTER AT A GLANCE

Research on the effects of relationships and social support began in the 1970s and evolved around the concept of social support, the belief that one "is cared for and loved, esteemed, and a member of a network of mutual obligations."[18] These early retrospective and prospective epidemiologic studies strongly suggested that the quantity and quality of relationships—marriage and friends—and social interaction—church and social activities—have powerful implications for morbidity and mortality.

Later research emphasized the assessment of biomedical variables (e.g., uric acid, cholesterol, and immune function [lymphocyte count, mitogen response, antibody titers]) and hormonal response (e.g., cortisol, norepinephrine [NEPI], epinephrine [EPI], growth hormone [GH], adrenocorticotropic hormone [ACTH]) as they relate to relationship passages (i.e., marital adaptation and disruption, spousal conflict, caregiving, bereavement). Psychologic mood state (i.e., depression, loneliness, hostility) was found to be correlated with immunologic and hormonal changes and health status, implicating a bi-directional response between mind and body. The biochemical, hormonal, and health effects of chronic stressors during relationship passages (e.g., caring for patients with Alzheimer's disease, bereavement, and fear of a nuclear accident) were topics of extensive research. Research on potential interventions was also conducted.

Acute stressors were assessed, in part, because researchers wanted to identify pathways by which biochemical and hormonal changes, if chronic, might alter health on a long-term basis. Academic stress and job-related stress were two areas of intense review because of the easy access to subjects and the ease of the study design.

> If we are a metaphor of the universe, the human couple is the
> metaphor par excellence, the point of intersection of all forces
> and the seed of all forms. The couple is time recaptured,
> the return to the time before time.
>
> OCTAVIO PAZ, MEXICAN POET, ALTERNATING CURRENT,
> ANDRÈ BRETON OR THE QUEST OF THE BEGINNING. (1967)

CHAPTER OBJECTIVES

After completing this chapter, you should be able to:

1. Describe how research on relationships and social support evolved.
2. Define stress and stressors.
3. Define, compare, and contrast social interaction and social support.
4. Summarize the findings of Berkman and Syme's study of social interactions and mortality. Clarify the weaknesses of the study.
5. Summarize the conclusions of the combined studies on social support.
6. Identify three biochemical indicators of health status that can be modified by stress.
7. Explain the limitations of perceived social support as a means of developing interventions for stress management.
8. Summarize the epidemiologic findings of the effects of social interaction, social support, and marital status on health.
9. Summarize the psychologic and biomedical findings from the clinical controlled trials on marital status and marital disruption.
10. Compare and contrast the outcomes of newlywed and marital disruption research. Explain how the outcomes differ and why.
11. Summarize the effects of bereavement on immune and hormonal function.
12. Describe the psychologic and biomedical effects of caring for the patient with Alzheimer's disease.
13. Compare and contrast the differences in health effects of caregivers of patients with Alzheimer's disease as compared with suffering bereavement.
14. Identify four other chronic stressors and hypothesize the biomedical and psychologic effects of these events.
15. Describe and summarize the psychologic and biomedical effects of short-term academic stress on medical students.

Social Interaction, Relationship Passages, Stress, and Health Outcomes

The epidemiologic studies of the 1960s and 1970s revealed that life stressors, that is, upsetting life changes such as divorce or job loss, conflicts, and the emotional conditions of unhappiness and depression, were markers of declining health. More specifically, these studies found that *social isolation was repeatedly associated with increased risk of mortality and morbidity* (Figure 4-1). It appears that we are benefited by social relationships with others, and yet it is this need for relationships that challenges both our adaptability and our health.

We strive for social connectedness and support. Often, however, we fail in our endeavors. When we fail (i.e., experience divorce, interpersonal conflict), our health often suffers. Issues of illness and relationship woes or lack of relationships are interwoven as significant and repeating threads in the tapestry of health research outcomes. Because of this, scientists have attempted to examine the connections between social relationships and health from a variety of different vantage points.

How Social Research Evolved

Four social research areas of interest have evolved. These include research studies on (1) social interaction and social support, (2) effects of relationship passages, (3) health effects of chronic stressors not directly related to relationships, and (4) health effects of short-term stressors (Box 4-1).

Research on *social interaction and social support* produced some of the first literature that

shed light on the health consequences of human interaction—or lack of interaction. In these studies the number of contacts with others (e.g., acquaintances, friends, family members, including spouses) were assessed as predictors of both physical and emotional health.

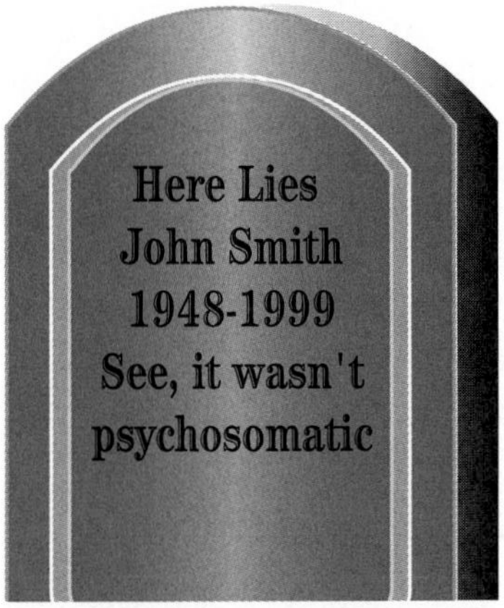

Next, the literature on *relationship passages,* or the stressors experienced because of failure to achieve or maintain intimate relationships, began to evolve. This research centered on relationship struggles that many, but not all persons, experience in their pursuit for or loss of connectedness. These passages included the following:

- Marital adjustment—newlywed period, marital adaptation, unhappy marriages
- Marital disruption—separation, divorce, widowhood
- Marital and family challenges—caregiving
- Social isolation or loneliness—school, separation, illness, or social maladjustment

These relationship passages became known as chronic stressors.

The third area of research assessed the *health effects of chronic stressors* brought about as a result of more indirect sources. For example, the fear of environmental disasters or other perceived threats could severely stress the individual, eliciting concern for the safety of self and others.

The fourth area of research evolved around the *health effects of short-term stressors* such as academic performance, loneliness, career challenges, and stress that followed the diagnosis and treatment of disease.

Research in these areas elicited enormous interest from investigators in a variety of fields. The goal of these researchers was to determine how this information could be applied to protect the quality of life and health. Questions posed by many health outcomes researchers included the following:

1. Does social interaction determine health and longevity? If so, what kind of social interactions are most important—organizations, friends, family, marriage? How much social interaction do we need?

Figure 4-1. Life stressors. Upsetting life changes, such as divorce or job loss, conflicts, and the emotional conditions of unhappiness and depression, are markers of declining health.

BOX 4-1 Evolution of Social Research

Health effects of relationship interaction and social support
Chronic stressors experienced during relationship passages
Perceived threats as chronic stressors
Short-term stressors

2. Do different stressful life events—bereavement, chronic caregiving, marital disruption—have unique effects on physiologic, hormonal, and immunologic responses, or are these effects essentially the same?

3. If different life events alter physiologic, hormonal, and immunologic responses, can we map out how these responses are altered and what pathways enable them?

4. If we can map out what types of physiologic, hormonal, and immunologic effects are produced by stressful life events and we know what pathways enable them, can we then create interventions that will protect us from some of the damage caused by these stressors?

5. If we can create interventions that offer protection from these life stressors, how should we implement them and motivate patients to participate in them?

6. How can we use this information to improve health care?

7. Can we use this information to lower or control our growing health care costs (Box 4-2)?

These are the questions that we explore in this chapter. As mentioned in previous chapters, it is not infectious diseases, physical deformities, or organ failures amenable to surgery that present challenges for medical science today. Indeed, it is chronic diseases, including autoimmune disorders, which challenge us and consume the majority of our health care dollars. In this chapter, we explore how psychosocial stress-inducing factors modulate physiology and biochemistry. We track the evolution of these bodies of research from their beginnings in the 1970s until today.

■ Social Interaction and Social Support: A Determinant of Health and Longevity

In the 1970s the early studies of social interaction and health were revitalized when new scientific research emerged around the concept of *social support*. This concept was first introduced in the mental health literature and was linked to physical health in a seminal article by Sidney Cobb, a physician and epidemiologist. In his 1976 article he defined social support as "information leading the subject to believe that he is cared for and loved, esteemed, and a member of a network of mutual obligations."[18]

Cobb reviewed numerous studies on stress and psychosocial factors leading to health or illness. He found that social support provided a protective factor for persons in crises. These crises included a variety of physiologic and pathologic conditions including low birth weight, arthritis, tuberculosis, depression, suicide, alcoholism, bereavement, and social change related to job loss and retirement. He also observed that when persons were ill, social support reduced the amounts of medication required, accelerated recovery rates, and facilitated compliance with prescribed medical regimens. Cobb concluded that social support acted as a buffer or a protective factor for a wide variety of transitions in the life cycle.

> **Points to Ponder**   Social support acts as a buffer or a protective factor for a wide variety of transitions in the life cycle. ■

Other researchers later questioned Cobb's conclusions because the evidence he reviewed was based on cross-sectional or *retrospective studies* (i.e., outcomes were determined from historical data) and because the data were gathered by self-reporting methods. However, data from long-term *prospective research* (i.e., studies that follow subjects for many years) soon provided supporting and additional evidence that a lack of social relationships constituted a major risk factor for *mortality* (death).

In a more comprehensive review of the epidemiologic and experimental literature, House and others concluded that there was solid scientific evidence to support the effects of social relationships on health.[62] The data, they believed, were sufficiently robust to demonstrate a causal connection between personal connectedness and health outcomes. Prospective studies controlled for baseline health status reliably demonstrated increased risk of death among persons with low quantity or quality of relationships, and social isolation was found to be a risk factor for mortality from a variety of causes. The prospective data

---

BOX 4-2 Lines of Thinking by Researchers of Health Outcomes

Social interaction ➡ Stressful passages ➡ Physiologic, hormonal, immunologic dysfunctions ➡
Creating interventions ➡ Motivating patients to change ➡ Improving health care ➡ Reducing health care costs

were made more compelling by the growing evidence of groundbreaking experimental and clinical trials on animal and human subjects. Experimental studies concluded that animals or persons exposed to social contact when being stressed received psychologic or physiologic benefits that prevented the serious illness and death experienced by more isolated animals or persons.

History of Research on Health, Social Interactions, and Social Support: An Overview

In this section we review the epidemiologic research on social interactions, isolation, marital disruption, and life span. We also follow five well-matched research subjects experiencing differing types of life challenges and describe how they, as individuals, fared physiologically and immunologically in the face of unique and different life stressors. You will note some obvious patterns of how the relationship and social support research evolved over time.

In the beginning, studies were actually more about social interactions than social support. *Social interactions* research assessed the quantity of time spent with other persons, the context of those interactions (e.g., leisure activities, church activities, formal or informal groups, friends and family, marriage partner), and the health effects of these interactions. The quality of those interactions was typically not assessed. *Social support* research assessed the health effects of time spent in relationships that are qualitatively meaningful and considered fulfilling or disturbing to the subject. This qualitative determination was not always adequately considered in earlier studies.

> **Points to Ponder** Social interactions research assessed the quantity of time spent with other persons, the context of those interactions (e.g., leisure activities, church activities, formal or informal groups, friends and family, marriage partner), and the health effects of these interactions. The quality of those interactions was typically not assessed. Social support research assessed the health effects of time spent in relationships that are qualitatively meaningful and considered fulfilling or disturbing to the subject. ∎

Later, the health effects of intimate relationships were analyzed on the basis of the quality of the relationship itself. Researchers began to focus on the positive effects of good relationships and the health consequences that accompanied negative or demanding relationships.

The research evolved from finding correlations between relationship quality and life span or health status to mapping the actual effects of relationship interactions on hormonal levels, biochemistry, and immune function. Studies were designed with biomedical measurements to evaluate the short-term biological effects of unhappy or disrupted relationships—separation, divorce, or death—and newlywed adjustment issues.

Finally, the actual pathways by which these effects occur were delineated, including how different systems in the body interact during times of stress. (These pathways, connecting the sympathetic nervous system, endocrine system, and immune system are outlined in previous chapters.)

In some cases, as with the caregiver of the person with Alzheimer's disease, health intervention measures were designed and assessed. In other cases, interventions were suggested, but not tested. Even in the case of successful interventions that were tested, most were not implemented as an integral part of our health care system.

Health Outcomes Research: Limitations

In a laboratory setting the effects of isolation, stress, and conditioning on animals can be studied and assessed with considerable control. When studying human beings, however, this task is more difficult. There are ethical constraints and the fortunate fact that human beings cannot be "sacrificed" for the sake of a clean research design. There is the problem of gathering research in a natural environment so that outcomes reflect real-world events. Finally, there are unlimited variables that affect the lives and health of persons every day—variables that can be observed, but not regulated. Because of these variables, outcomes from human studies cannot be applied absolutely to any one individual. Even so, well-designed studies provide a window to view the general factors that can support or hinder or provide unique challenges to the health and well-being of our human community. With this information, health organizations and individuals can make informed decisions about how to intervene or provide protective buffers for persons experiencing stressful life events. Perhaps the biggest challenge facing health care providers today is convincing organizational and governmental agencies to avail themselves of research information; to use intervention programs that apply such research in health-supporting ways; and to assess intervention outcomes as part of continuing medical care.

Points to Ponder   There are unlimited variables that affect the lives and health of persons every day—variables that can be observed, but not regulated.   ■

Defining Stress

Stress is defined as any physiologic, psychologic, or behavioral response within the organism elicited by evocative agents.[92] These evocative agents are called *stressors*. Stressors can have both a psychologic and a physical nature. Often, it is difficult to separate the two. For example, anorexia (i.e., an extreme fear of becoming obese, leading to an aversion to food) is a stressor brought on by psychologic factors that then impose physical stress (i.e., starvation). One must also keep in mind that what is stressful for one person may not be stressful for another. It is often the perception of an event that determines what is stressful.

■ Relationship Interaction and Social Support

Is the quantity of time spent in relationship interactions a critical factor in longevity and health? Is it simply the energy expended in relationship interactions that benefit health, or are the interactions themselves of specific benefit? Epidemiologic and prospective studies comparing relationship interactions and life span sought to answer these questions.

Berkman and Syme gathered data on subject demographics, health practices, and relationship interactions for 9 years.[7] At the end of the study, these data were used to find associations between relationship interactions and death rates (Table 4-1).

All of four variables of social relationships—marriage, close friends and relatives, church membership, informal and formal group membership—were found to predict mortality independently of one another, with the more intimate ties of marriage and contact with friends and relatives the biggest contributors to longevity.

It was concluded from this study that, in a general sense, marriage is a protective health factor, but interactions with friends and relatives also serve as protective factors and these differing forms of relationships are beneficial in their own right.

The major weaknesses of this study were the lack of other than self-reported baseline health information and the fact that satisfaction with intimate and other relationships was not adequately assessed.

In a second study, House, Robbins, and Metzner extended and replicated the Berkman and Syme study but with the addition of the biomedical measure of health and morbidity (disease state).[63] This study was done to determine how social networks affect the risk of death among otherwise healthy people as compared with persons with known chronic disease. Specifically,

TABLE 4-1	Social Interaction as a Determinant of Health and Longevity	
STUDY	**SUBJECTS**	**CONCLUSIONS**
Berkman and Syme	4775	Marriage, contacts with family and friends, church membership, and formal and informal groups predicted mortality 9 years later. Low-index score compared with high-index score doubled the risk of death.
House, Robbins, and Metzner	2745	Composite indices of social relationships and activities were inversely associated with mortality 10 to 12 years later. Adjusted for risk factors, low- versus high-index scores increased risk of death 2.0 to 3.0 times for men and 1.5 to 2.0 times for women.
Schoenbach et al.	2059	Adjusted for risk factors, an index similar to Berkman and Syme's instrument predicted risk for an 11- to 13-year period with similar outcomes.
Welin et al.	989	When controlled for age, coronary heart disease, and baseline health status, persons per household, outside activities, social activities, and marriage were significantly associated with mortality 9 years later.
Orth-Gomer and Johnson	17433	Swedish men, aged 29 to 74 years of age, were followed for 6 years. Study revealed that a total score for social network interactions predicted a relative risk of dying as 3.7 for the lowest tertile of social network interaction, compared with the upper two tertiles. Controlled for age, gender, and lifestyle, those with low social support still demonstrated an excess mortality risk of 50%.

the researchers wanted to know how social relationships actually contributed to a decrease in disease incidence and to higher survival rates. Were the effects on disease and survival the result of the diversion that relationships provide from daily life, the activity or functional capacity that they require, or the content and quality of the relationships?

Overall, this study concluded that the lack of meaningful social relationships or ties is most injurious to health. These findings suggest that formal and informal relationships are both important and may not be substitutes for one another.

In another replication of the Berkman and Syme's study of social networks, Schoenbach, Kaplan, Fredman, and Kleinbaum investigated the relationship between a new social network index modeled on Berkman's instrument and survivorship of Evans County, Georgia, residents between 1967 and 1980.[120] A sociability score, intimate contacts index, and seven-level social network were used to quantify relationship information.

The replication of Schoenbach and colleagues again confirmed the concept that social networks are predictive of survivorship. These and other studies report similar outcomes (see Table 4-1).[103,136]

Prospective Studies of Social Interaction and Mortality

The patterns of prospective association (e.g., the number and frequency of social relationships and contacts) and mortality were remarkably similar between studies. Most of the studies found that being married is more beneficial to health than being widowed, divorced, separated, or single, and that this association is greater for men than women. Women seem to benefit more successfully from social relationships with friends and relatives. However, unmarried persons still benefit from social contact with friends and relatives equal to that of isolated married persons. The study suggests that men benefit more from social relationships than women in cross-gender relationships. It can be concluded that social relationships predict mortality for men and women in a wide range of populations, after adjusting for biomedical factors of mortality.

> **Points to Ponder** Women seem to benefit more successfully from social relationships with friends and relatives. However, unmarried persons still benefit from social contact with friends and relatives equal to that of isolated married persons. ■

Social Interaction and Mortality Studies: Limitations

Differences in groups of individuals, such as those who are in abusive relationships, those living in long-term happy relationships but not legally married, or those who are very happy as single individuals, were not addressed. Further, the level of satisfaction derived from relationships—marital versus friend; family versus formal and informal groups—was not adequately assessed, again missing an opportunity to equate the degree of satisfaction or levels of intimacy with the outcomes. The findings that moderate levels of social interaction were more beneficial than excessive levels and that one meaningful relationship seemed to be a deciding factor in longevity suggest differences in the need for varying personality styles, that is, introversion versus extraversion, for example. However, these factors were not pursued. Therefore the outcomes as they relate to individuals are suggestive but not conclusive, and these findings do not represent or reflect the differing circumstances that are common in today's society.

Case Studies of Relationship Interaction and Health Outcomes

Keith, Carol, Louise, and Bob lived within 1 mile of one another in a Midwestern town (Figure 4-2).

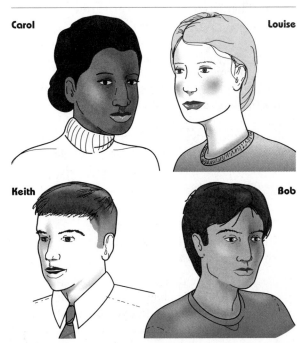

■ **Figure 4-2.** Carol, Keith, Louise, and Bob live within 1 mile of each other in a Midwestern town. They participated in a large (4000 subject) research project to evaluate the effects of relationships on long-term health.

In 1975 they agreed to participate in a large (4000 subject) research project to evaluate the effects of relationships on long-term health. At the beginning of the study, they were each 38 years old, were generally healthy with no known genetic predispositions to chronic disease, and practiced similar and moderate exercise and eating habits. Several times a year for 20 years, they submitted to medical reviews and physical examinations that included laboratory assessment of immune and hormonal function. Simultaneously, they completed written psychologic, relationship, and social interaction assessments. At the beginning of the study, all four reported satisfactory marriage relationships. As the study reached the 5-year mark (1980), the status of their marital relationships had changed.

- Keith's wife divorced him in 1980 and married a long-time family friend. Still in love with and attached to his wife, Keith seemed unable to adjust to the divorce and described himself as lonely and depressed.
- Carol remained married, although her annual scores reflecting marital satisfaction consistently deteriorated. He husband's infidelities and inattentiveness took a toll on the relationship and on Carol. Nonetheless, she was comfortable financially and continued in the relationship for religious and family reasons.
- Louise lost her husband in an automobile accident. Her children were grown, and she now faced a new life as a widow.
- In 1980, Bob's wife was diagnosed with early-stage Alzheimer's disease. He assumed the long-term role of caregiver.

Would the quality or loss of relationships affect the long-term health of these individuals? If so, how would these effects differ? Would individual short-term stressors affect health outcomes? We will follow these individuals throughout this chapter in the form of case studies to answer these questions.

■ Effects of Social Support on Stress-Related Biochemical and Immune Function

The epidemiologic data from the studies previously introduced in this chapter identified the health benefits of social interaction versus isolation, but in a very generalized sense. These studies also lacked the credibility of direct assessments of immune and biochemical effects as modulated by social interaction. Researchers could see that there were effects based on social interaction or the lack thereof, but what pathways accomplished these effects?

Effects of Stress on Neuroendocrine and Immunologic Responses

In his early works, Bovard described how stressful events or stimuli induce a complex cascade of neuroendocrine responses that lead to general *catabolism,* or a breaking down of bodily chemicals to liberate energy, and immunosuppression.[11,12] Supportive relationships, he theorized, must initiate a competing response that then modifies and neutralizes some of the harmful effects of stress. It therefore made sense to assess stress-related indicators and correlate these outcomes to the quantity or quality of social support.

Three well-documented indicators of stress that affect health status are *high level of serum uric acid* (i.e, poorly soluble white crystals that sometimes solidify into uric acid–based stones), *high level of cholesterol* (i.e, an important factor in coronary artery disease), and the *suppression of immune function.* The following research studies document effects of stress on biochemical and immune function:

- Friedman and colleagues found significant and large changes in serum cholesterol in accountants when comparing self-reported stressful career periods with more relaxed career periods.[33]
- Kasl and associates found that employee anticipation of plant shutdown and impending loss of job were associated with high levels of serum uric acid. These levels were the highest for those employees most stressed by the potential event.[68]
- Rahe and others found high levels of serum uric acid in Navy divers facing challenging training events.[105]
- Jemmott and colleagues reported physical or psychologic stress associated with immune suppression.[64]

These three indicators—high levels of serum cholesterol and uric acid and immune suppression—have repeatedly acted as independent predictors of subsequent morbidity and mortality. Therefore they are excellent markers for use in studies on the effects of stress on health.

Based on the demonstrated effects of these three independent predictors and Bovard's theoretical work, Thomas and others sought to remedy the shortcomings of the earlier epidemiologic studies by assessing associations between levels of stress indicators and true social support.[130] For this study, they defined social support as the presence of satisfying relationships with trusted individuals in whom the subjects could confide. The authors chose an older population to study for two reasons:

1. Older persons often suffer from the loss of significant relationships as a result of death or separation and therefore may be deprived of social support
2. Immune function is known to decline with age.

Effects of Social Support on Stress Indicators

Thomas and colleagues wanted to determine whether there was a relationship between the degree of social support and the stress indicators—high levels of serum cholesterol and serum uric acid and suppressed immune responses.[130] They hypothesized that individuals with confidant relationships will have lower uric acid and cholesterol levels and higher immune responses, including lymphocyte count and mitogen responsiveness, than those with poorer social support systems.

Method. The subjects consisted of 256 healthy adults, living independently, between the ages of 69 and 89. They were free of major illnesses and were taking no medications at the beginning of the study. Complete medical histories were taken, and the subjects underwent complete physical examinations. Social bonds were assessed using the "Interview Schedule for Social Interaction." The authors were only concerned with the scales that were related to frank and confiding relationships.

Outcomes

■ Correlations comparing social support with cholesterol and uric acid levels, lymphocyte count, and mitogen response revealed a significant inverse relationship. *Higher levels of social support were correlated with lower levels of uric acid and cholesterol* (p<0.01). The authors also found a *significant and positive relationship between social support and total lymphocyte count* (p<0.05).

■ The authors then controlled for the factors of smoking, body mass, age, alcohol intake, and stress and computed these independent variables separately for men and women. *Women demonstrated significant correlations between the degree of social support and uric acid level, mitogen response, and lymphocyte count* (p<0.05). Correlations between social support and serum cholesterol did not reach significance.

■ Men demonstrated a significant *inverse relationship between social support and serum cholesterol only* (p<0.05).

Conclusions and comments. Results were consistent with the hypothesis that *social support can reduce the physiologic response to stress.* The authors could only speculate about why physiologic variables differ between men and women, but these differences have health implications for men as related to coronary heart disease and for women as related to immune competence. Women overall had lower cholesterol and uric acid levels and better immune function than did the men. The authors suggested that the reasons might be because women appear to have greater sensitivity to close relationships and demonstrate more versatility in their choices of relationships. *These two factors may combine to produce greater survival adaptability among women as opposed to men.*

Conclusions from Epidemiologic Research on Social Support and Health Outcomes

The epidemiologic research indicates that generally social support can reduce the physiologic and immunologic response to stress and can potentially reduce morbidity and increase life span. Unfortunately, this conclusion has led many health care professionals to conclude that higher levels of social support should be virtually "prescribed" for individuals in certain stress-related disease categories or for those living through stressful life events.

Not all researchers agree with this approach. Coyne and DeLongis found that many health professionals believe therapeutic interventions are incomplete without a plan for increasing and strengthening social networks.[19] Yet, depending on the circumstances, this approach may actually increase anxiety and depression rather than decrease it.

> **Points to Ponder** Many health professionals believe therapeutic interventions are incomplete without a plan for increasing and strengthening social networks. Yet, depending on the circumstances, this approach may actually increase anxiety and depression rather than decrease it. ■

Limitations of Social Support

There are limitations to the concept of perceived social support as a coping mechanism. It is important to understand how and under what conditions social support may be beneficial to persons under stress. There are recurring themes in the literature concerning a *threshold effect.* Threshold effect refers to a maximal point beyond which no additional benefit can be received. In some instances, going beyond a threshold point can diminish positive outcomes. For example, too much social support could possibly induce rather than alleviate stress. The critical distinction, as related to health, seems to be between having at least one meaningful and supportive relationship as opposed to having none.

There are also negative outcomes related to the theory of social support. Fiore, Becker, and Coppel found that members of a social network can cause upset, especially for women who are more sensitive to network interactions.[30] The degree of upset associated with network members was found to be positively related to depression scores. Social involvement can become negative and overwhelming. Kessler and McLeod found that women are more vulnerable to life events because of their empathetic concern about crises in their social networks.[71] Fischer noted that many people are socially burdened by alcoholic husbands or wives, delinquent children, senile parents, and other intimate social contacts that are exhausting and stressful.[31] He concluded that we must not exaggerate the supportiveness of personal relationships. Efforts to increase social involvement for troubled or dysfunctional persons may expose these already stressed individuals to additional demands that are neither helpful nor beneficial.

Implications for Social Support Models as Health Interventions

Social support is best regarded as a personal experience rather than merely an interactional process. The diverse problems of individuals, as well as their personalities and coping styles, must be taken into account when discussing social networks or suggesting the expansion of social support networks. For some individuals, more supportive relationships may be healing; for others, such as individuals facing poverty and burdensome caregiving responsibilities, expanding the social network may only serve to provide additional stress and worry. There is also the personality issue to consider. Introverted persons often relax and feel energized by taking private time, whereas extroverted persons may find social involvement necessary to unwind.[88] It is important to remember that the circumstances of each individual must be considered before making global assumptions about the role of social support in his or her health and well-being. When these limitations are considered, it can then be concluded that, as a whole, some level of positive social support appears to be absolutely essential for optimal health and well-being. The amount

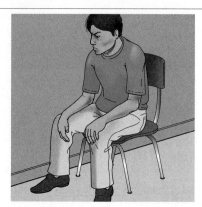

■ *Figure 4-3.* The stress of Keith's marital disruption contributed to decline in his overall health status.

and type of social support most beneficial will vary from person to person (Box 4-3) (Figure 4-3).

■ Effects of Marital Adjustment on Immune and Hormonal Reactivity

One may assume that immune response would be optimal for newlywed couples experiencing the bliss of a new-found love (Figure 4-4). However, the phase of marital adjustment often requires an intense negotiation and communication process. New couples must learn how to navigate through the daily details of living and set relationship boundaries that both can accept. This adjustment may create stress. Can the formulation of new relationships have implications for health? The following studies explore this question.

Newlyweds, Problem Solving, Sympathetic Drive, and Immune Function

Kiecolt-Glaser, Malarkey, and others chose to assess problem-solving behaviors and changes in immune function in 90 newlywed couples engaged in conflict discussions of martial problems.[83] They hypothesized that negative communication would be strongly related to immune function and immunologic changes over a 24-hour period and that support in other relationships would not fully compensate for marital distress.

Method

Subject selection. Subjects recruited for the study included those who had obtained marriage licenses in the previous 4 to 6 months, were 20 to 40 years of age with no children, and were in a first marriage. Further screening eliminated persons who had acute or chronic health problems, averaged more than ten alcoholic drinks per week, used street drugs, smoked, used caffeine exces-

---

BOX 4-3 Keith's After-Divorce Trauma

The day in 1980 when Keith's wife, Karen, told him she was leaving was by his own account "the day I died inside." The news came as a total surprise. Keith had no clue his wife and closest friend had been having an affair for over a year. Six weeks after the divorce, Keith's former wife and friend were married. Two months later, Keith was hospitalized for a short period after a suicide attempt. He was pharmacologically treated for depression for 18 months, but he refused to attend counseling sessions.

For the next 5 years, Keith made no effort to date or form new relationships, and he rebuffed attempts by single female co-workers to get to know him better. Instead, he made work his life, performing as many as 70 hours of work a week. He felt anything was better than going home to an empty house. He kept the house after the divorce because, as he explained it, he was sure that Karen would soon "come to her senses" and return to their marriage.

Denial turned into rage when Keith heard that Karen was expecting a child. He became hostile and accusatory with friends and co-workers. Soon after a company downsizing, Keith's job was selectively eliminated.

By this point (1986), Keith's blood pressure (BP) was 170/100, and medication was required. His pulse rate was rapid even at rest. He was diagnosed with an anxiety-related sleeping disorder. At his physician's insistence, Keith tried counseling. This time, he talked about his feelings and his reluctant acceptance that he and Karen would never be together again. For the first time, Keith cried openly in session and expressed his feelings honestly. After 3 months, Keith was able to locate another job with an acceptable salary. He contracted with his therapist to limit his work hours to no more than 50 hours a week. He still preferred to spend his time alone, however, and maintained no relationships outside his work environment. It was clear that Keith still grieved the loss of his wife.

In 1987, Keith had a heart attack. His widowed sister moved into his home, cared for him until he recovered, and encouraged him to take charge of his life and his health. In one sense, this illness was a "wake-up" call for Keith. He began attending classes on exercise and nutrition and slowly implemented lifestyle changes. In 1988, he joined a singles club and began to date.

Medical outcomes. In the years after Karen left, Keith's psychologic and social adjustment scores confirmed clinical depression, elevated distress and loneliness scores, and strong attachments to the former spouse. His albumin (protein) assessments demonstrated that he had developed extremely poor nutritional habits. When he learned about Karen's pregnancy and then lost his job, cortisol and EPI levels became chronically elevated. He visited his physician an average of six times a year for colds and influenza treatments, but he refused to take off work for adequate rest and recovery. He had significantly higher antibody titers to the Epstein Barr virus (EBV) and herpes simplex virus (HSV) as compared with levels recorded before his divorce, demonstrating that his body was not successfully controlling these latent viruses. Researchers recorded lower levels of helper or suppressor cells than had been assessed before his divorce. Approximately 8 years into the study (3 years after the divorce), medication was prescribed to control Keith's elevated BP, but his cholesterol levels consistently climbed throughout the years.

After his heart attack in 1987, Keith began to exercise, and, with his sister's help, he implemented healthier eating habits. He worked shorter hours and spent more time relaxing. Over a 2-year period with lifestyle changes, medication, and an improved social life, his BP, cholesterol, immune function, and psychologic assessments returned to healthier levels.

---

sively, were not within 20% of their ideal weight, and were taking medications other than birth control prescriptions. The Marital Adjustment Test (MAT) was administered to maximize marital satisfaction in the test sample. Detailed medical histories and lifetime psychiatric disorder data were obtained, and impaired individuals (vulnerable persons whose psychopathologic condition may produce marital discord) were eliminated from the study. Couples were also eliminated if they had any needle or hospital phobias. Therefore the study population consisted of very healthy newlyweds reporting moderate-to-high marital satisfaction with no identified psychopathologic conditions, a best-case scenario population.

Subject preparation. The subjects were admitted to the hospital for a 24-hour stay. A *heparin well,* also known as a heparin lock—an in-the-vein syringe for intermittent use—was inserted in the subjects' arms so that blood could be drawn regularly without discomfort. All couples were served the same food to control dietary factors and maintain caffeine-free intake. After the $1\frac{1}{2}$-hour adaptation period to the heparin well, the couples were positioned in chairs facing a curtain and were instructed to complete several questionnaires. For unobtrusive blood draws, a long polyethylene tube was later attached to the heparin well, so nurses could draw blood at set intervals and out of the subjects' sight.

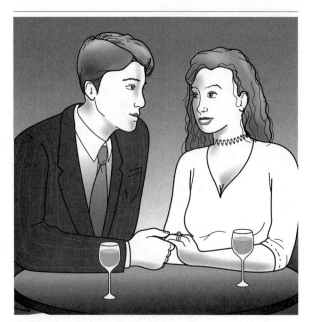

■ **Figure 4-4.** One may assume that immune response will be optimum for newlywed couples experiencing the bliss of a newfound love.

Subject interview and conflict resolution session. A postdoctoral fellow conducted an interview to identify negative and emotional topics for problem discussions. Based on this interview and the ratings from the Relationship Problem Inventory (RPI), the couples were asked to discuss and try to resolve three marital issues judged to be producing the greatest conflict. These discussions occurred during a 30-minute videotaped session. A 30-minute break followed the conflict session. The couples then responded to questions about the history of their relationships with the latter interview generally pleasant for most couples and lasting 30 to 45 minutes. The effects of conflict on heart rate and BP were determined by measurements taken immediately after the conflict session. Readings were recorded at the end of the 10-minute baseline, at the end of the conflict task (30 minutes later), at the end of the 30-minute break, and after the oral history interview. Couples were then assessed for cardiovascular reactivity during a 2-minute mental arithmetic serial subtraction task. This assessment took place in the late afternoon. The next morning, the couples completed self-report measures and discussed their reactions to the visit.

Immunologic assays. The blood samples used for immunologic assays were drawn at the beginning and end of the couples' 24-hour stay, both between 6 AM and 8 AM to control for diurnal (i.e., daylight hour) fluctuations in immune and hormonal responses.

Conclusions and comments

Persons who were more negative or hostile during the 30-minute conflict session showed greater immunologic change after 24 hours.

Diminished immune responses suggested that stress as a result of conflict impairs, at least temporarily, optimal immune functioning (Table 4-2). Across both high- and low-negative groups, the overall trend for immunologic change was for down-regulation after conflict, with low-negative persons more capable of buffering these effects of stress. Similar increases in lymphocyte numbers have been reported after mathematical stress tests, short-term laboratory stressors, and EPI injections. The newlywed couples in this study also produced significant changes in plasma EPI levels, with larger and more persistent elevations in high-negative subjects compared with low-negative persons.

The authors concluded *negative or hostile behavior is significantly related to physiologic change,* (e.g., BP, immune changes), but it is not related to avoidant, positive, or problem-solving behaviors. Neither the subject's reported marital quality nor support from other relationships moderated the effects; instead, *it was the hostility level during conflict that was the determinant factor.* The study concluded that women are more likely to show negative immunologic changes than men. These data provide information on the pathways by which close personal relationships may affect physiologic functioning and health. The authors concluded that *chronically abrasive relationships could potentially produce more frequent and pronounced immunologic, endocrinologic, and cardiovascular changes, leaving individuals in troubled relationships at greater risk over time* (see Table 4-2).

Newlyweds, Conflict, and Hormonal Changes

Evaluation of additional data gathered during the previous study resulted in a new piece of research that described the hormonal changes occurring in the participants during the above trial (Figure 4-5). The authors were interested in evaluating hormonal fluctuations for the following reasons:

■ Many diseases, including asthma, hypertension, ulcers, HSV, rheumatoid arthritis, and Graves disease, have been demonstrated to be induced or aggravated by stressful events.[138]

■ Stress is a stimulus for the release of pituitary and adrenal hormones that can alter humoral and cellular immune response.[113]

■ A variety of studies have found that NEPI, EPI, ACTH, cortisol, GH, and prolactin (PRL) influence quantitative and qualitative changes in

TABLE 4-2	Effects of Marital Conflict on Physiologic and Biochemical Conditions	
AUTHOR(S)	**TYPE OF STUDY**	**FINDINGS**
Kiecolt-Glaser, Malarkey et al.	Study assessed problem-solving behaviors and changes in immune function in newlywed couples engaged in conflict discussions of marital problems (N=90 couples).	Couples who were more negative or hostile during the 30-minute conflict session showed a decline in immune function 24 hours later. NK cell lysis; reductions in percentages of macrophages; poor proliferative responses to con A and PHA; and monoclonal antibodies to T3 receptors; and higher antibody titers to latent EBV were the findings. Hostile subjects also produced more neutrophils, had large increases in total T-lymphocytes and helper T-lymphocytes, and recorded in blood pressure.
Malarkey, Kiecolt-Glaser, Pearl, and Glaser	Study evaluated hormonal changes and problem-solving behaviors in the same 90 newlywed couples cited above. This additional paper was written on the basis of data gathered at the same time as the Kiecolt-Glaser study, but evaluated at a later time.	Hostile behaviors during the 30-minute marital conflict discussion produced, during the 24-hour period, a decrease in the PRL level and an increase in the levels of EPI, NEPI, GH, and ACTH. Differences in EPI were greater for hostile women than for hostile men. NEPI levels were sensitive only to the initial 15 minutes after conflict.
Carstensen, Levenson, and Gottmann	Long-term marriage partners in conflict were studied to determine whether predictability of a long-term relationship would blunt physiologic response to conflict. The identical method used in the previous two studies was employed, with the exception that the hospitalization period was 8 hours rather 24 hours. Couples were 55 to 75 years old and had been married an average of 42 years.	For wives, marital dissatisfaction and negative behavior during conflict had a strong relationship to endocrine changes, accounting for 16% to 21% of the variances in rates of change of cortisol, ACTH, and NEPI, but not EPI. By contrast, husband data demonstrated no significant relationship between negative behavior and marital satisfaction. For both wives and husbands, negative behavior during conflict led to poor response to PHA and con A stimulation, and both had higher antibody titers to EBV.

ACTH, Adrenocorticotropic hormone; *con A*, concanavalin A; *EBV*, Epstein-Barr virus; *EPI*, epinephrine; *GH*, growth hormone; *NEPI*, norepinephrine; *NK*, natural killer; *PHA*, phytohemagglutinin; *PRL*, prolactin.

cellular immunity.[1] Further, a bi-directional feedback system has been identified between the endocrine and immune systems.[128]

Malarkey, Kiecolt-Glaser, Pearl, and Glaser evaluated hormonal changes and problem-solving behaviors in the same 90 newlywed couples of the previous study during the same 24-hour period.[96] Endocrine assays had been performed to determine varying levels of GH, PRL, ACTH, cortisol, NEPI, and EPI.

Hostile behaviors during marital conflict were associated with decreased levels of PRL and increased levels of EPI, NEPI, GH, and ACTH. Differences of EPI levels between high- and low-hostile groups were higher for women than for men.

This study demonstrated that marital conflict and hostile or negative behaviors produce significant neuroendocrine consequences. EPI and NEPI are associated with immunologic down-regulation. These levels are higher in persons demonstrating the more hostile conflict behaviors.

PRL is immune enhancing, and the study noted that PRL levels are lower in the high-hostile group. In summary, the combination of elevated catecholamines (e.g., EPI, NEPI) and depressed PRL levels result in diminished immune function in the group with the most hostile behaviors.

If the endocrine system is involved in the pathogenesis of stress-related disease processes, it is possible that the mediators of these outcomes are the small, frequent, and day-to-day changes in hormonal levels after stressful events. Outcomes reflect a persistence of sympathetic stimulation after terminating the stressor.

Points to Ponder This study demonstrated that marital conflict and hostile or negative behaviors produce significant neuroendocrine consequences. EPI and NEPI are associated with immunologic down-regulation. These levels are higher in persons demonstrating the more hostile conflict behaviors.

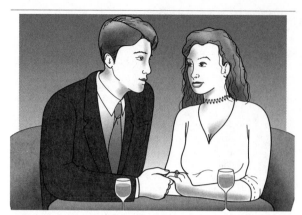

■ *Figure 4-5.* The conflict of the marital adjustment period may have biochemical and hormonal consequences.

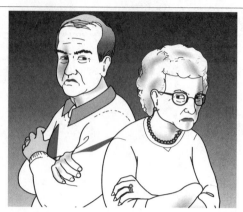

■ *Figure 4-6.* Even couples married for 40 years can experience negative physiologic or biochemical consequences of marital conflict.

Endocrinologic and Immunologic Effects of Long-Term Marriages on Partners

It is reasonable to expect that constant conflict can potentially lead to a down-regulation of immunity or degraded health—either short term or long term—in newlyweds, persons with dysfunctional marriages, and those undergoing marital disruption (Figure 4-6). However, most of us assume that couples married for 40 years or more have "settled in" to a more comfortable relationship that causes little negative physiologic or biochemical effects. After all, research strongly suggests that there is health protection in the marriage state, provided the marriage is a relatively beneficial one. Recent data suggest that older couples display less negative behavior and more affectionate interactions during conflict than middle-aged couples, representing the possibility that physiologic responses may be blunted as well.

One study, however, suggested that marital conflict, even in older adults in long-term relationships, can have physiologic consequences.[16] In this study the method was virtually identical to the one used to assess newlyweds, with one difference—the hospitalization time was shorter, only 8 hours. The subjects were 55 to 75 years of age. Selected couples were generally healthy and happy and their marriages had been stable and enduring, lasting an average of 42 years. Thus outcomes would again be best-case scenarios.

Escalation of negative behavior during conflict and marital satisfaction showed strong relationships to endocrine changes among the wives, accounting for 16% to 21% of the variance in rates of change of cortisol, ACTH, and NEPI, but not EPI. By contrast, the husbands' endocrine data

demonstrated no significant relationship between negative behavior and marital quality.

Both men and women who displayed more negative behavior during conflict demonstrated poorer blastogenic responsiveness to phytohemagglutinin (PHA) and concanavalin A (con A), and both demonstrated higher antibody titers to latent EBV. The same persons characterized their marital conflicts as more negative than individuals who demonstrated better immune responsiveness to these same assessments. The authors concluded that abrasive marital interactions can have physiologic consequences even among those long-married and in relatively happy relationships.

Conclusions and Limitations of Marital Adjustment Studies

It is reasonable to conclude from these data that immunologic and hormonal responses can and do occur in response to abrasive marital interactions. These responses can occur during virtually any stage of a marriage. Women seem to be more sensitive to abrasive interactions than men. However, do the physiologic and biochemical responses to marital conflict result in long-term health effects? Although the epidemiologic data have suggested that they do, we cannot, in fact, know for sure. Whether marital conflict leads to short- or long-term health degradation depends on (1) the quantity of abrasive interactions, (2) the intensity of the abrasive reactions, (3) the sensitivity of the persons involved, and (4) whether the persons are at risk as a result of existing immunologic or physiologic dysfunction. Nonetheless, the data suggest that chronic, intense, and abrasive marital interactions may have a significant effect on long-term health, especially for persons already at risk.

Implications for Marital Intervention

Avoidant, constructive, or problem-solving behaviors are not associated with negative modulation of endocrine and immunologic outcomes. Therefore the development of these skills early in a relationship may potentially offer a protective health factor during the marital adjustment periods. For persons already embroiled in an abrasive relationship, skills training in problem solving and constructive feedback may potentially improve the quality of life and offer a protective health measure.

■ Marriage versus Marital Disruption: Epidemiologic Studies

We now turn our attention to the more specific findings related to marital disruption. Previous research has strongly suggested that the marriage relationship is one of the most important relationships relevant to health and well-being. Many researchers wanted to know what specific factors produced in the marriage state would be beneficial or detrimental to overall health and what factors would reduce the risk of mortality. There was also interest in defining the physiologic mechanisms by which these benefits or detriments occurred. Some wanted to know whether just being married (i.e., having guaranteed companionship) was the beneficial factor or whether certain qualities found in marriage would prove more beneficial than others. Because of these questions, many epidemiologic and survey studies were performed to assess the effects of marital disruption on physical and psychologic health outcomes. *Marital disruption* is defined as the loss of a spouse as a result of divorce, separation, or death. Bloom, Asher, and White reviewed the studies exploring marital disruption as a major stressor.[9] They concluded that separated and divorced persons face profoundly stressful events that can lead to emotional disorders, increased injury rates, and health deterioration demonstrated by increased acute and chronic illnesses and premature death. We examine some of the studies of marital disruption and discuss their common findings in this text.

Morbidity Differences between Married and Unmarried Individuals

Verbrugge noted that a variety of U.S. studies found a high death rate for unmarried and formerly married persons compared with married ones.[44,45,61] However, little research had been done on marital differences as they relate to morbidity or disability and health behavior.[133]

Verbrugge posed the following questions: How do marital groups differ in rates of acute and chronic conditions, disability from these conditions, and use of health services? Which marital groups are more often committed to institutions for health problems? Do the marital groups with the highest mortality rate also have the highest morbidity rate, the greatest number of disabilities, and the highest use of health services?

Age-adjusted data were gathered from the Health Interview Survey, ongoing since 1957; from the Health Examination Survey, begun in the 1960s, which included a health examination; and from the 1960 and 1970 Censuses of population. Other federal health surveys from the National Center for Health Statistics, the Resident Places Survey, and the Hospital Discharge Survey were included. These data were used to evaluate institutionalized and long-term care adults.

The authors concluded that *formerly married persons demonstrated the most chronic conditions, single persons experienced an intermediate level of chronic disability, and married persons were the least disabled. Separated persons suffered the greatest number of short-term disabilities, followed by divorced and then widowed persons.* Single persons avoided short-term disability the most, but they differed little from married persons. *Although formerly married (i.e., separated, divorced) women were more affected by health limitations than formerly married men,* they still outlived formerly married men, a finding that was both of interest to the authors and confirmed previous studies.

Outcomes were potentially affected by marital roles and lifestyles that may have influenced health. For example, spouses may have observed and overseen the health condition of the other partner. Persons with spouses to care for them were less likely to be institutionalized. Marriage selectivity because of health was another factor that was considered. Chronically ill persons were less likely to meet and interact with a potential mate, and potential partners tended to select healthy counterparts. The stress of chronic illness may have also led to the dissolution of marriages. Individual inclinations to take health actions when feeling ill was also associated with better health outcomes (Table 4-3).

Health Effects of an Unhappy Marriage

Although marriage seems to provide a health benefit, this outcome may not always be the case. Persons who feel trapped in unhappy marriages may not enjoy the health benefits generally noted

TABLE 4-3	**Epidemiologic Studies of Marriage and Marital Disruption on Morbidity and Mortality**	
AUTHOR(S)	**TYPE OF STUDY**	**FINDINGS**
Verbrugge	Retrospective study that compiled data from ongoing Health Interview Surveys, which began in 1957; Health Examination Survey, which began in the 1960s; census data from the 1960s and 1970s; and federal health surveys.	Divorced and separated persons had more acute conditions than those who were married, widowed, or single. Separated and divorced persons had more permanently limiting chronic conditions, but separated persons had peak rates of limitation. Separated and divorced women were injured more often than those who were single, married, or widowed; and single men were injured more often than other male categories. Rates of institutionalization for health care were highest for single persons and lowest for married persons.
Renne	Marriage, as found in previous studies, appeared to be a benefit to health. Renne wanted to determine whether health effects differed for married persons, depending on whether they were happily or unhappily married. This study also evaluated the effects of divorce on health changes (N=5373 individuals).	One in five persons reported as being unhappily married. Marriage was associated with better health only when the relationship was satisfactory to the respondent. Unhappily married persons reported poorer health than those who had divorced and those who were happily married. Unhappily married persons had similar levels of neuroticism, isolationism, and depression of separated persons, but they had higher levels of neuroticism, isolationism, and depression than happily married persons. Previously divorced persons who were happily remarried reported health problems less often than other divorced persons.
Case et al.	This study evaluated the effects of a disrupted marriage or living alone with patients recovering from a major cardiac event. This study overcame the weaknesses of prior studies by using hard medical evidence in conjunction with self-reported data.	Living alone was an independent risk factor for recurrent cardiac events and death, even when age and beta-blocking agents were omitted from the models. Disruption of marriage was not found to be an independent risk factor to recurrent events. Simply living with someone was the protective factor, even when a disrupted marriage had previously occurred.

in the studies. The next study sought to determine whether health effects differ between unhappily married persons, happily married individuals, and divorced subjects.

Renne wanted to determine whether unhappily married persons are more susceptible than happily married or divorced persons to physical and psychologic health problems.[109] In 1965, probability samples from 4452 households in Alameda County, California, resulted in an analysis of 5373 currently married, separated, and divorced persons. Comparisons were then drawn between happily and unhappily married persons who had never been divorced, those who had remarried after divorce, and persons still divorced. Married persons answered nine questions about satisfaction with their marriage, and all respondents provided information about overall health status.

Unhappy marriages were correlated with poor health, social isolation, low morale, and emotional problems. Divorced persons were healthier physically and psychologically; they had higher morale and were less isolated than those who remained with an unsatisfactory mate. However, happily married persons and happily remarried persons reported less health problems than divorced persons. This study concluded that the *quality of the marriage determines whether a health benefit or health hindrance is conferred. The major limitation of this study was that the data were based on self-report information.* A pertinent question for investigation would be to determine whether marital status and satisfaction or disruption would contribute to the survival of or increased risk in persons recovering from a heart attack. The next study addressed this issue.

Major Cardiac Events, Disrupted Marriages, and Health Outcomes

In a more directed evaluation, Case, Moss, Case, McDermott, and Eberly assessed the health effects of a disrupted marriage or of living alone with patients recovering from a major cardiac event.[17] This study overcame some of the weaknesses of the prior study by using substantiated medical evidence in conjunction with self-report data. Surprisingly, the authors found that living alone was an independent risk factor for recurrent cardiac events and cardiac death, even when age and beta-blocking agents were omitted from the models. Disruption of marriage was not an independent contributing factor to recurrent events. Thus it seemed that simply living with someone was a protective factor, even when a disrupted marriage had occurred previously. This study did not assess the length of time since the disruption, however. The degree of attachment may not have been as significant an issue for many of these patients. Further, it was not determined who had severed the relationship—the patient or the former spouse—an issue that could affect outcomes. Potential support from significant others or spousal-equivalent relationships were also not considered.

Conclusions and Implications for Interventions in Unhappy Marriages

Although, in a general sense, being married appears to convey a health protection, it becomes clear that the quality of the relationship is indeed a determinant of the effects of the marital state on health. In one study, divorced persons fared better than their unhappily married counterparts.

Not all benefits of a marriage can be attributed to the quality of the relationship. Social control and the lack of financial stress may also be major contributors to the benefits of a marriage—happy or otherwise. The literature also suggested that in the face of marital stress, other relationships may not compensate for an unsatisfactory marriage. In relation to marital interventions, the research suggested that energy directed at increasing a social network may simply avoid the real issue—that the resolution of marital difficulties must be the focus of attention.

The Group for the Advancement of Psychiatry found that 87% of family therapists believe their primary goal is to improve the autonomy and individuation of family members, not strengthen the support system.[47] Therefore therapists' attempts to prevent over attachment to family members contradicts the stated goals of social support and may not be the best strategy for the patient. The individual goals of the patient must be paramount in making this decision. The following is an example of the need to integrate health concerns with patient needs (Box 4-4) (Figure 4-7).

■ Marital Disruptions: Clinical Trials

Prospective and epidemiologic research that suggests marital disruption (e.g., separation, divorce) is one of life's most stressful events, leading to suppressed immunity and a degradation of health, is often based on the *attachment theory*.[135] This theory is the primary concept used to explain why decreases in physiologic and psychologic well-being occur after separation. Attachment is defined as a bonding to a significant other. Once such bonds are formed, they are extremely diffi-

cult to break.[13] The inaccessibility to the spouse after marital disruption can lead to what is termed separation distress, characterized by increased symptoms.[14] Factors associated with less attachment are longer time periods since the separation, development of a new relationship, or being the initiator of the separation.[86] Data suggest that adaptation to the loss of a bonded relationship occurs slowly and over several years. In a longitudinal study, Wallerstein and Kelly found it took 3.3 years for the average woman's life to stabilize after separation.[134] It was also noteworthy that 5 years after separation, 42% of female subjects failed to adjust satisfactorily to the loss of their spouse.

The epidemiologic data, including those studies previously discussed, found that separation and divorce increased acute and chronic illnesses and decreased life span. Marital disruption was found to be the single most powerful sociodemographic predictor of stress-related physical illness, with separated individuals reporting 30% more acute illnesses and physician visits than their married counterparts.[126] With age, race, and income variables controlled, separated and divorced persons still obtained the highest rates of acute medical problems, chronic medical conditions limiting social activity, and disabilities as compared with married persons.[133] Separated and divorced individuals also had a higher rate of death from infectious diseases, including up to six times the number of deaths from pneumonia.[95] Researchers

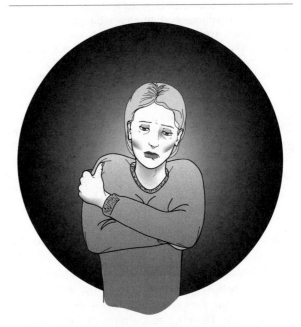

■ **Figure 4-7.** By the fifth year of the research study, Carol was experiencing clinical depression.

BOX 4-4 Carol's Coping Strategies

By the fifth year of the research study (1980), Carol (introduced earlier in this chapter) was experiencing clinical depression. Her husband, Steve, had admitted to an affair and made it clear to Carol that he intended to continue seeking relationships with other women. Carol was devastated, but she did not consider divorce as an option because of her religious convictions and her concern for her children. Carol's father and mother divorced when she was 9 years of age, leaving her mother with the difficult task of raising and supporting three children. As the oldest child when growing up, Carol bore the brunt of the hardships related to the breakup. She was responsible for many of the household tasks and served as surrogate mother for her brother and sister while her mother worked. When she was old enough, she helped buy clothes for herself and her siblings with money earned from babysitting and part-time jobs. When Carol was 16 years old, her mother was injured on the job—a situation that required the family to live on welfare for over a year.

Carol was determined that her children would never live with the pain, poverty, and stigma she experienced as a result of her parents' divorce. She decided to stay in her marriage at any cost. Nonetheless, the sense of betrayal and grief took its toll. Carol suffered from numerous colds and bouts of influenza. She retreated into herself and into her home, eliminating social interactions whenever possible. Her asthma, which had been minor during the early years of her marriage, became a serious health issue, with exacerbations following spousal arguments or the discovery of a new infidelity. By 1982, Carol was diagnosed with bleeding ulcers. Her physician referred her to a psychologist to help her sort her feelings and develop strategies for dealing with her stress.

Since Carol made it clear that she would not consider a divorce, her therapist suggested she work on her depression by becoming more involved in events outside her home. Over time, Carol became more active in her church, began taking art classes at the local university, and renewed some close relationships with female friends. Her depression became more manageable, and her general health seemed to improve. Her ulcers and asthma were still exacerbated by episodic marital difficulties, a response that researchers would see repeated

throughout the study. At the end of the study, an interviewer asked her if her decision to stay married had been a good one. "I simply had to choose which life would be the least stressful—living with an unfaithful husband or raising the children alone. I think for the children it was the right choice—but for me, I'm not so sure."

Medical outcomes. Carol's psychologic assessments indicated clinical depression for several years after her husband admitted his first affair. Carol's psychologic status then tended to move in and out of the depressive state, often reflecting new discoveries of affairs or emotional conflict situations. Her isolation scores climbed consistently between years 5 and 9 of the study, as did her anxiety reactions.

Carol was treated by physicians fourteen times during the first year after her husband's confession, receiving medications for asthma, colds, influenza, and stomach pain. EBV antibody titers were highest during that year; in subsequent years, titers were up and down. By year 9 of the study, EBV antibody titers were maintained at a consistently high and chronic level, demonstrating that her immune system was seriously compromised. Percentages of helper cells were low compared with levels during the first 5 years of the study. They remained low at different levels to the end of the study. Proliferation response to PHA was lower than before the conflict periods and remained low throughout the study. Her BP, cortisol, NEPI, EPI, GH, and ACTH levels were elevated during conflict periods, but they returned to normal levels as each crisis passed. Researchers observed that their interviews concerning changes in life events, performed before blood draws, potentially fueled the hormonal responses. Natural killer (NK) cell lysis was also consistently lower then before the conflict years.

Essentially, Carol's immune and biochemical responses were compromised, leaving her open to the expression of acute illnesses, such as influenza and colds, and the development of chronic problems of asthma and stomach ulcers. These problems, including depression, became more manageable as she began to take part in events outside the home. Even so, immunologic responses failed to return to a preconflict status. Although Carol "tolerated" her husband's affairs and their loss of intimacy, she was unable to come to terms with her life situation. Her health status reflected her internal conflict.

wanted to know how the stress that was related to martial disruption actually caused these effects. Some decided to evaluate the short-term effects of marital stress and marital disruption on immune and endocrine function. They were hopeful that assessing the interconnectedness of the immune and neuroendocrine systems could provide evidence concerning the pathways by which distressing marital events modulate immunity and affect long-term health outcomes. Researchers were also interested to know whether gender was a factor affecting which pathways would be most strongly influenced. We review some of these studies in the following text.

Points to Ponder Separated and divorced individuals also had a higher rate of death from infectious diseases, including up to six times the number of deaths from pneumonia.

Effects of Marital Satisfaction or Disruption on Immune Competence in Women

Kiecolt-Glaser and colleagues assessed the effects of marital disruption and marital satisfaction on psychologic and immunologic competence in women.[75]

Data were collected from 38 separated or divorced women and 38 married women. The subjects were recruited from similar sources—churches, universities, and newspaper advertisements—and the groups were matched by age, education, socioeconomic status of the ex-husband, length of marriage, and number of children.

The separated or divorced subjects were limited to those who separated from husbands within the previous 6 years. The separation date, not the divorce date, was considered the time of "marital disruption." *Research outcomes found that reported declines in marital satisfaction were strongly correlated with poorer health ratings at follow-up.*

Separation or divorce is a traumatic life event that can affect immune response and overall health. Research outcomes reported that the shorter the separation time, the greater the affect on immune function. However, the simple presence of a partner is not equivalent to a supportive relationship nor is it protective of immune competence. The quality of the marital relationship must be taken into account.

Effects of Marital Satisfaction or Disruption on Immune Competence in Men

Previous research emphasized the effects of marital disruption on women. Kiecolt-Glaser and colleagues wanted to assess, in specific detail, the effects of marital disruption on men.

These authors sought to determine immunologic and psychologic effects of marital disruption on men separated or divorced 3 years or less.[84] In this study, 32 separated or divorced men and 32 married men were matched for age, education, length of marriage, relative number of childless marriages, and number of children. Information was gathered concerning length of marriage, timing of separation or divorce, and frequency and degree of satisfaction with dating relationships since separation. Self-reporting tests were administered.

Separated or divorced men were significantly more distressed and lonelier than matched married men. They reported more recent illnesses and had significantly higher antibody titers to EBV and HSV-1 than married men, demonstrating poorer cellular immune system control over herpesvirus latency. Poor marital quality in married subjects was significantly related to greater depression and global distress and to greater loneliness. Marital quality in married subjects was significantly related to psychologic variables and immune function. Further, noninitiators demonstrated more illness and greater psychologic distress during the first year of separation compared with initiators. Unexpectedly, these outcomes were reversed for men separated for longer than 1 year.

As has been demonstrated in other studies, herpesvirus antibody titers seem to be sensitive to psychologic stressors and may reflect more general changes in functional or qualitative aspects of immunity. The findings of this study are consistent with the epidemiologic data that link marital disruption with high rates of psychologic and physical dysfunction, particularly for men (Table 4-4).

Conclusions from Clinical Studies of Marital Disruption

These studies and others suggest that marital disruption, marital dissatisfaction, and conflict can affect mood state, behavior, immune competency, and hormonal response. These responses affect health, both in the short-term basis (e.g., poorer control of viruses) and in the long-term (e.g., morbidity and mortality).

- Depression and loneliness are related to the degree of down-regulation of immunity (i.e., poor control of EBV; reduced NK cell lysis and proliferation response to con A, PHA, and monoclonal antibodies; increased neutrophils and absolute numbers of T_3 and T_4 lymphocytes).
- Hostility is related to down-regulation of immunity, increased BP and levels of stress hormones (e.g., NEPI, EPI, GH, and ACTH).
- Both men and women suffer from these effects, with women demonstrating the greater susceptibility.

These studies describe the effects of our most intimate relationships on health and quality of life and have implications for the need to refocus efforts on the marital state and the quality of relationships when considering such questions as therapeutic interventions, health care costs, and health management.

TABLE 4-4	**Clinical Studies of the Health Effects of Marital Disruption**	
AUTHOR(S)	**TYPE OF STUDY**	**FINDINGS**
Kiecolt-Glaser et al.	The study assessed the effects of marital disruption and satisfaction on psychologic and immunologic competence in women (N=38 divorced and 38 married women). Divorced women had separated from their husbands within the previous 6 years of the study.	Poor marital adjustment in married subjects was a strong predictor of depression and loneliness and an indicator of higher EBV antibody titers. For divorced women, the time since separation and attachment to former spouse was inversely related to psychologic and physiologic health. Compared with married counterparts, separated and divorced women had significantly higher EBV titers and significantly lower percentages of NK, helper T-cells, and responsivity to con A and PHA. Compared with married subjects, separated and divorced women had more depression, higher EBV titers, lower percentages of NK cells and helper T-lymphocytes, and lower proliferative response to PHA and con A.
Kiecolt-Glaser et al.	This study assessed the effects of marital disruption and satisfaction on psychologic and immunologic competence in men (N=32 married men and 32 divorced and separated men).	Separated or divorced men were significantly more distressed and lonelier than matched married men; they had more recent illnesses and higher antibody titers to EBV and HSV-1. In married subjects, poor marital quality was significantly related to greater loneliness, poorer control of HSV, and lower helper-suppressor ratios. Among separated and divorced men, those who did not initiate the separation had more illnesses and greater psychologic distress during the first year after separation than men who did not initiate separation.

con A, Concanavalin A; *EBV*, Epstein-Barr virus; *HSV*, herpes simplex virus; *NEPI*, norepinephrine; *NK*, natural killer; *PHA*, phytohemagglutinin.

Limitations of Studies of Marital Disruption

Although the findings are provocative, more research is needed to:

- Assess the subcategories of persons most affected by the observed biochemical and endocrine, mortality, and morbidity effects;
- Demonstrate a causal relationship between stress levels related to marital disruption and development of chronic disease;
- Assess interventions that may be effective in buffering those experiencing marital disruption;
- Determine how to motivate persons to participate in such interventions; and
- Demonstrate health care cost savings, which would likely guarantee funding of such programs.

Providing support to individuals experiencing marital disruption has become more difficult because of the reduction in insurance coverage for counseling services. Further, persons experiencing marital disruption are often reticent to seek therapeutic help. Support groups offered by well-trained peers may provide some benefit to individuals who are wary of counseling or unable to afford professional help.

In general, more diverse studies of larger populations and studies that follow subjects for longer time periods are needed to complete the "picture" of how relationships affect long-term health outcomes and health care costs.

■ What We Know and Do Not Know

What we know from the biochemical outcomes in relationship studies is that conflict, lack of social support, loss of meaningful relationships, stress of caregiving, and a variety of chronic and acute stressors can affect immunologic competence and hormonal balance. What we do not know is at what point these effects permanently impair health in individuals. The epidemiologic studies strongly suggest that stressors have both morbidity and mortality consequences. Researchers believe they have traced many of the basic pathways by which stress impairs immune function and health. In spite of a fairly formidably amount of research, we still cannot track how we "got from here to there." In other words, we need to track a large number of human beings through the majority of their lifetimes; assess the various stressors in their lives; consistently record their immunologic and hormonal responses to these stressors; document the development of short- and long-term illnesses; and quantify individual genetic risk for development of a variety of chronic diseases. Then and only then will we be able to accurately assess the effects of stress on morbidity and mortality. This task is relatively easy to accomplish with laboratory animals and virtually impossible to accomplish with human subjects. For now, we will have to settle for fitting together what pieces of the puzzle are available. The complete "picture" will no doubt remain a mystery for some time to come.

Still, there is the larger question. What if we knew, absolutely, that chronic stressors were responsible for a large chunk of all medical costs and significantly reduced both the quality and quantity of life? If we could absolutely document these effects, what would we as individuals, as governments, and as communities be willing to do to manage health and health care costs? Identifying the problem may prove to be the easy part. Implementing the kinds of changes that would be necessary to improve health will be the major challenge. In the 1990s, an obsessive work ethic, exhaustion, and the 70-hour work week have become our badges of honor. Family time, relaxation, and a balanced lifestyle have fallen victims to the push for success. If we are to improve the health of society as a whole, what we value, as a society, will need to be reframed.

■ Marital Challenges: Caregiving

Chronic Stress of Caregiving of the Patient With Alzheimer's Disease

It is not uncommon for a spouse in a marital relationship to become chronically ill, placing his or her partner in the position of caregiver (Figure 4-8). In the marriage relationship, responsibility for caring for an aged parent or ill child can also create stressors that place both the marriage and the health of the caregiver at risk. Although stressors related to caregiving can occur in response to any long-term family illness, the effects of Alzheimer's caregiving is a living laboratory for the exploration of chronic stress.

Caring for a relative with Alzheimer's disease has been described as an enduring form of living bereavement. The caregiver can only watch as the personality and intellect of their loved one disintegrates.[93] Those with Alzheimer's disease demonstrate behavioral problems such as wandering, inability to communicate or recognize family members, and incontinence. The length of illness can vary enormously, from 3 to 20 years, and the family members who must preside over the slow deterioration of those they love are often referred to as the "hidden victims."[52] The typical survival time from onset is 8 to 12 years, creating an enduring chronic stressor for the caregiver.[30] Adding to this stress is the information suggesting that the illness may be genetically transmitted.[60] Caregivers often wonder if they or their children will also face this debilitating illness, either as patient or caregiver for other family members. If institutionalization of the patient with Alzheimer's disease becomes necessary, this decision adds to the

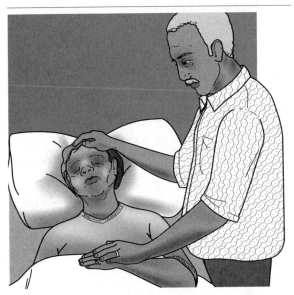

■ *Figure 4-8.* It is not uncommon for a spouse in a marital relationship to become chronically ill, placing his or her partner in the position of caregiver.

guilt and financial burden of caring for the family member.[20]

What health effects do the chronic stressors of caregiving provoke? Surprisingly, evidence from animal studies suggested that chronic stress might possibly lead to an enhancement of some immune functions. Studies with high-intensity noise found that the short-term consequence of sound stressors suppressed immunity, but more chronic stress seemed to enhance mitogenic response.[99] Similar studies with tumor-injected rats found those exposed to a single inescapable shock session increased tumor size and shortened survival time as compared with controls. However, mice that received ten daily shock sessions had tumor areas significantly smaller than control mice and survival times approximated that of the control group.[125] These data led some to hypothesize that there could possibly be adaptation or even enhancement of immunity in response to chronic stress. Scientists began to wonder whether these findings would extrapolate to human subjects. These issues fueled research on the health effects of chronic, as opposed to acute, stress in human subjects.

Would caregivers adapt to their chronic stress and maintain normal or even enhanced immune response—*the adaptation hypothesis*—or would their immune systems begin to fail under the chronic stress of caregiving—*the wear-and-tear hypothesis?* The following studies sought to explicate the answer to this question.

Immunologic and Psychologic Effects of Caregiving

Kiecolt-Glaser and colleagues studied the health of caregivers of patients with Alzheimer's disease using objective physiologic measures to determine the effects of chronic caregiving stress on immunologic and psychologic health.[81]

In this study, 34 Alzheimer's caregivers were matched with 34 noncaregivers. The subjects did not take immunosuppressive medication nor suffer immunologically based health problems. The subjects were matched for the presence or absence of beta-blockers and estrogen supplements, as well as for age, gender, and education. Data were gathered concerning depression ratings, health status, social contact levels, medical history, and functional level of the patient with Alzheimer's, and immunologic and nutritional assays were performed.

The percentages of total T-lymphocytes—helper-to-inducer T-cells and suppressor-to-cytotoxic T-cells—were determined using monoclonal antibodies. Immunofluorescence was used to determine antibodies to EBV viral capsid antigen (VCA). *Capsid* is the protein covering surrounding an elementary virus particle, called a virion, which is composed of a central core containing either deoxyribonucleic acid (DNA) or ribonucleic acid (RNA). Transferrin was determined by nephelometry procedure, and albumin was assessed by the bromcresol green dye-binding method. Analysis of variances (ANOVAs) based on group membership were used.

There were no reliable differences between caregivers and comparison subjects on the variables of age, education, or family income; matching was highly effective. Of the caregivers, there were twenty spouses, thirteen adult children, and one in-law. One half of the caregivers lived with their impaired relative.

The combined data supported the hypothesis that caregivers are more emotionally distressed and have poorer immune function than noncaregivers. Reported differences were important because these caregivers were well educated and had more financial resources than had been described in previous studies. These outcomes therefore represented "best-case" scenarios.

In general, the authors did not find that caregivers became isolated from companions and social activities except when impairment of the patient with Alzheimer's disease became great. Therefore relief that allows caregivers some social time when patients are greatly impaired may be a helpful strategy for maintaining caregiver health (Box 4-5) (Figure 4-9).

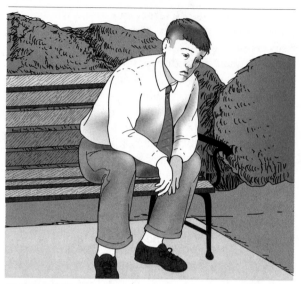

■ **Figure 4-9.** Bob experienced the consequences of caregiving-related stress.

Longitudinal Study of Caregivers

To provide more definitive and detailed data, Kiecolt-Glaser and others tracked caregivers and controls for 13 months and compared changes in health status. The authors assessed longitudinal changes in immunity, health, and depression as a result of chronic stress in spousal caregivers and controls.[74] In this study, 69 spousal caregivers—averaging 5.2 years of caregiving—and 69 sociodemographically matched control subjects were assessed. Each group contained 20 men and 49 women caregivers or controls. The average age, education, or income of the groups did not differ. At intake, caregivers reported spending an average of 8.26 hours per day in caregiving tasks; at follow-up, they averaged 7.04 hours of caregiving each day.

Caregivers demonstrated decreased immunocompetence on all three immunologic assays—proliferative response to con A and PHA, antibody titers to EBV, and leukocyte reaction to monoclonal antibodies. They reported an increase in illnesses, primarily upper respiratory infections, more physician visits, and greater prevalence of depressive disorders. EBV antibody titers showed the most dramatic changes, reflecting downregulation of cellular immunity. In conclusion, researchers found increasing time-related impairment of emotional well-being, immune function, and physical health of Alzheimer's caregivers. No evidence of physiologic adaptation to the stress of caregiving was observed. This raised the question of how long immune function and health would continue to decline and by what mechanisms this impairment would occur.

BOX 4-5 Bob's Challenge of Caregiving

Bob was not completely surprised when his wife, Lisa, was finally diagnosed with Alzheimer's disease. She had suffered from some memory loss and confusion for several years. It had been a joke between them—her absentmindedness, her inattentiveness. Bob had begun to suspect several months earlier that her memory problems could be an indicator of more than simple forgetfulness. He had insisted she see a specialist. Lisa was older than Bob by 7 years; they received the diagnosis on her fiftieth birthday.

They talked about how to cope with the deterioration that was to come. Lisa made it clear that she wanted the routine of their life to continue as much as possible. She asked Bob to keep her at home as long as possible, but she insisted on selecting an Alzheimer's care center where she would live when her health or behavior deteriorated beyond a manageable point. With this decision made, Bob and Lisa tried to simply get on with their life.

For 5 years, Lisa managed reasonably well at home. Bob was able to continue working. In the sixth year after her diagnosis, Bob began to find the stove or appliances left on or the water left running. At times, Lisa could not remember who Bob was. Lisa could no longer stay home alone. A caregiver was hired to stay with her during the day until Bob returned from work.

By the seventh year, Lisa became agitated and angry several times a day. During that summer while vacationing at their cabin, Lisa had a particu-larly bad day. She ran from Bob, screaming that she did not know him, yelling that he was trying to kidnap her. Fortunately for Bob, their neighbors knew of his wife's condition and helped to calm Lisa.

It was at this point that Bob knew he could never take Lisa outside of their home again.

Eight years after diagnosis, reluctantly and with great guilt, Bob placed Lisa in the Alzheimer's care center she had selected. He continued to visit her every evening and on weekends until her death. She died at the age of 63—13 years after diagnosis.

Medical outcomes. As expected, Bob's depression, anxiety, and exhaustion continued to climb during the years of caregiving. His responses to mitogen stimulation (e.g., con A, PHA) declined with time. His EBV titers were increasingly elevated as the years of caregiving progressed. The year before his wife was institutionalized, he developed pneumonia and was hospitalized for a short period. NK cells and cytokine function were impaired, and he continued to demonstrate immune suppression even after his wife's death. Bob's sense of isolation escalated during his wife's illness and, unfortunately, continued for 3 years after her death.

During the last 2 years of the study, Bob's daughter divorced and returned to live with Bob. Bob enjoyed his daughter's company and became involved with his three grandchildren and their social activities. His immune responses improved somewhat along with his mood state.

Points to Ponder   Researchers found increasing time-related impairment of emotional well-being, immune function, and physical health of Alzheimer's caregivers. No evidence of physiologic adaptation to the stress of caregiving was observed.

Cytokine Response, Natural Killer Cells, and Caregiving

The Kiecolt-Glaser study also addressed the issue of adaptation to chronic stress. Esterling, Kiecolt-Glaser, and Glaser wanted to know how long immunologic down-regulation would persist after the death of the Alzheimer's patient.[28] Most specifically they wanted to examine the effects on NK cell activity. In effect, this study bridges the gap between the immunologic effects of stressful caregiving and the immunologic effects of grief.

Natural killer cells. NK cells are vital for immune system surveillance. They protect us from viral infections, identify and eliminate tumor cells, and control metastases (i.e., spread of tumors or disease to other parts of the body).[57,58] Research has demonstrated that interleukin-2 (IL-2) and interferon-γ (INF-γ) modulate the effectiveness of NK cytotoxicity. For example, after NK cells are stimulated by IL-2, they acquire high affinity receptors and are then able to kill a much broader spectrum of tumor targets than the previously unstimulated NK cells could have killed. IL-2 also primes NK cells for cytokine secretion, including IFN-γ, and induces NK cells to become lymphokine-activated killer cells, resulting in enhanced cytotoxicity.[102] IFN-γ by contrast, increases the activity of NK cells, resulting in intense lysis of target cells and enhanced recruitment of pre-NK cells.[123]

There is strong evidence to suggest that stress can down-regulate NK cell activity and interfere with IFN-γ and IL-2 synthesis. This evidence led researchers to explore in greater depths the mechanisms underlying these previous findings. The authors wanted to explore the cellular and psychologic mechanisms underlying the previous finding that stress impairs NK cell functionality; they also wanted to determine to what degree depression and social support guide these mechanisms.

Experimental subjects for this study were part of a longitudinal study of caregiver stress. Caregiver subjects were or had been caring for patients with Alzheimer's disease on a weekly basis. Eleven enrollees were current caregivers, 17 were former caregivers who lost their spouses to Alzheimer's disease in the previous 6 years, and 29 were matched controls. Current caregivers had served their role for an average of 9.6 years, for an average of 4.2 hours a day. One half of the patients with Alzheimer's disease lived at home, and the remaining one half lived in nursing homes. For former caregivers, the average time since the death of their spouses was 36.6 months.

Although an average of more than 3 years had passed since the spouse's death, current and former caregivers did not differ in response of NK cells to IFN-γ or IL-2. However, both groups had significant cytokine impairment compared with noncaregiving controls. These findings suggested that the previously observed defect in NK cell response to these cytokines in family caregivers was related to direct effects on NK cells in response to the stress of caregiving. Consistent with previous research, there were no differences in NK cell cytotoxicity between current and former caregivers or control groups *in the absence of cytokine stimulation.* The authors concluded that down-regulation of NK cytokine-driven cellular cytotoxic responses is related to physiologic changes brought on by chronic stress—in this case, caregiving. *The fact that these effects continued for 3 years after the death of the patient with Alzheimer's disease suggests that chronic stress after the loss can have far-reaching and potentially important physiologic implications for health care.* These outcomes also suggest that after the death of the spouse, former caregivers are not reintegrating with society and are remaining separate from others. This persistent lack of social support has been found, in other studies, to sustain chronic stress in older adults by denying them the opportunities for support and reassurance of worth.[114,121] This study is the first to examine the impact of psychologic stressors on cytokine levels (Table 4-5).

Points to Ponder Although an average of more than 3 years had passed since the spouse's death, current and former caregivers did not differ in the response of NK cells to IFN-γ or IL-2. However, both groups had significant cytokine impairment compared with noncaregiving controls. ■

Summary of Effects of Chronic Stress on Caregivers

Data from these and other studies suggested that the persistent stress of caregiving produced degraded immune response and poorer physical health outcomes compared with demographically matched, noncaregiving controls. Caregivers had demonstrated impaired proliferative responses to con A and PHA and higher antibody titers to latent EBV. All of these responses demonstrated a down-regulation of cellular immunity, which seemed to result in greater susceptibility to viral infections. Caregivers were also found to suffer more days of infectious illnesses and more upper respiratory infections when compared with matched controls. Caregivers reporting the lowest levels of social support demonstrated the greater down-regulation of immune function at 1-year follow-up. Most surprising, the down-regulation of NK cells continued in caregivers several years after the death of the impaired family member.

In a more recent study comparing Alzheimer's caregivers with noncaregivers, subjects were given an influenza vaccination. Only 50% of the caregivers became vaccine responders, defined as a four-fold increase in antibody response, whereas 75% of the noncaregivers became responders.[79] Outcomes from these studies are consistent with other research linking chronic stress to impaired immune function.[27,97]

Caregiving of Patients with Alzheimer's Disease: Study Limitations

Although the information is provocative and clearly delineates an association between caregiving and physical and emotional health and immune impairment, the studies are few in number and use small numbers of subjects. Even so, the information was sufficient to strongly suggest that interventions should be provided to caregivers to help them cope, to improve the quality of their lives, and hopefully to prevent some of the health effects observed in these studies. A review of Alzheimer caregiver interventions follows.

Stress-Management Interventions for Caregivers of Patients with Alzheimer's Disease: Research Outcomes

A review of the literature by Bourgeois, Schulz, and Burgio[10] revealed 28 descriptive and 41 quantitative studies of caregiver interventions. Basically, Alzheimer's caregiver interventions consisted of (1) support groups, (2) individual or group counseling, (3) respite and day care services, (4) skills training, and (5) multicomponent programs using a combination of two or more of these strategies.

TABLE 4-5	Immunologic and Psychologic Effects of Caregivers of Patients with Alzheimer's Disease

AUTHOR(S)	TYPE OF STUDY	FINDINGS
Kiecolt-Glaser et al.	This study assessed the health of caregivers of patients with Alzheimer's disease using objective psychologic measures. The study objective was to determine the effects of chronic caregiving stress on immunologic and psychologic health. (N=34 Alzheimer's caregivers and 34 matched noncaregivers).	Caregivers had significantly higher depression scores, significantly lower life-satisfaction scores, and poorer health ratings compared with control subjects. Caregivers had higher antibody titers to EBV than matched control subjects, significantly lower percentages of helper T-lymphocytes and total T-lymphocytes, and significant differences in helper-to-suppressor ratios. Caregivers, whose relatives with Alzheimer's disease were institutionalized, had higher NK cell values than caregivers whose relatives lived with them and as compared with relatives caring for patients with Alzheimer's disease but living elsewhere.
Kiecolt-Glaser et al.	This study tracked caregivers of patients with Alzheimer's disease and controls for a long period (13 months). N=69 spousal caregivers and 69 sociodemographically matched control subjects. Each group contained 20 men and 49 women caregivers. Caregivers spend an average of 8.26 hours per day in caregiving tasks.	Caregivers demonstrated decreased immunocompetence in proliferative response to Con A, PHA, antibody titers to EBV and leukocyte reaction to monoclonal antibodies; caregivers had more illness days, primarily upper respiratory infections, more physician visits, and greater prevalence of depressive disorders.
Esterling, Kiecolt-Glaser, and Glaser	This study sought to determine whether immunologic down-regulation would persist after the death of the patient with Alzheimer's disease. They specifically evaluated the effects on NK cells. Eleven subjects were current caregivers, 17 former caregivers who lost their spouses in the last 6 years, and 29 matched controls (total N=58).	Although an average of more than 3 years passed since spousal death for prior caregivers, response of NK cells to interferon or interleukin-2 did not differ between former and current caregivers. Both groups had significant cytokine impairment compared with noncaregiving control subjects. There was no difference in NK cell cytotoxicity between former and current caregivers in the absence of cytokine stimulation.

Con A, concanavalin A; *EBV,* Epstein-Barr virus; *HSV,* herpes simplex virus; *NEPI,* norepinephrine; *NK,* natural killer; *PHA,* phytohemagglutinin.

Support groups. Support groups are based on the belief that when caregivers are provided with the knowledge of the patient's disease, information concerning available services, and an opportunity to share feelings and discuss problems with other caregivers, they are better able to meet the challenges of caring for the patient with Alzheimer's disease. Support groups provide information and informal support networking for caregivers that want this type of assistance, but study outcomes have been, at best, suggestive of improvements in areas such as locus of control, perceived burden, or emotional competence. Support groups have not been perceived by those in attendance as addressing the personal needs of caregivers, including unresolved feelings of guilt, anger, and fear of the future in relation to patient care.[3,8,35,51,53,89,101,106,112,115,119,124]

Individual or group counseling. When an individual caregiver has a particularly difficult time adjusting to or facing the burdens of caregiving, individual counseling sessions are often recommended. For specific subsets of caregivers, this intervention has been effective in reducing depression and improving caregiver-relative relationships. Specifically, daughters and daughters-in-law who care for frail elderly parents have made significant gains in psychologic functioning and well-being when they receive individual (not group) counseling. Group counseling, on the other hand, has been more effective in improving caregiver social support systems.[37,49,67,107,118,131,132]

Respite and day care services. The constant stress of caregiving is sometimes referred to as the "36-hour day." Respite interventions, including day care, home respite care, and institutional respite care, allow caregivers some relief from the constant responsibility for the patient. The modestly positive effects of respite programs include less stress and fewer reported caregiving problems. These effects increase as caregivers continue to use the programs, especially as cognitive ability of the patient significantly declines. Further, when caregivers make continual use of these programs, the patients remain in the community significantly longer than those whose caregivers do not make full use of respite services. Nonetheless, outcomes from the use of respite programs have not demonstrated large reductions in caregiver burden or improved physical or mental health.

Essentially, gains for the caregivers from respite care have been modest and have been realized by those caregivers inclined to use these services to their fullest.[15,21,38,90,94,100,116]

Skills training. Skills training includes teaching caregivers how to (1) develop and implement change in patient behavior, (2) monitor treatment, (3) provide corrective feedback, and (4) collect data used to evaluate and improve caregiver skills and to develop individualized programs. Significant changes in the behavior of patients have been accomplished from 73% to 76% of the time, and these changes have been maintained for 6 months after treatment 78% of the time. Caregivers have reported reduced stress and depression and increased morale. Although control caregivers have demonstrated increased burden as the patient deteriorated, caregivers receiving skills training have maintained their mental health status and have enhanced their coping abilities.[23,32,36,43,46,50,111]

Multicomponent programs. Although the literature suggests that "more is better," the components that have been most useful have depended on the characteristics of the caregiver and the special needs of both caregiver and patient. Since there is insufficient analyses to determine which components have been most used and most beneficial, and since multicomponent programs are more expensive, this approach may not be often prescribed because of its failure to demonstrate cost-effective outcomes.[29,98,122]

Summary of intervention programs. In a metaanalytic review, Knight, Lutzky and Macofsky-Urban concluded that individual counseling programs and respite programs were moderately effective, with group therapy sessions less valuable in alleviating caregiver distress.[87] As previously noted, skills training seems to provide significantly positive benefits when targeted toward specific goals, such as programs designed to change patient behavior.

Zarit and Teri emphasized that researchers may be overly optimistic when they expect to find positive outcomes from intervention programs. Intervention efforts may fail to reduce the burden of caregivers, with the exception of removing the caregiver responsibilities altogether.[139] In light of the constant and unrelenting stress created by the circumstances of caregiving for the patient with Alzheimer's disease, caregivers may not be resilient enough to prevent the significant health impairment that is the result of this stress.

In summary, it would appear that different interventions offer different levels of benefit to specific caregivers. Further, interventions must be tailored to the special needs of the Alzheimer's patient and the caregiver. More research, targeted at the needs of specific caregivers, should be performed. The chronic and debilitating nature of Alzheimer's caregiving presents unique challenges for health interventionists.

■ Effects of Bereavement on Immune and Hormonal Function

It is generally believed that with the exception of the loss of a child, no greater or more painful stressor occurs in life than the death of one's spouse. Some assert that the death of a spouse is the more painful and destructive experience from both a psychologic and immunologic point of view. Others argue that marital disruption caused by separation or divorce may be more difficult to overcome because the partner one longs for is still living, but not available. As with any area of research, the health effects depend on many factors related to the event itself and to the personality of the surviving partner. The researchers discussed in this text sought to shed light on the bereavement experience and its effects on health.

> **Points to Ponder**   It is generally believed that with the exception of the loss of a child, no greater or more painful stressor occurs in life than the death of one's spouse. ■

Bereavement and Immunologic and Hormonal Responsivity

Bartrop, Lazarus, Luckhurst, Kiloh, and Penny wanted to determine, prospectively, the behavioral, endocrinologic (hormonal), and immunologic consequences of bereavement.[4] In their study, 26 persons bereaved from the loss of spouses were matched with 26 nonbereaved hospital staff for age (20 to 65 years old), gender, and ethnicity. The subjects were excluded for any history of recent infection, allergic tendencies, or blood disorders. Blood was taken approximately 2 weeks after bereavement (sample 1) and again 8 weeks after the loss (sample 2). The control subjects had blood taken at the same times.

At 8 weeks, PHA responses were significantly different for the bereaved and control groups; the bereaved subjects demonstrated less responsiveness to PHA stimulation.

This study demonstrated that *severe psychologic stress as produced by bereavement can produce a measurable abnormality in immune function* (i.e., lymphocyte proliferative response) (Box 4-6) (Figure 4-10).

BOX 4-6 Louise Faces Her Grief

Louise and her husband had done everything together. They owned a consulting firm that specialized in team building and problem solving for government agencies and private businesses. They exercised together, vacationed together, even completed a Master's degree program together. To Louise, losing Jack meant that life as she had known it had died with him.

After the funeral, Louise decided that she needed time alone to sort things out. She selected a trusted employee to manage the firm and allowed herself the luxury of doing only what she wanted day to day. She reminded herself how difficult his death would have been if they were still raising their children. Their only child had completed college the year before.

Louise soon realized there were no support systems or sources of comfort or even hobbies in her life. Her son accepted work in another city, and her parents lived in another state. Work and Jack had been her existence. During the months that followed his death, Louise cried often, shopped occasionally, and mostly reflected on her life and her loss.

Louise realized that she and Jack had filled their lives with each other. Outside of business associates, they had socialized little. Louise now found herself isolated and lonely with no friends that she could talk with about personal matters, such as grief and rebuilding a life.

Approximately 9 months after Jack's death, Louise discovered that the firm was faltering. The employee who managed the business for her lacked the ability to solicit business in the way she and Jack had done. It soon became clear to her that it was her reputation—and Jack's—that kept the contracts flowing. She resumed management of the firm and soon found that her life once again had purpose. Her evenings and weekends were extremely lonely times, however, and she still felt a need for other friendships in her life—friends that were more than business associates.

She read in the newspaper that a woman she met years ago had also recently lost her husband. On a whim, she called Barbara and asked her if they could have lunch and share thoughts and feelings about the loss of their spouses. A supportive and warm friendship developed.

Louise began to think of spousal loss as a unique problem that was seldom addressed by society, a problem most individuals were sorely prepared to face. She decided to put her problem-solving and team-building skills to good use.

Months later, she and Barbara created a nonprofit support organization for widowed and divorced women. Events were scheduled where women could get together and participate in social activities—plays, opera, picnics, and sporting events. Financial counseling was made available, as well as "think-tank" sessions entitled, "Building a New Life Structure." Most important was the support and sharing that occurred for the individuals involved in the organization.

Approximately 14 months after Jack's death, Louise had found a new direction. Nothing would ever be the same with Jack gone—but there was still life.

Medical outcomes. As part of a study component on grief recovery, Carol agreed to give blood weekly for 2 months after her husband died and then twice monthly for 2 years. She also completed psychologic and social assessments once a month for 2 years.

Carol was clinically depressed for 7 months after her husband's death, but these scores improved consistently, however slowly, returning to acceptable limits within 11 months of bereavement. Isolation scores were initially high, but they began to improve when she went back to work. They returned to healthy levels after forming her nonprofit organization.

Her responses to mitogen stimulation with PHA, con A, and pokeweed were subnormal within 2 weeks of her husband's death and continued for many weeks at a low response level. Responses improved somewhat by week 18. T-cell function was also depressed for 3 months. By month 10, her immune responses were significantly improved, returning to their prebereavement status 16 months after her husband's death.

Immune Responsivity Before and After Bereavement

Although the Bartrop study demonstrated differences between the controlled and bereaved subjects in T-cell responsivity, many still questioned exactly when the impact on immunity had actually occurred. Had the T-cell differences originated during the stress of spousal illness or during the bereavement period? A study was conceived to explore this issue in greater detail.

Schleifer and colleagues were intrigued by epidemiologic studies suggesting increased mortality among bereaved widowers and widows.[54,55,117] They sought to determine whether lymphocyte responses were suppressed as a direct consequence of bereavement, or whether, as in the case of spousal preexisting illness, they may represent alterations of lymphocyte function occurring before loss during the caregiving period.

The authors compared the lymphocyte stimulation responses of 15 bereaved men before and after the death of their spouses; the deaths were caused by advanced breast cancer. The husbands were evaluated, and blood was drawn at 6- and 8-week intervals for the duration of the wives' illness and for up to 14 months after bereavement.

Responses to all three mitogens were lower during the first 2 months after bereavement as compared with the responses before bereavement. The differences found in immune levels before spousal death and during the 4- to 14-month follow-up period were intermediate when comparing the outcomes before bereavement and 2 months after bereavement.

Conclusions and Limitations of Bereavement Studies

This study demonstrated that suppression of mitogen-induced lymphocyte stimulation in these widowers was a direct consequence of the event of spousal loss. Preexisting suppressed immune states did not account for lymphocyte depression in response to bereavement; that is, *the stress of spousal illness did not lead to a habituation of lymphocyte stress response. A highly significant suppression of lymphocyte response occurred during the first month after spousal loss compared with measures taken before loss. Further, lymphocyte depression continued to month 2,* although there was some improvement of response. *The majority of subjects seemed to recover lymphocyte responsivity during the 4- to 14-month follow-up period.* Larger study samples are needed to determine whether some subjects recovered more quickly and effectively while others recovered less well or not at all (Table 4-6).

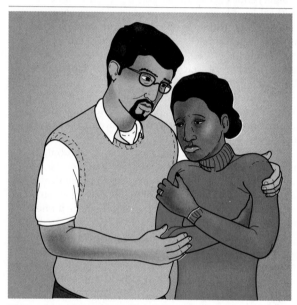

■ *Figure 4-10.* Louise was required to cope with the grief and stress-related consequences of bereavement.

Points to Ponder   A highly significant suppression of lymphocyte response occurred during the first month after spousal loss compared with measures taken before loss. The majority of subjects seemed to recover lymphocyte responsivity during the 4- to 14-month follow-up period. ■

TABLE 4-6	Bereavement and Immunologic and Hormonal Responsivity	
AUTHOR(S)	**TYPE OF STUDY**	**FINDINGS**
Bartrop et al.	In this study, behavioral, hormonal, and immunologic consequences of bereavement were assessed. Twenty-six persons bereaved from the loss of a spouse and 26 nonbereaved hospital staff were matched for age, gender, and ethnicity. Blood samples were taken 2 weeks and 8 weeks after bereavement. Control subjects donated blood at the same times.	At 8 weeks, bereaved subjects demonstrated less lymphocyte responsivity to PHA and con A stimulation than did control subjects. Hormonal assays were no different between bereaved and control persons.
Schleifer et al.	This study sought to determine whether lymphocyte responses were suppressed as a direct consequence of bereavement or whether suppression represented alterations that occurred during the illness period of the deceased spouse (N=15 bereaved men before and after the death of a spouse as a result of advanced breast cancer). Blood samples were taken at 6- and 8-week intervals for the duration of the wives' illnesses and for up to 14 months after spousal death.	Lymphocyte responsivity to stimulation with PHA, con A, and pokeweed were lower for the first 2 months after bereavement as compared with the responsiveness before bereavement. Differences between immune levels before spousal death and in the follow-up periods of 4 to 14 months were intermediate in strength between the outcomes before bereavement and those 2 months after bereavement.

Con A, Concanavalin A; *PHA,* phytohemagglutinin.

As with many studies related to relationship passages, the number of studies conducted are small and the populations studied are equally limited. The outcomes must therefore be considered suggestive until more studies with larger populations are undertaken. Personality styles, coping strategies, and support systems will vary from person to person. These variables, plus the general health status of the bereaved, will modify the emotional and physical effects and the recovery period related to loss.

■ Summary: Health Consequences of Relationship Passages

The relationship passages that have been reviewed in this chapter include the intimate conditions of newlywed and marital adaptation, disruption of the marital state (separation, divorce, death), and caregiving (patients with Alzheimer's disease). In evaluating the combined research on relationship passages, it became clear that certain relationship challenges produced specific, and often differing, changes in measurements of immune function. A lack of social support, conflict, disruption of the relationship, caregiving, and bereavement produced their own unique outcomes.

- Lack of social support resulted in lower lymphocyte counts, poorer mitogen responsivity, and higher cholesterol and uric acid levels.
- Newlyweds in conflict were associated with declines in NK cell lysis, reduced proliferative responses to con A and PHA, reduced macrophages, increased number of antibody titers to EBV, more neutrophils, higher BP, decreased level of PRL (immune-enhancing hormone), and increased levels of EPI, NEPI, GH, and ACTH (stress hormones).
- Marital disruption in women resulted in increased EBV antibody titers, an indication of compromised immune function; reduced NK cell activity, and lower proliferative responses to PHA and con A. Men in marital disruption experienced a greater number of illnesses, increased antibody titers to EBV and HSV-1, and a decline in the helper-suppressor ratio. These outcomes were strongest when the relationship loss had occurred in the recent past.
- Alzheimer's caregiving resulted in increased EBV antibody titers, decreased lymphocyte helper cells, and decreased NK cell-cytokine stimulatory effect, which appears to be the controlling factor responsible for the decline of NK cytotoxicity.

- Short-term bereavement (i.e., 8 weeks or less) resulted in reduced lymphocyte responsivity to con A, PHA, and pokeweed. These responses improved between 5 and 14 months after loss.

A pattern emerges when considering these outcomes. Although results varied somewhat depending on the population and the stress experience, relationship passages seemed to elicit the stress response in the short term in newlyweds, such as an elevated BP, an increase in stress hormones, and a temporary impairment of immune function. With more chronic stressors, the ability to control latent viruses became chronically impaired, representing a less-than-optimal immune response; proliferative responses were slowed; and illnesses increased. The pathways by which the immune impairments occurred appeared to be impairment of the messenger substances, which affected the cell's ability to become cytotoxic and to induce cytokine stimulatory effects. It has been suggested that emotional conditions related to relationship passages are communicated at the cellular level, affecting the functionality of the immune and hormonal systems.

■ Health Effects of Chronic Stress Other than Relationship Passages

Relationship passages are a major source of chronic stressors related to health outcomes. However, they are hardly the only sources of chronic stress with health consequences. One research area that has received ample attention is the health effects provoked by uncertainty and perceived threat. For example, in March 1979, a nuclear power station at Three Mile Island (TMI) was damaged and radiation was released. After the accident, radioactive gas was trapped in a containment building, it leaked periodically, and it was finally released into the air more than 1 year later. An evaluation advisory for pregnant women and families with young children escalated the residents' fears of radiation exposure, although the extent of that exposure was never clearly delineated.[22] Residents lived with an impending sense of threat. They did not know what effects the radiation exposure was likely to have on them or their loved ones, and there was also the possible risk of future leakage. This environmental stressor served as a "real world" laboratory in which researchers could evaluate the effects of stress on mental and physical well-being.

One study by Baum, Gatchel, and Schaeffer was particularly well done, using the TMI residents and three separate but demographically matched control groups (persons living near an undamaged reactor, persons living near a coal-fired power plant, and persons not living near any type of reactor).[5] Approximately 17 months after the event, research outcomes revealed greater symptom distress, greater sympathetic arousal, and poorer performance on stress-sensitive tasks by the TMI residents. Although the magnitude of these effects was mild, it represented a long-term stressor with potential cumulative consequences.

Fifty-eight months after the accident, Davidson and Baum demographically matched 52 residents of TMI with 35 subjects in a town 80 miles away.[22] Both groups were assessed on emotional, behavioral, and biochemical indicators of stress. TMI residents experienced more symptoms of chronic and posttraumatic stress than did the control group. TMI residents performed less well on behavioral measures of stress (e.g., proofreading tasks), exhibited higher levels of NEPI and cortisol (i.e., stress-related hormones), and demonstrated higher arousal on measures of cardiovascular function (i.e., higher resting systolic and diastolic BP levels and higher resting heart rate). Further, TMI residents were still bothered by intrusive thoughts about the nuclear accident almost 5 years after the event.

Clearly, the mere perception of danger can induce chronic stress in those who feel endangered. These studies have implications for persons experiencing any form of perceived threat. For example, victims of violent crime often live in fear that their abuser will harm them at some time in the future. Some patients who survive cancer live in fear that their cancer will reoccur. Similar emotional, behavioral, and biochemical responses, with their concomitant health effects, may occur in any situation that is perceived as a threat.

■ Short-Term or Acute Stress: Tracking the Pathways

Chronic stress can be defined as the accumulation of many short-term or acute stressors—over time. A negative life event that is constantly relived, such as rape or war memories, can also be considered a chronic stressor.

Researchers have been interested in studying short-term stressors as a way of evaluating the systemic mechanisms that lead to longer term health effects. By the 1980s, there was growing evidence that relatively minor life events could, temporarily, modulate physical and psychologic health. In fact, it appeared that minor events accounted for more of the variance in somatic and psychologic symptoms than did major life events.[24,66]

Kiecolt-Glaser and others were contributors to studies in this area. Their interest arose from animal experiments, which demonstrated that various stressors altered immune function. For example, though neither a stressful environment nor the inoculation of a virus was sufficient to produce clinical disease, when these two factors were combined, significant infection occurred.[34] In a mouse spontaneous tumor model, 7% of the control mice raised in a protected environment developed tumors by 1 year of age, whereas 92% of an experimental group exposed to a stressful environment developed tumors in the same time period.[110] There was clearly a need to further explore the effects of short-term or acute stressors on immunologic competence in human beings.

Medical and psychologic students are sometimes affectionately referred to as the "guinea pigs" of the research world. Many are willing to participate in research because of interest, for additional college credit, or for spending money. Their educational experiences provide a natural-occurring, short-term stress cycle, with vacations serving as relaxation periods, whereas preparation for and participation in final examinations create a temporary, but escalating, stress scenario. In 1982, Janice Kiecolt-Glaser and her husband, Ronald Glaser, began a series of studies on academic stress.[72] Every year for 10 years, medical students at Ohio State University were evaluated to determine the effects of academic stress on immune function and mood state. The students were literally tracked across the year in the context of a "real-world" situation. Much of the research on academic stress emphasized its effects on viral latency, the changes in NK cell function, and the contribution of loneliness or depression to the down-regulation of cellular activity. The following text provides a review of four of these studies.

Medical Students and Examination Stress, Immune Function, and Emotional Correlations

Kiecolt-Glaser and associates examined the effects of examination stress on NK cell activity, immunoglobulin levels, *C-reactive protein,* (i.e., a β-globulin found in the serum of persons with inflammatory, degenerative, or neoplastic diseases) and salivary IgA[76] (Figure 4-11).

In this study, 75 medical students (26 women, 49 men) gave blood samples 1 month before a series of final examinations for the first year of medical school. Samples were taken again

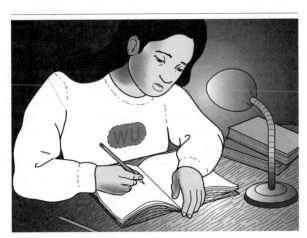

■ *Figure 4-11.* Examination stress on medical students can alter immunologic and short-term outcomes.

on the first day of final examination week and again after the students had completed their first two examinations.

There was a significant decrease in NK activity from the first to the second blood sample, with those scoring high for stressful life events demonstrating significantly greater decreases than the low scorers. High loneliness scorers also had lower levels of NK activity than did the low loneliness scorers.

Although IgG, IgA, and IgM plasma immunoglobulins increased from first to second blood draw, only IgA reached significance. There was not a significant change in salivary IgA between blood samples. Greater distress was reported on the brief symptom inventory (BSI) using the final blood sample with significant changes in the general symptom index (p<01).

Conclusions and Comments

The authors were somewhat surprised that healthy medical students who had previously distinguished themselves by their performance during examinations demonstrated significant decreases in NK cell activity in response to this mild form of stress. *There was a significant relationship between stressful life events, loneliness, and declines in NK activity, lending credence to the possibility that an accumulation of stressful life events may have negative consequences for health outcomes.*

Stress has been shown to have an impact on the activity of NK cells, and *since NK cells have an antiviral function, this suppression may explain the popular belief that viral illnesses, including upper respiratory illnesses, are more likely to follow stressful periods.*

Stress, Loneliness, and Changes in Herpesvirus Latency

Another assessment of immune competence is the level of antibody titers to one or more of the herpesviruses, including HSV-1, EBV, and cytomegalovirus (CMV). Persons who have been previously exposed to HSV-1, EBV, or CMV and are immune suppressed often show increases in antibody titers to these viruses. Although counter-intuitive, these increases are thought to reflect a weakened immune system; in other words, the latent viruses have become sufficiently reactivated to require an increased antibody response.

Glaser and associates probed possible mood state and stress-related changes in herpesvirus antibody titers.[39] This study hypothesized that a subjective quality of human relationships (i.e., loneliness) may have important consequences for health.

Blood samples and questionnaire data were gathered from 70 first-year medical students 1 month before and on the first day of final examinations and again on their return from summer vacation. Blood samples were taken mid-day to control for circadian effects.

Antibodies were assessed for EBV, CMV, and HSV. Antibody levels to a *recall antigen,* poliovirus type 2, were also assessed to determine whether herpesviral levels might simply be a reflection of more general changes in plasma IgG. Unlike latent herpesvirus infections, which are not eliminated from the immune system, the attenuated poliovirus used in vaccinations does not induce a latent infection and is cleared by the host. Therefore, in the study, the attenuated poliovirus provides a controlled response to determine whether, in fact, the herpesvirus data reflect stress-related changes in viral latency.

Significant changes in EBV, HSV, and CMV antibody titers, but not in poliovirus type 2, were found across sample points, suggesting that significant changes in cellular immune response (i.e., changes in herpesvirus antibody titers) are associated with everyday stressors in a healthy population. Subjects scoring high loneliness ratings demonstrated significantly higher *early antigen* (EA) and VCA titers than less lonely students. The product of early virus transcription, EA is synthesized independently of virus DNA synthesis. As a reminder, VCA is a late antigen-complex that is synthesized from new viral DNA. The increase in EBV and VCA IgG antibodies indicated a reactivation of the EBV from latently infected cells. Loneliness has been previously associated with immune suppression in medical students and in patients under psychiatric care, supporting the hypothesis that *loneliness has implications for health outcomes.*[77,85]

Effects of Stress on Interferon Production and Decreases in Natural Killer Cell Activity

There is strong evidence that NK cells are important in the body's defenses against cancer and viral infections.[56,127] Because interferon (IFN) affects both growth and differentiation of NK cells, it is considered to be a major regulator of NK activity. IFN activates the lysis activities of target-binding cells and increases the number of target cells that can be killed by an effector cell. There is also evidence that NK cells can produce IFN itself.

It was argued that stressors can reduce the ability of IFN to stimulate certain immune functions and can therefore have significant consequences for NK activity and overall health.[104] Based on their previous findings that NK cells were effected by academic stress, the authors wanted to identify the pathways by which NK cell competency was modulated.

Glaser and colleagues wanted to study changes in IFN production and NK cell numbers as related to examination stress.[41] Leukocytes were extracted from 40 second-year medical students 6 weeks before the examinations and again on the first day of the final examination.

This study demonstrated a large and significant decrease in the amount of con A–induced IFN production during an examination stress event, as compared with baseline values. Two assays used to quantify NK cells (percent Leu7+ cells and percent large granular lymphocytes) ruled out the possibility that only unique subsets of NK cells were being assayed. The data also suggested that a decrease in total number of NK cells may be the reason NK cell lysis was decreased by stress.

Effects of Relaxation on Medical Students' Immunity While Facing Examination Stress

Although it is helpful to identify the pathways and outcomes of stress-related immune suppression, the obvious next step is to determine how to neutralize the undesirable mental and physical effects. After the previous study, Kiecolt-Glaser and others decided to apply what they had learned by developing and testing a stress intervention. Could they produce the opposite effect of stress; that is, would relaxation provide a protective effect from the immunosuppression of a stressful event?

Kiecolt-Glaser and others[82] traced immunologic changes related to the stress of examination, specifically helper-induced cell and suppressor-cytotoxic cell ratios and NK cell activity while testing a stress-neutralizing intervention.

In this study, 34 first-year medical students (22 men, 12 women with a mean age of 23.5 years) submitted to blood draws 1 month before examinations (baseline data) and on the final day of semester examinations. One half of these subjects were randomly assigned to a hypnotic and relaxation group and were required to attend a minimum of five of a possible ten relaxation sessions in the $2^1/2$ weeks before the examinations.

For the relaxation group, each session began with the same deepening exercises. The middle portion of the sessions varied and included self-hypnosis, progressive relaxation, autogenic training, and imagery exercises. All sessions included the practice of deep relaxation with suggestions that the students experience deep relaxation throughout the day, enhanced comprehension and retention of academic material, and improved study habits. The subjects were strongly encouraged to practice relaxation techniques outside of class on a regular basis. The subjects rated the level of relaxation at the end of each session. Various methods of relaxation were used to allow subjects to identify the method most effective for them. No single method was emphasized over another, since available research at the time did not suggest that any single form produced more reliable physiologic effects than another.[6,25,26,91]

Baseline comparisons found no significant pretreatment differences in any assessment areas. Therefore the relaxation group versus the no relaxation group were well matched at the beginning of intervention.

The authors tested their hypothesis that relaxation practice will buffer stress-related changes in cellular immunity, with the magnitude of the relationship depending on the frequency of relaxation practice. There were large differences in the frequency of relaxation practice within the relaxation group, with the sum of group and home practice sessions ranging from 5 to 50. The average number of sessions was 12.07. *As hypothesized, the frequency of relaxation practice was a significant predictor of the percentage of helper-inducer cells during the examination period, after correcting for baseline levels. The more the subjects practiced, the higher the percentage of helper-inducer cells found. The frequency of practice was not a predictor of NK cell activity.*

Helper-inducer cell malfunction can lead to immune deficiencies. *Outcomes from this study demonstrated that relaxation frequency is related to improved helper-inducer cell function. This*

TABLE 4-7	Effects of Acute, Short-Term Stress on Immune Function

AUTHOR(S)	TYPE OF STUDY	FINDINGS
Kiecolt-Glaser et al.	This study sought to determine the effects of a short-term stressor (e.g., examination stress in medical students on immune function) (N=75; 26 women, 49 men). Blood was drawn 1 month before and on the first day of final examinations and again after completing the first two examinations (first year of medical school).	There was a significant decrease in NK activity from the first blood sample to the second, with these draws scoring higher for stressful life events, demonstrating significantly greater decreases than low scorers. High loneliness scorers also had lower NK activity than those scoring a low loneliness rating. IgA plasma immunoglobulins increased significantly from the first sample.
Glaser et al.	This study sought to determine the specific effects of loneliness on immune function (N=70 first-year medical students). Blood was taken 1 month before and on the first day of final examinations and on return from summer vacation.	Subjects with high loneliness rating demonstrated significantly higher early antigen and EBV-VCA titers than subjects with low loneliness rating.
Glaser et al.	This study evaluated changes in INF production and NK cell numbers related to examination stress in 40, second-year medical students 6 weeks before examinations and again on the first day of final examinations.	There was a large and significant decrease in the amount of con A–induced INF production during an examination stress event, as compared with baseline values.
Kiecolt-Glaser et al.	This study assessed immunologic changes in cellular immunity while testing a stress-neutralizing intervention (e.g., relaxation therapy). Thirty-four first-year medical students (22 men, 12 women) submitted blood samples 1 month before examinations and on final examination day. One half were assigned to a hypnotic and relaxation group.	Baseline comparisons showed the relaxation and non-relaxation groups well matched. The relaxation practice group maintained baseline psychologic status during the stress of examinations, whereas the nonrelaxation group demonstrated significant increases in anxiety, obsessive compulsivity, and global severity index. The frequency of relaxation practice was a significant predictor of the percentage of helper-inducer cells during the examination period. The more they practiced, the higher the percentages of helper-inducer cells.

Con A, Concanavalin A; *EBV,* Epstein-Barr virus; *HSV,* herpes simplex virus; *INF,* interferon; *NEPI,* norepinephrine; *NK,* natural killer; *PHA,* phytohemagglutinin; *VCA,* viral capsid antigen.

finding has implications for the use of stress-reduction interventions as a method for modulating the effects of stress and ultimately influencing the incidence and course of disease (Table 4-7).

Summary of Research on Short-Term Academic Stress

The outcomes from the academic stress studies revealed the following:

■ *During short-term examination stress, antibody titers to EBV, CMV, and HSV significantly increased, reflecting a loss of immune competence (i.e., these latent viruses were poorly controlled as compared with baseline levels).* Herpesviruses have the ability to produce multiple diseases. For example, HSV-1 is responsible for common cold sores, but it can also lead to generalized infections, such as encephalitis, and to death. CMV infections can produce mononucleosis, which typically resolves in 3 to 6 weeks. However, in those with compromised immunity, primary or secondary infections from reactivated CMV can

lead to interstitial pneumonia, the largest source of death in bone marrow transplants.[129] Therefore stress can be a critical factor for morbidity and mortality, especially in persons who may already have impaired immune function.

■ *Significant declines were found in percentages of helper-inducer cell and helper-suppressor cell ratios during the examination period* as compared with the month before. This finding may have important implications for other aspects of immune response. Larger reductions in the percentages of helper-inducer cells can produce immunodeficiency, and large changes in the percentages of suppressor-cytotoxic cells are associated with autoimmune disorders.[108] Helper-inducer cells induce B-lymphocyte proliferation and differentiation necessary for the synthesis of the immunoglobulins that provide defenses against infectious invaders. The optimal development of cytotoxicity requires the presence of helper-inducer cells, which play a critical role in interactions between T-cells and macrophages.

■ *Significant declines were found in IFN production and NK cell activity during examination periods.* NK cells are immune cells with specific and preprogrammed antitumor and antiviral activities. They are vitally important in preventing the development and growth of tumors. Alterations in NK activity may suggest a pathway by which stress can increase the risk of malignancies. The modified theory of immune surveillance suggests that cancer cells develop in the body spontaneously, but they are destroyed by the immune system. The changes in IFN and NK data in relationship to a commonplace stressor, such as academic stress, may have important health implications for control of cancerous cells.

■ *Loneliness was found to be a contributing factor to immune suppression.* This finding has implications for the development of meaningful psychosocial relationships as a protective factor of immune competence. The reader is reminded that the social support literature found that each person's individual needs in this area are unique. One meaningful, sharing relationship that is available to the person is often sufficient, although other individuals may feel a need for many such relationships. Simply thrusting a relationship on a person may add stress, rather than relieve it. Nonetheless, the issue of loneliness, as it relates to the individual, must be addressed when any form of psychosocial intervention is attempted.

■ *In summary, the effects of stress on viral latency, as well as the poorer destruction of mutated cells caused by IFN and NK cell lysis alteration, and the effects of stress on T-cell helper-inducer and helper-suppressor ratios strongly suggest that stress has implications for health management, especially for those who may already have impaired immune function,* such as those in the older population who experience declines in immune competency as a result of age and those experiencing illness who are already at risk for increased morbidity and mortality.

■ *Relaxation training and practice may buffer some of the effects of stress-induced immune suppression.* In the previous study, helper-inducer cell function was improved with relaxation practice. An issue that is further explored in this text is the potential for effective stress intervention with relaxation, imagery, hypnosis, biofeedback, and meditation. We can conclude that both short- and long-term stress modulate immunity and that optimal health requires the evaluation and systematic management of stress.

An Expert Speaks: Dr. Janice Kiecolt-Glaser

Janice Kiecolt-Glaser, PhD, is professor and director of the Division of Health Psychology, Department of Psychiatry, at Ohio State College of Medicine. For nearly 2 decades, she has vigorously researched and published human subject outcomes concerning the effects of stress and emotion on immunity, hormonal responsivity, morbidity, and mortality. In this text she discusses how she became involved in this type of research and how individuals and the health care industry can apply its outcomes.

Question. How did you first become involved in research on the health effects of stress and emotion?

Answer. Early human PNI [psychoneuroimmunology] research focused on the effects of very novel and very intense events on the immune response. Researchers showed that astronauts had poorer immune function after splashdown than before liftoff, volunteers in a Swedish study had poorer immune function at the end of 77 hours of noise and sleep deprivation than before they began their ordeal, and bereaved spouses had poorer immune function than nonbereaved control subjects. These findings were interesting, but most of us do not experience such extreme events with any regularity. When we began our PNI research program in 1982, we were struck by the paucity of human studies (compared with the research on rodents); we could count the number of well-designed studies that used human subjects on both hands. We reasoned that if stress-related immune suppression was indeed a risk factor of any importance in the incidence of infectious disease—and perhaps cancer as well—then we should find immunologic changes associated with more commonplace stressful events, as well as intense and novel events. To address this question, we began conducting annual studies with medical students; we compared immunologic and psychologic data collected from the students during a 3-day examination block with baseline (or lower stress) blood samples collected a month previously when they did not have any scheduled examinations. [Note: See the review of these studies in this chapter.]

Question. What do you think are the most meaningful findings from your years of research?

Answer. The most meaningful findings are the demonstrations of how important personal relationships are linked to alterations in immune function. For example, lonelier medical students had lower NK cell activity than fellow students who were not as lonely. Medical students who reported better social support mounted a stronger immune response to a hepatitis B vaccine than those with less support. Married couples whose disagreements were most hostile or nasty showed subsequent downward changes in immune function.

Question. How should or could that information be used by the health industry and by individuals to improve health outcomes?

Answer. Recent data on wound healing clearly point to the importance of presurgical interventions. Your readers may want to review the article in the American Psychologist [Kiecolt-Glaser JK et al: Psychologic influences on surgical recovery: perspectives from psychoneuroimmunology, *Am Psychologist* 53:1209, 1998.] In addition, we now have good evidence that stress alters response to vaccines and, by analogy, to challenges by infectious agents.

Question. Can you tell us a little about the research you are currently working on?

Answer. Wound healing! Stress can slow wound healing significantly. Among students taking examinations, for example, the difference in time to heal is averaging 40% longer than during a low-stress period for the same student.

▪ Findings from Other Studies of Stress and Health Outcomes

Stress and DNA Repair

It appears that stress may contribute to cancer directly through impairments in the DNA repair process. This outcome was previously demonstrated in animal studies. Forty-four rats were given the carcinogen, dimethylnitrosamine, in drinking water; one half were stressed by a rotational stress model, and the control rats were not. The levels of methyltransferase, a DNA-repair enzyme induced in response to carcinogen damage, was significantly lower in the spleens of the stressed animals, as compared with the control rats.[42]

Stress, Social Support, and the Epstein-Barr Virus

Memory T-cell response to EBV was impaired by examination stress in another study.[40] In 25 healthy medical students, proliferative response to five of six EBV polypeptides significantly decreased during the final examination period.

The subjects dissatisfied with current levels of support had the lowest responses to three EBV polypeptides and higher levels of antibody titers to EBV-VCA. The authors tested a variety of polypeptides (antigens) to EBV in this study, because prior evidence concluded that only some EBV polypeptides may be synthesized under times of stress, suggesting that stress may not contribute to the expression to all viral genes.[73] It would appear from this study that the effects of stress extend to the majority of viral genes.

Stress, Relationships, Inhibited Power Needs, and Secretory Immunoglobin A

Jemmott and associates[65] found secretory IgA significantly lowered during high-stress academic times as compared with low-stress periods. Individuals unfulfilled by personal relationships or with a high-inhibited need for power produced significantly lower levels of secretory IgA and recovered less readily than persons not reporting these characteristics. In a West Point study of cadets, the incidence of infectious mononucleosis was highest among those experiencing academic difficulty and with those whose parents were most invested in their success.[69] These studies again support previous finding that stress and poor social support impair immune function.

Recurrent Herpes Simplex Virus, Depression, and CD4 and CD8 Cells

In patients with recurrent HSV, those reporting higher levels of stressful events over a 6-month period had lower proportions of CD4 and CD8 cells, whereas those reporting high levels of depressive mood had the highest rate of HSV recurrence.[70] A model was proposed linking depressive mood, CD8+ cells and HSV recurrence.

Stress and Hepatitis B Vaccine Seroconversion

In a more recent study by Kiecolt-Glaser and colleagues,[72] the authors sought to determine whether stress during examinations affects a student's immunologic response to a vaccine. Hepatitis B vaccine was administered in the normal way, except that it was given during the most stressful examination period. During the first and second inoculation, only 12 of 48 students seroconverted (i.e., developed measurable levels of antibody.) The students that demonstrated seroconversion experienced significantly less stress and anxiety than the students who did not convert. Further, students who converted reported more satisfying personal relationships, which correlated with higher antibody titers and enhanced T-cell immunity. In another study, caregivers of patients with Alzheimer's disease were less likely to show a significant increase in antibody titers 4 weeks after receiving an influenza virus vaccine than the matched controls who were not caregivers.[80] These studies have implications for the timing of vaccinations, especially in the older population who may already have impaired immunity. Vaccinations should, ideally, be administered during low-stress periods.

Stress and Serum Cholesterol Levels

The effects of academic examinations on serum cholesterol levels were studied on two groups of medical students. A significant increase in mean total serum cholesterol was recorded during examination periods as compared with control periods of relaxation (the middle of two quarters).[48] In a study of occupational stress involving accountants with routine schedules interrupted by high-stress, tax-deadline periods, blood was taken biweekly, for 6 months. The highest serum cholesterol levels consistently occurred during high-stress workload weeks, and the lowest cholesterol levels were recorded during low-stress workload weeks. These results were not attributable to weight, exercise, or diet. Marked acceleration of blood clotting also occurred during high-stress weeks. The average cholesterol level of the accountants self-reported during the most stressful period averaged 252 mg per 100 ml, whereas the average level self-reported during the least stressful time was 210 mg per 100 ml[33]—a 42-point mean difference.

Stress and Immune Response of the Patient with Cancer

Finally, one of the most provocative studies relates to disease-induced stress and its effects on immune function. In a recent study, 116 patients treated surgically for invasive breast cancer, but not yet receiving adjuvant therapy, completed a validated questionnaire (Impact of Event Scale), which assessed the stress induced by being a patient with cancer.[2] Approximately 70% of patients had reached stage II, and 30% were at stage III. The authors controlled for other variables exerting stress effects on responses and ruled out confounding variables such as nutritional differences and sleep patterns.

Blood samples were subjected to a panel of NK cell and T-lymphocyte assays. NK cell lysis was assessed because these cells are believed to act early in the immune response and because they play an important role in immune surveillance against tumors and viral-infected cells.[58,59] The ability of NK cells to respond to recombinant IFN-γ and IL-2 was assessed because lymphokine-activated NK cells are highly cytotoxic against a wider variety of tumor cells than those lysed by resting NK cells.[137] Finally, T-cell activity was assessed by the responsiveness of peripheral blood leukocytes to PHA and con A. Proliferation was induced by stimulating T-cells with a monoclonal antibody to the T-cell receptor.

For both in-group and between-group assessments, the authors found that stress levels significantly predicted (1) lower NK cell lysis, (2) diminished response of NK cells to IFN-γ, and (3) decreased proliferative response of blood lymphocytes to PHA and con A and to a monoclonal antibodies directed against the T-cell receptor. The authors concluded that data demonstrated the finding that the physiologic effects of stress (i.e., being diagnosed with cancer) inhibit cellular immune responses, which are relevant to cancer prognosis, including NK cell toxicity and T-cell responsiveness.

■ Chapter Review

The magnitude of change after an acute stressor typically lasted 60 to 120 minutes, although more intense stressors such as shock and noise may have longer lasting effects. Some immunologic parameters change rather quickly, whereas others have well-defined time courses. For example, degradation of IgG to a vaccine or to latent herpesvirus cannot change over a few hours and changes in gene expression are not transient.[78] When short-term stressors occur repeatedly (e.g., continuing examination stress, which occurs over a period of 1 week or more), the effects may lead to a greater likelihood of illness. In some instances, what starts as a series of acute stressors will eventually merge into a long-term chronic stressor; an example of this type of progression occurs in the caregivers for patients with Alzheimer's disease. In scenarios like this, health effects of caregiving can be influenced by other variables. For example, caregivers with little social support often display different patterns of age-related heart rate reactivity and BP than their counterparts with high social support. In essence, the magnitude of health degradation is determined by the differences among people who vary in their autonomic reactivity, the intensity of the stressor, the length of time under stress, and other variables such as social support and quality of relationships.

In summary, this literature should serve as a wake-up call to the health care industry. Psychosocial challenges have both health and health care dollar consequences. No responsible health care program can afford to overlook the importance and implications of this literature. When illness strikes—especially chronic illness—the psychologic stressors in the life of the individual and his or her family need to be assessed and potential interventions and strategies for stress reduction need to be discussed as part of the health care plan.

Matching Terms and Definitions

Match each numbered definition with the correct term. Place the corresponding letter in the space provided.

_____ 1. Assessing the quantity of time spent with other persons and the context of that time (e.g., leisure activities, church, formal and informal groups, friends and family, and spouse)

_____ 2. Relationships that are qualitatively meaningful or fulfilling

_____ 3. Any physiologic, psychologic, or behavioral response within an organism elicited by evocative agents

_____ 4. Evocative agents

_____ 5. Long-term studies that follow subjects for many years

_____ 6. Death

_____ 7. Diseased state

_____ 8. Breaking down of bodily chemicals to liberate energy

_____ 9. Maximal point beyond which no benefit can be received

_____ 10. Loss of a spouse as a result of divorce, separation, or death

_____ 11. Bond to a significant other that is extremely difficult to break

_____ 12. Inaccessibility to a spouse after marital disruption, leading to increased symptoms

_____ 13. Maintenance or enhancement of normal immune response when experiencing stress

_____ 14. Degradation of immune function when experiencing stress

_____ 15. Outcome or event being investigated

_____ 16. Antibodies directed against one's own healthy tissues

_____ 17. Anxiety that is part of one's natural state

_____ 18. Anxiety in response to a short-term event

_____ 19. Studies based on the evaluation of historical data

a. Marital disruption
b. Stressors
c. Retrospective studies
d. Mortality
e. Trait anxiety
f. Autoantibodies
g. Social interaction
h. Morbidity
i. Catabolism
j. Stress
k. Social support
l. Adaptation hypothesis
m. Wear-and-tear hypothesis
n. Prospective studies
o. Threshold effect
p. Separation distress
q. Dependent variable
r. Attachment theory
s. State anxiety

Multiple Choice

Circle the letter(s) for the most accurate response(s). Most statements will require more than one response.

1. Interventions for the caregivers of patients with Alzheimer's disease include which of the following?
   a. Respite care
   b. Art therapy
   c. Hypnosis training
   d. Individual or family counseling
   e. Support groups
   f. Skills training

2. Which one of the following is *not* a hormone assessed for stress reactivity?
   a. ACTH
   b. Cortisol
   c. CMV
   d. GH
   e. PRL
   f. EPI
   g. NEPI

3. Which of the following are three indicators of health status that are well-documented as to be modified by stress?
   a. Uric acid
   b. Albumin
   c. Cholesterol
   d. Immune function
   e. Serotonin

4. Elevated antibodies to which of the following viruses indicate compromised immune function?
   a. VCA
   b. HSV-1
   c. CMV
   d. EBV
   e. REA

CRITICAL THINKING AND CLINICAL APPLICATION EXERCISES

1. Summarize the findings of the Berkman and Syme study, and the two replication studies that followed. Explain the differences found between the effects of certain kinds of social interactions on men and women. Discuss why you think these differences exist. Describe how this information can be applied to health care management.

2. Summarize the immunologic and hormonal data explored in the marital disruption studies for (a) unhappily married persons, (b) divorced and separated persons, and (c) bereaved spouses. In your opinion, which of these disruptors has the most destructive and long-term health effects? What purpose may this information serve in the management of stress and health outcomes?

3. Summarize the psychologic and biomedical effects of caregiving for the patient with Alzheimer's disease. Compare these findings with the outcomes related to bereavement. How do they differ? How are they similar? Why do you think this is so? What implications do these findings have for health care outcomes?

4. Review the basic findings related to stress. If you were given unlimited funds to improve the overall health status of those in your community, what types of interventions would you implement, where would you implement them, and what outcomes would you expect? Consider all levels of your population (e.g., children, adults, older adults). Explain what consequences our society faces if it fails to successfully implement similar protective measures.

References

1. Ader R, Felten Dl, Cohen N, editors: *Psychoneuroimmunology,* ed 2, New York, 1991, Academic Press.
2. Anderson BL, Farrar WB, Golden-Kreutz D, Kutz LA, MacCallum R, Courtney ME, Glaser R: Stress and immune responses after surgical treatment for regional breast cancer, *J Natl Cancer Inst* 90:30, 1998.
3. Aronson M, Levin G, Lipkowitz R: A community-based family/patient care group program for Alzheimer's disease, *Gerontologist* 24:339, 1984.
4. Bartrop RW, Lazarus L, Luckhurst E, Kiloh LG, Penny R: Depressed lymphocyte function after bereavement, *Lancet* 16:834, 1977.
5. Baum A, Gatchel RJ, Schaeffer MA: Emotional, behavioral, and physiological effects of chronic stress at Three Mile Island, *J Consult Clin Psychol* 51(4):565, 1983.
6. Benson H, Frankel FH, Apfel R, Daniels MS, Schniedwind HE, Nemiah JC et al: Treatment of anxiety: a comparison of the usefulness of self-hypnosis and a meditation relaxation technique, *Psychother Psychosom* 30:229, 1978.
7. Berkman LF, Syme SL: Social networks, host resistance, and mortality: a nine-year follow-up study of Alameda County residents, *Am J Epidemiol* 109(2):186, 1979.
8. Bernstein H: An Alzheimer's family support group project, *J Jewish Communal Ser* 61:160, 1984.
9. Bloom BL, Asher SJ, White SW: Marital disruption as a stressor: a review and analysis, *Psychol Bull* 85(4):867, 1978.
10. Bourgeois MS, Schulz R, Burgio L: Interventions for caregivers of patients with Alzheimer's disease: a review and analysis of content, process and outcomes, *Int J Aging Hum Dev* 43(1):35, 1996.
11. Bovard EW: The balance between negative and positive brain system activity, *Perspect Biol Med* 6:116, 1962.
12. Bovard EW: Psychology: the effects of social stimuli on the response to stress, *Psychol Rev* 66:267, 1959.
13. Bowlby J: *Attachment and loss,* New York, 1975, Basic Books.
14. Brown P, Felton BJ, Whiteman V, Manela R: Attachment and distress following marital separation, *J Divorce* 3:303, 1980.
15. Burdz MP, Eaton WO, Bond JB: Effects of respite care of dementia and nondementia patients and their caregivers, *Psychol Aging* 3:38, 1988.
16. Carstensen LL, Levenson RW, Gottman JM: Emotional behavior in long-term marriage, *Psychol Aging* 10:140, 1995.
17. Case RB, Moss AJ, Case N, McDermott M, Eberly S: Living alone after myocardial infarction, *JAMA* 267(4):515, 1992.
18. Cobb S: Social support as a moderator of life stress, *Psychosom Med* 38(5):300, 1976.
19. Coyne JC, DeLongis A: Going beyond social support: the role of social relationships in adaptation, *J Consult Clin Psychol* 54:454, 1986.
20. Crook TH, Miller NE: The challenge of Alzheimer's disease, *Am Psychol* 40(11):1245, 1985.
21. Crossman L, London C, Barry C: Older women caring for disabled spouses. A model for supportive services, *Gerontologist* 21:464, 1981.
22. Davidson LM, Baum A: Chronic stress and posttraumatic stress disorders, *J Consult Clin Psychol* 54(3):303, 1986.
23. Davies H, Priddy JM, Tinklenberg JR: Support groups for male caregivers of Alzheimer's patients, *Clin Gerontologist* 5:385, 1986.
24. DeLongis A, Coyne JC, Dakof G, Folkman S, Lazarus RS: Relationship of daily hassles, uplifts, and major life events to health status, *Health Psychol* 1:119, 1982.
25. Edmondston WE: *Hypnosis and relaxation,* 1981, New York, John Wiley.
26. English EH, Baker TB: Relaxation training and cardiovascular response to experimental stressors, *Health Psychol* 2:239, 1983.
27. Esterling BA, Kiecolt-Glaser JK, Bodnar J et al: Chronic stress, social support, and persistent alterations in natural killer cell response to cytokines in older adults, *Health Psychol* 13:291, 1994.
28. Esterling BA, Kiecolt-Glaser JK, Glaser R: Psychosocial modulation of cytokine-induced natural killer cell activity in older adults, *Psychosom Med* 58:264, 1996.
29. Ferris S, Steinberg G, Shulman E, Kahn R, Reisberg B: Institutionalization of Alzheimer's disease patients: reducing precipitating factors through family counseling, *Home Health Care Serv Q* 8:23, 1987.
30. Fiore J, Becker J, Coppel DB: Social network interactions: a buffer or a stress? *Am J Community Psychol* 11(4):423, 1983.
31. Fischer CS: *To dwell among friends: personal networks in town and city,* Chicago, 1982, University of Chicago Press.
32. Fox M, Lithwick M: Groupwork with adult children of confused institutionalized adults, *Long Term Care Health Care Adm* 2:121, 1978.
33. Friedman M, Rosenman RH, Carroll V: Changes in serum cholesterol and blood-clotting time in men subjected to cyclic variation of occupational stress, *Circulation* 17:852, 1958.
34. Friedman SB, Ader R, Glasgow LA: Effects of psychologic stress in adult mice inoculated with Coxsackie B viruses, *Psychosom Med* 27:361, 1965.
35. Fuller J, Ward E, Evans A, Kay M, Gardner A: Dementia: supportive groups for relatives, *BMJ* 1:1684, 1979.
36. Gallagher-Thompson D, DeVries HM: Coping with frustration classes: development and preliminary outcomes with women who care for relatives with dementia, *Gerontologist* 34:548, 1994.
37. Gallagher-Thompson D, Steffen AM: Comparative effects of cognitive/behavioral and brief psychodynamic psychotherapies for the treatment of depression in family caregivers, *J Consult Clin Psychol* 62:543, 1994.
38. Gilleard CJ, Belford H, Gilleard E, Whittick JE, Gledhill K: Emotional distress amongst the supporters of the elderly mentally infirm, *Br J Psychiatry* 145:172, 1984.
39. Glaser R, Kiecolt-Glaser JK, Speicher CE, Holliday JE: Stress, loneliness, and changes in herpesvirus latency, *J Behav Med* 8(3):249, 1985.
40. Glaser R, Pearson GR, Bonneau RH, Esterling BA, Atkinson C, Kiecolt-Glaser JK: Stress and the memory T-cell response to the Epstein-Barr virus in healthy medical students, *Health Psychol* 12(6):435, 1993.
41. Glaser R, Rice J, Speicher CE, Stout JC, Kiecolt-Glaser JK: Stress depress interferon production by leukocytes concomitant with a decrease in natural killer cell activity, *Behav Neurosci* 100(5):675, 1986.
42. Glaser R, Thorn BE, Tarr KL, Kiecolt-Glaser JK, D'Ambrosio SV: Effects of stress on methyltransferase synthesis: an important DNA repair enzyme, *Health Psychol* 4(5):403, 1985.
43. Glosser G, Wexler D: Participants evaluation of education/support groups for families of patients with Alzheimer's disease and other dementias, *Gerontologist* 24:576, 1985.
44. Gove WR: Sex, marital status, and mortality, *Am J Sociol* 79:45, 1973.
45. Gove WR: Sex, marital status, and suicide, *J Health Soc Behav* 13:204, 1972.
46. Greene VL, Monahan DJ: The effect of a support and education program on stress and burden among family caregivers to frail elderly persons, *Gerontologist* 29:472, 1989.
47. Group for the Advancement of Psychiatry: *Treatment of families in conflict,* New York, 1970, Science House.
48. Grundy SM, Griffin AC: Effects of periodic mental stress on serum cholesterol levels, *Circulation* 14:496, 1959.
49. Gwyther L: Letting go: separation-individuation in a wife of an Alzheimer's patient, *Gerontologist* 30:698, 1990.

50. Haley WE: Group intervention for dementia family care-givers: a longitudinal perspective, *Gerontologist* 29:481, 1989.

51. Hartford ME, Parsons R: Groups with relatives of dependent older adults, *Gerontologist* 22:394, 1982.

52. Heckler MM: The fight against Alzheimer's disease, *Am Psychol* 40(11):1240, 1985.

53. Helphand M, Porter CM: The family group within the nursing home: maintaining family ties of long-term care residents, *J Gerontol Soc Work* 4:51, 1981.

54. Helsing KJ, Szklo M: Mortality after bereavement, *Am J Epidemiol* 114(1):41, 1981.

55. Helsing KJ, Szklo M, Comstock GW: Factors associated with mortality after widowhood, *Am J Public Health* 71:802, 1981.

56. Herberman RB: Possible effects of central nervous system on natural killer (NK) cell activity. In Levy SM, editor: *Biological mediators of health and disease: neoplasia,* New York, 1982, Reed Elsevier.

57. Herberman RB: Tumor immunology, *JAMA* 268:2935, 1992.

58. Herberman RB, Ortaldo JR: Natural killer cells: their roles in defenses against disease, *Science* 214:24, 1981.

59. Hersey P, Edwards A, Honeyman M, McCarthy WH: Low natural-killer-cell activity in familial melanoma patients and their relatives, *Br J Cancer* 40:113, 1979.

60. Heston LL, Mastri AR, Anderson VE, White J: Dementia of the Alzheimer type: clinical genetics, natural history, and associated conditions, *Arch Gen Psychiatry* 38:1085, 1981.

61. Holmes TH, Masuda M: Life change and illness susceptibility. In Dohrenwend BS, Dohrenwend BP, editors: *Stressful life events,* New York, 1974, John Wiley.

62. House JS, Landis KR, Umberson D: Social relationships and health, *Science* 241:540, 1988.

63. House JS, Robbins C, Metzner HL: The association of social relationships and activities with mortality: prospective evidence from the Tecumseh Community Health Study, *Am J Epidemiol* 116(1):123, 1982.

64. Jemmott JB, Borysenko JZ, Borysenko M et al: Academic stress, power motivation, and decrease in secretion rate of salivary secretory immunoglobulin A. *Lancet* 1:1400, 1983.

65. Jemmott JB, Borysenko M, Chapman R, Borysenko JZ, McClelland DC, Meyer D, Benson H: Academic stress, power motivation, and decrease in secretion rate of salivary secretory immunoglobulin A, *Lancet* 1(8339):1400, 1983.

66. Kanner AD, Coyne JC, Schaefer C, Lazarus RS: Comparison of two modes of stress measurement: daily hassles and uplifts versus major life events, *J Behav Med* 4:1, 1981.

67. Kaplan CP, Gallagher-Thompson D: The treatment of clinical depression in caregivers of spouses with dementia, *J Cogn Psychother Int Q* 9:35, 1995.

68. Kasl SV, Cobb S, Brooks GW: Changes in serum uric acid and cholesterol level in men undergoing job loss, *JAMA* 206:1500, 1968.

69. Kasl SV, Evans AS, Niederman JC: Psychosocial risk factors in the development of infectious mononucleosis, *Psychosom Med* 41:445, 1979.

70. Kemeny ME, Cohen F, Zegans LS, Conant MA: Psychologic and immunological predictors of genital herpes recurrence, *Psychosom Med* 51:195, 1989.

71. Kessler RC, McLeod JD: Social support and mental health in community samples. In Cohen S, Syme SL, editors: *Social support and health,* New York, 1985, Academic Press.

72. Kiecolt-Glaser JK: Immunological changes in Alzheimer caregivers. In Hall N, Altman F, Blumenthal S, editors: *Mind-body interactions and disease and psychoneuroimmunological aspects of health and disease. Proceedings of a conference on stress, immunity and health sponsored by the NIH,* Celebration, FL, 1996, Health Dateline Press.

73. Kiecolt-Glaser JK, Dura JR, Speicher CE, Trask OJ, Glaser R: Spousal caregivers of dementia victims: longitudinal changes in immunity and health, *Psychosom Med* 53:345, 1991.

74. Kiecolt-Glaser JK, Dura JR, Speicher CE, Trask OJ, Glaser R: Spousal caregivers of dementia victims: longitudinal changes in immunity and health, *Psychosom Med* 53:345, 1991.

75. Kiecolt-Glaser JK, Fisher LD, Ogrocki P, Stout JC, Speicher CE, Glaser R: Marital quality, marital disruption, and immune function, *Psychosom Med* 49(1):13, 1987.

76. Kiecolt-Glaser JK, Garner W, Speicher CE, Penn GM, Holliday J, Glaser R: Psychosocial modifiers of immunocompetence in medical students, *Psychosom Med* 46(1):7, 1984.

77. Kiecolt-Glaser JK, Garner W, Speicher CE, Penn GM, Holliday J, Glaser R: Psychosocial modifiers of immunocompetence in medical students, *Psychosom Med* 46:15, 1984.

78. Kiecolt-Glaser JK, Glaser R: Stress and immune function in humans. In Ader R, Felten D, Cohen N, editors: *Psychoneuroimmunology,* San Diego, 1991, Academic Press.

79. Kiecolt-Glaser JK, Glaser R, Gravenstein S, Malarkey WB, Sheridan J: Chronic stress alters the immune response in influenza virus vaccine in older adults, *Proc Natl Acad Sci U S A* 93:3043, 1996.

80. Kiecolt-Glaser JK, Glaser R, Gravenstein S, Malarkey WB, Sheridan J: Chronic stress alters the immune response in influenza virus vaccine in older adults, *Proc Natl Acad Sci U S A* 93:3043, 1996.

81. Kiecolt-Glaser JK, Glaser R, Shuttleworth EC, Dyer CS, Ogrocki P, Speicher CE: Chronic stress and immunity in family caregivers of Alzheimer's disease victims, *Psychosom Med* 49:523, 1987.

82. Kiecolt-Glaser JK, Glaser R, Strain EC, Stout JC, Tarr KL, Holliday JE, Speicher CE: Modulation of cellular immunity in medical students, *J Behav Med* 9(1):5, 1986.

83. Kiecolt-Glaser JK, Malarkey WB, Chee M, Newton T, Cacioppo JT, Mao H, Glaser R: Negative behavior during marital conflict is associated with immunological downregulation, *Psychosom Med* 55, 395, 1993.

84. Kiecolt-Glaser JK, Newton T, Cacioppo JT, MacCallum RC, Glaser R, Malarkey WB: Marital conflict and endocrine function: are men really more physiologically affected than women? *J Consult Clin Psychol* 64(2):324, 1996.

85. Kiecolt-Glaser JK, Ricker D, George J, Messick G, Slpeicher CE, Garner W, Glaser R: Urinary cortisol levels, cellular immunocompetency, and loneliness in psychiatric patients, *Psychosom Med* 46:15, 1984.

86. Kitson GC, Raschke HJ: What we know: what we need to know, *J Divorce* 4:1, 1981.

87. Knight BG, Lutzky SM, Macofsky-Urban F: A meta-analytic review of interventions for caregiver distress: recommendations for future research, *Gerontologist* 33:240, 1993.

88. Kroeger O, Thuesen JM: *Type talk: the 16 personality types that determine how we live, love, and work,* New York, 1988, Dell Publishing.

89. LaVorgna D: Group treatment for wives of patients with Alzheimer's disease, *Soc Work Health Care* 5:219, 1979.

90. Lawton MP, Brody EM, Saperstein AR: A controlled study of respite service for caregivers of Alzheimer's patients, *Gerontologist* 29:8, 1989.

91. Lehrer PM, Schoickett S, Carrington P, Woolfolk RL: Psychophysiological and cognitive responses to stressful stimuli in subjects practicing progressive relaxation and clinically standardized meditation, *Behav Res Ther* 18:293, 1980.

92. Levi L: Stress and distress in response to psychosocial stimuli: laboratory and real life studies on sympatho-adrenomedullary and related reactions, *Acta Med Scand Suppl* 528:1, 1972.

93. Light E, Lebowitz BD, editors: *Alzheimer's disease treatment and family stress: directions for research,* Rockville, MD, 1989, National Institute of Mental Health.
94. Lundervold D, Lewin LM: Effects of in-home respite are on caregivers of family members with Alzheimer's disease, *J Clin Exp Gerontol* 9:201, 1987.
95. Lynch J: The broken heart, New York, 1977, Basic Books.
96. Malarkey WB, Kiecolt-Glaser JK, Pearl D, Glaser R: Hostile behavior during marital conflict alters pituitary and adrenal hormones, *Psychosom Med* 56:41, 1994.
97. McKinnon W, Weisse CS, Reynolds CP et al: Chronic stress, leukocyte subpopulations, and humoral response to latent viruses, *Health Psychol* 8:389, 1989.
98. Mohide EA, Pringle DM, Streiner DL, Gilbert JR, Muir G, Tew M: A randomized trial of family caregiver support in the home management of dementia, *JAGS* 38:446, 1990.
99. Monjan AA, Collector MI: Stress-induced modulation of the immune response, *Science* 196:307, 1977.
100. Montgomery RJ, Borgatta EF: The effects of alternative support strategies on family caregiving, *Gerontologist* 29:457, 1989.
101. Nathan PK: Helping wives of Alzheimer's patients through group therapy, *Soc Work Groups* 9:73, 1986.
102. Oppenheim JJ, Roscetti FW, Faltynek C: Cytokines. In Stites DP, Terr AI, Parslow TG, editors: *Basic and clinical immunology,* Norwalk, Conn, 1994, Appleton & Lange.
103. Orth-Gomer K, Johnson JV: Social network interaction and mortality: a six year follow-up study of a random sample of the Swedish population. *J Chronic Dis* 40(10):949, 1987.
104. Pavlidis N, Chirigos M: Stress-induced impairment of macrophage tumoricidal function, *Psychosom Med* 42:47, 1980.
105. Rahe RH, Arthur RJ: Stressful underwater demolition training: serum uric rate and cholesterol variability, *JAMA* 202:1052, 1967.
106. Reever KE: Self-help groups for caregivers coping with Alzheimer's disease: the ACMA model, Pride Institute, *J Long Term Health Care* 3:23, 1984.
107. Reifler BV, Eisdorfer C: A clinic for the impaired elderly and their families, *Am J Psychiatry* 137:1399, 1980.
108. Reinherz EL, Schlossman SF: Current concepts in immunology: regulation of the immune response-inducer and suppressor T-lymphocyte subsets in human beings, *N Engl J Med* 303:370, 1980.
109. Renne KS: Health and marital experience in an urban population, *J Marriage Fam* 338, 1971.
110. Riley V: Mouse mammary tumors: alteration of incidence as apparent function of stress, *Science* 189:465, 1975.
111. Ritchie K, Ledesert B: The families of the institutionalized dementing elderly: a preliminary study of stress in a French caregiver population, *Int J Geriatr Psychiatry* 7:5, 1992.
112. Roozman-Weigensberg C, Fox M: A groupwork approach with adult children of institutionalized elderly: an investment in the future, *J Gerontol Soc Work* 2:355, 1980.
113. Rose RM: Overview of endocrinology of stress. In Brown GM, Kosllow SH, Reichlin S, editors: *Neuroendocrinology and psychiatric disorder,* New York, 1984, Raven Press.
114. Russell D, Cutrona CE, Rose J et al: Social and emotional loneliness: an examination of Weiss's typology of loneliness, *J Pers Soc Psychol* 46:1313, 1984.
115. Safford F: A program for the families of the mentally impaired elderly, *Gerontologist* 20:656, 1980.
116. Scharlach A, Frenzel C: An evaluation of institution-based respite care, *Gerontologist* 26:77, 1986.
117. Schleifer SJ, Keller SE, Camerino M, Thornton JC, Stein M: Suppression of lymphocyte stimulation following bereavement, *JAMA* 250(3):374, 1983.
118. Schmidt GL, Bonjean JJ, Widem AC, Schefft BK, Steele DJ: Brief psychotherapy for caregivers of demented relatives: comparison of two therapeutic strategies, *Clin Gerontologist* 7:109, 1988.
119. Schmidt GL, Keyes B: Group psychotherapy with family caregivers of demented patients, *Gerontologist* 25:347, 1985.
120. Schoenbach VJ, Kaplan BH, Fredman L, Kleinbaum DG: Social ties and mortality in Evans County, Georgia, *Am J Epidemiol* 123(4):577, 1986.
121. Scradle SB, Dougher MJ: Social support as a mediator of stress: theoretical and empirical issues, *Clin Psychol Rev* 5:641, 1985.
122. Seltzer MM, Ivry J, Litchfield LC: Family members as case managers: partnership between the formal and informal support networks, *Gerontologist* 27:722, 1987.
123. Silva A, Bonavide B, Targa S: Mode of action of interferon-mediated modulation of natural killer cytotoxic activity: recruitment of pre-NK and enhanced kinetics of lysis, *J Immunol* 125:479, 1980.
124. Simank MH, Strictland KJ: Assisting families in coping with Alzheimer's disease and other related dementias with the establishment of a mutual support group, *J Gerontol Soc Work* 9:49, 1986.
125. Sklar LS, Anisman H: Stress and coping factors influence tumor growth, *Science* 205:513, 1979.
126. Somers AR: Marital status, health and the use of health services, *JAMA* 241:1818, 1979.
127. Spector NH: Can hypothalamic lesions change circulating antibody or interferon responses to antigens. In Chernukh AM, Pytskii VI, editors: *The pathogenesis of allergic processes in experiment and in the clinic,* Moscow, 1979, Meditsina.
128. Sternberg EM, Chrousos GP, Wilder RL, Gold PW: The stress response and the regulation of inflammatory disease, *Ann Intern Med* 117:854, 1992.
129. Sullivan JL, Hanshaw JB: Human cytomegalovirus infections. In Glaser R, Gottlieb-Stematsky T, editors: *Human herpesvirus infections: clinical aspects,* New York, 1982, Marcel Dekker.
130. Thomas PD, Goodwin JM, Goodwin JS: Effect of social support on stress-related changes in cholesterol level, uric acid level, and immune function in an elderly sample, *Am J Psychiatry* 142(6):735, 1985.
131. Toseland RW, Rossiter CM, Peak T, Smith GC: Comparative effectiveness of individual and group interventions to support family caregivers, *Soc Work* 35:209, 1990.
132. Toseland RW, Smith GC: Effectiveness of individual counseling by professional and peer helpers for family caregivers of the elderly, *Psychol Aging* 5:256, 1990.
133. Verbrugge LM: Marital status and health, *J Marriage Fam* 41:267, 1979.
134. Wallerstein JS, Kelly JB: *Surviving the breakup: how children and parents cope with divorce,* New York, 1980, Basic Books.
135. Weiss RS: *Marital separation,* New York, 1975, Basic Books.
136. Welin L, Tibblin G, Svardsudd K, Tibblin B, Ander-Peciva S, Larsson B, Wilhelmsen L: Prospective study of social influences on mortality: the study of men born in 1913 and 1923, *Lancet* 915, 1985.
137. Whiteside TL, Herberman RB: Characteristics of natural killer cells and lymphocyte-activated killer cells, *Immunol Allergy Clin North Am* 10:663, 1990.
138. Wilson JD, Braunwalk E, Isselbacher KJ et al, editors: *Harrison's principles of internal medicine,* ed 12, New York, 1991, McGraw-Hill.
139. Zarit S, Teri L: Interventions and services for family caregivers. In Schaie KW, Lawton P, editors: *Annual review of gerontology and geriatrics,* vol 11, New York, 1992, Springer.

Mind-Body
Interventions

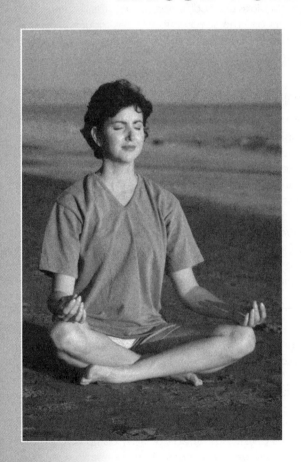

5

Relaxation Therapy

Lyn W. Freeman

WHY READ THIS CHAPTER?

We live in a highly stressful culture that has contributed to the development or exacerbation of stress-related illnesses. Stress-related diseases include cardiovascular disease, hypertension, gastrointestinal disorders, anxiety, and depression. When stressed, we also experience pain more intensely because we block our body's natural opioids. Learning to relax on command can reduce the destructive effects and the symptoms of stress-induced illnesses and improve the quality of life. This chapter describes the somatic methods of deep relaxation that were originally developed as medical interventions.

CHAPTER AT A GLANCE

In 1905, Edmund Jacobson discovered that being very relaxed hindered the elicitation of the startle reaction, which is the sudden jerking reaction to loud noises. His discovery proved to be the first systematic study of the effects of relaxation on the body. In 1938, Jacobson further noted that chronic sustained tension of skeletal muscles increased the amplitude of reflexive responses while decreasing their latency. Jacobson eventually concluded that detailed observation and introspection of the body's kinesthetic sensations and the mental processes accompanying them were necessities for accomplishing complete relaxation.

Jacobson developed a systematic method for relaxing all the muscles of the body. This somatic relaxation method, called **Jacobson's Progressive Relaxation Therapy** (JPRT), was very time consuming, often requiring 100 or more practice sessions to master. Students targeted one major group of muscles at a time, learning to recognize—more and more—subtle tension cues and relax them away.

Because the time commitment was not palatable for most persons in need of training, Joseph Wolpe developed a method called **Abbreviated Progressive Relaxation Training** (APRT), which focused on relaxing several muscle groups simultaneously during one session. Wolpe's method allowed practitioners to become reasonably proficient at relaxation in as few as ten training sessions.

In opposition to the teachings of Jacobson, Wolpe taught students to tense muscles and then relax them, as opposed to simply observing existing tension and then relaxing it away. Other researchers eventually developed more abbreviated methods of their own that varied in application, sometimes adding strong cognitive components to the relaxation protocol.

Research on the physiologic effects of APRT demonstrated that relaxation practice blunted the excitatory autonomic changes experienced in response to everyday life events. APRT accomplished this effect by modulating both arms of the autonomic cardiovascular control systems (i.e., sympathetic and vagal). Relaxation also induced the release of endogenous opioids. These opioids are partially responsible for the reduction of circulatory stress reactivity that occurs in response to relaxation practice. The practice of relaxation was discovered to improve immune competence, especially in older populations, who often experience a loss of immune function.

APRT has been effectively used as an intervention for a variety of medical conditions, including chemotherapy-induced nausea and vomiting, hypertension, pain control, mood state management, and epilepsy.

CHAPTER OBJECTIVES

After completing this chapter, you should be able to:

1. Describe how JPRT was developed.
2. Explain in detail the philosophy underlying Jacobson's method.
3. Describe Wolpe's APRT method.
4. Compare and contrast the methods of Jacobson and Wolpe, and outline the strengths and weaknesses of both methods.
5. Summarize the effects of relaxation on autonomic response and immune function.
6. Summarize the findings of APRT as an intervention for chemotherapy-induced nausea and vomiting.
7. Summarize the findings of APRT as an intervention for hypertension.
8. Compare and contrast the effectiveness of relaxation therapy for the various forms of pain reviewed in this chapter.
9. Outline the indications for using JPRT and APRT.
10. Outline the contraindications for using JPRT and APRT.
11. Describe the limitations of the relaxation studies.

■ History of Relaxation Therapy

In this chapter, we review the development and current use of relaxation techniques typically referred to as somatic relaxation methods. Other relaxation techniques, essentially considered to be cognitive in nature, are reviewed in Chapter 6. *Somatic relaxation* refers to a method that emphasizes muscle relaxation through detailed observation and introspection of the body's kinesthetic sensations (i.e., purposeful relaxation of the muscles). *Cognitive relaxation* refers to the use of a mental device (e.g., word, thought, sound, breathing) and the practice of a passive or non-judgmental attitude to induce relaxation in the mind and body. In this chapter we discuss two somatic relaxation methods, JPRT and APRT. JPRT is a systematic but lengthy method of becoming aware of and relaxing all the muscles in the body. APRT is a shortened version of JPRT and differs from JPRT in its basic principles of application.

■ Jacobson's Progressive Relaxation Therapy

In 1905, Edmund Jacobson, the originator of JPRT, entered graduate school at Harvard. He had no idea that a seemingly negative educational event would provide an opportunity that would shape the rest of his life.

At Harvard, Jacobson was a research assistant to Hugo Munsterberg, a professor who was considered to be one of the great minds of the day. Munsterberg became unhappy when data collected by Jacobson supported theories in opposition to Munsterberg's own hypotheses. Munsterberg summarily discharged Jacobson. With time on his hands, Jacobson turned to the study of the startle response, a sudden jerking or startle reaction that naturally occurs in response to unexpected loud noises. He discovered that deeply relaxed students demonstrated no obvious startle response to a sudden noise. Jacobson's discovery proved to be the first systematic study of the effects of relaxation on the body and eventually led to the birth of JPRT as an intervention.[32]

While working at the University of Chicago, Jacobson found that the amplitude (strength) of knee-jerk reflexes varied with the tenseness of the patient. As patients practiced relaxation, knee-jerk reflexes decreased. Research performed by Jacobson in 1938 demonstrated that chronic, sustained tension (tonus) of skeletal muscles increased the amplitude of reflexes while decreasing their latency.[33] Relaxation produced the opposite effects.

With the aid of other scientists, Jacobson was able to develop a method to measure this tension in more direct terms. He was able to record electrical muscle action potentials in a unit as little as a microvolt. This was the first use of quantitative electromyography (EMG) in research. With objective measures to assist him, Jacobson then devoted himself to the further development and validation of JPRT.

■ Philosophy of Progressive Muscle Relaxation Therapy

Jacobson would eventually conclude that (1) detailed observation and introspection of the body's kinesthetic sensations and the mental processes that accompany them were necessities if one were to accomplish complete relaxation; and (2) localized body tensions occur as meaningful acts that originate in one's imagination and thoughts. For example, just the thought of moving a limb produces measurable EMG responses in that limb.

Jacobson concluded that all thought is followed by musculoskeletal activity, even though the response amplitude may be nearly undetectable. Conversely, mental processes diminish or disappear as muscle relaxation reaches its maximum levels. In other words, although we may not "think" with our muscles, our muscles are involved in the thinking process. Jacobson believed cognitive activities were identical to the energies expended when neuromuscular circuits resonate. Therefore if neuromuscular circuits become completely relaxed (i.e., are silenced), then cognitive activity will also be silenced.

Jacobson argued that it was impossible to experience emotion while being totally relaxed. Thus the key to developing emotional control, he believed, was to learn progressive relaxation. Relax the muscles, which embodies an undesired emotion, he instructed, and the emotion can be contained or eliminated. This embodiment of the mind and emotions in the musculature was an essential part of Jacobson's teachings. Tension was the "process" by which the emotions were embodied; the purpose of the tension was the "meaning." The two concepts—the tension process and the purpose of the tension—became the foundation of his future relaxation research. For the next 70 years, Jacobson tested his basic concepts and the foundational principle—to relax the mind and body, one must relax all skeletal musculature.

Jacobson believed that to remain healthy, a person must develop habits of effective rest. If these habits were learned and practiced, tension maladies could be avoided and bodily energy would be used more efficiently. He noted that normally a startle response (i.e., a fight-or-flight effect) results in persons hunching forward, rising to the balls of their feet, and preparing for battle.[14] This startle reaction naturally elicits a cascade of autonomic and endocrine responses that help the person survive. However, if this condition becomes chronic and if relaxation fails to follow, a continued state of hyperactivity occurs in the body that can result in pathologic abnormalities. Successful application of progressive muscle relaxation returns the body to a healthier state. Accomplishing progressive relaxation meant literally getting in touch with and learning to control the tension levels in all the striated muscles in the body.

■ Mechanisms of Relaxation

Jacobson's Progressive Relaxation Therapy

To practice the method known as JPRT, a person learns to identify very sensitive sensory observations of what occurs beneath the skin. This is considered a form of physiologic introspection. Whereas *tension* is a contraction of muscle fibers that elicit a tension sensation, *relaxation* is the lengthening of those fibers that then eliminates the tension sensation. The process of observing the tension, relaxing it away, and observing the difference in a muscle before and after relaxation is then systematically applied to all major muscle groups. With practice, one can "fine tune" the ability to recognize sensory tension signals and then, at will, to relax away any tension not desirable in the body. The final goal of JPRT is to develop what is known as *automaticity*—a state where one automatically and unconsciously monitors and eliminates unwanted bodily tensions.[48]

Learning progressive relaxation involves detecting the faintest of tension signals. Often one starts with obvious signals, such as raising the hand at a 90-degree angle. Then, the person experiences the effects of tension in the forearm and carefully observes and notes the sensations. The person then moves on to more subtle tension cues, such as raising the hand to a 45-degree angle, then to a 20-degree angle, and so on. When the student is proficient at this practice, he or she can identify a tension signal of perhaps one–one thousandth (1/1000), the intensity of the signal experienced in the first exercise. This level of signaling is common in muscles of the tongue and eyes. Requesting an individual to generate and experience high intensity tension is, Jacobson believed, counterproductive since the purpose of

JPRT is to learn control of more and more subtle tension points. Therefore no purposeful tensing of muscles should occur while practicing JPRT.

JPRT is quite different from hypnosis because practitioners avoid the use of suggestion, that is, telling students their muscles are getting heavy or warm. Jacobson was careful to note that he intended students to learn physiologic control leading to changes in the body different from those that occur in response to suggestion.[5,33] He believed that suggestion could lead the person to believe relaxation had occurred when, in fact, it had not. Others have pointed out that the words relaxation *exercise* or *relaxation response* are inappropriate in the context of Jacobsonian progressive relaxation. JPRT was intended to be delivered in a scientific and clinical context, and since relaxation is the opposite of work, the terms *exercise* and *response* are contradictory to the intended outcome. One cannot make an *effort to relax, because effort guarantees failure.*[48]

Initially, the required time investment to learn JPRT seemed extreme to many. For example, practicing in one position might take as long as 3 hours. Jacobson eventually shortened his methods to allow practice of three positions in 1 hour. However, he felt there were no true shortcuts to learning to relax a body that had been in a state of tension for decades. Because of the time commitment of Jacobson's sessions, experimental and controlled trials that have remained true to his original method are virtually nonexistent. A review of the literature reveals that when the term *progressive relaxation* is applied to a relaxation method, the process has typically been shortened to such an extent that it is often contradictory to Jacobson's intent of intense observation and introspection. In other cases, the process has been confused with hypnotic procedures or lumped in with other interventional forms so that no conclusions can be drawn from the outcomes as they relate to the original JPRT.[50,57] There is, however, a body of experimental literature using APRT, and there are clinical, uncontrolled studies of the effectiveness of JPRT.

Learning Jacobson's Progressive Relaxation Method

To learn JPRT, the skeletal muscles in the body are studied in progressive groups. First, the muscles in the arms are studied, and then the legs, followed by the trunk, neck, and eye region, and finally, the all-important speech muscles, are studied. Each of the major muscle groups is broken down into localized groups. For example, there are six localized muscle groups in the arm.

Sessions are started by lying down, and typically only one position is practiced during each hour session; each position is repeated three times. For example, the first practice position entails bending the hand back at the wrist to produce tension in the upper surface of the forearm. This tension is carefully sensed and studied as the student holds this position for 2 minutes or more. Then the student is instructed to let the "power go off," and total letting go occurs. The tension felt is called a *control signal,* and this is what the practitioner learns to recognize so that the opposite, complete relaxation, can be experienced. In each session, the practitioner recognizes a control signal and then relaxes it away. For a typical second session, the student practices bending the left hand forward rather than backward. The entire practice sequence consists of the following:

Left arm	7 days
Right arm	7 days
Left leg	10 days
Right leg	10 days
Trunk	10 days
Neck	6 days
Eye region	12 days
Visualization	9 days
Speech region and speech imagery	19 days
TOTAL:	**90 days**

After all of these positions are practiced lying down, they are repeated and practiced sitting up. The time commitment is extensive. The original course frequently required 100 or more sessions for the practitioner to become proficient, and took from several months to several years to master.

Wolpe's Abbreviated Progressive Relaxation Training

Many individuals found it impossible to make the time commitment required for the full JPRT technique. For this and other reasons, APRT was developed by Joseph Wolpe. He designed this condensed version as part of his counter-conditioning methods for fear reduction.[65]

Wolpe viewed relaxation as valuable in a slightly different context than did Jacobson. He saw relaxation as but only one of many responses that are capable of inhibiting anxiety. He shortened Jacobson's method and inserted it into a framework called *systematic desensitization.* Systematic desensitization refers to a process whereby patients, while in a state of deep relaxation, are exposed to stimuli that historically induced anxiety or fear. Since relaxation is incompatible with anxiety, patients desensitized their anxiety and fear responses.

Whereas Jacobson's program focused on only a single muscle group for several sessions, Wolpe taught patients to relax several of the sixteen major muscle groups each session, completing the training process in ten or fewer sessions. Unlike Jacobson, Wolpe thought that suggestion and instructions were a necessary part of the relaxation process. During the 1960s and 1970s, Wolpe's methods were modified by others, making the training requirements even shorter and, in some cases, working all sixteen major muscle groups in one session. In contradiction to Jacobson's methods, instructions regarding strong tensing (e.g., make a tight fist) followed by sudden release of tension were included as part of the relaxation instructions. Strong tensing and letting go is called a *tension-release cycle.*[8] In some instances, relaxation imagery was also introduced into the sessions.[6,17]

Proponents of APRT acknowledge that their methods are not unique, but they are simply one of many that can induce relaxation (e.g., biofeedback, autogenic training, meditation). The choice of APRT is based on its adaptability and its convenience for patient and therapist. In the research literature, when the phrase "progressive relaxation" is used, it typically refers to one of the abbreviated versions that are offshoots of Jacobson's original model.

Following an Abbreviated Progressive Relaxation Format

In the first three sessions of a typical APRT session, practitioners strive to achieve deep relaxation by tensing and relaxing all 16 muscle groups. When this is achieved, a shorter procedure, using seven muscle groupings, is used to accomplish deep relaxation. Clients then move on to an even shorter method that uses four muscle groups to achieve deep relaxation. In essence, although all muscles are fully relaxed in all sessions, the practitioner learns to relax more and more groupings of muscles simultaneously. At the four-muscle-group level, relaxation can be accomplished in 10 minutes or less.

After 10 minutes of relaxation is accomplished, releasing tension by recall is employed. In this procedure, the client becomes capable of complete relaxation without the use of muscle tensing. The client is capable of inducing complete relaxation by recalling the sensations associated with the release of tension. This allows the client to induce relaxation, at will, at any point throughout a busy day. The final step in APRT is recall with counting. At this stage, the client should achieve such muscular control as to induce complete relaxation by simply counting from 1 to 10.

Although an exact timetable for training will vary, depending on the APRT practitioner and client progress, the following ideal case scenario was suggested by Bernstein and Borkovec, the method most consistently used in the APRT research literature.[7]

Method	Session
16 muscle groups, tension-release	Sessions 1,2,3
7 muscle groups, tension-release	Sessions 4,5
4 muscle groups, tension-release	Sessions 6,7
4 muscle groups, recall	Session 8
4 muscle groups, recall and counting	Session 9
Counting	Session 10

■ How Progressive Relaxation Benefits Health

You may wonder how the process of progressive relaxation actually conveys health benefits. Essentially, benefits are bestowed in three ways: (1) modulating affects of relaxation on autonomic responses, (2) increased opioid responsivity, and (3) support for optimal immune function. First, we examine the effects of relaxation on the cardiovascular system.

During the day, periods of rest are typically interspersed with periods of moderate physical (e.g., eating, moving, standing) and mental or emotional arousal activities. A sympathetic cardiovascular response has previously been shown to contribute to *myocardial ischemia* (i.e., reduced flow of blood to the heart muscle) in persons so predisposed. Prior research had found that mental activities are as likely to trigger a cardiac event as mild physical activity.[23]

In one groundbreaking study, the authors wanted to determine whether relaxation therapy had the potential for protecting those at risk of cardiac events by reducing the sympathetic response throughout the day. However, since various disease states alter autonomic response, researchers decided it would be wise to first test healthy students to see whether their autonomic responses could be buffered.

Effects of Progressive Relaxation on Autonomic Excitatory Response In Human Subjects

Purpose and Hypothesis

The purpose of the study was to assess the effects of a 3-month APRT and breath-training program on autonomic responses in healthy subjects unaffected by confounding disease states.[41] Autonomic pathways carry information to the autonomic or visceral effectors, which are the smooth muscles, cardiac muscle, and glands (Figure 5-1). There was no stated hypothesis.

Method

Three groups were assessed: (1) subjects trained for 3 months in APRT relaxation and breathing techniques (N=13); (2) subjects who received sham training for 3 months (N=12); and (3) subjects who received a 4-day treatment of β-adrenergic blockers, drugs known to blunt sympathetic drive (N=12).

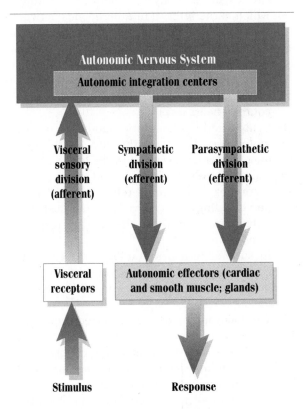

■ *Figure* 5-1. **Autonomic Nervous System.** In the autonomic nervous system, visceral sensory pathways conduct information toward central nervous system integrators, whereas the sympathetic and parasympathetic pathways conduct information toward autonomic effectors. *Modified from Thibodeau GA, Patton KT:* Anatomy and physiology, *ed 4, St Louis, 1999, Mosby.*

■ The relaxation-training group was structured in weekly group meetings, which included teaching, discussions, and practice sessions. The practice sessions emphasized muscle relaxation and breathing exercises. The students were then asked to practice relaxation at home for 30 to 60 minutes per day.

■ The sham group was given instructions on behavioral health and asked to rest for 30 to 60 minutes per day while reading or listening to music.

■ The beta-blocker group received 50 mg of atenolol once daily, a drug that alters β-adrenergic receptor–mediated mechanisms. This dosage is considered to be a small one, but it is significant enough to induce a 25% reduction in resting heart rate.

Subjects were assessed in the laboratory before and 3 months after training and intervention. During assessment, an electrocardiogram (ECG) was recorded continuously, as was respiration and arterial pressure.

Cross-spectral analysis of both the RR interval, which is the interval in milliseconds between two successive ECG complexes, and variability of systolic arterial pressure (SAP) provided the following quantitative markers:

■ Sympathetic-vagal balance modulating the sinoatrial node of the heart (the vagus nerve controls heart rate)

■ Sympathetic vasomotor modulation (the motor nerves activate the muscles that produce movement, such as in the legs)

■ Gain of arterial pressure and heart period baroreflex index α (a reflex stimulated by nerve endings in the auricles of the heart that reduce pressure within the heart in response to pressure)

In simpler terms, the ability to affect heart rate, the activation of muscles, and the pressure-balance controls in the heart were all being monitored.

The following recordings occurred sequentially: reclining baseline for 10 minutes; active unaided standing for 7 minutes; another reclining break; and finally, mental arithmetic exercises for 7 minutes. The mental arithmetic exercises consisted of subtracting two-digit numbers from four digit numbers as fast as possible. Both standing and arithmetic exercises were used to excite cardiovascular responses with different mechanisms. Standing produces sympathetic activity by arterial baroreceptor uploading, whereas the arithmetic stressor acts by modifying "central command" processes.

Outcomes

Higher heart rate and arterial pressure were induced by both standing and arithmetic exercises. Using cross-spectral analysis of RR interval and SAP variability, the authors found that both beta-blocker drugs and 3 months of relaxation training significantly reduced sympathetic excitation in response to simple physical (standing) and mental (arithmetic) laboratory stressors. These stressors were chosen because they represented common everyday occurrences. Simultaneously, measurements of baroreflex gain and vagal modulation were increased. No changes occurred as a result of sham training.

Conclusions and Comments

Frequency domain analysis of cardiovascular variability indicated that relaxation training significantly blunted the excitatory autonomic changes produced by common everyday activities. This study provided direct evidence that relaxation training can modulate both arms of autonomic cardiovascular control (sympathetic and vagal-parasympathetic). The sympathetic system evokes the "fight-or-flight" response; and the vagus cranial nerve affects organ sensation and movement, and most of its motor fibers are parasympathetic. After relaxation training, markers indicated a less intense modulation during both physical and mental stimulation than was observed before training alone. It must be noted that chronic treatment with β-adrenergic blocker drugs still produced a more potent effect than relaxation training.

Relaxation Therapy and Opioid Responsivity

Most of the research on relaxation therapy has focused on its ability to blunt the drive of the sympathetic nervous system. Although these mechanisms are important during stress, recent work has suggested that endogenous opioids may also be important players in modulating stress responses.[42] Endogenous opioid peptides can counter-regulate neurohormones released during intense stress and limit the action of visceral excitatory mechanisms.

Opioids, (endorphins and enkephalins) make up a complex system of neurotransmitters and hormones. These substances bind to multiple receptor subtypes. Research has demonstrated a diminished opioid inhibition of stress reactions in monkeys at risk for coronary heart disease, in young adults with mildly elevated blood pressure (BP), and in persons with low levels of aerobic fitness.[43-45] These and other studies have led to hypotheses that behavioral enhancement of opioid responsiveness that may occur in relaxation therapy can have potentially important therapeutic or preventative effects for stress-induced circulatory disorders.

In response to these hypotheses, a study tracked the effects of relaxation practice on endogenous opioids.[46] McCubbin and colleagues recruited 32 young men with mildly elevated arterial BP for placebo-controlled naltrexone stress tests and relaxation training. Naltrexone is a drug that blocks opioid receptors.

The subjects practiced a 25-minute APRT relaxation procedure just before exposure to a laboratory stressor. The relaxation procedure significantly reduced the diastolic BP response to mental arithmetic stress tests of constantly escalating difficulty. By contrast, opioid receptor blockage with naltrexone reversed the protective effects of the relaxation procedure. These outcomes suggested that relaxation is accompanied by a release of endogenous opioids and that these opioids are at least partially responsible for the relaxation-induced reduction of circulatory stress reactivity, in this case, diastolic BP.

Relaxation Therapy and Strengthening Immune Function in an Aging Population

We have seen that relaxation training has the potential to modulate sympathetic drive and opioid pathways in response to stressors. Can relaxation also have implications for the health of the immune system? Kiecolt-Glaser wanted to know whether relaxation therapy would enhance immunity in a population known to be at risk for immune impairment. As we grow older, our immune systems become less competent. Therefore testing the effect of relaxation on the older adult would provide valuable data for potentially improving immunocompetence in this population. Since "baby boomers" are entering this category at an ever-increasing number, methods for enhancing immunity in the older adult would be a valuable tool for health care management and for containment of health care dollars (Figure 5-2).

Purpose
The purpose of the Kiecolt-Glaser study was to assess the effects of relaxation training and social contact on immunocompetence in geriatric residents of independent-living facilities.[37]

Hypothesis
Relaxation training and social contact will produce significant increases in natural killer (NK)

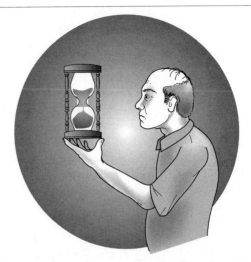

■ *Figure 5-2. Relaxation and immune function in the older population.* Relaxation training has been demonstrated to improve immune competence in the older population. Most specifically, improved natural killer cell function was demonstrated, an immune parameter that is particularly important since natural killer cells provide antitumor and antiviral functions. Natural killer competence typically declines with age.

cell activity and mitogen responsiveness and significant decreases in herpes simplex virus (HSV) antibody titers after intervention. Changes will persist only in the relaxation group.

Method
Forty-five older adults, average age of 74, were randomly assigned (1) APRT training conducted by a trained medical or graduate student; (2) social contact with an undergraduate student selected for his or her social skills, during which the older adult and student discussed whatever they wished; or (3) no contact. The older adults randomized to the relaxation and social contact groups were seen for 45 minutes, three times a week for 1 month. Self-report data and blood samples were obtained before the study, after 1 month of intervention, and 1 month after completion of the study.

Outcomes
■ The Hopkins Symptom Checklist (HSCL) assessed psychologic symptoms of distress (e.g., depression, anxiety, somatization, obsessive-compulsive symptoms, interpersonal sensitivity) and a total distress score. When baseline scores were compared with postintervention and follow-up scores, the relaxation group demonstrated a significant drop in psychologic distress ($p < 0.05$ and $p < 0.05$, respectively).

- The Life Satisfaction, the UCLA Loneliness Scale, and the Desired Control Interview, were administered before and after intervention. The Life Satisfaction Index-Z measures morale or life satisfaction in geriatric populations. The UCLA Loneliness Scale assesses the effects of interpersonal contact or lack of contact. The Desired Control Interview provides information on geriatric patients' perceptions of environmental constraints or loss of control. No significant differences were found between the groups or in groups before to after intervention on any of these assessments.
- NK cell target/effector ratio demonstrated significant changes in the relaxation group (p<0.05) but not in the social contact or no-contact groups.
- Similar significant interactions were found between group memberships and change over trials in the HSV antibody data (p<0.05).

Conclusions and Comments

- The data, demonstrating that relaxation training produced significant increases in NK cell

target/effector ratio and a decrease in HSV antibody titers and improved immune function, strongly suggest that relaxation training can increase immune competence in the older adult. The improved NK cell function is particularly important since NK cells provide antitumor and antiviral functions.
- The authors did not find consistent significant change associated with the social contact intervention, even though other studies have suggested that social contact improves immune function. However, the importance of the relationship may be the decisive factor of whether benefit is conveyed. Undergraduate students may not have provided an emotionally meaningful interaction for the older adults in this study.
- It is of interest that although the relaxation group did not report significant changes in feelings of control, life satisfaction, or loneliness, an immunologic benefit was still conveyed from relaxation practice.

■ Application of Relaxation Therapy as Medical Intervention

Progressive relaxation training has been used as a medical intervention for a variety of conditions. These include: (1) chemotherapy-induced nausea and vomiting; (2) hypertension; (3) pain control; (4) mood state management; and (5) epilepsy. In the following text, we review the effectiveness of relaxation therapy as treatment for these conditions.

Relaxation Therapy and Chemotherapy-Induced Nausea and Vomiting

Patients with cancer receiving chemotherapy often experience unpleasant side effects that compromise their quality of life. Symptoms may become so severe that physicians resort to suboptimal drug dosages, rather than have patients discontinue treatment altogether. Relaxation therapy has been used as a modulating intervention for the physiologic symptoms of nausea and vomiting and the psychologic symptoms of anxiety and depression accompanying chemotherapy. APRT methods, with the addition of guided imagery, have typically been the intervention of choice (Figure 5-3).

Over a 10-year period, Burish, Lyles, and others conducted a series of research projects at Vanderbilt University on chemotherapy-induced nausea and vomiting. In 1992, Burish and Tope performed a synthesis and review of a decade of this work.[12] They found that conditioned side effects related to chemotherapy are developed as a form

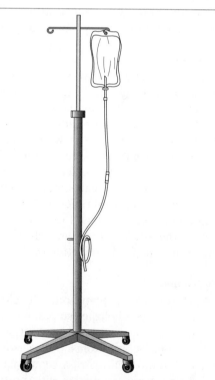

■ *Figure 5-3.* **Chemotherapy, nausea, and relaxation therapy.** Relaxation therapy has been used as a modulation intervention for the physiologic symptoms of nausea and vomiting and the psychologic symptoms of anxiety and depression accompanying chemotherapy.

of associative learning and that the environment and the anxiety associated with chemotherapy can become conditioning cues. They arrived at four basic conclusions:

1. Progressive muscle relaxation therapy can be effective in reducing the distress of chemotherapy, including conditioned nausea and vomiting, negative effect, and physiologic arousal.

2. If taught before chemotherapy begins, progressive muscle relaxation can prevent or significantly delay the onset of conditioned symptoms. Strongest results were obtained when the intervention was administered before the start of chemotherapy.

3. Other approaches, such as preparation training before chemotherapy begins and simple distraction techniques, can also help alleviate symptoms. For some patients or for practical reasons related to treatment, these techniques may be required in addition to or instead of relaxation therapy.

4. Although the results of research are generally positive, no single relaxation treatment appears to work uniformly for all patients.

In a follow-up self-report study, Burish and others sent anonymous questionnaires to 58 patients with cancer who had been taught progressive muscle relaxation as an intervention for reducing the side effects of chemotherapy. Of the 68% who responded, 65% reported that they continued to practice progressive relaxation after chemotherapy had ended and reported that they used APRT for a wide variety of stress-related problems.[13]

Progressive muscle relaxation had its limitations, however. It did not work for all patients and did not alleviate pharmacologically induced side effects. Overall, it was effective as an adjunct to antiemetic (antinausea) medications. Some antiemetic medications compromised patient ability to learn and practice progressive muscle relaxation, because they interfered with patient alertness or ability to concentrate and focus.

Apparently, high levels of anxiety also interfered with the patients' abilities to learn and perform APRT. This suggested that patients receiving chemotherapy who perhaps had the greatest need for an effective intervention might be the least likely to benefit from it. Highly anxious patients required more time, practice, and training effort to learn and use the method effectively. EMG tracings and thermal biofeedback was used as methods for improving the effectiveness of relaxation therapy. Although they reduced some measurements of physiologic arousal, they did not ameliorate other measurements of stress. Generally, biofeedback alone was not effective in reducing the conditioned side effects of chemotherapy.[12]

Patients had to desire to learn APRT for the method to be effective, and patient desire for control was a positive indicator that APRT would be applied and would help alleviate chemotherapy side effects. Further, if a spouse learned relaxation with the patient, progressive relaxation was practiced more often, resulting in optimal benefits for both patient and spouse. Researchers were particularly interested to find that many patients continued to use progressive muscle relaxation after chemotherapy. This was an important finding since it was often a challenge for researchers to motivate patients to continue practice after chemotherapy had ended. This was based on self-report information, however, and patients may have over reported their practice levels (Table 5-1).

Relaxation Therapy and Hypertension

The Joint National Committee (JNC) on Detection, Evaluation, and Treatment of High Blood Pressure determined that a diagnosis of hypertension is confirmed when diastolic BP is consistently 90 mm Hg or higher.[36] As determined by this definition, approximately 25% of American adults have hypertension. Approximately 70% of these are categorized as having mild essential hypertension, with diastolic BP averaging 90 mm Hg to 104 mm Hg (Figure 5-4). Over the past 30 years, numerous reports have demonstrated that relax-

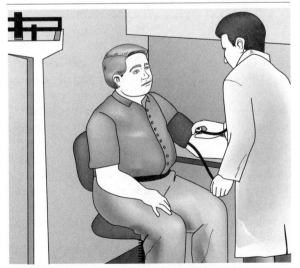

▪ *Figure 5-4. Relaxation therapy and hypertension.* Over the past 30 years, numerous reports have demonstrated that relaxation training can decrease blood pressure in hypertensive patients.

TABLE 5-1	Effects of Progressive Relaxation on Chemotherapy-Induced Nausea and Anxiety	
AUTHOR(S)	**DESIGN**	**FINDINGS**
Burish TG, Lyles JN: Effectiveness of relaxation training in reducing adverse reactions to cancer chemotherapy, *J Behav Med* 4:65, 1981.	(1) No treatment control (2) APRT plus guided imagery Practiced before and after chemotherapy treatment N=16 Number of sessions: 2	With APRT, less distress and nausea, lower heart rate than controls both before and after relaxation sessions; no difference between groups with vomiting
Lyles JN, Burish TG, Korzely MG, Oldham RK: Efficacy of relaxation training and guided imagery in reducing the aversiveness of cancer chemotherapy, *J Consult Clin Psychol* 50(4):509, 1982.	(1) No treatment control (2) APRT plus guided imagery (3) Therapist support N=50 Number of sessions: 3	Reduced pretreatment nausea and anxiety; lower heart rate and systolic BP; less after-treatment anxiety, nausea, depression
Carey MP, Burish TG: Providing relaxation training to cancer chemotherapy patients: a comparison of three delivery techniques, *J Consult Clin Psychol* 55(5):732, 1987.	APRT, guided imagery, delivered by: (1) Professional (2) Volunteer (3) Professional audiotape No treatment control N=45 Number of sessions: 3	Professionally administered APRT significantly reduced emotional distress, physiologic arousal, and increased food intake as compared with audiotape and volunteer training; last two did not reduce symptoms more than standard treatment (antiemetic only)
Morrow GR: Effect of the cognitive hierarchy in the systematic desensitization treatment of anticipatory nausea in cancer patients: a component comparison with relaxation only, counseling, and no treatment, *Cogn Ther Res* 10(4):421, 1986.	(1) APRT plus systematic desensitization (2) APRT only (3) Rogerian counseling (4) No treatment control Number of sessions: 2 1-hr sessions between successive chemotherapy treatments for groups 1, 2, 3 N=92	Group 1 (APRT plus systematic desensitization) produced significant decrease in severity and intensity of anticipatory nausea as compared with groups 2 and 3; groups 1 and 2 produced significant decreases in duration and severity of after-treatment nausea as compared with groups 3 and 4
Burish TG, Carey MP, Krozely MG, Greco FA: Conditioned side effects induced by cancer chemotherapy: prevention through behavioral treatment, *J Consult Clin Psychol* 55(1):42, 1987.	(1) No treatment control (2) APRT plus guided imagery N=24 Number of sessions: 1 to 3 per chemotherapeutic visit	APRT produced less nausea and vomiting, lower BP, heart rate, and anxiety

APRT, Abbreviated progressive relaxation training; *BP,* blood pressure.

ation training can decrease BP in patients with hypertension. In 1984 the JNC report recommended consideration of behavioral therapies, including relaxation therapies, as parts of a comprehensive hypertension treatment program, noting that these therapies may be particularly relevant for mild hypertension. The recommendations were prompted by evidence suggesting that behavioral treatment produced modest but significant reductions in elevated BP in selected groups of individuals with hypertension.[64] Of particular interest was a study demonstrating that relaxation training reduced systolic and diastolic BP levels assessed in the working environment itself.[59]

Not all studies have found relaxation more effective than BP monitoring. Chesney and associates found it more beneficial for systolic but not diastolic BP when a cognitive restructuring component was added.[18] Jacob and colleagues observed that patients who participated for 6 months in a relaxation and a weight- and salt-reduction program obtained significant reductions in the levels of systolic and diastolic BP, but the reductions were no greater than those recorded by the BP-monitoring control group.[31] Goldstein and others found no significant differences in reducing BP among a relaxation group, a relaxation and biofeedback group, and a BP-monitoring group.[25] One explanation offered for these findings is that repeated BP assessment may result in habituation to having BP taken by others in a clinic or laboratory. Another possible explanation is that nonspecific effects of participating in a BP-monitoring program may exert treatment effects. Further, patients with mild hypertension have been observed to have elevated BP in clinics as opposed to readings obtained in home settings.

There is evidence to support the hypothesis that efficacy of behavioral interventions for hypertension depends on the level of the pretreatment BP. It has been demonstrated that there is a linear relationship between systolic pretreatment BP and treatment change.[30] However, individuals in hypertension studies are typically randomized into experimental groups that are then checked for equivalency by assessing an average pretreatment BP. Susceptibility of individuals to treatment based on the degree of hypertension is then masked in the outcomes. This method may account for the contradictory findings among studies that are otherwise well designed and well controlled. The same basic flaw is found in studies when age is not controlled, because older patients with hypertension may respond more or less effectively to relaxation methods than do younger patients.

Effects of Somatic versus Cognitive Relaxation on Hypertension

It would seem to be important to determine exactly what elements of relaxation training provide the most benefit in the treatment of hypertension. To date, this determination has been difficult because most clinical relaxation techniques include an adulteration of relaxation techniques. Many interventions that use progressive muscle relaxation (i.e., a somatic technique) also focus attention on verbal suggestions of relaxation that are cognitive techniques.[7,16,55] On the other hand, relaxation methods reported as cognitive in nature often require clients to perform muscle relaxation.[19] Accurate descriptions of various relaxation techniques require a statement addressing which method (cognitive or somatic) is emphasized the most, since both are invariably used to some degree in relaxation protocols.

There was one study that attempted to definitively assess the differences between somatic and cognitive techniques.[67] Yung and Keltner assigned thirty borderline patients with hypertension to one of the following five groups: (1) muscle tense-release training, (2) muscle stretch-release training, (3) cognitive relaxation training, (4) placebo medication, and (5) test-only control. Great pains were taken to ensure that instructions for each of the relaxation methods remained purely cognitive or somatic. Patients were orthogonally matched among groups with respect to pretreatment BP levels and ages.

Both cognitive and muscle relaxation procedures proved more effective than control (placebo-medication and test-only) groups in reducing BP, but the muscle tense-release training proved most effective. The authors argued that these findings dispelled the common assumption that a mixture of the two components—somatic and cognitive—is most effective; they asserted that a bare-bones muscular relaxation method without cognitive suggestions was more effective for the treatment of hypertension.

Although this was a well-designed study, the small number of subjects in each group (6) and the lack of any replications of this study does not allow the discerning reader to draw this conclusion. The findings of this study are suggestive, however, and similar research with larger numbers should be attempted. It was of interest that in this study the placebo-medication and test-only control groups also demonstrated reductions in BP, demonstrating the power of expectancy to affect health outcomes. The potency of expectation to alter actual health effects and outcomes should never be underestimated in a health care intervention program.

The length of practice in this study was 20 minutes per session. Patients reported practicing more often, and attrition rates were relatively low. A low attrition rate was not a surprising finding with this study design. Other researchers have observed that patients will dedicate no more than 30 minutes per day to the practice of a relaxation component. The 20- to 30-minute practice sessions seemed to be ideal for providing a health effect without overburdening patient time.

Factors Affecting Outcomes of Hypertension

Researchers hypothesize that muscle-oriented methods may work more effectively for hypertension that is driven by somatic problems, and cognitive-oriented methods may be more effective for cognitive and behavior-driven problems.[40] Personality style may contribute strongly to which method is most effective for the individual patient.

While using the Myers-Briggs Personality Inventor (MBPI), the author of this chapter (Dr. L. Freeman) has observed that those typed as sensing individuals seem to prefer a somatic method, whereas those typed as intuitive individuals often respond more favorably to the cognitive approaches. Other issues (e.g., degree of hypertension, age, somatic versus cognitive techniques, motivational imperatives, personality style, length of practice, outcome expectancy, and over reporting) must also be considered when developing an effective intervention.

In summary, combining techniques makes it difficult, if not impossible, to ascertain which method—somatic or cognitive—is most effective for varying populations of patients with hypertension. This, in combination with confounding procedural variables related to the degree of hypertension and age, leads to conflicting outcomes and an inability to assess the most efficacious components for intervention. There is also the issue of a high rate of attrition, the over reporting of practice, and the problem of motivating patients to continue practice.[35,54,60] Nonetheless, we can conclude that relaxation has great potential in the management of hypertension. To date, the most effective method for reducing hypertension in subpopulations, including components that increase motivation and practice compliance, has yet to be delineated (Table 5-2).

Relaxation Therapy and Pain Control

The International Association for the Study of Pain has defined *pain* as an unpleasant sensory and emotional experience associated with actual or potential tissue damage described in terms of such damage.[52] Pain is typically classified as (1) acute, (2) cancer related, or (3) chronic nonmalignant. *Acute pain* is associated with a noxious event; its severity is generally proportional to the degree of tissue injury and is expected to diminish with healing and time. *Cancer-related pain* has both acute and chronic episodes, because of its malignant nature and long duration. *Chronic nonmalignant pain* frequently develops from an injury, but it persists long after a reasonable healing time. Its causes are not necessarily discernible, and the pain is often disproportionate to identifiable tissue damage. Chronic nonmalignant pain frequently leads to alterations in sleep, mood, and sexual and vocational and avocational function (Figure 5-5).

A non-Federal, nonadvocate, 12-member panel representing the fields of family, social, and psychiatric medicine, psychology, public health, nursing, and epidemiology reviewed and assessed all Medline data relevant to behavioral and relaxation approaches in the treatment of pain.[51] Relaxation techniques were first categorized in a general sense as methods with the primary objective to achieve nondirected relaxation, rather than directed achievement of a specific therapeutic goal. These cognitive techniques were found to share two basic components: (1) the repetitive focus on a word, sound, prayer, phrase, body sensation, or muscular activity; and (2) the adoption of a passive attitude toward intruding thoughts and a return to focus. It was determined that

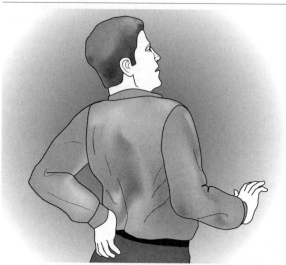

■ *Figure 5-5.* **Relaxation and control of pain.** The U.S. Agency for Health Care Policy and Research has determined that the evidence is strong that relaxation techniques are effective in reducing chronic pain in a variety of medical conditions.

these techniques induce a common set of physiologic changes that result in a decrease in metabolic activity. These methods were found to be beneficial for the management of generalized stress, and this form of relaxation is reviewed in detail in Chapter 6.

Relaxation techniques were then subdivided into two methods: deep and brief. Deep methods included progressive muscle relaxation and the full-version autogenic training. Brief methods included the shortest versions of progressive muscle relaxation, short autogenic training methods, and paced respiration breathing. The definition of *brief* as presented here is different from the abbreviated versions previously described. A committee of the National Institutes of Health (NIH) used the word "brief" to define the very shortest interventions, such as deep breathing methods or self-control (e.g., counting) that can be accomplished in a matter of minutes. The most abbreviated progressive relaxation methods, for example, are classified as *deep* by the committee's definition, because they still require weeks of training to master.

The U.S. Agency for Health Care Policy and Research developed a four-point scale for assessing the strength of evidence supporting or refuting interventional methods for pain control. The panel used this scale to draw certain conclusions. Based on strong scientific evidence presented in an open forum and from the scientific literature, the panel concluded six points.

TABLE 5-2	Effects of Progressive Relaxation on Hypertension

AUTHOR(S)	DESIGN	FINDINGS
Southam MA, Agras WS, Taylor CB, Kraemer HC: *Arch Gen Psychiatry* 39:715, 1982.	(1) APRT (2) No treatment control Number of sessions: 8 N=42	APRT produced lower systolic and diastolic BP during workday (in the natural environment) than controls Benefits continued at 6-month follow-up
Agras WS, Schneider JA, Taylor CB: Relaxation training in essential hypertension: a failure of retraining *Behav Ther* 1:191, 1984.	(1) APRT (2) BP monitoring (3) APRT subset monitored secretly Number of sessions: 10 N=22	Subjects, who had already been trained, successfully lowered BP, but later experienced returns to pretraining levels They were therefore retrained No significant benefit of retraining was found Home practice was adequate, suggesting relapse prevention, not retraining, is more beneficial after relapse because of life disruptions (e.g., family disruption, job loss) that occurred with these patients
Jacob RG, Shapiro AP, Reeves RA, Johnson AM, McDonald RH, Coburn PC: Relaxation therapy for hypertension: comparison of effects and beta-blocker, *Arch Intern Med* 146:2335, 1986.	All patients sequentially received the following: (1) Placebo pill (4 wks) (2) Placebo and APRT (8 wks) (3) Atenolol only (6 wks) (4) Atenolol and APRT (8 wks) (5) Atenolol only (6 wks) (6) Atenolol and APRT (6 wks) (7) Chlorthalidone (6 wks) (8) Chlorthalidone and APRT (6 wks) N=30	Effects of APRT on BP were clinically modest with average reduction of 2 to 3 mm Hg There was no generalization of the effect to environment with concomitant placebo, diuretic Atenolol was significantly more effective than relaxation in reducing systolic and diastolic BP Chlorthalidone was significantly more effective than APRT in reducing systolic BP, but not diastolic BP Long-term APRT effects were independent on drug use
Hoelscher TJ, Lichstein KL, Rosenthal TL: Home relaxation practice in hypertension treatment: objective assessment and compliance induction, *J Consult Clin Psychol* 54:217, 1986.	(1) Individualized APRT (2) Group APRT (3) Group APRT and contingency contracting for home practice (4) Wait-list control Number of sessions: 4 plus home practice N=50	All relaxation therapies reduced systolic and diastolic BP significantly as compared with controls, but it did not differ from each other Gains were maintained 16 weeks after training began Those who contracted for rewards or punishments based on 5-day per week practice did worse than any other group
Chesney MA, Black GW, Swan GE, Ward MM: Relaxation training for essential hypertension at the worksite. I. The untreated mild hypertensive, *Psychosom Med* 49:250, 1987.	(1) APRT (2) APRT and cognitive restructuring (3) APRT and biofeedback (4) APRT, biofeedback, and cognitive restructuring (5) BP monitoring Number of sessions: 13 with five follow-up visits over the 9 months after training N=158	Both APRT and BP monitoring equally and significantly reduced systolic and diastolic BP at the worksite and at the clinic Improvements were maintained for 1 year In each case, the addition of cognitive restructuring to relaxation or relaxation and biofeedback reduced systolic BP at the worksite by an additional 5.4 mm Hg (p<0.05)
Hoelscher TJ, Lichstein KL, Fischer S, Hegarty TB: Relaxation treatment of hypertension: do home relaxation tapes enhance treatment outcome? *Behav Ther* 18:33, 1987.	(1) APRT, no audiotapes (2) APRT and audiotapes (3) Wait-list control Number of sessions: 4 N=48	APRT and APRT with audiotape demonstrated significant decreases in systolic and diastolic BP compared with controls 47% reduced BP to less than 140/90 mm Hg at follow-up compared with 19% for controls Results maintained at 2-month follow-up Home use audiotapes did not provide a significant improvement

APRT, Abbreviated progressive relaxation training; *BP,* blood pressure.

Continued

TABLE 5-2	Effects of Progressive Relaxation on Hypertension—cont'd	
AUTHOR(S)	**DESIGN**	**FINDINGS**

Agras WS, Taylor CB, Kraemer HC, Southam MA, Schneider JA: Relaxation training for essential hypertension at the worksite. II. The poorly controlled hypertensive, *Psychosom Med* 49(3):264, 1987.	(1) APRT
	(2) BP monitoring
	Number of sessions: 8
	N=137 hypertensives with BP poorly controlled by medication
		APRT provided modest results of short duration compared with monitored group; however, large numbers of APRT subjects came into good control
		Control group compared with BP-monitoring group
		Advantage continued for 24-month follow-up
		No difference was found at 30 months
		  BP monitoring also produced significant BP lowering
		  Diastolic BP was most controlled by APRT
		  BP was most controlled by APRT

Blanchard EB, McCoy GC, Wittrock D, Musso A, Gerardi RJ, Pangburn L: A controlled comparison of thermal biofeedback and relaxation training in the treatment of essential hypertension. II. Effects on cardiovascular reactivity, *Health Psychol* 7:19, 1988.	(1) APRT
	(2) Thermal biofeedback
	  Number of sessions:
	  Biofeedback: 16 sessions
	APRT: 8 sessions
	N=73 for Phase I-II
	N=44 for Phase III
		Effects of biofeedback resulted in a downward shift of basic heart rate and systolic BP, but reactivity to stressors was not controlled for systolic BP or heart rate
		APRT produced modest effect on systolic BP, all values than biofeedback
		Diastolic BP significantly less reactive to stress for APRT group
		  Biofeedback group showed no change
		  Authors conclude both treatments equivalent to substitution with a second-stage antihypertensive medication, but relaxation is a better strategy for reducing cardiovascular reactivity

Adsett CA, Bellissiom A, Mitchell A, Wilczynski N, Haynes RB: Behavioral and physiological effects of a beta-blocker and relaxation therapy on mild hypertensives, *Psychosom Med* 51:523, 1989.	(1) APRT and beta-blocker
	(2) APRT and placebo pill
	(3) Education and beta-blocker
	(4) Education and placebo pill
	Number of sessions: 8
	N=47
		Beta-blocker was more effective than placebo in lowering BP
		APRT was no more effective than education in lowering BP
		APRT and beta-blocker was no more effective than beta-blockers alone
		  Authors concluded pharmacologic treatment is superior to APRT for BP management
		  Outcomes were consistent at 1-mo after treatment and 3-mo follow-up

MIXED METHODS RELAXATION		
Wadden T: Relaxation therapy for essential hypertension: specific or nonspecific effects? *J Psychosom Res* 28(1):53, 1984.	(1) Individual relaxation training consisting of relaxation response, APRT, passive muscle relaxation and imagery techniques (2) The same training as above, but with spouse (3) General information on stress, cognitive restructuring and assertiveness training Number of sessions: 8 N=48	All three groups achieved significant reductions in systolic and diastolic BP, which were maintained 1 and 5 months after treatment No significant differences were found between groups Authors concluded positive expectancy may be a sufficient condition for BP reduction, not relaxation

APRT, Abbreviated progressive relaxation training; *BP*, blood pressure.

■ Relaxation techniques are effective in reducing chronic pain in a variety of medical conditions.

■ Relaxation techniques, as a group, generally alter sympathetic activity as indicated by decreased oxygen consumption, slower respiration, decreased heart rate, and lower BP. Relaxation interventions clearly reduce arousal.

■ Increased electroencephalographic slow wave activity is part of a relaxation response.

■ One may infer from indirect evidence that decreased arousal as a result of alterations in catecholamines or other neurochemical systems plays a key role in relaxation effects.

■ One barrier to the integration of relaxation techniques in standard medical care is the sole emphasis on the biomedical model, which

TABLE 5-2	Effects of Progressive Relaxation on Hypertension—cont'd	
AUTHOR(S)	**DESIGN**	**FINDINGS**
Avazyan TA, Zaitsev VP, Salenko BB, Yurenev AP, Patrusheva IF: Efficacy of relaxation techniques in hypertensive patients, *Health Psychol* 7(suppl):193, 1988.	(1) Autogenic training (2) Thermal biofeedback (3) Breathing relaxation (APRT and meditation) (4) No-treatment control resistance (5) Psychologic placebo (told to practice relaxation, but not trained) Number of sessions: 14 to 16	After treatment and at 12-month follow-up, treatment groups had significant reduction in diastolic and systolic BP, peripheral vascular resistance, and hypertensive response to stress Profile of subjects who most significantly reduced BP were those with highest BP and shortest illness duration Groups 2 and 3 were most effective in reducing BP
Van Montfrans GA, Karemaker JM, Wieling W, Dunning AJ: Relaxation therapy and continuous ambulatory blood pressure in mild hypertension: a controlled study, *BMJ* 300:1368, 1990.	(1) Hatha yoga breathing and postures, APRT, autogenic training, Benson's relaxation response (2) Nonspecific counseling Number of sessions: 8 N=35	Diastolic BP was assessed in this study and it was not significantly reduced for either group after treatment or at 1-yr follow-up Authors concluded relaxation was ineffective for lowering 24-hour BP, being no more effective than nonspecific advice and support, which, in itself, was ineffective
Irvine MJ, Logan AG: Relaxation behavior therapy as sole treatment for mild hypertension, *Psychosom Med* 53:587, 1991.	(1) Muscle contraction relaxation with biofeedback, one session Systematic muscle relaxation without muscle contraction phase, with biofeedback, 4 sessions Mental imagery and meditation, 4 sessions (2) Support therapy N=110	Subjects in both groups showed similar reductions in BP and alcohol consumption after treatment and at 6-mo follow-up Alcohol reduction was positively correlated with the change in diastolic BP at outcome

defines disease in anatomic and pathophysiologic terms to the exclusion of the biopsychosocial model that emphasizes the patient's experience of disease. A balance must be drawn between these two models.

■ Because of the variability among relaxation methods and the differences within the same methods used in experimental research, the data are currently insufficient to conclude that one technique is more effective than another for a given condition. For any patient, one approach may indeed prove more beneficial than another. Research is reviewed in the categories of headache, back, menstrual, orthopedic postoperative, and rheumatic pain (Table 5-3 on page 156).

An Expert Speaks: Dr. G. Frank Lawlis

Dr. G. Frank Lawlis has focused on mind-body clinical and research methods since 1968 when he received his PhD in Counseling Psychology with an emphasis in medical psychology and rehabilitation. Dr. Lawlis was awarded Diplomate in both Counseling Psychology and Clinical Psychology (ABPP). He received status of Fellow from the American Psychological Association for his scientific contributions to the field of clinical psychology and behavioral medicine, as well as other awards for his pioneering research in the mind-body field. Having served on five prestigious medical school facilities in the Departments of Psychiatry, Orthopedic Surgery, and Rehabilitation Medicine, Dr. Lawlis has blazed new studies and approaches in the care of patients with chronic and acute pain and cancer and psychosomatic problems. He is the author or co-author of more than 100 articles and chapters on mind-body medicine, as well as three textbooks: *Imagery and Disease, Bridges of the Bodymind,* and *Transpersonal Medicine.* Dr. Lawlis is President and Chief Operating Officer of the Santa Fe Institute of Medicine and Prayer and Director of Psychological Services, New Mexico Cancer Care Associates.

Question. Dr. Lawlis, please describe your clinical work with progressive relaxation as an intervention for pain.

Answer. Basically, my work with progressive relaxation methods started in 1967 when I was an intern at New York Medical School, Rusk Institute. We were charged with the responsibilities of helping patients with brain injuries deal with pain, and the only tool available at that time was the relaxation method. People who suffer spinal cord injuries have numerous muscle spasms as a result of the reactive process of the injury. We found the progressive relaxation method to be effective for two reasons. It was structured enough to grasp the attention of the patient, and it gave the patient a valuable tool for control.

Later, when I became Co-Director of the Spinal-Pain Program in Dallas, Texas, we initiated progressive relaxation programs for patients with chronic low back pain. Again, the instructions were straightforward, and we developed audiotapes for home use. We noticed that patients would find some relief from the practice of these approaches, so we studied them to determine their effectiveness. As you would probably guess, there were some people who really benefited from them and some who did not. The ones who did not tended to have reactions to the structure, the authoritarian approach of, "You will do this," or "You will do that." But the ones who found progressive relaxation most useful were the novices to body-mind approaches. These people wanted methods on "how" to help themselves, not "why."

Question. What do you see is the future for the use of progressive relaxation techniques?

Answer. The future of progressive relaxation is probably somewhat limited because it has served its purpose clinically. Several people have built upon progression relaxation in their own theories and applications. I suppose progressive relaxation belongs to those approaches that serve as springboards to others. We will always be grateful for the pioneers who developed these techniques. The field of medical psychology has gone on to be more specific to medical conditions and protocols. Progressive relaxation has become so general that simply learning to relax is not enough. We have learned that we need to be more specific for maximal benefit. For example, using progressive relaxation for presurgery can be helpful for those patients who are having stress attacks. But it is even more helpful to add specific imagery for the surgical process, such as "making the blood flow slow in the area of the surgery," or "seeing the healing power of the body perform its rehabilitation." In fact, some studies found that if the progressive relaxation is too general, the patients may become too passive

in their treatment. These [imagery] reactions serve to promote healing.

Question. Specifically, how should this method be used in health care settings?

Answer. As I indicated, progressive relaxation is a generic skill and can be utilized best with those patients and programs for beginning to develop skills. It is almost a foregone conclusion that relaxation helps almost anything. And remember that medicine treats all patients, not just the sophisticated ones that are used in experiments. I think that the simple instructions are going to be very important if we are to move into a true body-mind protocol for medicine in general. And, although these methods were researched many years ago and are not particularly interesting for modern day scientists, they are very "usable" today. So I suspect that the uses of progressive relaxation will be as a basic technique for the public, especially for those patients who need and desire structure.

Relaxation Therapy and Mood State Management

Relaxation therapy has been used successfully to reduce the symptoms of depression. There is an abundance of evidence linking depression to stress, supporting the concept of relaxation therapy as a treatment method for depressive disorders.[2,58] Further, relaxation training provides individuals with coping strategies for dealing with stress and may provide relief for the stress-related neurochemical changes that are linked with the depressive state.[3,24] A 1979 outcome study found relaxation therapy as effective as psychotherapy and the pharmacotherapy interventions of that era.[9,49] Relaxation as therapy has also been incorporated as a component into a number of depression treatment packages[10,68] (Figure 5-6).

Although relaxation training is a routine part of childbirth education classes, few realize that it can also be a useful intervention for treating postpartum depression. Postpartum depression or "maternity blues" occurs in approximately 80% of women giving birth and typically strikes between the third and tenth postpartum days.[66] In some cases, the symptoms can escalate into the more serious condition known as postpartum psychosis that requires immediate medical intervention.

Even mild symptoms can affect the mother-child bonding relationship and reduce the quality of life for both mother and child. One study (Table 5-4 on page 159) compared groups with (1) progressive relaxation training, (2) progressive relaxation training with systematic desensitization,

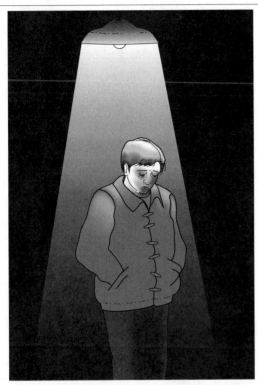

■ *Figure 5-6. Relaxation and depression.* Relaxation therapy has been used successfully to reduce the symptoms of depression. Abundance evidence links depression to stress, supporting the concept of relaxation therapy as a treatment method for depressive disorders.

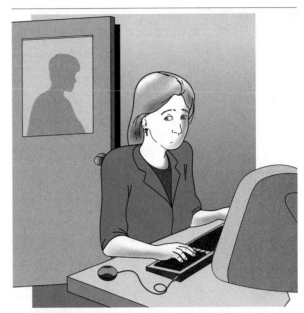

■ *Figure 5-7.* Relaxation therapy has been important in the treatment of generalized anxiety disorders, for which no apparent triggering cues have been identified for desensitization training.

(3) systematic desensitization only, and (4) discussion-only control to assess which of these interventions would prove beneficial in the treatment of postpartum depression. Both relaxation conditions reduced postpartum depression, but exposure to postpartum stressors as part of the systematic desensitization experience reduced the reported elation mood state that can occur postpartum.

Relaxation therapy has been effective in treating both depressed adults and adolescents. In adolescents, relaxation therapy was found as effective as cognitive-behavioral therapy in reducing depressive symptoms, and moderately depressed adolescents moved into nondepressed levels at posttest and follow-up.[56]

Anxiety is often associated with depression, a condition that relaxation therapy is also capable of modulating.[4] Cognitive behavioral therapies that include relaxation components have been successful in the treatment of a variety of anxiety disorders. The relaxation component has been particularly important in the treatment of generalized anxiety disorders in which no apparent triggering cues could be identified for desensitiza-

tion training[15,34,39] (Figure 5-7). In an effort to sort out the separate effects of cognitive therapy and relaxation training, Borkovec and others randomized subjects into an APRT program plus cognitive therapy or an APRT program with nondirective therapy in which the facilitator offered only reflections of the subject's experiences. Although both groups improved anxiety scores, the combination of APRT and cognitive therapy produced better results on some, but not all, measures of anxiety.[11]

Many of the studies of relaxation for the treatment of depression or anxiety contain methodologic flaws including inadequate diagnostic methods, use of audiotape recorded training, therapy trials that were too brief, absence of instructions for application of skills, lack of follow-up, weak outcome results, or small subject numbers. Well-operationalized treatment packages with self-assessing quality control components could add credibility to the research in this field. Nonetheless, results do strongly suggest that APRT interventions are beneficial in the treatment of depression and anxiety. As with other relaxation studies, the same issues of subject motivation and over reporting of practice apply (see Table 5-4).

Relaxation Therapy and Epilepsy

Epilepsy has been treated with interventions based on relaxation therapy, classical conditioning, and systematic desensitization in which hier-

TABLE 5-3	Effects of Progressive Relaxation on Headache, Menstrual, and Back Pain	

AUTHOR(S)	DESIGN	FINDINGS
HEADACHE PAIN		
Blanchard EB et al: Biofeedback kinds of headache: and relaxation training with three treatment effects and their prediction, *J Consult Clin Psychol* 50:562, 1982.	(1) APRT and subjects with tension headache (2) APRT and subjects with migraine headache (3) APRT with subjects with combined headache Number of sessions: 10 APRT, 12 biofeedback, if required	With only APRT, subjects with tension headache improved 64%; subjects with migraine improved 53%; subjects with combined headache improved 54%; (if patients did not improve with APRT alone, 12 sessions of biofeedback [thermal or EMG] was implemented) Overall, 73% and 52% of patients with tension and vascular headache, respectively, improved 32% of variance predicted by APRT; 44% predicted by psychologic tests if biofeedback was required
Williamson DA et al: Relaxation for the treatment of headache, *Behav Modif* 8(3):407, 1984.	(1) Written SHRTP (2) Therapist-assisted APRT relaxation program (3) Attention wait-list control Number of sessions: 4 for groups 1 and 3 8 for group 2 N=41 Note: SHRP included	At 1-mo follow-up, both SHRTP and APRT superior to control Only therapist-assisted APRT made significant progress in within-groups analysis APRT: 39.3%, 50.6%, and 52.8% improvement after treatment and 1 and 4 month later audiotapes and manual SHRTP: 19.4%, 31.7%, and instructions 13.9% same time periods
Teders SJ et al: Relaxation training for tension headache: comparative efficacy and cost-effectiveness of a minimal therapist contact versus a therapist-delivered procedure, *Behav Ther* 15:59, 1984.	(1) APRT (clinic program) (2) APRT (home-based program) N=35 Number of sessions: Clinic based: 10 Home based: 3	Both improved significantly on headache index, headache peak, headache-free days, and medication use, with no difference between methods Authors concluded home-based treatment is as effective as clinic treatment and more cost effective, reducing therapist time by 59%
Larsson B et al: A school-based treatment of chronic headaches in adolescents, *J Pediatr Psychol* 12(4):553, 1987.	(1) SHRTP (3 hrs) (2) Problem discussion group (7 hrs total) (3) Self-monitoring condition N=36 high school students Program time over 5 wks Note: SHRP included audiotapes and an instruction manual	SHRPT group significantly reduced headaches (all dimensions) more than problem-solving or self-monitoring groups
Attansio V et al: Cognitive therapy and relaxation training in muscle contraction headache: efficacy and cost-effectiveness, *Headache* 27:254, 1987.	(1) APRT and cognitive therapy (office) (2) APRT and cognitive therapy (home) (3) APRT only (home) Number of sessions: 11 sessions for office-based 5 sessions for home-based 3 sessions for APRT only N=25	Self-practice at home was as effective as office treatment All subjects reported less headache at 1 mo Slight benefit was demonstrated for cognitive groups and therapist contact 71.4% for group 1, 62.2% for group 2, and 50.0% for group 3 demonstrated clinical improvements of 50%+ symptom reduction
McGrath PJ et al: Relaxation prophylaxis for childhood migraine: a randomized placebo-controlled trial, *Dev Med Child Neurol* 30:626, 1988.	(1) APRT (2) Therapist-attention placebo-control Own best-effort record-keeping Number of sessions: 6 for groups 1 and 2 1 for group 3 N=99	All three groups showed significant reduction in headaches after treatment and at 12-mo follow-up, equally Authors concluded APRT is no more effective than own best efforts

APRT, Abbreviated progressive relaxation training; *BP*, blood pressure; *EMG*, electromyogram; *SHRTP*, self-help relaxation training program.

TABLE 5-3	Effects of Progressive Relaxation on Headache, Menstrual, and Back Pain—cont'd	

AUTHOR(S)	DESIGN	FINDINGS

Blanchard EG et al: Two studies of the long-term follow-up of minimal therapist contact treatments of vascular and tension headache, *J Consult Clin Psychol* 56:427, 1988.	(1) APRT (clinic program) patients with vascular headache received thermal biofeedback
	(2) APRT (home program)
	Number of sessions:
	  Clinic program:
	    10 with tension headache
	    16 with vascular headache thermal biofeedback
	  Home based program: 3
	N=58
		81% of patients with vascular headache, who clinically improved at end of treatment 50% or more improvement after 1 year, 75% after 2 years
		Of those not clinically improved, 56% and 47% had improved by year 1 and 2
		For patients with tension headache, 78% improved at end of treatment and maintained improvement at year 2
		50% of unimproved patients improved by end of year

Wisniewski JJ et al: Relaxation therapy and compliance in the treatment of adolescent headache, *Headache* 28:612, 1988.	(1) APRT (children 12-17 yrs) (2) Wait-list control Number of sessions: 8 N=10 Note: audiotape use was secretly monitored	APRT significantly reduced headache index score compared with controls Headache-free days, peak rating, and medication index did not significantly improve Subjects overreported practice by 70% 6 patients improved 50% or more; 2 improved 20% to 49%
Blanchard EB et al: Placebo-controlled evaluation of abbreviated with progressive muscle relaxation and of relaxation combined cognitive therapy in the treatment of tension headaches, *J Consult Clin Pathol* 58:210, 1990.	(1) APRT (2) APRT and cognitive therapy (3) Attention-placebo (pseudomeditation) (4) Headache monitoring (general control) Number of sessions: 10 N=66	APRT equal to APRT and cognitive Both produced significant reductions on headache Index and med use as compared with both controls APRT and cognitive therapy demonstrated a trend for superior treatment as compared with APRT alone
Blanchard EB et al: The role of regular home practice in the relaxation treatment of tension headache, *J Consult Clin Psychol* 59(3):467, 1991.	(1) APRT, home and clinic (2) APRT, clinic only (3) Headache monitoring Number of sessions: 10 N=33	APRT reported less headache activity than controls Home practice marginally more beneficial than clinic only p=.056)
Larsson B, Carlsson J: A school-based, nurse-administered relaxation training for children with chronic tension-type headache, *J Pediatr Psychol* 21(5):603, 1996.	(1) APRT (2) No-treatment control Number of sessions: 10 N=26 school children	Headache activity in APRT was significantly more reduced than in control after treatment (69%) and 6 months later (73%) For controls, improvement was 8% and 27%, respectively
BACK PAIN		
Turner JA: Comparison of group progressive-relaxation training and cognitive-behavioral group therapy for chronic low back pain, *J Consult Clin Psychol* 50:757, 1982.	(1) APRT (2) Cognitive behavioral therapy and APRT (3) Wait-list control Number of sessions: 5 N=36	APRT was equal to cognitive therapy and APRT for reduced depression, disability, and pain Cognitive and APRT provided more pain tolerance as compared with APRT alone At 1 month, both groups maintained depression and disability improvements, but subjects with cognitive therapy and APRT had more pain tolerance and were better able to participate in normal activities than those in APRT only At 1-2 yrs, both groups reported less health care use and decreased pain intensity compared to pretreatment
MENSTRUAL PAIN		
Sigmon ST, Nelson RO: The effectiveness of activity scheduling and relaxation training in the treatment of spasmodic dysmenorrhea, *J Behav Med* 11:483, 1988.	(1) APRT (2) Activity scheduling (3) Wait-list control Number of sessions: 6 N=40	APRT and activity scheduling both significantly reduced discomfort ratings before and after testing and as compared with wait-list control group Both treatments effectively reduced both spasmodic and general measures of pain

Continued

| TABLE 5-3 | Effects of Progressive Relaxation on Headache, Menstrual, and Back Pain—cont'd |

AUTHOR(S)	DESIGN	FINDINGS
Borkovec TD, Mathews AM: Treatment of nonphobic anxiety disorders, a comparison of nondirective, cognitive, and coping desensitization therapy, *J Consult Clin Psychol* 55:883, 1988.	(1) APRT and cognitive therapy (2) APRT and nondirective therapy (3) APRT and coping desensitization Number of sessions: 12 N=30	All treatments equally effective in reducing state and trait anxiety, depression, reactions to relaxation, and to arousal as assessed by heart rate, respiration, and skin conductance in response to stressors
Long BC, Haney CJ: Coping strategies for working women: aerobic exercise and relaxation interventions, *Behav Ther* 19:75, 1988.	(1) APRT (2) Aerobic exercise Number of sessions: 8 N=61	APRT equal to aerobic exercise for decreasing trait anxiety and increasing self-efficacy Significant improvements were maintained at follow-up Coping strategies did not change over treatments
ORTHOPEDIC AND POST-OPERATIVE PAIN		
Flaherty GG, Fitzpatric JJ: Relaxation technique to increase comfort level of postoperative patients: a preliminary study, *Nurs Res* 27(6):353, 1978.	(1) Jacobson relaxation of mouth, throat, jaw, tongue (2) No-treatment control Number of sessions: 1 hour N=42 surgical patients matched for procedure	Note: Pain was assessed after first attempt to get out of bed Incisional pain, body distress, 24-hr narcotics use, and respiratory rates were significantly less for relaxation group
Ceccio CM: Postoperative pain relief through relaxation in elderly patients with fractured hips, *Orthop Nurs* 3(3):11, 1984.	(1) Jacobson relaxation of mouth, throat, jaw, and tongue (2) No-treatment control Number of sessions: 3 including coaching when being turned N=20	Relaxation subjects reported significantly lower levels of pain and distress when turned and took significantly less analgesics 24 hrs after surgery
Lawlis GF et al: Reduction of postoperative pain parameters by presurgical relaxation instructions for spinal pain patients, *Spine* 10(7):649, 1985.	(1) Brief progressive relaxation, deep breathing, distraction (2) No-treatment control Number of sessions: 1 N=10	Relaxation group had significantly less days of hospitalization, nurse complaints, and medication use (primarily demerol and phenaphen)
Achterberg J et al: Behavioral strategies for the reduction of pain and anxiety associated with orthopedic trauma, *Biofeedback Self Regul* 14(2):101, 1989.	(1) EMG biofeedback-assisted relaxation (2) Relaxation audiotape (3) Attention-control (4) No-treatment control Number of sessions: 6+ N=64 patients with multiple fractures	Both the biofeedback-assisted relaxation and audiotape groups demonstrated significant and equivalent reductions in peripheral temperature, pain discomfort, anxiety, and systolic BP No changes occurred for the two control groups
RHEUMATIC PAIN		
Stenstrom CH et al: Dynamic training exercise for patients versus relaxation training as home with inflammatory rheumatic diseases, *Scand J Rheumatol* 25:28, 1996.	(1) Muscle strength, mobility training (2) APRT training (3) Individual instruction N=54	APRT significantly improved health profile, energy, Ritchie's auricular index, muscle function, arm endurance Strength training significantly improved exertion on-walking test Authors concluded APRT was superior to strength training in improving muscle function of lower extremities

APRT, Abbreviated progressive relaxation training; *BP,* blood pressure; *EMG,* electromyogram; *SHRTP,* self-help relaxation training program.

TABLE 5-4	Effects of Progressive Relaxation on Anxiety and Depression	
AUTHOR(S)	**DESIGN**	**FINDINGS**
Halonen JS, Passman RH: Relaxation training and expectation in the treatment of postpartum distress, *J Consult Clin Psychol* 53: 839, 1985.	(1) APRT (2) APRT plus exposure (3) Exposure to postpartum stressors only (4) Discussion Number of sessions: 2 N=48	Both relaxation groups reported less postpartum distress compared with stressor only and discussion groups Exposure to stressors reduced elation for groups 2 and 3 Authors conclude relaxation practice after childbirth can reduce postpartum distress
Reynolds WM, Coats KI: A comparison of cognitive-behavioral therapy and relaxation training for the treatment of depression in adolescents, *J Consult Clin Psychol* 54:653, 1986.	(1) APRT (2) Cognitive behavior (3) Wait-list control Number of sessions: 10 N=30 moderately depressed adolescents	APRT and cognitive behavior both superior to controls for reduced depression Improvement was maintained at 5-week follow-up Improvement in anxiety and academic self-concept also demonstrated
Borkovec TD et al: The effects of relaxation training with cognitive or nondirective therapy and the role of relaxation-induced anxiety in the treatment of generalized anxiety, *J Consult Clin Psychol* 55, 883, 1987.	(1) APRT plus cognitive therapy. (2) APRT plus nondirective therapy Number of sessions: 12 N=30	Both groups demonstrated significant improvement in anxiety scores but APRT plus cognitive therapy produced significantly greater improvement on several but not all assessments of anxiety
Rasid ZM, Parish TS: The effects of two types of relaxation training on students' levels of anxiety, *Adolescence* 33:(129), 99, 1998.	(1) Cognitive relaxation (2) APRT	Both groups demonstrated significant reductions in state but not trait anxiety scores

APRT, Abbreviated progressive relaxation training.

archies of anxiety provoking situations associated with seizures were explored. Much of this research was case study reports that used no statistical analysis. Three studies used an experimental design and allowed evaluation of the treatment itself. Those studies are summarized in Table 5-5.

Overall, studies on relaxation therapy and desensitization for the control of epilepsy contained small sample sizes, were few in number, and included only one long-term evaluation of 8 years, allowing no final conclusions to be drawn as to the effectiveness of this type of intervention.[20] However, the results are promising, especially for patients who are uncontrolled by medications and have seizures triggered in response to stress (see Table 5-5).

Relaxation Therapy for Other Medical Conditions

Alcoholism

Thirty-five severe alcoholic men were detoxified and received either cue exposure or APRT training. *Cue exposure* is based on the following conditioning model: repeated exposure to preingestion cues in the absence of drug ingestion will lead to extinction of conditioned responses, thus reducing the likelihood of relapse to drug-taking behavior. In this study, cue exposure consisted of 400 min-

utes of exposure to the sight and smell of preferred drinks over 10 days in a laboratory setting. Subjects in the relaxation group received 6 hours of relaxation training and only 20 minutes of cue exposure. Subjects in the cue exposure group had more favorable outcomes as compared with APRT-trained subjects in terms of latency (length of time) to relapse of drinking and total alcohol consumption. In this case, researchers concluded that cue exposure, a conditioning to extinction model, is a more effective treatment for addictive alcohol behavior than relaxation therapy.[21]

Gastroesophageal Reflux

Gastroesophageal reflux is a backflow of stomach contents upward into the esophagus. Twenty subjects with documented gastroesophageal reflux disease were assessed during psychologically neutral and stressful tasks. Before the stressful task, subjects were intubated with a probe that passed through the nasopharynx and was positioned 5 cm above the lower esophageal sphincter. They were then fed a high-fat meal consisting of 12 ounces of Classic Coke and two pieces of pizza with extra cheese and pepperoni—a diet proven to induce reflux. After 1 hour, subjects were exposed to a 45-minute neutral task (watching a videotape on America's National Parks or on the National Aeronautics and Space Administration)

TABLE 5-5	EFFECTS OF PROGRESSIVE RELAXATION ON EPILEPTIC SEIZURES	
AUTHOR(S)	**DESIGN**	**FINDINGS**
Dahl J et al: Effects of a broad-spectrum behavior modification treatment program on children with refractory epileptic seizures, *Epilepsia* 26(4):303, 1985.	(1) APRT and recognition of preseizure events and stimuli (2) Attention-control support therapy (3) No-treatment control Number of sessions: 6 N=18 children whose epilepsy was uncontrolled by medication	At 10 weeks and 1 year follow-up, there was a significant reduction in seizure index only for children in group 1 (seizure index consisted of the number of seizures and seizure duration) Number of seizures did not change significantly
Dahl J, Melin L, Lund L: Effects of a contingent relaxation treatment program on adults with refractory epileptic seizures, *Epilepsia* 28(2):125, 1987.	(1) APRT+seizure stimuli signal and recognition training (2) Attention-control supportive therapy sessions (3) No-treatment control Number of sessions: 6 N=18 adults whose epilepsy was uncontrolled by medication	Results of 10-week follow-up demonstrated that only group 1 significantly reduced seizures (66% reduction), group 2 increased seizures (68%), and group 3 remained the same At 10 weeks, groups 2 and 3 were then also trained in APRT and seizure stimuli recognition Once trained, all three groups demonstrated highly significant reductions in seizures at 10- and 30-week follow-up (p<0.001)
Puskarich CA et al: Controlled examination of effects of progressive relaxation training on seizure reduction, *Epilepsia* 33(4):675, 1992.	(1) APRT (2) Quiet sitting Number of sessions: 6 N=24	APRT decreased seizures 29% (p<0.001); quiet sitting reduced seizures 3%

APRT, Abbreviated progressive relaxation training.

followed by a stressful task (a high-stress, fast-paced computer game or timed arithmetic problems). The subjects then participated in either a (1) 45-minute APRT training group or (2) 45-minute attention-placebo control group (a videotape on gastrointestinal reflux). Before intervention, stressful tasks produced significant increases in BP, anxiety ratings, and reports of reflux symptoms. Even though symptom reports increased, stressful tasks did not significantly increase objective measures of esophageal acid exposure. The subjects who received APRT training after the stressful tasks had significantly lower heart rates and lower ratings of anxiety, reflux symptoms, and total esophageal acid exposure as compared with attention-placebo subjects. The authors concluded that APRT may be a useful adjunct to antireflux therapy in patients experiencing increased symptoms during stress.[47]

Irritable Bowel Syndrome

A study of 102 patients with the diagnosis of irritable bowel syndrome who had medically uncontrolled symptoms for 6 months or longer were randomized into one of two groups: (1) psychotherapy, relaxation training, and standard medical treatment; or (2) continuation of standard medical treatment alone. At 3 months, the treatment group demonstrated significantly greater improvement, as compared with the control group, on physicians' and patients' ratings of diarrhea and abdominal pain. Constipation was unaltered. Positive predictions of success with treatment included overt psychiatric symptoms or intermittent pain exacerbated by stress. Those with constant abdominal pain were helped very little by the intervention. The authors concluded that this form of intervention would prove effective for approximately two thirds of patients with irritable bowel syndrome who were unresponsive to medical treatment.[26]

Myocardial Infarction

A study randomly assigned 156 patients who experienced myocardial infarctions to one or two groups: (1) rehabilitation plus relaxation therapy (six sessions of breathing and relaxation instruction), or (2) cardiac rehabilitation alone. At 5-year follow-up, 20% of the relaxation group and 33% of the control group had another cardiac event (e.g., death, reinfarction, or cardiac surgery). Patients in the relaxation group were hospitalized a total of 476 days, and those in the control group were hospitalized a total of 719 days, reducing hospitalization by 31% for those practicing relaxation. The authors concluded that the disease course after myocardial infarction is influenced favorably by adding relaxation instruction to cardiac rehabilitation.[63]

◼ Indications and Contraindications of Progressive Relaxation

McGuigan has stated that, where rest is prescribed, progressive relaxation is indicated.[48] In all his years of experience, Jacobson reported no contraindications for the use of progressive relaxation. Although other forms of relaxation-induced anxiety have been reported, (e.g., fear of sensations, fear of losing control, anxiety), these were not reported when the Jacobsonian method was applied as designed.[27,38] Some subjects reported feelings of floating, but these sensations caused no undue discomfort. However, the reader must recall that JPRT has not been adequately tested in experimental trials; the briefer and more intense APRT method is often referred to as "progressive relaxation," but it is not based on the full JPRT method and is what is more typically used in relaxation therapies.

Although adverse reactions are rare, some have been reported with the more rapid paced APRT. Edinger and Jacobsen surveyed 116 clinicians who conducted relaxation practice with an estimated 17,542 clients. They found that the most common side effects were intrusive thoughts (15%), fear of losing control (9%), upsetting sensory experiences (4%), muscle cramps (4%), sexual arousal (2%), and psychotic symptoms (0.4%).[22] In those patients suffering from generalized anxiety disorder, 30% experienced an increase in tension while practicing APRT.[28] Adverse reactions to relaxation practice have been described as *relaxation-induced anxiety* (RIA) or *relaxation-induced panic* (RIP). RIA is described as a gradual increase in behavioral, physiologic, and psychologic anxiety, whereas RIP is severe anxiety of rapid onset.[1] Persons with a history of generalized anxiety disorder or panic disorder and persons with a history of hyperventilation are those most likely to experience these adverse effects. Although the risk is small, persons with these histories should be carefully monitored during relaxation practice.

Contraindications for success with any of the relaxation therapies are found in those who are:

- Unwilling or lacking the time to devote to learning the technique
- Unable to maintain focused attention
- Have secondary gains from tension states
- Not motivated to continue to practice at home once the technique is mastered

As noted, individuals with a history of severe anxiety, panic disorder, or hyperventilation may not be good candidates for this intervention. Patients fitting this profile should be informed of the potential complications, and efforts should be made to avoid these problems. For example, teaching patients deep breathing before APRT has been reported to reduce adverse reactions. Changing to an alternative relaxation technique may also reduce adverse reactions.

In some cases, medical status may suggest that it is better to practice muscle strengthening rather than muscle relaxation, such as occurs with lower back problems. In these cases, APRT can be altered to delete or modify the procedure for problematic muscle groups.[7] The same advice applies for persons with neuromuscular disability that renders them unable to exercise voluntary control over all muscles in the body.[17] Further, if a client is taking medication on a regular basis for such conditions as diabetes and hypertension, medical consultation is required before beginning APRT, because regular relaxation practice induces biochemical changes in the body that can result in a change in the amount of medication required.

◼ Summary of Relaxation Training as a Medical Intervention

Ost performed a review of 18 controlled outcome studies that found APRT effective for the treatment of phobias, panic disorder, headache, pain, epilepsy, and tinnitus. Studies encompassed as few as 7 and as many as 66 subjects who attended between 6 and 25 sessions. The results demonstrated that APRT was significantly more effective than no-treatment or attention-placebo conditions, and as effective as other behavioral methods with which it was compared. At follow-up (5 to 19 months), improvements were maintained; in nine studies, further improvements were noted.[53] There were few side effects, and in no case did it become necessary to abandon treatment.

◼ Study Limitations

There was considerable variability in procedures across studies in relation to the number of sessions used, whether videotaped or live instructions were given, and the elements related to home practice. These types of differences produced great variability in study quality and made it impossible to draw generalized conclusions. Detailed descriptions of methodology were often absent. Most troubling was the fact that no objective methods were used to measure home practice, although home practice contributed to the majority of the intervention effects. In some cases, only one session was held and home practice was relied on for all subsequent intervention effects.

By contrast, a study by Taylor and associates used audiotape recorders with hidden microelectronic systems to store a real-time record of relaxation practice to recordings. They found that although 71% of patients reported full compliance (five times per week of relaxation practice), only 39% actually practiced as instructed.[61] In a study by Hoelscher and others, a similar electronically monitored compliance method was used. Of the subjects who self-reported, 91% exceeded the actual amount of practice and only 32% averaged one practice session per day.[29] These studies suggest that noncompliance and over reporting of practice are commonplace.

There were differences in outcomes across varying clinical populations and conditions, again making generalized conclusions impossible. Standardized methods of assessing physiologic and cognitive changes in populations are needed, particularly in populations being treated for anxiety, a syndrome involving physiologic arousal and cognitive and behavioral symptoms.

In many studies, the "kitchen soup" approach was used, lumping combinations of APRT, meditation, biofeedback, hypnosis, and distraction into intervention techniques. For example, a study intended to measure the effects of stress management on men who tested positive for human immunodeficiency virus (HIV) used five subjects each in the treatment and control group. The subjects were then trained in APRT, meditation, and hypnosis with the addition of imagery.[62] The small subject number and multiple interventions make it impossible to draw conclusions about any of these interventions as independent contributing factors.

■ Chapter Review

There are significant methodologic and design flaws in the available studies of progressive muscle relaxation. It is, nonetheless, still clear that for many patients, though not all, progressive relaxation may be an effective intervention for chemotherapy-induced nausea and vomiting, chronic and acute pain, hypertension, cardiovascular disorders, epilepsy, anxiety and depression, and other conditions that are exacerbated by stress.

In Chapter 6, we review the outcomes of cognitive-based relaxation interventions commonly referred to as meditation.

Matching Terms and Definitions

Match each numbered definition with the correct term. Place the corresponding letter in the space provided.

_____ 1. Use of a mental device such as a word, a thought, a sound, or the breath and the practice of a passive attitude to induce relaxation of the mind and body

_____ 2. Emphasis of muscle relaxation through detailed observation and introspection of the body's kinesthetic sensations

_____ 3. Relaxation method originally developed by Edmund Jacobsen; systematic method of becoming aware of and relaxing all the major muscle groups

_____ 4. Instrument used to measure electrical muscle action potentials in microvolts; first quantitative measurement of muscle tension

_____ 5. Contraction of muscle fibers that elicits a tension sensation

_____ 6. Lengthening of muscle fibers that eliminates muscular tension sensation

_____ 7. State wherein one unconsciously and automatically monitors and eliminates unwanted body tension

_____ 8. Blunts excitatory autonomic changes, increases opioid output, potentially strengthens immunity

_____ 9. Two arms of autonomic cardiovascular control

a. Sympathetic and vagus
b. Cognitive relaxation
c. EMG
d. Relaxation
e. Somatic relaxation
f. Automaticity
g. Three effects of progressive relaxation
h. Progressive muscle relaxation
i. Tension

SHORT ANSWER ESSAY QUESTIONS

Define the difference between somatic and cognitive relaxation methods. Discuss which method you think you may prefer and why.

1. Explain the basic philosophy of Edmund Jacobson and how this philosophy led to the development of progressive relaxation.
2. Describe Wolpe's APRT and discuss the main differences between his method and JPRT.
3. What are the advantages and disadvantages of APRT?
4. What are the advantages and disadvantages of JPRT?

CRITICAL THINKING AND CLINICAL APPLICATION EXERCISES

1. APRT can be an effective treatment for the management of chemotherapy-induced nausea and vomiting. Some patients respond less effectively than others, for example, highly anxious or poorly motivated patients. Describe how you would work with these patients to implement an effective and specialized relaxation protocol.
2. You have been asked to design a research-based relaxation program for the treatment of hypertension. Discuss the issues that must be considered when developing an effective program design, and then use these factors to describe the "ideal" hypertension program.
3. Which is most effective for patients with hypertension—muscle tense-release training, tense-stretch training, or cognitive training? Why?
4. Relaxation seems to be effective in reducing perceived pain. What pathways do you think allow this to occur? Describe them and their chemical messengers.
5. Discuss indications and contraindications for progressive relaxation training. Now, as an instructor of a relaxation program, how would you screen patients to ensure relaxation therapy is appropriate and safe? How would you monitor patient participation to ensure that RIA and RIP were not becoming problems?
6. Discuss how progressive relaxation affects autonomic, opioid, and immune responses. What implications do these responses have for cardiovascular disease and other disorders?

References

1. Adler CM, Craske MG, Barlow DH: Relaxation-induced panic (RIP): When resting isn't peaceful, *Integr Psychiatry* 5:94, 1987.
2. Aneshensel CS, Stone JD: Stress and depression: a test of the buffering model of social support, *Arch Gen Psychiatry* 39:1392, 1982.
3. Anisman H, Lapierre YD: Neurochemical aspects of stress and depression: formulations and caveats. In Neufeld RWJ, editor: *Psychological stress and psychopathology,* New York, 1982, McGraw-Hill.
4. Beck AT, Rush AJ, Shaw BF, Emergy G: *Cognitive therapy of depression,* New York, 1979, Guilford Press.
5. Benson H, Greenwood MM, Klemchuk H: The relaxation response: psychophysiologic aspects and clinical applications, *Int J Psychiatry Med* 6(1/2):87, 1976.
6. Bernstein DA, Borkovec TD: Cognitive therapy and relaxation training in muscle contraction headache: efficacy and cost-effectiveness, *Headache* 27:254, 1973.
7. Bernstein DA, Borkovec TD: *Progressive relaxation training: a manual for the helping professions,* Champaign, IL, 1973, Research Press.
8. Bernstein DA, Carlson CR: Progressive relaxation: abbreviated methods. In Lehrer PM, Woolfolk RL, editors: *Principles and practice of stress management,* ed 2, New York, 1993, Guilford Press.
9. Biglan A, Dow MG: Toward a second-generation model: a problem-specific approach. In Rehmb LP, editor: *Behavior therapy for depression: present status and future directions,* New York, 1981, Academic Press.
10. Blaney PH: The effectiveness of cognitive and behavior therapies. In Rehm LP, editor: *Behavior therapy for depression: present status and future directions,* New York, 1981, Academic Press.
11. Borkovec TD, Mathews AM, Chambers A, Ebrahimi S, Lytle R, Nelson R: The effects of relaxation training with cognitive or nondirective therapy and the role of relaxation-induced anxiety in the treatment of generalized anxiety, *J Consult Clin Psycho* 55:883, 1987.
12. Burish TG, Tope DM: Psychological techniques for controlling the adverse side effects of cancer chemotherapy: findings from a decade of research, *J Pain Symptom Manage* 7(5):287, 1992.
13. Burish TG, Vasterling JJ, Carey MP, Matt DA, Krozely MG: Posttreatment use of relaxation training by cancer patients, *Hospice J* 4(2):1, 1988.
14. Cannon WB: *Bodily changes in pain, hunger, fear, and rage,* New York, 1929, Appleton-Century.
15. Canter A, Kondo CY, Knott JR: A comparison of EMG feedback and progressive relaxation training in anxiety neurosis, *Br J Psychiatry* 127:470, 1975.

16. Carlson CR, Ventrella MA, Sturgis ET: Relaxation training through muscle stretching procedures: a pilot case, *J Behav Ther Exp Psychiatry* 18:121, 1987.

17. Cautela JR, Groden J: *Relaxation: a comprehensive manual for adults, children, and children with special needs,* Champaign, IL, 1978, Research Press.

18. Chesney MA, Black GW, Swan GE, Ward MM: Relaxation training for essential hypertension at the worksite. I. The untreated mild hypertensive, *Psychosom Med* 49:250, 1987.

19. Crowther JH: Stress management and relaxation imagery in the treatment of essential hypertension, *J Behav Med* 6:169, 1983.

20. Dahl J, Melin L, Brorson L, Schollin J: Effects of a broad-spectrum behavior modification treatment program on children with refractory epileptic seizures, *Epilepsia* 26(4):303, 1985.

21. Drummond DC, Glautier S: A controlled trial of cue exposure treatment in alcohol dependence, *J Consult Clin Psychol* 62(4):809, 1994.

22. Edinger JD, Jacobsen R: Incidence and significance of relaxation treatment side effects, *Behav Ther* 5:137, 1982.

23. Gabbay FH, Krantz DS, Kopp WJ et al: Triggers of myocardial ischemic during daily life in patients with coronary artery disease: physical and mental activities, anger and smoking, *J Am Coll Cardiol* 27:585, 1996.

24. Goldfried MR, Trier CS: Effectiveness of relaxation as an active coping skill, *J Abnorm Psychol* 83:348, 1974.

25. Goldstein IB, Shapiro D, Thananopavaran C: Home relaxation techniques for essential hypertension, *Psychosom Med* 46:398, 1984.

26. Guthrie E, Creed F, Dawson D, Tomenson B: A controlled trial of psychological treatment for the irritable bowel syndrome, *Gastroenterology* 100:450, 1991.

27. Heide FJ, Borkovec TD: Relaxation-induced anxiety: mechanisms and theoretical implications, *Behav Res Ther* 22:1, 1984.

28. Heide FJ, Borkovec TD: Relaxation-induced anxiety: paradoxical anxiety enhancement due to relaxation training, *J Consult Clin Psychol* 51:171, 1983.

29. Hoelscher TJ, Lichstein KL, Rosenthal TL: Home relaxation practice in hypertension treatment: objective assessment and compliance induction, *J Consult Clin Psychol* 54(2):217, 1986.

30. Jacob RG, Chesney MA, Williams DM, Ding Y, Shapiro AP: Relaxation therapy for hypertension: design effects and treatment effects, *Ann Behav Med* 13:5, 1991.

31. Jacob RG, Fortmann SP, Kraemer HC, Farquhar JW, Agras WS: Combined behavioral treatments to reduce blood pressure: a controlled outcome study, *Behav Modif* 9:32, 1985.

32. Jacobson E: The origins and development of progressive relaxation, *J Behav Ther Exp Psychiatry* 8:119, 1977.

33. Jacobson E: *Progressive relaxation,* ed 2, Chicago, 1938, University of Chicago Press.

34. Jannoun L, Oppenheimer C, Gelder M: A self-help treatment program for anxiety state patients, *Behav Ther* 13:103, 1982.

35. Johnston DW: How does relaxation training reduce blood pressure in primary hypertension? In Schmidt T, Dembroski T, Blumchen G, editors: *Biological and psychological factors in cardiovascular disease,* Berlin, 1986, Springer.

36. The Joint National Committee: The 1984 Report of the Joint National Committee on Detection, Evaluation, and Treatment of High Blood Pressure, *Arch Intern Med* 44:1045, 1984.

37. Kiecolt-Glaser JK, Glaser R, Williger D, Stout J, Messick G, Sheppard S, Ricker D, Romisher C, Briner W, Bonnell G, Donnerberg R: Psychosocial enhancement of immunocompetence in a geriatric population, *Health Psychol* 4(1):25, 1985.

38. Lazarus AA, Mayne TJ: Relaxation: some limitations, side effects and proposed solutions, *Psychotherapy* 27:261, 1990.

39. LeBoeuf A, Lodge J: A comparison of frontalis EMG feedback training and progressive relaxation in the treatment of chronic anxiety, *Br J Psychiatry* 137:279, 1980.

40. Lehrer PM, Carr R, Sargunarraj D, Woolfolk RL: Stress management techniques: are they all equivalent, or do they have specific effects? *Biofeedback Self Regul* 19:353, 1994.

41. Lucini D, Covacci G, Milani R, Mela GS, Malliani A, Pagani M: A controlled study of the effects of mental relaxation on autonomic excitatory responses in healthy subjects, *Psychosom Med* 59:541, 1997.

42. McCubbin JA: Stress and endogenous opioids: behavioral and circulatory interactions, *Biol Psychol* 35:91, 1993.

43. McCubbin JA, Cheung R, Montgomery TB, Bulbulian R, Wilson JF: Aerobic fitness and opioidergic inhibition of cardiovascular stress reactivity, *Psychophysiol* 29:687, 1992.

44. McCubbin JA, Kaplan JR, Manuck SB, Adams MR: Opioidergic inhibition of circulatory and endocrine stress responses in cynomolgus monkeys: a preliminary study, Psychosom Med 55:23, 1993.

45. McCubbin JA, Surwit RS, Williams RB, Nemeroff CB, McNeilly M: Altered pituitary hormone response to naloxone in hypertension development, *Hypertension* 7(14):636, 1989.

46. McCubbin JA, Wilson JF, Bruehl S, Ibarra P, Carlson CR, Norton JA, Colclough GW: Relaxation training and opioid inhibition of blood pressure response to stress, *J Consult Clin Psychol* 53(3):593, 1996.

47. McDonald-Haile J, Bradley LA, Bailey MA, Schan CA, Richter JE: Relaxation training reduces symptom reports and acid exposure in patients with gastroesophageal reflux disease, *Gastroenterology* 107:61, 1994.

48. McGuigan FJ: Progressive relaxation: origins, principles, and clinical applications. In Lehrer PM, Woolfolk RL, editors: *Principles and practice of stress management,* ed 2, New York, 1993, Guilford Press.

49. McLean PD, Hakstian RA: Clinical depression: comparative efficacy of outpatient treatments, *J Consult Clin Psychol* 47:818, 1979.

50. Murphy AI, Lehrer PM, Jurish S: Cognitive coping skills training and relaxation training as treatments for tension headaches, *Behav Ther* 21:89, 1990.

51. NIH Technical Assessment Panel: Integration of behavioral and relaxation approaches into the treatment of chronic pain and insomnia, *JAMA* 276:313, 1996.

52. NIH Technical Assessment Panel: Integration of behavioral and relaxation approaches into the treatment of chronic pain and insomnia, *JAMA* 276:314, 1996.

53. Ost, Lars-Goral: Applied relaxation: description of a coping technique and review of controlled studies, *Behav Res Ther* 25(5):397, 1983.

54. Patel C: Psychological and behavioral treatment of hypertension. In Byrne DG, Rosenman RH, editors: *Anxiety and the heart,* New York, 1990, Hemisphere Publishing Corporation.

55. Patel C, Marmot MG, Tertry DJ, Carruthers M, Hunt B, Patel M: Trial of relaxation in reducing coronary risk: four year follow up, *BMJ* 290:1103, 1985.

56. Reynolds WM, Coats KI: A comparison of cognitive-behavioral therapy and relaxation training for the treatment of depression in adolescents, *J Consult Clin Psychol* 54:653, 1986.

57. Schaer B, Isom S: Effectiveness of progressive relaxation on test anxiety and visual perception, *Psychol Rep* 63:511, 1988.

58. Shaw BF: Stress and depression: a cognitive perspective. In Neufeld RWJ, editor: *Psychological stress and psychopathology,* New York, 1982, McGraw-Hill.

59. Southam MA, Agras S, Taylor CB, Kraemer C: Relaxation training: blood pressure lowering during the work day, *Arch Gen Psychiatry* 39:715, 1982.

60. Steptoe A, Patel C, Marmot M, Hunt B: Frequency of relaxation practice, blood pressure reduction and the general effects of relaxation following a controlled trial of behaviour modification for reducing coronary risk, *Stress Med* 3:101, 1987.

61. Taylor CB, Agras WS, Schneider JA, Allen RA: Adherence to instructions to practice relaxation exercises, *J Consult Clin Psychol* 51:952, 1983.

62. Taylor DN: Effects of a behavioral stress-management program on anxiety, mood, self-esteem, and T-cell count in HIV-positive men, *Psychol Rep* 76:451, 1995.

63. Van Dixhoorn J: Favorable effects of breathing and relaxation instructions in heart rehabilitation: a randomized 5-year follow-up study (abstract), *Ned Tijdschr Geneeskd* 141(11):530, 1997.

64. Wadden TA, Luborsky L, Greer S, Crits-Christopher P: The behavioral treatment of essential hypertensions: an update and comparison with pharmacological treatment, *Clin Psychol Rev* 4:403, 1984.

65. Wolpe J: *Psychotherapy by reciprocal inhibition*, Stanford, CA, 1958, Stanford University Press.

66. Yalom ID, Lunde DT, Moos RH, Hamburg DA: "Postpartum blues" syndrome: a description and related variables, *Arch Gen Psychiatry* 18:16, 1968.

67. Yung PMB, Keltner AA: A controlled comparison on the effect of muscle and cognitive relaxation procedures on blood pressure: implications for the behavioural treatment of borderline hypertensives, *Behav Res Ther* 34(10):821, 1996.

68. Zeiss AM, Lewinsohn PM, Munoz RF: Nonspecific improvement effects in depression using interpersonal skills training, pleasant activity schedules or cognitive training, *J Consult Clin Psychol* 47:427, 1979.

6

Meditation

Lyn W. Freeman

WHY READ THIS CHAPTER?

In these times of chronic stress, it is often our cognitive processes—what we think, our interpretation and reinterpretation of events—that fuel the biochemical responses that can impair or improve our health. Meditation offers the opportunity to quiet our minds, to rest from the constant "marathon" of thinking, and to provide an opportunity to restructure ingrained and often unconscious emotional response patterns. This chapter introduces you to four different meditation approaches and explains how meditation can contribute to improved health and a higher quality of life.

CHAPTER AT A GLANCE

There are four forms of meditation that have received attention from researchers. These forms are: transcendental meditation, created by Maharishi Mahesh Yogi; Herbert Benson's respiratory one method; clinically standardized meditation, developed by Carrington and others; and mindfulness meditation, a Buddhist form of meditation.

Meditation essentially induces a deep state of restfulness and elicits different physiologic responses, depending on the method and the length of time one meditates. Oxygen consumption, heart and respiratory rates, and electrical skin resistance are lowered; hormone levels are modulated; and electroencephalographic patterns are altered, modulating alpha and theta brain wave patterns.

Meditation can be described as a wakeful, hypometabolic state. Mechanisms that may explain meditative effects include the blank-out phenomenon—rhythm, desensitization, balancing cerebral hemispheres, and reorganizing mental constructs.

Meditation has been reported to reduce health care costs, strengthen immune function, modulate mood states of anxiety and depression, lower blood pressure, reverse some components of cardiovascular disease, reduce the frequency and duration of epileptic seizures, improve coping skills for chronic pain, and lower the rates of substance abuse.

Meditation is contraindicated for some persons, including those with a history of schizophrenia or psychosis and those that are hypersensitive to meditation. In some healthy persons, meditation may unveil traumatic memories or emotions.

CHAPTER OBJECTIVES

After completing this chapter, you should be able to:

1. Explain the difference between concentrative and nonconcentrative methods of meditation.
2. Describe the history and name the founders of the four meditation methods discussed in this chapter.
3. Compare and contrast the differences among the four meditation methods.
4. Summarize the physiologic and biochemical effects of meditation.
5. Describe the underlying mechanisms believed to explain the effects of meditation.
6. Discuss the signs and symptoms of persons most likely to benefit from meditation.
7. Explain the effects of meditation on sympathetic drive.
8. Discuss the research outcomes of meditation for anxiety and depression.
9. Compare and contrast the research outcomes of meditation as intervention for hypertension and cardiovascular disease.
10. Discuss the research outcomes of meditation and epilepsy.
11. Describe the outcomes of meditation as intervention for chronic pain.
12. Discuss the findings of the effects of meditation on the use of addictive substances.
13. Explain, in detail, the contraindications and side effects of meditation.

■ Meditation and its Forms

Although spiritual forms of meditation have been around for thousands of years, it has only been in the last 25 years that meditation has been researched as a medical intervention in the Western cultures (Figure 6-1). Technically, meditation forms can be classified as concentrative or nonconcentrative. *Concentrative techniques* limit stimuli input by instructing the meditator to focus attention on a single unchanging or repetitive stimulus (e.g., sound, breathing, focal point). If the meditator's attention wanders, he or she is directed to bring the attention gently back to the focal object. By contrast, *nonconcentrative techniques* expand the meditator's attention to include the observation, in a nonjudgmental way, of his or her mental activities and thoughts.

Meditation Research

Generally, four forms of meditation have received varying levels of attention from Western researchers. These forms are:

- Transcendental meditation (TM)
- Herbert Benson's respiratory one method (ROM)
- Clinically standardized meditation (CSM), which is clinically oriented meditation techniques developed by Carrington and others[11,21]
- Mindfulness meditation (MM)

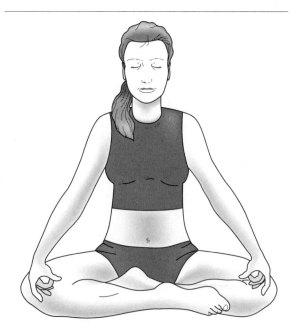

■ **Figure 6-1.** Although spiritual forms of meditation have been around for thousands of years, it is only in the last 25 years that meditation has been researched as a medical intervention in the West.

The TM movement does not invite mental health practitioners to teach its methods unless they are approved TM teachers. Because of this, TM was not initially used as a treatment for disease nor was it applied practically in clinical settings. The physiologic effects of TM were extensively researched, however, and from this literature comes information on the effects of meditation on consciousness and its general effects on physiology. In the last decade, researchers have begun to evaluate TM as a potential health intervention.

The ROM and CSM techniques, modifications of other meditative forms, were specifically designed for use as therapeutic interventions for disease management. They were designed to be "noncultish," so as not to offend religious preferences and to be clinically oriented.

The MM technique, a nonconcentrative method, differs significantly from the other three. MM has also been researched as a health intervention. It has been particularly effective as an intervention for emotional and psychologic dysfunction.

The methods of TM, ROM, CSM, and MM differ. The following text reviews these methods and their differences.

Transcendental Meditation

TM is described as a mental technique that allows the mind to experience progressively finer levels of thought until the source of thought—pure consciousness—is experienced. In TM, a mantra is chosen specifically for the individual's level of consciousness. TM instructors believe that the proper selection of the mantra is of utmost importance in obtaining optimal results and that elevation of consciousness is the primary goal of meditation, with health benefits considered an important and positive side effect of meditation practice. Meditating for 20 minutes, twice a day, is encouraged.

Clinically Standardized Meditation

A practitioner of the CSM technique selects a sound from a list of standard sounds and is instructed to select the one that sounds most appealing. No importance is placed on the need for the mantra to "match" the individual's state of consciousness. The goal of CSM meditation is to gain health benefits—physical and/or psychologic. The client is instructed to repeat the selected sound mentally without linking the sound to breathing patterns or pacing the sound in any structured way. Because of this lack of structure, CSM is considered the most permissive form of meditation.

Respiratory One Method

ROM requires the meditator to repeat the word "one" or another phrase repeatedly while intentionally linking the word or phrase with each exhalation. ROM uses two meditation objects—the chosen word or phrase and the breath—and is therefore considered a structured and rigorous form of meditation. ROM requires more mental effort than CSM.

Mindfulness Meditation

One nonconcentrative method of meditation that has received attention as a medical intervention is the less standardized Buddhist MM. This meditation form has been used as intervention for chronic pain, for drug abuse, and for the treatment of posttraumatic stress syndrome. MM practitioners are encouraged to observe thoughts and images in a nonjudgmental way. MM is different from the other three forms of meditation, all of which suggest that thoughts and images be released or gently pushed aside to allow the mind to become more quieted. This method has been shown to increase cognitive ability in older populations. (MM is discussed in greater detail later in this chapter.)

Physiologic Effects of Meditation

Essentially, the different meditative techniques described in this chapter induce a deep state of restfulness that elicits certain physiologic responses. These physiologic effects vary with the technique practiced and the experience of the meditator. The following is a summary of physiologic effects of the meditative forms:

- Oxygen consumption is lowered to a degree ordinarily reached only after 6 to 7 hours of sleep.[112]
- Heart and respiration rates decrease with meditation, and electrical skin resistance increases, suggesting a low level of anxiety.[4,110,111]
- Blood lactate levels, an indicator of stress, sharply decline.[112]
- Compared with nonmeditators, experienced practitioners become "habituated" (i.e., less reactive) to emotional stressors experienced outside the meditative condition, as demonstrated by heart rate, skin conductance responses, and less anxiety.[48]
- Long-term TM meditation practitioners demonstrate serum dehydroepiandrosterone sulfate (DHEA-S) levels equivalent to those of nonmeditating-matched subjects 5 to 10 years younger. Some techniques of meditation seem to modify the age-related deterioration of DHEA-S, a hormone secreted by the adrenal cortex.[44] The level of DHEA-S is correlated with aging, reducing to 20% its normal level by the eighth decade of life. Increased levels are associated with reduced age-related disorders, including ischemic heart disease and all cardiovascular diseases.
- Meditation has been found to result in significant elevation of positive mood state and significant decreases of corticotropin-releasing hormone (CRH).[53] The physiologic, as opposed to the psychologic, definition of stress is any stimulus that results in the neurons of the hypothalamus releasing CRH. CRH is a trigger that initiates diverse changes in the body, and these changes constitute the syndrome known as the stress response.[107]
- Meditators of CSM who experience the physical stress of a running competition demonstrate less suppression of immunity than matched nonmeditators, as demonstrated by less of an increase in CD8+ (a T and natural killer [NK] cell surface antigen) after maximum volume of oxygen per minute (VO_{2max}) is consumed.[104]
- Compared with practitioners of abbreviated muscle relaxation training (APRT) (see Chapter 5), subjects practicing CSM meditation produce more frontal alpha and fewer symptoms of anxiety when exposed to loud tones; subjects also demonstrate greater cardiac decelerations after each tone. Researchers have found that frontal alpha, as produced during meditation, is a marker for the absence of anxiety.[69]
- Yogic meditators demonstrate persistent alpha activity with increased amplitude modulation during the state of bliss known as "samadhi." This alpha activity cannot be blocked by various sensory stimuli (e.g., light, sound, hot glass, vibration) during meditation, supporting the yogi's claims that they are oblivious to outside influences while in this state of meditation. Yogis who are able to control pain sensations to cold water also demonstrate persistent alpha activity during experiments.[5]
- In novice subjects practicing ROM, EEG topographic mapping reveals that beta activity is greatly reduced, producing significant reductions in cortical activation in anterior brain regions from the first time subjects practice ROM.[60]
- EEG patterns also demonstrate high alpha and occasional theta wave patterns, as well as unusual patterns of fast shifts from alpha to

theta and back again. These patterns suggest a fluid state of consciousness composed of both sleep and wake components.[8,54,112]

■ Meditation has been demonstrated to exert a positive influence on the hormones implicated in stress-related diseases. Meditation for as little as 4 months has been demonstrated to affect cortisol, thyroid-stimulating hormone (TSH), and growth hormone (GH) responses to chronic and acute stress. These changes are demonstrated to be in the opposite direction of the hormonal profile related to poor health outcomes.[74]

The combined research suggests that meditation induces a deep state of relaxation similar to the deepest phase of non–rapid-eye-movement sleep, but in a wakeful state. This phase has been referred to as a "wakeful, hypometabolic state" and a "state of trophotropic dominance."[43,112] Jevning and others argued that meditation is a unique state of consciousness—a wakeful hypometabolic-integrated response—with peripheral circulatory and metabolic changes that induce, simultaneously, both a very relaxed and a very alert state of consciousness.[61]

Contradictory Findings

Although an abundance of literature concludes that meditation induces unique physiologic and biochemical changes, not all authors agree with these findings. In an earlier study, Fenwick and others found that oxygen consumption and carbon dioxide production dropped during meditation, but no more so than during muscle relaxation. No evidence for a hypometabolic state beyond that which is produced by muscle relaxation was found, and no evidence that EEG changes were different from that which is observed in stage "onset" sleep was recorded.[36] Pagano and others reported that a considerable part of the meditation time was composed of various sleep stages.[85]

In an attempt to put the debate to rest, Stigsby and others recorded TM meditators' EEGs when they meditated and when they did not and compared these with various stages of consciousness including wakefulness, drowsiness, sleep onset, and sleep. TM practitioners were compared with age-matched, nonmeditator control subjects and with their own waking outcomes. Authors found the EEG studies to be clearly different from those recorded during sleep onset and sleep patterns.[105] The frequency spectra demonstrated that experienced meditators were at a quantitative level,

characterized as a state between wakefulness and drowsiness in EEG studies. Further, experienced meditators were able to maintain this state virtually unchanged during each 20-minute meditation period, a phenomenon quite different from one of normal relaxation patterns. In comparing their outcomes with other studies, Stigsby and associates noted that changes in response to meditation in short- and long-term meditators differ—an issue to be considered when discussing the EEG effects of meditation.

With meditation, long-term changes beyond those experienced during the meditation practice may occur. Regular meditation practice has been found to alter behavior occurring outside of the meditative state, and therein may lie the most important difference between relaxation practice alone and meditation.[23]

■ Mechanisms Underlying the Effects of Meditation

The following five mechanisms have been suggested as the reasons cognitive methods of meditation induce deep relaxation:

1. Blank-out phenomenon
2. Effects of rhythm
3. Effects of desensitization
4. Balancing cerebral hemispheres
5. Reorganizing mental constructs

Blank-Out Phenomenon

When stimulus input is intentionally limited as occurs with focused meditation, this limitation may create a situation similar to what occurs when the eye is limited in its ability to scan an image. The eye can be artificially prevented from constantly scanning the surface of a visual field. For example, this occurs when an image is painted onto a contact lens because the lens follows the movement of the eye, making the image absolutely stable. In this scenario, the image soon becomes invisible. Without the constant scanning phenomenon, the person can no longer register the object mentally. This is referred to as the *blank-out phenomenon*. During this period, prolonged bursts of alpha waves are recorded in the occipital cortex.[84]

The central nervous system (CNS) operates in such a manner; we remain acutely aware only of changing sources of stimulation. This limitation provides survival value so that we do not become overwhelmed with the common elements of life but are alerted to danger or change in the environment. If we continually recycle the same input, as occurs with mantra meditation, we may induce a similar form of blank-out effect, because the CNS will eventually refuse to attend to this stable form of stimulation. This mental state temporarily clears the mind of thought, creating an aftereffect in a sense. This results in a renewed enthusiasm for new stimuli, similar to what occurs in the maximally receptive attitude of young children. The clearing of the mind that can occur in meditation may serve to break up mental sets that are unproductive. Meditators often describe the experiences after meditation as "sensing the world more vividly," and this awareness may explain the reason meditation has an antidepressive effect on practitioners.[23]

Effects of Rhythm

The repetition of a mantra in a chanting or sing-song style brings the effects of rhythm into play. The stilling of the mind and body also allows the practitioner to become aware of his or her own internal rhythms—breathing patterns, heart rate, or pulse rates are experienced consciously. Zen meditation and MM, for example, use concentration on breathing as part of the focus of meditation. This attention to rhythm induces a calming effect and serves as a natural tranquilizer, as occurs when a parent rocks and sings rhythmically to a child. For example, Salk found that newborn infants responded to recorded heartbeat sounds by crying less than control infants that were not exposed to the sounds.[91] Contacting our own natural rhythms may serve to provide us with a sense of constancy and dependability in a world full of chaotic and competing fast-paced rhythms.

Effects of Desensitization

In systematic desensitization behavior therapy, patients are systematically counter-conditioned by pairing a state of deep relaxation with exposure to the object of their anxiety or fear.[24] Meditation induces deep relaxation and a permissive attitude with respect to thoughts, images, and sensations. This may allow relaxation and objects of anxiety to be paired in a similar manner but in a naturally unrehearsed part of the meditation process. The soothing effect of the meditative mental state may then neutralize disturbing thoughts as the mind initiates a rapid review of a wide variety of mental constructs—verbal and oral, positive and negative, and visual and kinesthetic. Therefore the meditative process may serve as a miniform of desensitization to release the "charge" from anxiety or fear-producing mental constructs.

Balancing Cerebral Hemispheres

Researchers have found that meditation works to equalize the workload between the two cerebral hemispheres[8] (Figure 6-2). Verbal, linear, and time-based thinking is processed through the left hemisphere in most right-handed people. During meditation, this form of thinking is lessened. Holistic, intuitive, and wordless thinking, typically processed through the right hemisphere, becomes more pronounced. A shift in balance between the two hemispheres occurs during the meditation process. This balancing may contribute to the therapeutic effects of meditation. Beginning meditators access the right hemisphere more readily and shift away from left hemisphere activity—the hemisphere that is dominant during waking hours. It is almost as if this shift is needed to balance the typically over-stimulated left hemisphere.[26] Advanced meditators demonstrate EEG readings that are different from those of beginners. The advanced meditator's EEGs reflect more of a balancing of the two hemispheres during meditation.[31] The shifting away from left-dominant hemispheric activity minimizes verbal-conceptual experience and may afford practitioners temporary relief from derogatory thoughts. This

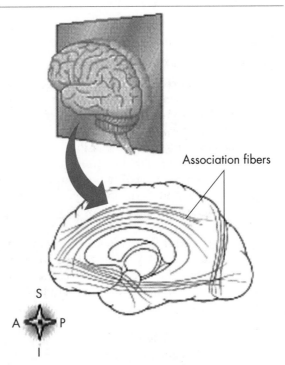

Association fibers

S
A ✦ P
I

■ *Figure 6-2.* **Meditation and cerebral hemisphere synchrony.** Researchers have found that meditation works to equalize the workload between the two cerebral hemispheres.

reduction in internal self-criticism may move from meditative practice to an experience in everyday life.

Reorganizing Mental Constructs

Kelly postulated that our perception of reality is a result of our personal *constructs* or our way of organizing mental events so we can predict future events.[65] Meditators may successfully reorganize some of their constructs by constricting some of them, as occurs in concentrative meditation; or they may broaden the perceptual field to include new elements in a construct, as can occur in non-concentrative meditations, such as Zen Buddhism. The results are a production of less cognitive and more nonverbal constructs, with a change in perception of the reality.

We first focus attention on the meditative practices designed specifically as health interventions—Benson's ROM and the CSM methods. Then, this text reviews the TM and MM research.

It should be noted that Benson, (the creator of ROM), Wallace and Carrington (the developers of CSM), along with other well-known researchers such as Charles Tart, were all initially interested in, studied, and wrote about the methods and outcomes of TM.[102] Their methods therefore may reflect various evolutions of their original experiences with TM.

■ Herbert Benson's Relaxation Response

History of the Relaxation Response

In the 1960s the practice of TM gained popularity in the West, attracting famous proponents like the Beatles and Mia Farrow. Maharishi Mahesh Yogi, a follower of Shri Guru Deva and the founder of TM, had studied physics early in his life. This influenced his decision to eliminate from Yoga certain elements that he considered nonessential. Having developed a revised form of Yoga, Maharishi decided to leave India and bring his new teachings to the West.

In 1968, Herbert Benson was performing animal studies at Harvard Medical School to assess the relationship between behavior and BP. Practitioners of TM heard of these studies and asked Dr. Benson to allow them to demonstrate their ability to lower BP with TM. Although they were initially turned away, the practitioners persisted and Dr. Benson finally agreed to test them.[11]

Before beginning the research, Dr. Benson met with Maharishi Mahesh Yogi to ascertain his level of cooperation and to pose a question. Would the Maharishi continue to cooperate with the research and accept the findings of the research, even if they proved detrimental to his movement? The Maharishi agreed that he would cooperate regardless of the outcomes. Volunteers were then readily obtained from the TM movement. Volunteers ranged from 17 to 41 years of age and with experience in meditation ranging from 1 month to 9 years. The majority had been practicing from 2 to 3 years.

In research protocols, measuring devices were attached or inserted into subjects and 30 minutes elapsed so subjects could become accustomed to the devices. Measurements were then started and continued for three periods: (1) 20 to 30 minutes of quiet sitting; (2) 20 to 30 minutes of meditation; and (3) another 20 to 30 minutes of quiet sitting without meditating. Initial findings confirmed that meditators were able to markedly decrease the body's oxygen consumption, decrease metabolic rate (hypometabolism), and experience a profound sense of restfulness. It was then questioned whether meditation may be a form of "mini-hibernation." In hibernation, rectal temperature decreases. Rectal probes were therefore added to the research protocol, and it was determined that meditation was definitely not a hibernation-like condition. Was meditation a sleeplike phenomenon? During sleep, oxygen consumption slowly decreases until, 4 or 5 hours later, it is as much as 8% lower than the waking state. Meditation decreased average oxygen consumption from 10% to 20%—and during the first 3 minutes of meditation. Meditation was clearly not like sleep. EEG measurements also found differences between meditation and sleep. Meditation produced a predominance of alpha waves—a measurement of deep relaxation, but not sleep. None or few of the characteristic EEG signals indicating rapid eye movement were found in meditators.

Meditation also produced a marked drop in blood lactate, a substance produced by the metabolism of skeletal muscles. This reduction was particularly interesting because of its association with anxiety. Heart rate decreased an average of three beats per minute from a resting state, and respiration slowed. BP did not change in practiced meditators, however. BP was low before, during, and after meditation. This led Benson to wonder whether meditation was a natural form of treatment for hypertension.

R. Keith Wallace, a PhD candidate in physiology at the University of California, Los Angeles, performed similar studies. Although these two sets of studies were originally performed independently, Dr. Wallace eventually joined the research team at Harvard's Thorndike Memorial Laboratory of the Boston City Hospital. A series of ongoing research experiments then ensued.

A study was designed to answer the question, "Can meditation reduce the BP level of subjects who already have high BP?" Would-be initiates of TM who were diagnosed with high BP were recruited for the research. Eighty-six subjects, who tested and consistently demonstrated high BP for 6 weeks were entered into the study. The subjects were taught TM. Once they demonstrated proficiency, their BP was measured at random times throughout the day, but never while they were meditating. At the end of the study, only 36 of the subjects had consistently maintained medication, diet, or smoking habits and had practiced regularly—all factors that had to be considered in interpreting the results. These 36 subjects had lower systolic BP from an average of 146 to 137 and lower diastolic BP from 93.5 to 88.9. Improvements were maintained only as long as the subjects continued to practice. Based on these early experiences, Benson decided to develop a meditation protocol of his own. He called this meditation technique ROM. This technique was based on an effect referred to as the *relaxation response.*

Philosophy of the Relaxation Response

Whereas the JPRT and APRT methods can be considered to be somatically oriented techniques that focus almost exclusively on muscle relaxation, Benson's relaxation response method can be considered the antithesis of that approach. Benson argued that, in human beings, all relaxation techniques produce a single relaxation response. This response results in diminished sympathetic arousal. Benson stated that, in his opinion, all relaxation methods involve oral repetition and a passive attitude; therefore all relaxation methods produce similar results.[12]

Eliciting the Relaxation Response

According to the teachings of Benson, there are four basic elements that are typically necessary to elicit a relaxation response. These elements are:

- *Mental device.* A device that provides constant mental stimulus (e.g., sound, word, phrase) repeated either silently or audibly is the first basic element. The purpose of this device is to free the person from logical, externally oriented thought by providing the mind a device on which to dwell.

- *Passive attitude.* If distracting thoughts occur during the repetition of the sound, word, or phrase, practitioners attempt to disregard the distraction and gently redirect attention back to the mental device. Practitioners are instructed not to worry or be judgmental about how well they are performing the technique; instead, they are simply encouraged to continue the practice.

- *Decreased muscle tone.* Practitioners find a comfortable posture that requires minimal muscular work to maintain the meditative posture. Often supine or sitting postures are selected.

- *Quiet environment.* Quiet surroundings with minimal environmental stimuli provides an optimal relaxation experience. During practice, the practitioner is usually instructed to close his or her eyes.[15]

Mechanisms of the Relaxation Response

Based on these four elements, Benson designed a simple method for eliciting the relaxation response. The instructions for his technique are the following:

1. Sit quietly in a comfortable position.
2. Close your eyes.
3. Deeply relax all your muscles, beginning at your feet and progressing to your face.
4. Breathe through your nose, becoming aware of your breathing. As you breathe out, say the word "ONE" silently to yourself.
5. Continue for 20 minutes. Sit quietly for several minutes after the meditation period is completed.
6. Do not worry about succeeding; simply maintain a passive attitude and permit relaxation to come at its own pace. Ignore distracting thoughts. Practice the technique twice daily, but not within 2 hours of any meal.[16]

These same elements are common as part of many spiritual disciplines. Benson argued that the practice of his relaxation response technique produced the same hypometabolic respiratory changes observed during the practice of other meditational techniques.[10]

Elements of the Relaxation Response in Early Religious Practices

Practices using these principles have existed within a religious context for centuries and in almost every culture. They have been used in the practices of Christian and Jewish mysticism and in Eastern religions such as Zen, Yoga, Hinduism,

Shintoism, and Taoism.[14] In the fourteenth century at Mount Athos in Greece, Gregory of Sinai described a prayer that was referred to as a secret meditation and was transmitted to new monks during initiation.

> Sit down alone and in silence. Lower your head, shut your eyes, breathe out gently, and imagine yourself looking into your own heart. Carry your mind, your thoughts from your head to your heart. As you breathe out, say "Lord Jesus Christ, have mercy on me." Say it moving your lips gently, or simply say it in your mind. Try to put all other thoughts aside. Be calm, be patient and repeat the process very frequently.[37]

■ Clinically Standardized Meditation

The CSM method was devised as a scientifically developed form of meditation intended to be "noncultish" in nature to avoid violating any religious convictions of the practitioners. It was also developed to be easy to learn, and it does not require intense mental concentration. For type-A patients, it is often suggested that they learn CSM by performing "mini-meditations" as short as 2 to 3 minutes.[21] For other patients, 20 to 30 minutes a day is recommended. CSM has been successfully combined with solitary but repetitive physical activities, such as jogging, walking, or swimming.

Participants receiving personal instruction select a mantra from a list of 16 mantras in a workbook. They are asked to choose the one that is most pleasant and soothing to them, or they are instructed to make up a mantra that is personally pleasing. The mantras in the workbook have resonant sounds, often ending in "m" or "n" because these sounds have been shown to be calming. The words have no meaning in English, but they are created for their soothing sound alone. The instructor repeats the mantra with the participant in a rhythmic manner to help him or her develop a "feel" for the harmony of the word. Unlike Benson's ROM, the mantra is *not* associated with breathing. The participant repeats the word with the instructor, and then he or she is asked to first whisper the word and then to "think it to yourself" silently with eyes closed. The participant and instructor meditate together for 10 minutes. The participant is then questioned about his or her meditation technique, and the instructor attempts to correct any misconceptions the participant may have about how to practice CSM. The participant then meditates for 20 minutes alone. After meditation, the participant completes a questionnaire and reviews the responses with the instructor. An interview is then conducted to clarify procedures for home meditation practice. The participant is apprised of possible side effects of tension release and limitations of the method and is told how to handle side-effect reactions, should they occur. Individual follow-up interviews are held at intervals, and group meetings can be scheduled that allow new meditators to share their experiences.

Participants are helped to adjust their techniques to their individual needs and life styles. Close clinical supervision and follow-up programs support maximal participation in meditation. The success of this method, Carrington believes, is based on continually working with the meditator so that the method is constantly fine-tuned to meet the changing needs and life styles of the client.[23]

■ Signs and Symptoms of Persons Who May Benefit from Meditation

Clinicians often suggest that cognitive relaxation methods such as meditation work more effectively for persons with symptoms of cognitive anxiety, whereas progressive relaxation works best for those with somatic symptoms.[26,96] Currently, there are insufficient data to substantiate these claims.[70] A suggested avenue for assessing whether meditation is indicated for a patient involves determining whether the patient demonstrates one or more of the following meditative-responsive symptoms:

- Chronic fatigue symptoms
- Tension or anxiety states
- Psychophysiologic disorders
- Abuse of alcohol or tobacco
- Insomnia or hypersomnia
- Excessive self-blame
- Chronic low-grade depression or subacute reaction depression
- Irritability and low tolerance for frustration
- Strong submissive tendencies, difficulties with self-assertion, poorly developed psychologic differentiation
- Pathologic bereavement reactions
- Separation anxiety
- Blocks in productivity or creativity
- Inadequate eye contact with low effect
- Need to shift emphasis from reliance on therapist to self-reliance[23]

If the patient possesses one or more of these symptoms, the therapist must then decide whether he or she is an appropriate candidate for meditation. The therapist must consider the following:

1. *Lack of time and moderate self-discipline.* Since meditation does not require great mental effort and the process is easy to learn and

follow, only 20 to 30 minutes a day are necessary to benefit from the meditation process. Therefore meditation may be an effective intervention for clients with limited time and moderate self-discipline,

2. *Self-reinforcing properties.* The peaceful mental state induced by meditation provides a built-in, self-reinforcing effect. When client motivation is minimal, meditation may be the most effective strategy for involving the patient in a relaxation method.

3. *Meditative skills.* The ability to focus and to let go of unnecessary goal-directed and analytical activities and the skill of receptivity—the willingness to tolerate and accept subjective experiences that may seem unfamiliar and paradoxical—are all required.

■ Effects of Meditation on Sympathetic Drive, Mental Functionality, Health Care, and Survival Rates

As discussed in previous chapters, research has found that acute or chronic stress affects immune function and overall health. Continuous behavioral adjustment has been associated with the pathogenesis of several diseases, including hypertension and sudden coronary death.[52,63,75] The role that prolonged stimulation of the sympathetic nervous system plays in the elevation of serum cholesterol levels has been clearly determined.[7,38,50] Situations that require constant adjustment, as measured by physiologic responsivity, stimulate an integrated hypothalamic response. This hypothalamic

response has been labeled, the "fight-or-flight response." The "fight-or-flight" response, also referred to as the ergotropic response, is activated by increased activity of the sympathetic nervous system and results in increases in catecholamine production, oxygen consumption, heart and respiratory rates, arterial blood lactate, and skeletal muscle blood flow.[1,43] A second hypothalamic response compensates for the emergency response. This response is often referred to as trophotropic or relaxation.[17] It results in decreased activity of the sympathetic nervous system leading to decreased oxygen consumption, lower heart and respiratory rates, and reduced arterial blood lactate, as well as increased frequency and intensity of EEG alpha- and theta-wave activity.[112]

It is believed that meditation is capable of blunting the excitatory autonomic responses brought on by stress and by sudden excitatory events. Stress-related diseases, correlated with continuous behavioral adjustment, can often be prevented. Either reducing the emergency response or increasing the relaxation response can reduce the excitatory autonomic response (Boxes 6-1 and 6-2).

■ Meditation and Health Care Costs

Researchers have consistently hypothesized that when meditation is practiced on a regular basis, it will provide protection from disease states induced by stressful life events. One study compared 5 years of medical insurance utilization statistics of approximately 2000 practitioners of TM with a

---

BOX 6-1 Stimulation of Ergotropic (Fight-or-Flight) System

Autonomic effects: sympathetic discharge resulting in:
  Increased cardiac rate
  Elevated blood pressure
  Sweat secretions
  Pupil dilation
  Inhibition of gastrointestinal motor and secretory
    functions
Somatic effects:
  Desynchrony of electromylogram
  Increased skeletal muscle tone
  Elevation of the hormones epinephrine, norepinephrine,
    adrenocortical steroids, and thyroxin
  Decreased skin resistance
Behavioral effects:
  Arousal/tension
  Increased activity
  Emotional responsivity
  Heightened alertness/focus

BOX 6-2 Stimulation of the Trophotropic (Rest-and-Digest) System

Autonomic effects: parasympathetic discharge
resulting in:
  Reduction in cardiac rate
  Reduction in blood pressure
  Pupil constriction
  Increased gastrointestinal motor and secretory
    function
Somatic effects:
  Synchrony of electromyogram
  Loss of skeletal muscle tone
  Blocking of shivering response
  Increased secretion of insulin
  Increased skin resistance
Behavioral effects:
  Inactivity
  Drowsiness
  Deep relaxation

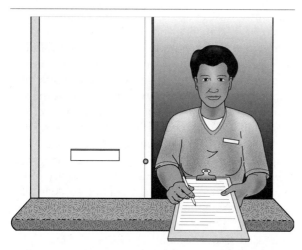

■ **Figure 6-3.** When compared with five other health insurance groups, the TM group still demonstrated 53.3% fewer inpatient admissions and 44.4% fewer outpatient visits.

normative database of approximately 600,000 members of the same insurance carrier. Benefits, deductible, co-insurance terms, and distribution by sex of the TM group were similar to the normative insurance sample. TM practitioners had lower medical utilization rates in all categories. When comparing inpatient stays for meditators in age categories with those in the normative sample, there were 50.2% fewer days for children, 50.1% fewer days for young adults, and 69.4% fewer days for adults aged 40 plus years (Figure 6-3).

Outpatient visits for meditators, as compared with the normative sample, were 46.8% fewer for children, 54.7% fewer for young adults, and 73.3% fewer for adults aged 40 plus years. When compared with five other health insurance groups, the TM group still demonstrated 53.3% fewer inpatient admissions per 1000 patients and 44.4% fewer outpatient visits per 1000. TM group's admissions for childbirth were similar to the normative sample.[81]

Studies have found that patients with high levels of anxiety run greater surgical risks because they require higher doses of anesthesia.[62] Further, psychologic stress has provoked ventricular arrhythmias, exacerbated diabetes, altered blood-clotting mechanisms, and increased the risk of gastric ulceration.[39,73] Surgery-related benefits of anxiety-reducing interventions are decreased postoperative use of narcotics and shortened hospital stays, reducing hospitalization by an average of 1½ days per person.[29,77]

Meditation may have implications for well-being in the older population.[2] In an interesting study, 73 older adults living in seven different

retirement and nursing homes and one apartment complex were randomly assigned to one of four groups: (1) TM meditation; (2) mindfulness training (not MM, but a guided-attention technique involving structured word production and a creative task in which participants were asked to think of a topic in new and creative ways); (3) mental relaxation (passive repetition of a client-chosen word, referred to as "low mindfulness"; or (4) no treatment. Both TM and mindfulness training groups produced significant improvements on paired associate learning, two measures of cognitive flexibility, mental health, systolic BP, ratings of behavioral flexibility, and treatment efficacy, as compared with the relaxation and control groups. Compared with mindfulness training, TM produced the greatest improvements in these categories. Both TM and mindfulness training demonstrated significantly greater improvements than both the relaxation and control groups on perceived control and word fluency, with the mindfulness-training group out performing the TM group in these categories. At 3 years, the survival rates per group were 100% (TM), 87.5% (mindfulness), 65.0% (relaxation), and 77.3% (control). The average survival rate for remaining populations in the same institutions not assigned to any group was 62.6%.

■ Role of Stress in Psychiatric and Somatic Disorders

MacLean and others have emphasized the role of chronic stress in psychiatric and somatic disorders.[74] Chronic stress appears to elevate baseline cortisol, but it reduces cortisol short-term responsiveness to acute stressors—a profile associated with poor health. Glucocorticoid regulation through the hypothalamic-pituitary-adrenal (HPA) cortisol axis is one of the clearest and best-studied pathways for the effects of stress on disease and aging.[32,92]

While elevating baseline cortisol, chronic stress simultaneously decreases testosterone titers and inhibits GH secretion.[3,67] In human beings, short-term stress, such as strenuous exercise or a stressful job interview, appears to increase TSH and GH release.[79,90,94] In other words, chronic stress tends to elevate hormonal levels as a function of baseline, but it makes "bursts" of these hormones less available when they are needed to respond to an acute stressor.

In one study, effects of laboratory short-term stressors on plasma hormones were assessed in TM practitioners who had meditated for 4 months

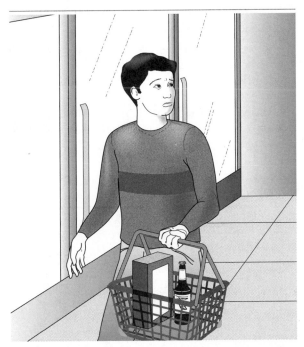

■ **Figure 6-4.** As an intervention, meditation may initially be less effective for patients with long-term and severe anxiety disorders or for those suffering from panic disorders.

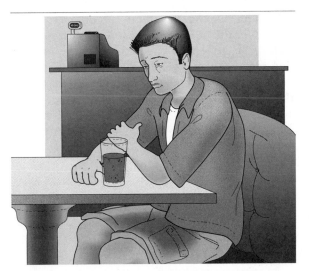

■ **Figure 6-5.** Meditation is often helpful to those suffering from chronic low-grade depression or subacute reaction depressions. Benefits may include a reduced need for anti-depressive medications.

(N=16) and in persons who attended a stress education class (N=13). Three stressors—mental arithmetic, mirror star-tracing task, and isometric hand gripping—were used. Before and after testing, TM practitioners significantly decreased baseline cortisol and overall cortisol average (p=0.04), whereas cortisol response increased after testing compared with the cortisol response before testing—a profile exactly the opposite of the chronic stress hormonal profile (p=0.02). Changes in TSH and GH responses in the TM group to stress before and after testing differed from the stress education group (p=0.02 and 0.05, respectively), as did testosterone baseline changes before and after testing (p=0.05), again in the direction opposite to a chronic stress hormonal profile. The results suggested that meditation alters acute response of four prominent hormones to laboratory stresses in the direction of more optimal function. The authors suggested that hormonal response to stressors may be the result of alterations in hippocampal neurons caused by frequent stress-induced elevations of glucocorticoids.[74] Other studies have suggested that similar mechanisms may explain the effects of stress on human health.[93,98] Meditation has implications for the regulation of hormonal homeostasis outside of the practice experience, especially in the regulation of cortisol and TSH.

Meditation for the Treatment of Mood State Disorders

As previously discussed, there is evidence that practicing meditation on a regular basis can reduce anxiety for individuals with clinically elevated levels of anxiety. However, there is a "floor effect" (i.e., meditators with preexisting low scores for anxiety are unable to alter scores appreciably, a phenomenon that is consistent with the "wisdom of the body" homeostasis theory discussed in earlier chapters)[28] (Figure 6-4 and 6-5).

As an intervention, meditation may initially be less effective for patients with long-term and severe anxiety disorders or for those suffering from panic disorders. These patients may have trouble focusing long enough to practice the procedure and may cease practice out of frustration. In a study with a group of psychiatric inpatients, Glueck found that dosages of psychotropic medication and sedatives could be reduced if patients were first stabilized and then taught to meditate.[45] This strategy may have implications for the use of meditation with inpatients in treatment for mood disorders.

The calming effects of meditation differ considerably, however, from the calming effects of psychotropic drugs. Drugs bring the side effects of grogginess and loss of energy, whereas meditation actually sharpens alertness, increases the speed of reaction times, and allows practitioners to perform perceptual motor tasks with greater speed and accuracy.[6,87,89] Meditation may therefore be indicated for the treatment of anxiety if the patient is sufficiently stable to concentrate. The lack of negative side effects induced by meditation may allow the patient to perform more productively during the day. In Table 6-1, we review the findings of meditation as a mood modulator and as a treatment for emotional and mental dysfunction.

Effects of Progressive Relaxation versus Meditation on Anxiety

As noted, Benson believed that all relaxation methods produce essentially the same results. He argued that the effects of ROM are equivalent to more complex techniques, such as progressive relaxation, and that ROM is preferable because it is easy to learn and practice.[49] He also suggested

TABLE 6-1	Effects of Progressive Relaxation on Mood State Disorders	
AUTHOR(S)	**DESIGN**	**FINDINGS**
Smith JC: Psychotherapeutic effects of transcendental meditation with controls for expectation of relief and daily sitting, *J Consult Clin Psychol* 44(4:630, 1976.		
Experiment 1	(1) TM (2) PSI—twice-daily sitting placebo with no meditation (3) No-treatment control N: 100 Number of sessions: 4	At 6 months, TM and PSI were equally effective for reducing anxiety, muscle tension, and autonomic arousal symptoms
Experiment 2	(1) TM-like exercise (2) CMS, the generation of many thoughts—the antithesis of meditation N=54 Number of sessions: 4	At 11 weeks, both treatments were equal in effectiveness—for reducing anxiety, muscle, tension, and autonomic arousal symptoms Authors concluded TM was no more effective than sitting, no meditation, or than the antithesis of meditation; the crucial component of TM is not the TM exercise
Benson H et al: Treatment of anxiety: a comparison of the usefulness of self-hypnosis and a meditational relaxation technique, *Psychother Psychosom* 30:229, 1978.	(1) ROM (2) Hypnosis/relaxation N=32 Number of sessions: 2	Psychiatric assessment demonstrated 34% improvement; self-report, 63% There were no differences between groups for outcome efficacy
Carrington P et al: The use of meditation-relaxation techniques for the management of stress in a working population, *J Occup Med* 22:221, 1980.	(1) CSM (2) ROM (3) APRT (4) Wait-list control N=154 Number of sessions: Data not provided	At 5.5 months, ROM and CSM, but not APRT, subjects demonstrated significantly reduced symptoms compared with control groups 78% of meditators practiced, with improvement found whether subjects practiced frequently or occasionally
Raskin M et al: Muscle biofeedback and Transcendental Meditation: a controlled evaluation of efficacy in the treatment of chronic anxiety, *Arch Gen Psychiatry* 37:93, 1980.	(1) TM (2) Muscle biofeedback (3) APRT N=31 Number of sessions: 18 for groups 2 and 3 4 consecutive days of lecture/practice for group 1	40% of subjects had clinically significant decrease in anxiety No difference between treatments in efficacy, symptom reduction, and 18-mo maintenance gains Profoundly deep relaxation was not necessary to significantly reduce anxiety
Brooks JS et al: Transcendental meditation in the treatment of post-Vietnam adjustment, *J Counseling Dev* 64:212, 1985.	(1) TM (2) Psychotherapy N=18 Number of sessions: TM: 15 Psychotherapy: 11 and family/group counseling for some clients	TM significantly reduced degree of post-traumatic stress, emotional numbness, anxiety, depression, alcohol consumption, family problems, and insomnia compared with psychotherapy TM also increased habituation response to stressful stimuli

APRT, Abbreviated progressive relaxation therapy; *PHEP,* personal happiness enhancement program; *PSI,* periodic somatic inactivity; *ROM,* respiratory one method; *TM,* transcendental meditation; *CMS,* cortically mediated stabilization.

that prayer or other oral distractions can be substituted for the word "one."[19]

Other authors did not agree and found differences in the effects of relaxation methods and meditation. Norton and Johnson identified cognitive-somatic differences. They compared progressive relaxation with Agni yoga, which uses imaginal meditative exercises. Snake phobias were studied using the two techniques, and the authors found that subjects scoring high on cognitive anxiety were able to approach the snakes more closely after practicing Agni yoga than after progressive relaxation. By contrast, patients scoring high on somatic anxiety approached the snakes more closely after practicing progressive relaxation. In this study, the type of anxiety

TABLE 6-1	Effects of Progressive Relaxation on Mood State Disorders—cont'd	
AUTHOR(S)	**DESIGN**	**FINDINGS**
Domar AD et al: The preoperative use of the relaxation response with ambulatory surgery patients, *J Hum Stress* 13(3):101, 1987.	(1) ROM (2) Reading for relaxation N=42 Number of sessions: 1 Given instruction on the use of a cassette for practice or reading instructions—no actual practice session was conducted for either group, a potential confounding variable for practice effect	Neither group demonstrated increased anxiety immediately before nor after surgery; on psychologic nor physiologic measures Self-report anxiety patterns found ROM clients with highest anxiety before entering study and lowest anxiety several days before surgery Controls experienced highest anxiety levels before and during surgery
Kabat-Zinn J et al: Effectiveness of a meditation-based stress reduction program in the treatment of anxiety disorders, *Am J Psychiatry* 149(7):936, 1992.	(1) Mindfulness (2) No control group N=22 Number of sessions: 8 2-hour sessions +1 7.5-hr intensive meditation	Medical outpatients received clinically and statistically significant reductions in anxiety and depression at 3-mo (p<0.0001) for Beck and Hamilton Depression/Anxiety scales
Miller J et al: Three-year follow-up and clinical implications of a mindfulness meditation-based stress reduction intervention in the treatment of anxiety disorders, *Gen Hosp Psychiatry* 17:192, 1995.	This is a 3-year follow-up of the Kabat-Zinn study described above	The outcomes described at 3 months maintained at 3 yrs
Smith WP et al: Meditation as an adjunct to a happiness enhancement program, *J Clin Psychol* 51(2):269, 1995.	(1) PHEP (2) PHEP and ROM (3) Control group N=36 Number of sessions: PHEP: 12 PHEP and ROM: 13	On subjective measures of happiness, state, and trait anxiety, and depression, groups 1 and 2 improved significantly more than controls; group 2 also improved significantly more than group 1 on happiness, depression, and trait anxiety Authors concluded ROM enhances states of happiness
MENOPAUSAL SYMPTOMS		
Irvin JH et al: The effects of relaxation response training on menopausal symptoms, *J Psychosom Obstetr Gynecol* 17:202, 1996.	(1) ROM (2) Reading control (3) No-treatment control N=33 Number of sessions: 1 and audiotape	ROM group produced significant reductions in hot flash intensity, tension anxiety, and depression (p<0.05) Reading group produced significant improvement in trait anxiety and confusion bewilderment (p<0.05) Control group had no changes

(somatic or cognitive) determined which method was most effective for the individual.[80]

Meditation Forms: Differences in Outcomes

Stanford University researcher Kenneth Eppley performed a well-designed and thorough meta-analysis study of the effects of relaxation techniques on trait anxiety.[34] *Trait anxiety* refers to the general tendency to be anxious. *State anxiety* is an assessment of an individual's anxiety level at any given moment. Using 109 studies, effect sizes were calculated by population, age, sex, experimental design, duration, hours of treatment, pretest anxiety, demand characteristics, experimenter attitude, type of publication, and attribution. Only population, duration, hours of treatment, and attrition influenced effect size, whereas confounding variables did not. The authors found that APRT, EMG biofeedback, and various forms of meditation produced similar effect sizes with one exception; TM produced significantly larger effect sizes ($p < 0.005$). Relaxation produced an effect size of 0.39, whereas TM produced an effect size of 0.70. When concentrative meditation forms were assessed separately, other concentrative methods including CSM and ROM produced an effect size of approximately 0.28. The authors concluded that even if TM practitioners meditated more consistently; if their teachers were more experienced or if motivation was higher because of a sense of "tradition," the result was that TM still produced larger and more consistent effects in relaxation as a treatment of anxiety.

Meditation and Relaxation: Differences in Outcomes

Why are there differences in the results between meditation and relaxation? Differences in the cognitive effects of meditation as compared with APRT have been reported. Mantra meditation appears to produce a lack of synchrony between cortical and somatic indices of arousal, specifically as they relate to EEG readings. Reviews have found that meditative ecstasy is accompanied by increases in beta rhythms and suppressions of alpha, whereas alpha activity is enhanced in the deep relaxation states that occur in meditation.[27,117,119] APRT, on the other hand, does not seem to produce consistent effects of EEG activity.[68,72]

In one study, 83 black college students were tested on EEG coherence, skin potential, habituation to a series of loud tones, psychometric measures of mental health, and intelligence quotient (IQ) scores. The students were then assigned to six training sessions of TM, APRT, or cognitive-

behavioral strategies. Approximately 1 year later, the students were tested again. Those practicing either TM or APRT recorded significantly improved scores for overall mental health factors ($p < 0.04$) and anxiety ($p < 0.0006$). TM produced a greater reduction in neuroticism than either APRT or cognitive behavioral methods ($p < 0.03$). TM also produced global increases in alpha and theta coherence among frontal and central leads during TM meditation, as compared with having eyes closed but not meditating ($p < 0.02$). Neither APRT nor cognitive intervention produced EEG state changes. Coherence among frontal and central areas in the alpha band is positively correlated with creativity and concept learning efficiency; and it is negatively correlated with neuroticism.[30,82,83] TM also produced faster skin potential habituation after meditation than before ($p < 0.05$).[41]

Not all studies found meditation an effective technique. In one double-blind, placebo-controlled study, TM taught by a TM trainer was compared with a placebo identical to the TM process (sitting twice daily with eyes closed), but with no meditation.[103] The interventions were assessed for their ability to reduce anxiety. A TM-like exercise was also compared with a procedure that was the antithesis of meditation—generating as many positive thoughts as possible. All treatments produced essentially the same effective outcomes, suggesting that the TM method was not the responsible component leading to reduced anxiety. The authors concluded it was the expectation of relief that produced the results, not TM itself.

Effects of Meditation versus Relaxation on Blood Pressure and Cardiovascular Disease Outcomes

Several authors have found that meditation with its cognitive focus is not as effective as other relaxation techniques or biofeedback in reducing BP. They concluded that other relaxation techniques have more of an autonomic focus, making them more effective tools for the management of hypertension (Figure 6-6). Hefner found meditation to have weaker effects on BP than EMG and galvanic skin resistance (GSR) biofeedback. Similarly, Cohen and Boxhill found meditation less effective than EMG biofeedback for the reduction of BP. English and Baker's results demonstrated meditation to be less effective for hypertension than progressive relaxation, whereas Cohen and Sedlacek obtained better results with a combination of progressive relaxation, autogenic training, relaxation training, and biofeedback than with meditation alone.[25,33,55,97]

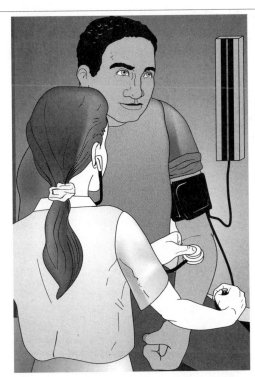

■ *Figure 6-6.* The black population suffers from high blood pressure more than other populations. Recent studies using meditation as hypertensive intervention with black patients have demonstrated significantly reduced levels of systolic and diastolic blood pressure and more effective results than APRT.

Evidence supports the possibility that progressive relaxation produces greater reduction in somatic tension than does meditation. Resting heart rates were found to be lower among long-term practitioners of APRT when compared with long-term practitioners of TM; and APRT had produced greater decreases in systolic BP than did ROM.[33,116]

More recently, studies of TM meditation as an intervention for hypertension in black Americans have produced promising results. These are important findings because, as compared with Caucasian populations, black Americans are more likely to develop hypertension at a young age, to suffer from more severe forms of hypertension, to be under-controlled for longer periods, and to develop hypertension that progresses more rapidly with age.[20,35,56,58] Recent studies targeting this population and using meditation as hypertensive intervention have demonstrated reduced levels of systolic and diastolic BP as compared with BP levels in those participating in APRT and in those assigned to control groups.[9,95] These studies are ongoing and will continue to gather data on the long-term effects of meditation as an intervention for hypertension.

Meditation may decrease premature ventricular contraction in patients with ischemic heart disease. In one study, 11 ambulatory patients with proven, stable ischemic heart disease and premature ventricular contractions (PVCs) were taught Benson's ROM relaxation response and practiced for 4 weeks.[13] The frequency of PVCs was measured by computer analysis tapes for 2 complete days before beginning practice and at the end of the 4 weeks of practice. Of the 11 patients, 8 had reduced frequencies of PVCs. This effect was especially striking during sleeping hours. In one study, meditation reduced postoperative supraventricular tachycardia (ST).[71] In another study, meditation increased exercise duration and maximal workload, delayed onset of ST depression, and reduced rate pressure products in patients with cardiovascular disease[120] (Tables 6-2 and 6-3).

An Expert Speaks: Dr. Robert H. Schneider

Robert H. Schneider, MD, is Co-Director, Doctoral Program in Physiology, Department of Physiological and Biological Sciences, and Dean, College of Maharishi Vedic Medicine, Maharishi University of Management, Fairfield, Iowa. He is a fellow of the American Heart Association. Currently, Dr. Schneider is the principal investigator of eight National Institutes of Health (NIH) grants researching TM as an intervention for hypertension and cardiovascular disease in black Americans and for health promotion and disease prevention in the older population. He has served as principal investigator, co-investigator, or coordinator for nine earlier studies on the effects of meditation on hypertension, lipid levels, cardiovascular disease, disease prevention, stress reduction, and treatment of Type-A behavior.

Question. Dr. Schneider, can you describe your work with meditation as an intervention for hypertension and cardiovascular disease?

Answer. The history of our work started in the late 1980s. We began a series of randomized controlled trials on the effects of TM and compared it with the most widely used relaxation technique of the time—progressive muscle relaxation—and with a health education control. The literature of the time showed that cognitive behavioral techniques, when studied in controlled settings, were on average no more effective than placebo. However, in randomized controlled settings, our studies demonstrated that TM was significantly more effective than muscle relaxation and much more effective than atten-

TABLE 6-2	Effects of Meditation on Hypertension and Cholesterol	
AUTHOR(S)	**DESIGN**	**FINDINGS**
YOGIC-BASED MEDITATION		
Patel CH: Yoga and biofeedback in the management of hypertension, *Lancet* II:1053, 1973. Patel CH: 12 month follow-up of yoga and biofeedback in the management of hypertension, *Lancet* I:62, 1975.	(1) Yoga-based meditation with relaxation/biofeedback (2) Matched controls N=40 Number of sessions: 36	Initial study, 1973 Follow-up, 1975 In Group 1, systolic BP reduced 20.4 mm Hg and diastolic BP 14.2 mm Hg (p<0.001) Drug requirements fell 41.9% No significant changes were found in the control group Results maintained at 12-month follow-up
Patel C et al: Controlled trial of biofeedback-aided behavioural methods in reducing mild hypertension, *BMJ* 282:2005, 1981. Patel C et al: Trial of relaxation in reducing coronary risk: our year follow-up, *BMJ* 290:1103, 1985.	(1) Yoga-based meditation with relaxation/biofeedback (2) Controls given informational health leaflets N=192 Number of sessions: 8	On completion of training, 6 months and 4 years after intervention, group 1 still maintained significantly lower systolic and diastolic BP than controls After 4 years, controls had more angina and treatment for hypertension, ischemic heart disease treatments, fatal myocardial infarction, or EEG evidence of ischemia than treatment group
Hafner RJ: Psychological treatment of essential hypertension: a controlled comparison of meditation and meditation plus biofeedback, *Biofeedback Self Regul* 7:305, 1982.	(1) Yoga-based meditation (2) Meditation and biofeedback (3) No-treatment control Number of sessions: 8	Statistically significant falls in systolic and diastolic BP occurred for groups 1 and 2, but not statistically more than control group Group 2 produced falls in diastolic BP earlier than group 1
Patel C et al: Can general practitioners use training in relaxation and management of stress to reduce mild hypertension? *BMJ* 296:21, 1988.	(1) BP-controlled patients discontinued on active drug (2) BP-controlled patients still taking active drug N=103 Number of sessions: 8 Note: In this part of the hypertension trial, patients were given cassettes for practice Sessions were physician/nurse lectures on research and stress management strategies and also included meditation protocol with biofeedback	At 1 year, patients who discontinued drugs maintained their improvements Those who continued drug therapy reduced BP even more (patients in both groups practiced a yogic-based form of meditation, which emphasized deep breathing, muscle relaxation, biofeedback, and concentrative meditation Controls who discontinued drugs increased BP

APRT, Abbreviated progressive relaxation therapy; *BP*, blood pressure; *PMR*, progressive muscle relaxation; *TM*, transcendental meditation.

tion control. This was the first time, to my knowledge, in a strongly controlled clinical trial design that any behavioral or meditation-type approach was shown to be highly effective. In this case, the reductions that we saw, at least in older black Americans, were as great as the average reduction reported in metaanalyses of drug treatment for mild hypertension. Those original findings were published in the American Heart Association's journal, *Hypertension*, in a series of two papers.

Based on those early findings, the NIH supported a series of several follow-up trials. We are conducting these trials with collaborators at major medical centers around the country. We assess the effects of TM on end-organ damage from hypertension, on health care costs related to the treatment of cardiovascular disease, and on cardiovascular morbidity and mortality in high-risk populations. The first studies were technically in the area of secondary prevention, treating the risk factor. Then we moved into tertiary prevention—working with individuals who already had the disease clinically. The stage we are on now is in primary prevention, using this approach with individuals who do not have the risk factor or the disease, but who are at high risk for developing the risk factor of hypertension and the subsequent disease.

We have some exciting preliminary findings also. One of our graduates, Dr. Kofi Kondwani, in his dissertation has found in an important pilot study that those individuals who practiced TM had regression of left ventricular mass and

TABLE 6-2	Effects of Meditation on Hypertension and Cholesterol—cont'd	
AUTHOR(S)	**DESIGN**	**FINDINGS**
TRANSCENDENTAL MEDITATION		
Cooper MJ et al: A relaxation technique in the management of hypercholesterolemia, *J Hum Stress* 5:24, 1979.	(1) TM (2) No-treatment control N=23 Number of sessions: 4	In TM practitioners, serum cholesterol was significantly reduced (p<0.005) at 11-month follow-up (29 points) Reduction was also significantly less than controls (p<0.05) Results were independent of dietary changes
Schneider RH et al: A randomized controlled trial of stress reduction for hypertension in older African Americans, *Hypertension* 26:820, 1995.	(1) TM (2) APRT (3) Lifestyle modification education program N=111 Number of sessions: approximately 6	TM practitioners reduced systolic BP 10.7 mm Hg (p<0.0003) and diastolic by 6.4 mm Hg (p<0.00005) APRT lowered systolic/diastolic BP by 4.7 & 3.3 (p<0.05 and 0.02) TM reduced systolic/diastolic BP significantly more than APRT (p=0.02 and 0.03)
Barnes V et al: Stress, stress reduction and hypertension in African Americans: an updated review, *J Natl Med Assoc* 89:464, 1997.	(1) TM (2) PMR (3) Lifestyle modification N=127 Number of sessions: 6	Compared with controls, TM reduced systolic BP by 10.7 mm Hg (p<0.0005) and diastolic BP 6.4 mm Hg (p<0.00005) at 3-month follow-up PMR lowered systolic BP 4.7 mm Hg (p<0.054) and diastolic 3.3 mm Hg (p<0.025) TM reduced systolic (p<0.025) and diastolic (p<0.05) more than PMR

improvements in the function of their heart or essentially a reversal of the damage to the heart caused by hypertension. Those results in some ways were equivalent to health education about diet and exercise, but the results were also broader; that is, the TM group also showed improvements in the quality of life in the area of psychologic and social health not seen in the health education group. They showed improvements in these areas, as well as in their heart function, which was not seen in the comparison group. We then performed some long-term follow-up studies, pioneered by a graduate student here, Vernon Barnes. We followed subjects for 5 or 7 years—actually in one group [for] 15 years. Their mortality rates showed substantially reduced death rates; that is, there was a lower mortality rate from heart attack and stroke in those who practiced TM, as compared with behavioral controls. There was also lower mortality for all causes.

And there are some very exciting unexpected findings. When we followed up our mortality records from our cardiovascular trials and looked at cause of death, we found that there were reduced mortality rates from cancer. Cancer is the number two cause of death in the population and much higher in black Americans, specifically, so we are also following that up now.

Question. Did you assess specific biochemical alterations resulting from meditation?

Answer. In collaboration with the neurochemistry laboratory here directed by Dr. Ken Walton and the University of Iowa Clinical Research Center, we conducted a randomized controlled trial funded by the NIH where we looked at several biochemical parameters. This trial generally confirmed findings from observational studies. We found improvements in serum DHEA-S and in cortisol levels, showing capacity to buffer reactivity to stress. There were also pilot findings with a trend toward lower levels of catecholamines at baseline.

Question. When can we expect results from your ongoing studies?

Answer. The study on morbidity and mortality will be finished in about 3 years. [This study] is currently ongoing in collaboration with Dr. Clarence Grim of the Medical College of Wisconsin. The large trial on hypertensive heart disease, which followed up the pilot findings I just told you about, just finished this summer [1999]. We are analyzing that data now. In that trial, we are not only measuring left ventricular hypertrophy and cardiac function, but we are also measuring carotid atherosclerosis, which is highly correlated with coronary atherosclerosis. Everyone is measuring the carotid [artery] by noninvasive means rather than sticking catheters in the heart, at least in many prevention studies following changes in coronary heart disease.

TABLE 6-3	Effects of Meditation on Cardiovascular Disease	
AUTHOR(S)	**DESIGN**	**FINDINGS**
ROM MEDITATION		
Benson H et al: Decreased premature ventricular contractions through use of the relaxation response in patients with stable ischemic heart-disease, *Lancet* 380, 1975.	(1) ROM (no other groups) N=11 Number of sessions: 1	Reduced frequency of PVSs was documented in 8 of 11 patients with stable ischemic heart disease
Leserman J et al: The efficacy of the relaxation response in preparing for cardiac surgery, *Behav Med* 15(3):111, 1989.	(1) ROM (2) Education information N=27 Number of sessions: 6 1 session initially; nurse helped with practice after training Days of postsurgical practice varied (2 to 7)	ROM groups had less postoperative SVT, less tension and anger than education group (p<0.04 for all three) Authors concluded ROM reduces SVT, anger, and tension in cardiac surgery
TRANSCENDENTAL MEDITATION		
Zamarra JW et al: Usefulness of the transcendental meditation program in the treatment of coronary artery disease, *Am J Cardiol* 77:867, 1996.	(1) TM (2) Wait-list control N=21 Number of sessions: 10 hrs	At 7.6 months, TM increased exercise duration by 14.7% (p=0.013) and maximal workload 11.7% (p=0.004) and delay of onset of SVT depression 18.1% (p=0.029) TM reduced rate pressure products at 3 and 6 min of exercise and at maximal exercise (all p=0.016) Wait-list demonstrated no improvements

PVCs, premature ventricular contractions; *ROM*, respiratory one method; *SVT*, supraventricular tachycardia.

It is quite possible, based on preliminary findings, that there may be regression of athelosclerosis with this consciousness-based approach, I would like to say, because it is even more than stress reduction. Nevertheless, this is quite remarkable, very significant for the field. Of course, diet and other lifestyle factors are important, but for an approach of consciousness to show slowing or regression of athelosclerosis is quite amazing.

Our NIH-supported study on primary prevention of hypertension is also starting now in Milwaukee and will be over in 5 years. Observational studies indicate a primary prevention of hypertension with a TM-practicing group.

Question. How can meditation as a health intervention be applied by health care professionals?

Answer. The TM technique is already being applied. Several large corporations, Fortune 500 corporations, are already paying for their employees to learn the TM program as an educational and preventative health measure and also to improve their job performance. When persons are less stressed, they often perform better on the job.

We have been collaborating with several hospitals and medical centers [in Milwaukee, Los Angeles, Oakland, and Atlanta] with the TM program. At least in a research setting it is incorporated into the clinical treatment arm. The method we have found most helpful—any doctor or health professional can do this—we ask patients to continue their usual medical care with their usual health care providers. As adjunctive therapy or complementary therapy, you could say, patients who have high BP or coronary heart disease or [who are] at risk for these conditions can begin the TM program. Then, what we find is that over time many of the patients taking hypertensive medications can taper them off with their health care providers' approval. This [practice of the TM program] may prevent the need for medications in some cases or may help reduce the need for other invasive cardiovascular interventions. So, the main idea is that there is no conflict at all with conventional medical care. What seems to be the easiest and most effective is for the health care provider to refer their patients to a qualified instructor or hire or have as a consultant a qualified instructor of the program in their health care facility. Just like you would refer a patient for physical therapy or nutrition or any other specialty therapy, the hypertensive or at-risk patient can be referred to a TM class, and the physician can continue to work with the patient on their standard medical care.

TABLE 6-4   Effects of Meditation on Epilepsy Outcomes

AUTHOR(S)	DESIGN	FINDINGS
Deepak KK et al: Meditation improves clinicoelectro-encephalographic measures in drug-resistant epileptics, *Biofeedback Self Regul* 19(1):25, 1994.	(1) Classical Indian meditation with mantra (2) Wait-list controls Number of sessions: 12 N=20	20 drug-resistant, uncontrolled epileptics of 3 years or more At 6 months duration, meditators had significant reductions in seizure frequency duration, ($p<0.01$), increased dominant EEG frequency ($p<0.0001$); controls experience no change Between 6 months and 1 year, seizure reduction and duration again reduced Ability to meditate deeply was confirmed by EEG reading and microswitch responses and compared with visual analog scale
Panjwani U et al: Effect of Sahaja yoga practice on stress management in patients with epilepsy, *Indian J Physiology Pharmacol* 39(2):111, 1995.	(1) Sahaja yoga meditation (2) Placebo-yoga meditation (3) No-treatment control Number of sessions: 60 N=32	At 3 and 6 months, GSR and U-VMA levels and blood lactate were significantly reduced in group 1 but not group 2 or 3

EEG, Electromyographic; *GSR*, galvanic skin response; *U-VMA*, urinary vinyl mandelic acid.

TABLE 6-5   Meditation for the Treatment of Chronic Pain

AUTHOR(S)	DESIGN	FINDINGS
Kabat-Zinn J et al: Four-year follow-up of a meditation-based program for the self-regulation of chronic pain: treatment outcomes and compliance, *Clin J Pain* 21:159, 1987.	(1) Mindfulness and breathing and hatha yoga linked to mindfulness meditation No control group	Follow-up times ranged from 2.5 to 48 months; program was offered in rotational cycles 30%-55% of patients' pain was "greatly improved" in each cycle; 60%-72% of patients' pain was moderately improved; 1%-25% received no relief or worsened, depending on the cycle Improvements related to physical and psychologic status; the McGill Melzack Pain Rating Index tended to revert to preintervention levels after intervention
Kaplan KH et al: The impact of a meditation-based stress reduction program on fibromyalgia, *Gen Hosp Psychiatry* 15:284, 1983.	(1) Mindfulness meditation No control group N=59 Number of sessions: 10	51% of patients were defined as "responders" (25% improvement in at least 50% of 10 instruments) 19% of the 51% were "marked responders," showing a 50% plus improvement in 50% of instruments

Effects of Meditation on Chronic Disease States

Meditation has been used as an intervention for other chronic conditions such as asthma, psoriasis, and menopause.[40,57,59] Results have been generally positive. Meditation has also been used in the treatment of epilepsy, chronic pain, and alcohol and drug addiction. Table 6-4 reviews data on two studies for epilepsy, Table 6-5 reviews the research on chronic pain, and Table 6-6 outlines the research on addictive behaviors.

Sahaja Yoga Meditation and Epilepsy

It has been suggested by research studies that epilepsy might be a behavioral and neurologic problem rather than purely one of a neurologic origin;

as a result, reduction in stress might be an important factor in seizure control.[88] Stress precipitates seizures in some predisposed persons, and daily stress has been reported to be a significant predictor of seizure activity.[106]

Interest in finding complementary methods for controlling epilepsy has resulted, in no small part, because drug therapy often fails to provide complete seizure control in approximately 20% of drug-resistant patients with epilepsy.[76] An early study of Yogic-based meditation found that meditation reduced the frequency and duration of seizures.[51] This finding inspired researchers to investigate the effects of yoga meditation on GSR, blood lactate levels, levels of tension and relaxation, and EEG readings to define more clearly the

TABLE 6-6	Meditation as Therapy for Addictive Behaviors	
AUTHOR(S)	**DESIGN**	**FINDINGS**
ALL ADDICTIVE SUBSTANCES		
Benson H et al: Decreased drug abuse with transcendental meditation: a study of 1,862 subjects. In Zarafonetis CJD, editor: *Drug abuse: proceedings of the International Conference*, Philadelphia, 1972, Lea and Febiger.	N=1862 meditators Survey results by independent data processing company Usage before and during specified time periods after were assessed	Meditation decreased use of marijuana, hallucinogens, narcotics, amphetamines, barbiturates, hard liquor, cigarettes, and prescribed medication after an average of 21 months of meditation
ALCOHOL USE		
Shafii M et al: Meditation and the prevention of alcohol abuse, *Am J Psychiatry* 132:942, 1975.	(1) TM (2) Matched control N=216 Note: Survey study	No control subjects reported discontinuation of beer/wine 40% of those meditating for 2 years or more reported discontinuation of wine/beer within 6 months of beginning practice Within 2 and 3 years of practice, this figure increased to 60% 54% of meditators vs 1% of nonmeditators stopped drinking hard liquor
Murphy TJ et al: Lifestyle modification with heavy alcohol drinkers: effects of aerobic exercise and meditation, *Addict Behav* 11(2):175, 1986.	(1) CSM (2) Exercise (3) No treatment control N=43 Number of sessions: 24	Subjects in the exercise group significantly reduced alcohol consumption compared with no-treatment controls

CSM, Clinically standardized meditation; *TM,* transcendental meditation.

mechanisms by which meditation affects seizure rate. The two studies that follow confirmed that yogic meditation was effective in reducing the correlates of stress in those with epilepsy. Panjwani and colleagues suggested it was possibly the "conditioning" of the limbic system via meditation that leads to clinical improvement[86] (see Table 6-4).

Mindfulness Meditation and Chronic Pain

Relaxation techniques are currently being taught in clinical settings to help patients cope with chronic pain (Figure 6-7). Most of these exercises are derived from meditation techniques and are often applied in clinical settings as strategies for pain management. These methods have been incorporated into multi-disciplinary pain clinic treatment programs and into cognitive-behavioral approaches to pain management.[18,108,109] Many studies have reported short-term improvement in the pain, but few have provided data on the effectiveness of the meditation technique on a long-term basis. The following Kabat-Zinn study describes outcomes 4 years after chronic pain intervention with MM.

Fibromyalgia is a chronic illness characterized by widespread pain, fatigue, sleep disturbance, and resistance to treatment. In randomized, controlled trials using tricyclic and other CNS medications, a clinically significant response is reported in less than one third of the patients. Further, other interventions such as cardiovascular fitness training, biofeedback, and hypnotherapy still leave patients with persistent pain, fatigue, and sleep disturbances.[64] The Kaplan study, also discussed in the following text, is important because fibromyalgia causes pain that is difficult to treat, and because outcomes of program responders versus nonresponders are reported.

Neither the Kabat-Zinn nor the Kaplan study contained a control group—a flaw in many studies of pain. Researchers find it unethical to withhold treatment from patients with pain, and other comparative forms of intervention are often not included as part of the design. Further, outcome data are essentially self-reported. Nonetheless, these two studies provide important information about the use of meditation as a pain control strategy.

It has been suggested that MM combines the benefits of meditation with cognitive therapy (i.e., it induces the relaxation response while involving the participant in the observation of his or her

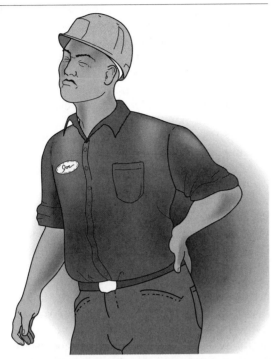

■ *Figure 6-7.* Relaxation techniques are currently being taught in clinical setting to help patients cope with pain. Most of these exercises are derived from meditation techniques and are often applied in clinical settings as strategies for pain management.

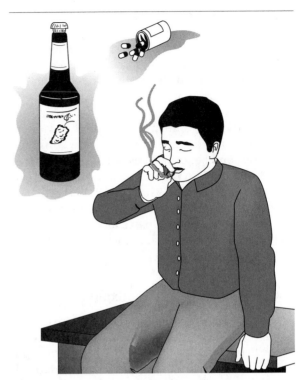

■ *Figure 6-8.* Meditation has been found effective in reducing use of addictive substances because of the biochemical and physiologic affects of meditation on serotonin and cortisol levels.

own cognitive processes). This combination has both positive and potentially negative aspects. Although MM has been used successfully for treating posttraumatic stress syndrome, it has also been reported to unexpectedly unveil traumatic memories and emotions in individuals during the practice of meditation. It may, however, be this cathartic and therapeutic effect (i.e., the revealing of suppressed memories and emotions) that allows MM to improve the capacity to cope with pain, even if pain itself is not significantly relieved long term. Outcomes suggest that MM is more effective for the management of chronic pain than other forms of intervention, such as cognitive therapy or concentrative forms of meditation alone (see Table 6-5).

Meditation and Addictive Behaviors

In a seminal article by Walton and Levitsky, chronic stress was postulated as a potent exacerbator of addictive behaviors[115] (Figure 6-8). The authors hypothesized that meditation had been effective in reducing the use of addictive substances because of the biochemical and physiologic effects of meditation on serotonin and cortisol levels. The mechanism by which meditation serves to reduce or prevent addictive behaviors was hypothesized in this manner as displayed in Box 6-3.

In a review of 24 studies assessing the effects of meditation on substance abuse, the authors found that meditation was an effective intervention for the treatment and prevention of abuse of chemical substances.[42] Studies covered noninstitutionalized users, participants in treatment programs, and prisoners with histories of heavy drug use (see Table 6-6).

■ Making the Choice: Relaxation or Meditation?

The effectiveness of both relaxation and meditation interventions will vary depending on factors pertinent to the individual. Only a method that is consistently practiced will benefit the client. An associate of the author of this text, who is an analytical thinker, is comfortable with the systematic and scientific approach of progressive relaxation, but the thought of cognitive meditation methods leaves her frightened and concerned that she will lose control. Some clients have objected to any form of meditative relaxation, considering it in opposition to their spiritual beliefs. A health professional finds meditation an excellent method for relaxation because it is simple and easy to apply and because her meditative experiences are interpreted as emotionally rewarding. She has no patience for the concepts of progressive relaxation, referring to APRT as "that anal-retentive method."

For any intervention to be effective, it must be incorporated into the lifestyle, thinking processes, and belief systems of the patient. What will the patient find rewarding, and what will he or she practice? Under what conditions will the patient practice? Are short meditations all that can be expected from a particular client? In the end, these are some of the most important questions that must be answered.

■ Contraindications of Meditation

A contraindication for all forms of cognitive meditation is a client with an excessive need to control. Clients who fear loss of control may equate meditation with mind control. Once experienced, they may consider meditation a form of punishment or loss of supremacy and may soon refuse to practice because they experience meditation as a loss of self.

Persons with psychiatric history are at risk, and the commencement of meditation training for these persons can result in psychotic episodes.[46,66] Meditation is therefore contraindicated unless it is introduced as a form of therapy in a clinical setting and with close supervision. Dosages of psychotropic medications may need to be adjusted as meditation is introduced to the patient. Meditation, especially in doses of more than 30 minutes a day, may enhance the effects of certain medications, requiring lower doses of antianxiety, antidepressive, antihypertensive, and, in some cases, thyroid-regulating medications. Lower doses of these medications may be prescribed after meditation has become part of the lifestyle.[23]

Even in otherwise healthy clients, meditation has been reported to unveil previously repressed traumatic memories and painful emotions. As the background "chatter" of the mind quiets, a common experience is the recall of traumatic or abusive events in earlier life. If the event is significant, it may not be possible for the meditator to release the memory. The unveiling of such memories can be quite traumatic to the individual. Although this has occurred with all forms of meditation, MM, with its emphasis on the observation of thoughts, has been more often reported to elicit this response. This effect can be quite helpful as part of a therapeutic process, and, indeed, many therapists suggest meditation as an adjunct to therapy. However, for unprepared individuals and for those without professional guidance, this response can pose certain dangers. It is strongly suggested that because of these occurrences during meditation, an informed consent should be sought as part of the prescreening process for any meditation intervention.[78]

Side Effects: All Forms of Cognitive Meditation

Meditation can help balance an intellectually driven thinking process, but extreme amounts of meditation can unbalance an individual's equilibrium. The release of emotional context in amounts too intense to handle can occur in persons meditating for long hours, over periods of days or weeks.

Several side effects have been noted with cognitive meditative forms. There are side effects from tension release and the potential for rapid behavioral changes. Occasionally, a person may be hypersensitive to meditation. Even for healthy individuals, long hours of meditation can be dangerous. There have been reports of adverse effects from meditation that include depersonalization, altered reality testing, and appearance of previously repressed but highly charged memories—although these instances appear to be rare.

Side Effects: Excessive Meditation

In one study, adverse side effects of MM in 27 long-term meditators during attendance at a meditation

---

BOX 6-3 How Meditation Affects Drug Abuse Outcomes

Reduced Stress

Reduced Cortisol

Lowered Tryptophan Pyrrolase and Increased Tryptophan

Increased Serotonin Availability

More Effective Adaptive Mechanisms (including HPA axis)

More Optimum Homeostasis

Decreased Drug Abuse

retreat were assessed 1 and 6 months after the retreat. The study reported that 62.9% of the practitioners experienced at least one adverse effect and 7.4% suffered profound adverse effects. Years of meditation practice (i.e., 17 to 105 months) did not determine who would experience adverse effects.[99]

Walsh and others reported only three psychotic episodes while observing several thousand persons in intensive and long-term meditation training.[113] Other researchers have reported cases of individuals whose depressive effects were exacerbated by intensive meditation during meditation retreats; some meditators have reported that mantra meditation may heighten ongoing tension and restlessness. These effects seem to manifest in persons who are "abnormally sensitive" to meditation rather than in the general population.[66]

Lazarus observed that TM seemed to be effective with obsessive-compulsive individuals whose levels of anxiety and tension were moderate rather than severe. Persons with hysterical tendencies or strong depressive reactions, as well as schizophrenics who were reported to experience increased depersonalization and self-preoccupation, were contraindicated for meditation. Disturbed patients with serious psychiatric disorders should only be taught to meditate under the supervision of a health professional and only after stabilization with medication.

Side Effects: Tension Release

In novice but otherwise healthy meditators, temporary symptoms may occur. These symptoms appear to be produced by the release of deep-seated tensions.[22] Although it is generally considered a sign of health to be able to release tensions, a too-rapid release can discourage and frighten a new meditator. Tension release can be controlled by careful adjustments of meditation time and, in some cases, adjustment of the technique. It is important to remember that all forms of relaxation therapy can and should be modulated as needed to meet the special needs of the practitioner.

Side Effects: Rapid Behavioral Change

Meditation often results in the practitioner becoming less rigid in his or her lifestyle and thinking patterns. Although this is considered a healthy trend, these changes can frighten family members or interfere with career goals if these goals require an unrelenting schedule. Some of the most typical behavioral changes include the following: (1) a new found sense of self-assertion and less self-effacement, (2) an increase in the feelings of well-being and optimism; (3) the pleasurable feelings that accompany meditation inducing anxiety in the person with deeply formed guilt complexes, and (4) a lessening of life's pace that may be incompatible with current career goals or the demands and expectations of others. These changes do not occur at a pace that is uncomfortable for most patients. In those who do have difficulty adapting, the pace of the meditation practice can be slowed as new attitudes are more slowly integrated into the lifestyle.

Side Effects: Hypersensitivity to Meditation

A very few persons are hypersensitive to meditation, finding even 20 to 30 minutes a day too taxing. In these cases, the amount of meditation can be divided into 3- to 5-minute sessions throughout the day or limited even further. The client can increase meditation slowly over many months until a typical 20-minute session is comfortable.

■ Reasons for Meditation, Compliance, and Outcomes

Meditation is currently used for three different purposes: (1) self-regulation as occurs for stress and pain management and for relaxation in relation to stress-related diseases; (2) self-exploration, a psychobiologic form of introspection, used as psychotherapy or for self-understanding; and (3) spiritual self-liberation as occurs in the context of many religious disciplines. Most of the interventional research literature has focused on meditation for self-regulation and self-exploration, with evaluation of the outcomes lasting for short periods (e.g., 6 to 8 weeks) and with novice meditators. Researchers often took pains to operationalize the content and components of meditation so that it would be separated from its spiritual context. Many felt this separation a necessary requirement so as to remove meditation intervention from the definition of "occult" and to avoid any clashes clients may feel between meditation and their religious ideology.

Currently, researchers are suggesting that there is much to be learned from examining long-term meditators, their goals for meditation, the thoughts (cognitions) associated with meditation practice, and the importance of a spiritual context in meditation as these issues relate to outcomes and long-term compliance.[47,100,101,118] Historically, meditation has been a central theme and essential element in nearly all contemplative religious and spiritual traditions, including Eastern Hindu/Vedic and Buddhist traditions, Judaism, Christianity, and Islam. The goal of meditation in these disciplines has been the liberation of the ego, developing a sense of harmony with the universe, and the ability to increase one's compassion, sensitivity, and sense of service to others.[114] It has been suggested that it is important to consider this self-liberation and compassionate service aspect of meditation as part of meditative interventions.

One study sought to evaluate the importance of goals, religious orientation, and cognitions in long-term meditators and to determine how these elements related to the effects and outcomes of meditation.[100] In this study, 27 long-term meditators (mindfulness or Vipassana meditation) who signed up for a 2-week or 3-month meditation retreat were evaluated before the retreat and at 1 and 6 months after the retreat. Average length of prior meditation practice was 4.27 years, and 81% meditated regularly for 45 minutes to 1 hour each day. Of the 27 meditators, 63% were men; 50% were in professional careers, and 70% had college degrees. They were divided into three groups: (1) group 1 was made up of those who were the short-term meditators (i.e., had mediated less than 2 years), averaging only 16.7 months of practice; (2) group 2 were meditators of moderate length (i.e., more than 2 and less than 7 years), and they averaged 47.1 months of meditation; and, (3) group 3 included long-term meditators of 8 years or longer, and they averaged 105 months of meditation. Meditation practice during the retreat occurred for 16 hours a day, both sitting and walking meditation, and complete silence was maintained during the retreat. The groups were assessed on the basis of their years of practice, meditation motivation, and expectation of and adherence with practice. The authors' held two primary hypotheses: (1) the goals and expectations related to meditation will "shift" along a continuum, and the greater the number of years of practice, the more the continuum will move from the direction of self regulation (SR) to self exploration (SE) and then toward self liberation (SL); and (2) the effects of meditation will be related to the goals and expectations for meditation; that is, what the meditator receives will be related to what he or she wants and is seeking. There were three secondary hypotheses: (1) religious orientation will be significantly related to length of practice; (2) cognitions made when the meditator does NOT practice will be significantly related to the length of practice; and (3) cognitions before beginning practice will be significantly related to adverse effects of meditation. Of those in Group 3, 75% had goals and

expectations of SL and none had only SL hopes. By contrast, in Group 1, only 30% had SL hopes and 50% had SR goals. The differences were significant (p=<0.05), and the first primary hypothesis was confirmed. The expectations and goals related to meditation shifted along the SR-SE-SL continuum in direct proportion to the length of practice. The second primary hypothesis was partially confirmed. Of the 27 meditators, 67% reported positive effects of meditation congruent with their reasons for beginning, confirming that the goal of SR produced a positive SR outcome at the completion of the retreat. At 1- and 6-month follow-up, a continuing trend for positive SR outcomes was reached (p=0.081). The relationship between religious orientation (Buddhist or universal) and the length of practice was significant (p=0.05), as were cognitions when the meditators failed to practice. Approximately 80% of the cognitions of Group 1 and 66.6% of the cognitions of Group 2 blamed external events or others or blamed self (anger, I should have) if meditation was missed. However, in Group 3, only 12.5% blamed self, events, or others; instead, they reported using nonmeditation as something to learn from—an opportunity to, without judgment, observe the self and its reasons for not meditating. Cognitions made before beginning practice were significantly related to adverse effects, both retrospectively and prospectively. Approximately 56% of the patients (15 meditators) reported positive cognitions occurring just before sitting down to meditate ("pleased with myself"; desire to come into God's presence") as compared with 7 meditators who reported either varying cognitions or cognitions they could not recall and 5 meditators who reported negative or mixed cognitions.

The authors concluded that although meditation for SL and stress management can be an end unto itself, meditation might accomplish more. Further, this "more" is related to believing that meditation is a rewarding experience and a practice with which meditators will comply for long periods. Both retrospectively and prospectively, positive SL effects increased with length of practice, following the hypothesized continuum. The authors concluded that although the generic, secular approach to meditation as a technique devoid of context may be effective and appropriate in some settings and for short-term interventions, when meditation is to be practiced as a long-range strategy, a spiritual orientation and context may be important as motivational factors for some patients.

This study, although small, suggested the following:

- Cognitions are critical in relation to emotional and behavioral change.
- Adherence and compliance is linked both to these cognitions, the emotional experience of meditation and a potential spiritual context.
- Emphasizing noncompliance as an educational and learning method may prevent dropping out as a result of condemnation and frustration.

The issues of positive cognitions and meditation as a rewarding experience can be addressed as part of the preparatory and follow-up phases of health care. The motivational aspects of meditation can then be reinforced. The spiritual aspects are a personal matter for the patient and simply should not be negated if they occur.

■ Chapter Review

The benefits of meditation are outlined in this chapter. As intervention for cardiovascular disease and for general health, TM meditation is an excellent intervention. As part of treatment for chronic pain, posttraumatic stress syndrome, and as an adjunct to psychologic therapy, MM is a good choice. MM is also beneficial for maintaining cognitive sharpness with the older adult. For individuals "put off" by methods with any traditional or spiritual underpinnings, CSM and the ROM method are good alternatives. Ultimately, the most important factor for selecting the form of meditation is the personality of the individual and his or her preference. In the end, benefit can come only from those methods that are practiced on a regular basis.

Matching Terms and Definitions

Match each numbered definition with the correct term. Place the corresponding letter in the space provided.

_____ 1. Side effects of meditation practice (pick 4)
_____
_____
_____
_____ 2. Buddhist meditation form
_____ 3. Method developed by Maharishi Mahesh Yogi
_____ 4. Hormone modulated by meditation
_____ 5. Developed by Carrington and others
_____ 6. Herbert Benson's method
_____ 7. Brain patterns altered by meditation

a. Concentrative
b. Hypersensitivity to meditation
c. Nonconcentrative
d. Excessive meditation
e. CSM
f. TM
g. Tension release
h. MM
i. ROM
j. Rapid behavior changes
k. DHEA-S
l. Alpha and theta

SHORT ANSWER ESSAY QUESTIONS

1. Define the differences between concentrative and nonconcentrative meditation methods, and discuss which method you think you would prefer and the reasons why.
2. Explain the basic philosophy of Herbert Benson and how his philosophy led to the development of ROM.
3. Describe TM, and discuss the main differences between this method and Benson's method.
4. Compare and contrast CSM and the TM and ROM methods.
5. List and define the potential side effects of meditation.

CRITICAL THINKING AND CLINICAL APPLICATION EXERCISES

1. Under what conditions might MM be more effective than TM and why? Argue your position based on the research.
2. Under what conditions might TM be the most effective intervention and why? Argue your position based on the research.
3. What are the advantages of CSM for health intervention?
4. Describe how the individual's personality can be a factor in determining which meditation form will be most effective. Describe two very different personality styles, and select the method potentially best suited for each.
5. What meditative method would you prefer and why? Explain your preference in terms of your personality, lifestyle, and medical history.
6. Describe, in physiologic terms, the effects of meditation on the sympathetic drive and how this effect alters health outcomes.
7. Describe the differences between outcomes for APRT and meditation. Explain, specifically, why these differences may exist.
8. You must interview persons before they can enroll in your meditation class. Describe, in detail, your screening procedure to ensure no persons contraindicated for meditation are enrolled.
9. Even healthy persons indicated for meditation can experience side effects. Describe how you would prepare your class to ensure that potential side effects are identified and managed as quickly as possible.

References

1. Abrahams VC, Hilton SM, Zybrozyna AW: Active muscle vasodilation produced by stimulation of the brain stem: its significance in the defense reaction, *J Physiol* 154:491, 1960.
2. Alexander CN, Chandler HM, Langer EJ, Newman RI, Davies JL: Transcendental meditation, mindfulness, and longevity: an experimental study with the elderly, *J Pers Soc Psychol* 57(6):950, 1989.
3. Allen PIM, Batty KA, Dodd CAS, Herbert J, Hugh CJ, Moore GF, Seymour MJ, Shiere HM, Stacey PM, Young SK: Dissociation between emotional and endocrine responses preceding an academic examination in male medical students, *J Endocrinol* 107:163, 1985.
4. Allison J: Respiratory changes during the practice of transcendental meditation, *Lancet* 7651:833, 1970.
5. Anand BK, Chhina GS, Singh B: Some aspects of electroencephalographic studies in Yogis, *Electroencephalogr Clin Neurophysiol* 13:452, 1961.
6. Appelle S, Oswald LE: Simple reaction time as a function of alertness and prior mental activity, *Perceptual Motor Skills* 38:1263, 1974.
7. Arguelles AE, Martinez MA, Hoffman C, Ortiz GA, Chekherdemian M: Corticoadrenal and adrenergic overactivity and hyperlipidemia in prolonged emotional stress, *Hormones* 3:167, 1972.
8. Banquet JP: Spectral analysis of the EEG in meditation, *Electroencephalogr Clin Neurophysiol* 35:143, 1973.
9. Barnes V, Schneider R, Alexander C, Staggers F: Stress, stress reduction and hypertension in African Americans: an updated review, *J Natl Med Assoc* 89:464, 1997.
10. Beary JF, Benson H: A simple psychophysiologic technique which elicits the hypometabolic changes of the relaxation response, *Psychosom Med* 36:115, 1974.
11. Benson HB: *The relaxation response,* New York, 1975, Morrow.
12. Benson HB: The relaxation response and norepinephrine: a new study illuminates mechanisms, *Integr Psychiatry* 1:15, 1974.
13. Benson H, Alexander S, Feldman CL: Decreased premature ventricular contractions through use of the relaxation response in patients with stable ischaemic heart disease, *Lancet* 380, 1975.
14. Benson HB, Beary JF, Carol MP: The relaxation response, *Psychiatry* 37:37, 1974.
15. Benson HB, Greenwood MM, Klemchuk H: The relaxation response: psychophysiologic aspects and clinical applications, *Int J Psychiatry* 6(1/2):90, 1975.
16. Benson HB, Greenwood MM, Klemchuk H: The relaxation response: psychophysiologic aspects and clinical applications, *Int J Psychiatry Med* 6(1/2):87, 1976.
17. Benson H, Greenwood MM, Klemchuk H: The relaxation response: psychophysiologic aspects and clinical applications, *Int J Psychiatry Med* 6(1/2):87, 1976.
18. Benson H, Pomeranz B, Kutz I: The relaxation response and pain. In Wall PD, Melzack R, editors: *Textbook of pain,* New York, 1984, Churchill Livingstone.
19. Benson H, Proctor E: *Beyond the relaxation response,* New York, 1985, Berkeley.
20. Berenson GS, Voors AW, Dalferes ERJ, Webber LS, Schuler SE: Creatinine clearance, electrolytes, and plasma renin activity related to blood pressure of black and white children—The Bogalusa Heart Study, *J Lab Clin Med* 93:535, 1979.
21. Carrington P: *Clinically standardized meditation (CSM) instructor's kit,* Kendall Park, NJ, 1978, Pace Educational Systems.
22. Carrington P: *Freedom in meditation,* Garden City, NY, 1977, Doubleday/Anchor.
23. Carrington P: Modern forms of meditation. In Lehrer PM, Woolfolk RL, editors: *Principles and practice of stress management,* New York, 1993, Guilford Press.

24. Carrington P, Ephron HS: Meditation as an adjunct to psychotherapy. In Arieti S, editor: *New dimensions in psychiatry: a world view*, New York, 1975, Wiley.

25. Cohen J, Sedlacek K: Attention and autonomic self-regulation, *Psychosom Med* 45:243, 1983.

26. Davidson R, Goleman D, Schwartz G: Attentional and affective concomitants of meditation: a cross-sectional study, *J Abnorm Psychol* 85:235, 1976.

27. Delmonte MM: Electrocortical activity and related phenomena associated with meditation practice: a literature review, *Int J Neurosci* 24:217, 1984.

28. Delmonte MM: Personality and meditation. In West M, editor: *The psychology of meditation*, New York, 1987, Oxford Press.

29. Devine E, Cook T: A meta-analytic analysis of effects of psychoeducational interventions on length of postsurgical hospital stay, *Nurs Res* 32:267, 1983.

30. Dillbeck MC, Orme-Johnson DW, Wallace RK: Frontal EEG coherence, H-reflux recovery, concept learning, and the TM-Sidhi program, *Int J Neurosci* 15:151, 1981.

31. Earle JB: Cerebral laterality and meditation: a review of the literature, *J Transpersonal Psychol* 13:155, 1981.

32. Elliot GR, Eisendorfer C, editors: *Stress and human health: analysis and implications of research*, New York, 1982, Springer Publishing.

33. English EH, Baker TB: Relaxation training and cardiovascular response to experimental stressors, *Health Psychol* 2:239, 1983.

34. Eppley KR, Abrams AI, Shear J: Differential effects of relaxation techniques on trait anxiety: a meta-analysis, *J Clin Psychol* 45(6):957, 1989.

35. Falkner B: Characteristics of prehypertension in black children. In Fray JCS, Douglas JG, editors: *Pathophysiology of hypertension in blacks*, New York, 1993, Oxford University Press.

36. Fenwick PBC, Donaldson S, Gillis PI, Bushman L, Bushman J, Fenton GW, Perry I, Tilsley C, Serafinowicz H: Metabolic and EEG changes during transcendental meditation: an explanation, *Biol Psychol* 5:101, 1977.

37. French RM: *The way of a pilgrim (translation)*, New York, 1968, Seabury Press.

38. Friedman M, Byers SO, Rosenman RH: Coronary-prone individuals (type A behavior pattern): some biochemical characteristics, *JAMA* 212:1030, 1970.

39. Furst J: Emotional stress reactions to surgery. A review of some therapeutic implications, *New York State J Med* 78:1083, 1978.

40. Gaston L: Efficacy of imagery and meditation techniques in treating psoriasis, *Imagin Cogn Personality* 8(1):25, 1988.

41. Gaylord C, Orme-Johnson D, Travis F: The effects of the transcendental meditation technique and progressive muscle relaxation on EEG coherence, stress reactivity, and mental health in black adults, *Int J Neurosci* 46:77, 1989.

42. Gelderloos P, Walton KG, Orme-Johnson DW, Alexander CN: Effectiveness of the transcendental meditation program in preventing and treating substance misuse: a review, *Int J Addictions* 26(3):293, 1991.

43. Gellhorn E, Kiely WF: Mystical states of consciousness: neurophysiological and clinical aspects, *J Nerv Ment Dis* 154(6):399, 1972.

44. Glaser JL, Brind JL, Vogelman JH, Eisner MJ, Dillbeck MC, Wallace RK, Chopra D, Orentreich N: Elevated serum dehydroepiandrosterone sulfate levels in practitioners of the transcendental meditation (TM) and TM-Sidhi programs, *J Behav Med* 15(4):327, 1992.

45. Glueck BC: *Current research on transcendental meditation*, Paper presented at the Rensselaer Polytechnic Institute, Hartford, CT, 1973, Hartford Graduate Center.

46. Glueck BC, Stroebel CF: Biofeedback and meditation in the treatment of psychiatric illness, *Comp Psychiatry* 16:302, 1975.

47. Goleman D: *The meditation mind*, Los Angeles, 1988, Tarcher.

48. Goleman DJ, Schwartz GE: Meditation as an intervention in stress reactivity, *J Consult Clin Psychol* 44(3):456, 1976.

49. Greenwood MM, Benson H: The efficacy of progressive relaxation in systematic desensitization and a proposal for an alternative competitive response, *Behav Res Ther* 15:337, 1977.

50. Grundy SM, Griffin AC: Relationship of periodic mental stress to serum lipoprotein and cholesterol levels, *JAMA* 171:1794, 1959.

51. Gupta HL, Dudani U, Singh SH, Surange SG, Selvamurthy W: Sahaja Yoga in the management of intractabl-epileptics. *JAPI* 39(8):649, 1991.

52. Gutmann MC, Benson H: Interaction of environmental factors and systematic arterial blood pressure: a review, *Medicine* 50:543, 1971.

53. Harte JL, Eifert GH, Smith R: The effects of running and meditation on beta-endorphin, corticotropin-releasing hormone and cortisol in plasma, and on mood, *Biol Psychol* 40:251, 1995.

54. Hebert R, Lehmann D: Theta bursts: an EEG pattern in normal subjects practicing transcendental meditation technique, *Electroencephalogr Clin Neurophysiol* 42:397, 1977.

55. Hefner RJ: Psychological treatment of essential hypertension: a controlled comparison of meditation and meditation plus biofeedback, *Biofeedback Self Regul* 7:305, 1982.

56. Hildreth CJ, Saunders E: Hypertension in blacks, *Maryland Med J* 40:213, 1991.

57. Honsberger RW, Wilson AF: Transcendental meditation in treating asthma, *Resp Ther J Inhalation Technol* 3:79, 1973.

58. Hypertension Detection and Follow-Up Program Cooperative Group: Race, education, and prevalence of hypertension, *Am J Epidemiol* 106:351, 1977.

59. Irvin JH, Domar AD, Clark C, Zuttermeister PC, Friedman R: The effects of relaxation response training on menopausal symptoms, *J Psychosom Obstretr Gynecol* 17:202, 1996.

60. Jacobs GD, Benson H, Friedman R: Topographic EEG mapping of the relaxation response, *Biofeedback Self Regul* 21(2):121, 1996.

61. Jevning R, Wallace RK, Beidebach M: The physiology of meditation: a review. A wakeful hypometabolic integrated response, *Neurosci Biobehav Rev* 16:415, 1992.

62. Johnston M: Anxiety in surgical patients, *Psychol Med* 10:145, 1980.

63. Julius S: Changing role of the autonomic nervous system in human hypertension, *J Hypertens Suppl* 8:59, 1990.

64. Kaplan KH, Goldenberg DL, Galvin-Nadeau M: The impact of a meditation-based stress reduction program on fibromyalgia, *Gen Hosp Psychiatry* 15:284, 1993.

65. Kelly GA: *The psychology of personal constructs*, New York, 1955, Norton.

66. Lazarus AA: Psychiatric problems precipitated by transcendental meditation, *Psychol Rep* 10:39, 1976.

67. Leedy MG, Wilson MS: Testosterone and cortisol levels in crewmen of US Air Force fighter and cargo planes, *Psychosom Med* 47:333, 1985.

68. Lehrer PM: Psychophysiological effects of progressive relaxation in anxiety neurotic patients and of progressive relaxation and alpha feedback in nonpatients, *J Consult Clin Psychol* 46:389, 1978.

69. Lehrer PM, Schoicket S, Carrington P, Woolfolk RL: Psychophysiological and cognitive responses to stressful stimuli in subjects practicing progressive relaxation and clinically standardized meditation, *Behav Res Ther* 18:293, 1980.

70. Lehrer PM, Woolfolk RL: Specific effects of stress management techniques. In Lehrer PM, Woolfolk RL, editors: *Principles and practice of stress management,* New York, 1993, Guilford Press.

71. Leserman J, Stuart EM, Mamish ME, Benson H: The efficacy of the relaxation response in preparing for cardiac surgery, *Behav Med* 15(3):111, 1989.

72. Lindholm E, Lowry S: Alpha production in humans under conditions of false feedback, *Bull Psychosom Soc* 11:106, 1978.

73. Lown B, Verrier R, Rabinowitz S: Neural and psychologic mechanisms and the problem of sudden cardiac death, *Am J Cardiol* 39:890, 1977.

74. MacLean CRK, Walton KG, Wenneberg SR, Levitsky DK, Mandarino JP, Waziri R, Hillis SL, Schneider RH: Effects of the transcendental meditation program on adaptive mechanisms: changes in hormone levels and responses to stress after 4 months of practice, *Psychoneuroendocrinology* 22(4):277, 1997.

75. Malliani A, Pagani M, Lombardi F et al: Spectral analysis to assess increased sympathetic tone in arterial hypertension, *Hypertension* 17(3):36, 1991.

76. Masland RI: Epidemiology and basic statistics of epilepsies: where are we? In Laidlaw J, Richens A, editors: *Textbook of epilepsy,* New York, 1982, Churchill Livingstone.

77. Matthews A, Ridgeway V: Personality and surgical recovery: a review, *Br J Clin Psychol* 20:243, 1981.

78. Miller JJ: The unveiling of traumatic memories and emotions through mindfulness and concentration meditation: clinical implications and three case reports, *J Transpersonal Psychol* 25(2):169, 1993.

79. Mougey EH, Oleshansky MA, Meyeroff JL: *Soc Neurosci Abs* 17(1):145, 1991.

80. Norton GR, Johnson WE: Characteristics of subjects experiencing relaxation and relaxation-induced anxiety, *J Behav Ther Exp Psychiatry* 16:211, 1983.

81. Orme-Johnson D: Medical care utilization and the transcendental meditation program, *Psychosom Med* 49:493, 1987.

82. Orme-Johnson DW, Hayes CT: EEG phase coherence, pure consciousness, creativity, and TM-Rishi experiences, *Int J Neurosci* 13:221, 1981.

83. Orme-Johnson DW, Wallace RK, Alexander CN, Ball OE: *Factor analysis of EEG coherence parameters,* Steamboat Springs, CO, 1982, Fifteenth annual winter conference on brain research.

84. Ornstein R: *The psychology of consciousness,* San Francisco, 1972, WH Freeman.

85. Pagano RR, Rose RM, Stivers RM, Warrenberg S: Sleep during transcendental meditation, *Science* 191:308, 1976.

86. Panjwani U, Gupta HL, Singh SH, Selvamurthy W, Rai UC: Effect of Sahaja yoga practice on stress management in patients with epilepsy, *Indian J Physiol Pharmacol* 39(2):111, 1995.

87. Pirot M: The effects of the transcendental meditation technique upon auditory discrimination. In Orme-Johnson DW, Farrow JT, editors: *Scientific research on the transcendental meditation program: collected papers,* vol 1, Livingston Manor, NY, 1978, Maharishi European Research University Press.

88. Puskarisch CA, Whitman S, Dell J, Hughes JR, Rose AJ, Hermann BP: Controlled examination of effects of progressive relaxation training on seizure reduction, *Epilepsia* 33(4):675, 1992.

89. Rimol AGP: The transcendental meditation technique and its effects on sensory-motor performance. In Orme-Johnson DW, Farrow JT, editors: *Scientific research on the transcendental meditation program: collected papers,* vol 1, Livingston Manor, NY, 1978, Maharishi European Research University Press.

90. Rolandi EE, Reggiani R, Franceschini G, Bavastro V, Messina G, Odaglia G, Barreca T: Comparison of pituitary responses to physical exercise in athletes and sedentary subjects, *Hormone Res* 21:209, 1989.

91. Salk L: The role of the heartbeat in the relations between mother and infant, *Sci Am* 228:24, 1973.

92. Sapolsky RM: The endocrine stress-response and social status in the wild baboon, *Horm Behav* 16:279, 1990.

93. Sapolsky RM: When stress is bad for your brain, *Science* 272:749, 1996.

94. Sapolsky RM: In Becker JB, Breedlove SM, Crews D, editors: *Behavioral neuroendocrinology,* Cambridge, MA, 1993, MIT Press.

95. Schneider RH, Staggers F, Alexander CN, Sheppard W, Rainforth M, Kondwani K, Smith S, King CG: A randomized controlled trial of stress reduction for hypertension in older African Americans, *Hypertension* 26:820, 1995.

96. Schwartz G, Davidson R, Goleman D: Patterning of cognitive and somatic processes in the self-regulation of anxiety: effects of meditation versus exercise, *Psychosom Med* 40:321, 1978.

97. Sedlacek K, Cohen J, Boxhill C: *Comparison between biofeedback and relaxation response in the treatment of hypertension,* (paper presented at the annual meeting), San Diego, 1979, Biofeedback Society of America.

98. Seeman TE, Robbins JR: Aging and hypothalamic-pituitary-adrenal response to challenge in humans, *Endocrine Rev* 15:233, 1994.

99. Shapiro DH: Adverse effects of meditation: a preliminary investigation of long-term meditators, *Int J Psychosom* 39:62, 1992.

100. Shapiro DH: A preliminary study of long-term meditators: goals, effects, religious orientation, cognitions, *J Transpersonal Psychol* 24(1):23, 1992.

101. Shapiro DH, Walsh RN, editors: *Meditation: classic and contemporary perspectives,* New York, 1984, Aldine.

102. Smith JC: *Cognitive behavioral relaxation training: a new system of strategies for treatment and assessment,* New York, 1990, Springer Publishing.

103. Smith JC: Psychotherapeutic effects of transcendental meditation with controls for expectation of relief and daily sitting, *J Consult Clin Psychol* 44(4):630, 1976.

104. Solberg EE, Halvorsen R, Sundgot-Borgen J, Ingjer F, Holen A: Meditation: a modulator of the immune response to physical stress? A brief report, *Br J Stress Med* 29(4):255, 1995.

105. Stigsby B, Rodenberg JC, Moth HB: Electroencephalographic findings during mantra meditation (transcendental meditation). A controlled, quantitative study of experienced meditators, *Electroencephalogr Clin Neurophysiol* 51:434, 1981.

106. Temkin NR, Davis GR: Stress as a risk factor for seizures among adults with epilepsy, *Epilepsia* 25:450, 1984.

107. Thibodeau GA, Patton KT: *Anatomy and physiology,* St Louis, 1996, Mosby.

108. Turk DC, Meichenbaum D: A cognitive-behavioral approach to pain management. In Wall PD, Melzack R, editors: *Textbook of pain,* New York, 1984, Churchill Livingstone.

109. Turk DC, Meichenbaum D, Genest M: *Pain and behavioral medicine,* New York, 1983, Guilford Press.

110. Wallace RK: Physiological effects of transcendental meditation, *Science* 167:1751, 1970.

111. Wallace RK, Benson H: The physiology of meditation, *Sci Am* 226:84, 1972.

112. Wallace RK, Benson H, Wilson AF: A wakeful hypometabolic state, *Am J Physiol* 221:795, 1971.

113. Walsh R, Roche L: Precipitation of acute psychotic episodes by intensive meditation in individuals with a history of schizophrenia, *Am J Psychiatry* 136(8):1085, 1979.

114. Walsh RN, Vaughan F, editors: *Beyond ego,* Los Angeles, 1980, Tarcher.
115. Walton KG, Levitsky D: A neuroendocrine mechanism for the reduction of drug use and addictions by transcendental meditation, *Alcoholism Treat Q* 11(1/2):89, 1994.
116. Warrenberg S, Pagano RR, Woods M, Hlastala MA: Comparison of somatic relaxation and EEG activity in classical progressive relaxation and transcendental meditation, *J Behav Med* 3:73, 1980.
117. West MA: Meditation and the EEG, *Psychol Med* 10:369, 1980.
118. West MA, editor: *The psychology of meditation,* Oxford, 1987, Clarendon Press.
119. Woolfolk RL: Psychophysiological correlates of meditation, *Arch Gen Psychiatry* 32:1326, 1995.
120. Zamarra JW, Schneider RH, Besseghini I, Robinson DK, Salerno JW: Usefulness of the transcendental M\meditation program in the treatment of coronary artery disease, *Am J Cardiol* 77:867, 1996.

7

Biofeedback

G. Frank Lawlis

WHY READ THIS CHAPTER

Although biofeedback is a relatively new medical therapy, people have been essentially practicing forms of biofeedback for generations. When my neighbor taught himself how to wiggle his ears while looking into a mirror, he was using the mirror as a source of feedback while practicing body control. Dancers also learn to achieve various movements by monitoring their actions through mirrors. Biofeedback, the current technology for assessing physiologic responses, functions like a highly sophisticated mirror.

Sports-related research helps identify the processes leading to the development of specific physical skills. Many of the world's spiritual practices teach that, with disciplined concentration, physical changes can be achieved that enhance health of both the mind and body. Biofeedback is a way of applying these same kinds of skills to achieve optimal health in specific physiologic systems. Cardiovascular changes in blood pressure, alterations in brain waves, and specific muscle groups can be controlled.

The most exciting outcome of biofeedback is the empowerment of the individual to teach himself or herself internal control. With the application of biofeedback techniques and continued practice, lifetime health improvements can be the result.

CHAPTER AT A GLANCE

Biofeedback is a therapeutic model for medical care, enabling patients to participate in their own healing. It teaches them to regulate their physiologic functions in healthy ways. Biofeedback allows immediate monitoring of skin temperature, muscle tension, brain waves, and skin conductance. The type of feedback will depend on the disease state and which physiologic parameter is most closely related to symptoms of the disease. The patient learns to control these functions in subtle ways, thereby readjusting their psychologic and physiologic responses.

Patients can also learn to change their reactions to stressful or challenging events, creating more balanced behavioral responses. Biofeedback offers patients a way to develop more wholesome lifestyles.

Biofeedback has been used to successfully treat migraine headache pain, low back pain, temporomandibular joint pain, neuromuscular and gait dysfunctions, incontinence, hypertension, and Raynaud's disease. Biofeedback is also used as a research strategy.

There are indications and contraindications for biofeedback interventions. Nonetheless, the possibilities for gaining such physiologic control are limited only by the advances of technology, therapist creativity, and patient motivation and interest.

> The spirit is the master, imagination the tool, and the body the plastic material...The power of the imagination is a great factor in medicine. It may produce diseases in man and animals, and it may cure them...ills of the body may be cured by physical remedies or by the power of the spirit acting through the soul.
>
> JOSÉ ORTEGA Y GASSET, MEDITATIONS ON QUIXOTE, "PRELIMINARY MEDITATION" (1914) PARACELSUS, FATHER OF MODERN MEDICINE

CHAPTER OBJECTIVES

After completing this chapter, you should be able to:

1. Describe the operational definitions of biofeedback.
2. Describe the philosophic dimensions underlying biofeedback.
3. Discuss the historical perspectives related to the development of biofeedback.
4. Describe the effectiveness and limitations of biofeedback for low back pain.
5. Discuss the use of biofeedback for temporomandibular jaw pain.
6. Compare and contrast the system effects of biofeedback for relief of migraine pain as opposed to tension headache.
7. Discuss how biofeedback is used for the treatment of incontinence.
8. Describe thermal biofeedback.
9. Explain how skin conductance activity is related to biofeedback, name the biofeedback method related to skin conductance, and describe the use of the method.
10. Discuss how the electroencephalogram is used as a biofeedback method, and discuss the disease states that are treated with the use of this tool.
11. Explain the indications for the use of biofeedback.
12. Explain the contraindications for the use of biofeedback.
13. Describe some of the new areas being explored for biofeedback intervention.

■ Historical Perspectives

Biofeedback is a product of the 1970s when a variety of forces came together to provide the technology and the culture for its introduction. Frustration with and distrust of the Vietnam War led to disillusionment with authoritarian rule. Civil Rights activists were challenging the spiritual moralities of the land. Faith that medical science would soon conquer illness was eroded by the ongoing fact that disease, especially chronic illness, was increasing. The country was embracing a philosophy of a humanistic source of power, as reflected by the human potential movement; and the emphasis was on personal creativity and alternative lifestyles. The "God is dead" discussions were indicative of the people's loss of faith in orthodox religion, as well as science. Yet, interest ran high in Eastern religions and philosophy. In essence, the country was ready for a therapy that embraced a concept of self reliance.

With rapid advances in the computer field, the technology of monitoring ongoing physiologic parameters made biomedical engineering available to the clinician. Before World War II, available equipment was not sufficiently sensitive to measure body functions without the use of invasive procedures that could leave the patient at risk of permanent damage. In the 1960s, even the skin temperature, measured in intervals required for feedback, required extensive space for equipment.

Research prepared the medical establishment for a new theory of medicine that reconnected the mind and body. Walter Cannon's pioneering research articulated the theory that stress was a critical factor in all disease.[8] This concept raised the question of whether the germ was the "cause" of disease or whether the "cause" was the vulnerability of the host. Cannon named the natural physiologic responses to stress the "flight-or-fight" response. If this response is triggered excessively, as occurs with chronic stress, homeostasis is impaired and disease susceptibility is increased.

Hans Selye broadened the concept of stress as the central feature of health by defining the responses as alarm, resistance, and exhaustion. We first experience stress as a challenge to our system—the alarm phase (Figure 7-1). The next phase is one of adaptive resistance, followed by a condition in which our bodies can no longer stand up to the challenge—exhaustion. It is usually in this last stage that we are most vulnerable to disease, and it is stress that is the greatest culprit. In essence, the diagnosed disease reflects which organ or system was vulnerable at the exhaustion phase.

It was not long before scientists became extremely intrigued with stress management as a treatment for mental and physical illness, and the development of the electroencephalogram (EEG) served as a doorway for continued exploration (Figure 7-2). In the late 1960s, researchers demonstrated relationships between EEG alpha-wave activity (8 Hertz [Hz] to 12 Hz) and emotional states of relaxation.[6,16,19,22] Moreover, they were showing that certain individuals could voluntarily control their alpha waves, a feat previously thought impossible.

There was a proliferation of relaxation training methods, the majority of which were mental techniques. Islamic Sufis, Hindu yogis, Christian contemplatives, and Hasidic Jews have practiced religious meditation for centuries. Thus the connection between a new era of spiritual practice and health was formed and embraced. In fact Herbert Benson had consistently argued that the mind and body are hard wired into a state of "remembering peace," and that this state is what we associate with God and comfort.[3-5]

Many forms of mind training became institutionalized. Meditation became popular in the United States with the introduction of transcendental meditation (TM) as practiced and promoted by a teacher from India named Maharishi Mahesh Yogi.[12] Strobel's "Quieting Reflex," Fehmi and Fritz's "Open Focus" techniques, Jose Silva's

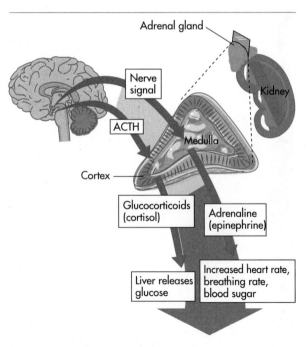

■ **Figure 7-1. The alarm phase.** Note the interaction of the nervous and hormonal responses.

"Silva Mind Control," and Norman Shealy's "biogenics" all focused on wellness and disease prevention.

However, the practice of mind control was still a domain of the gurus of mental disciplines, and no acceptable links existed between these forms of stress management and orthodox medicine. There were no mind control studies demonstrating the remediation of disease in any form, and the mental disciplines listed previously often required motivation or ability that exceeded the comfort level of the ordinary person.

The stage was set for the research findings of Neal Miller who demonstrated that rats could perform psychophysiologic feats through the application of learning theory—specifically, operant conditioning. These results impressed those in the scientific domains of stress management and of medicine for the following two reasons:

1. The method of operant conditioning had been well-established through other forms of psychophysiologic dimensions; as a result, "scientific" logic could be easily applied in basic science.
2. Mental applications could potentially begin with individuals who had the interest and resources to pursue locally available mental disciplines. Applications could then be extended to larger populations.

Operant conditioning functions at a lower conscious process in which the individual is encouraged to perform tasks or to decrease performance through the use of reward or punishment. For example, a rat may be given food pellets each time it selects the color red or pushes a bar down. Neal Miller stimulated a pleasure zone in the rat's brain as the reward for a behavior, in many cases changing the blood flow to a particular

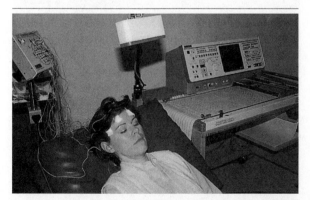

■ **Figure 7-2. Person undergoing electroencephalographic assessment.** Notice the scalp electrodes that detect voltage fluctuations within the cranium.

part of the body.[21] He demonstrated that rats could raise and lower blood pressure (BP), increase and decrease heart rates, and even increase vascular dilation in one ear as opposed to the other. In fact, he reported that some of the rats died from lowering their heart rate in an effort to be reinforced by pleasure zone stimulation.

The research, which was related to instrumental conditioning of visceral responses and was mediated by the autonomic nervous system, gave major impetus to the development of clinical biofeedback. If monitoring of physiologic functions could be immediate enough to allow learned responses and if significant reinforcements could be found, the applications for biofeedback would appear unlimited.

■ Definition of Biofeedback Therapy: Underlying Assumptions

Operational Definitions of Biofeedback

There are several definitions of biofeedback. Operational definitions (i.e., how biofeedback is actually accomplished) emphasize the processes or procedures involved. The objectives and goals of biofeedback are stated in more philosophic terms. The following are operational definitions of biofeedback:

1. "Biofeedback is a recently coined term that refers to a group of experimental procedures in which an external sensor is used to provide the organism with an indication of a state of bodily process, usually in an attempt to affect a change in the measured quantity."[24]
2. "The term biofeedback has gone into widespread use to designate the process. A more precise term would be external psychophysiologic feedback."[14]
3. Kamiya suggested three procedural requirements for biofeedback training, "First, the physiologic function to be brought under control must be continuously monitored with sufficient sensitivity to detect moment-by-moment changes. Second, changes in the physiologic measure must be reflected immediately to the person attempting to control the process. Third, the person must be motivated to learn to affect the physiologic changes under study."[19]

Philosophy Underlying Biofeedback

Some of the more philosophic definitions of biofeedback are the following:

1. "The primary goal of biofeedback has been to promote the acquisition of self-control of physiologic processes."[23]

2. "A tentative definition is that biofeedback is the process or technique for learning voluntary control over automatically, reflexively regulated body functions."[6]

3. "Biofeedback is a tool for learning psychosomatic self-regulation."[15]

Theoretically and philosophically, biofeedback has been consistently grounded in operant learning theory. Researchers have assumed that the reward of accomplishing the assigned task or of seeing that a physical function was changed by subject control would serve as sufficient reinforcement to result in continued effort. For example, when the client sees that his finger temperature increases or decreases at his will or ability, there is a pleasure in experiencing control. The consequential alleviation of the symptom, such as headache pain, would obviously also serve as a reinforcing component.

The ability to learn a conditioned response depends on the technology available. For example, no existing technology exists that can provide immediate feedback of the reactivity of immune function. Technologies currently used with biofeedback include the assessment of muscle activity (measured by the electromyogram [EMG]), of vascular changes (measured by thermal changes), of brain waves (measured by the EEG), of skin conductance, and respiration rate (see Figure 7-2). P cuffs and innovative posture devices have also been used for feedback, although these are not common.

Although these technologies are limited, they have been effectively applied in significant numbers of clinical syndromes. The methods have grown beyond the general stress-disease model; consequently, many of the applications are more specific to cause, although many of the protocols still focus on the reduction of stress. For example, muscle strengthening using the EMG is a treatment of choice for neuromuscular reeducation and gait training, which extends beyond stress reduction as its major focus. These approaches are discussed with greater specificity in the following section.

■ General Descriptions of Biofeedback Modalities

Electromyography

The EMG has been the workhorse of biofeedback. According to Basmajian, EMG instrumentation grew out of the studies and diagnostic work related to neuromuscular and spinal cord functions.[2]

Current biofeedback equipment differs from those early technologies in that there is no invasive administration (Figure 7-3).

EMG biofeedback procedures are based on the fact that muscles produce an instantaneous electric discharge when they are activated. Typically, two electrodes and one reference electrode are attached to the skin in close proximity to the muscular activity, usually pasted or held with straps. The level of activity is usually read in microvolts (mv) of electrical output within a range of 100 Hz to 200 Hz. A measurement of 5 mv or higher is defined as a stressed or spastic muscle; 2 Hz to 4 Hz defines an active muscle; and 0.5 Hz to 1.5 Hz defines a relaxed or flaccid muscle (peak-to-peak). For example, if a patient's measurement for the frontalis muscle (forehead) is 9.8 mv, then the clinician will assume significant muscle tension and will provide feedback for the reduction of muscular tension. This approach is common for tension headaches.

EMG biofeedback is most beneficial when the associated symptoms or medical problem can be related to some level of muscular activity. Several neuromuscular syndromes have been successfully treated through EMG biofeedback. These include tension headache, low back pain, temporomandibular jaw (TMJ) pain, and incontinence.

Tension Headaches

As previously described, sensor electrodes are applied to the muscles that appear to be associated with pain inductions. The most typical muscles have been the frontalis muscles (forehead) and the cervical insertion points or the TMJ muscles. The patient learns to relax these muscles through

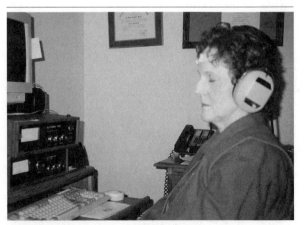

■ *Figure 7-3.* Electromyographic therapy using audio feedback for muscle control on frontalis muscles.

instrument feedback by watching a meter or listening to a sound that is correlated to the intensity of the signal. Listed in Table 7-1 is a brief overview of some of the research efforts for this method.

Low Back Pain

EMG applications for low back pain have many strategies for treatment, depending on the type of muscular dysfunction. Most of the clinical work involves the reduction of muscular spasms in a particular area, thus direct feedback from those muscle groups is beneficial. However, many patients with low back pain have some muscles that are in spasm because other muscles are weak or under used. In these cases, one set of EMG measurements may be used to teach the patient to relax one set of muscles while another set of EMG measurements engages the patient in strengthening and balancing other muscles. This approach develops a better, more efficient, and concerted effort of the back muscles. A list of studies for EMG biofeedback syndromes are presented in Table 7-2.

Case study: EMG biofeedback

Larry is a 50-year-old truck driver who injured his back while reaching down to pick up a napkin. (Most back injuries involve picking up objects weighing less than 10 pounds.) When evaluated for a ruptured disk, physicians found a significant bulge in the L-5/S-1 and L-4/L-5 disk spaces. Surgical removal of disk sections was performed. The pain did not resolve itself; instead, it grew worse. Larry consulted a chiropractor who manipulated his spine. Although he felt some immediate relief, the pain returned in a few days. Physical therapy worsened his pain, especially the day after therapy.

Larry was reluctant to return to work because he was afraid that he would be fired for his lack of ability to do his work, although he felt well enough on some days to perform the duties he knew he had to accomplish. He became irritable with family members and was defensive with friends when asked about his use of the medical disability system. Within 6 months, Larry became depressed and began to self-medicate with alcohol for his pain and depression. He drank in spite of the fact that he was taking heavy doses of pain medications.

Although Larry was not eager to see a psychologist, he agreed to submit to a psychophysio-logic profile. Several causes were revealed. Larry had a severe imbalance of muscle strength with a spastic bundle in the upper right side of his back and another spastic bundle in the lower side with weaknesses in the other areas. When he strained his muscles asymmetrically, the muscles would go into spasms, creating a torque and increasing his pain.

Through EMG biofeedback monitoring, Larry taught himself to relax the muscle spasms and coordinate the back spasms evenly, even through the lifting process. In 1 month of intense therapy, he returned to his work without the need to continue medication or therapy. After 2 weeks of light duty, work restrictions were lifted and he continued to work without incident. His depression soon lifted and his abuse of drugs ceased.

Temporomandibular Jaw Pain

Pain associated with the TMJ radiates from the joint of the jaw. It is usually a result of muscle spasm or muscle imbalance. Often treated in dental offices with splints and dental medicine (even when the "cause" is remedied), the pain cycle persists because of the continuing pain response.

Biofeedback can often relieve the pain associated with TMJ. Typically two EMG instruments are used, one for each side of the head. Electrodes are attached to the skin over the respective joints, enabling the client to monitor the muscular activity on both sides. The therapy helps the patient relax the muscles and eventually use them in harmony while moving the jaw. Anxiety and anger are often associated with this condition, underlying dynamics that must be addressed during therapy.

Neuromuscular Dysfunction and Paralysis

Most of us assume there is a thorough understanding of how motor control of our limbs is activated through the central nervous system (CNS). In reality, there is more mystery than fact, especially in relationship to rehabilitation needs. Underlying dimensions leading to the effects of stroke, head trauma, cardiovascular events, and even genetic conditions often defy scientific understanding. Serious injury to neurologic tissue can occur, causing loss of function in arms, legs, and even facial muscles. Fortunately, there is abundant evidence to demonstrate that these functions can be restored through physical therapy, occupational therapy, and biofeedback.

EMG electrodes can be attached to flaccid muscles, which are essentially considered to be totally paralyzed. However, a "flicker" of activity

TABLE 7-1	Summary of Biofeedback Treatment Studies for Tension Headaches

STUDY	PATIENTS	BIOFEEDBACK TREATMENT	SYMPTOMS	BIOLOGICAL FUNCTIONS
Budzynski TH et al: EMG biofeedback and tension headache: a controlled outcome *Psychosom Med* 35:484, 1973.	2 males 16 females Average age: 35 yr Range: 22-44 yr	Auditory feedback of frontal EMG during 30-min sessions, twice weekly for 9 wk	Average hourly headache activity, subjectively rated from 0 to 5, decreased from 0.5 during the baseline to 0.2 at the end of training to 0.1 at 3-mo follow-up	Average microvolt levels of EMG: baseline, 10; training, 3.9; 3-mo follow-up, 3.9 Weekly headache activity was correlated (0.90) with frontal EMG levels
Chesney MA, Shelton JL: A comparison of relaxation and electro-myogram biofeedback treatments for muscle contraction headache, *J Behav Ther Exp Psychiatry* 7:221, 1976.	22 females 2 males	Auditory and visual feedback of frontal EMG during eight, 30-min feedback sessions, twice weekly for 4 wks	Average levels during first and fourth weeks: headache frequency, 4.8 and 2.8; duration, 5.3 and 6.3 hr; severity on a scale of 1 to 100, 52.3 and 32.5	Data unavailable
Cox DJ et al: Differential effective-ness of reductions in EMG and feedback, verbal relaxation instructions, and medication placebo with tension head-aches, *J Consult Clin Psychol* 43:892, 1975.	20 females 7 males Age range: 16-64 yr Symptom duration: 1-39 yr Average age: 11 yr	Auditory analogue feedback to frontal EMG during 20-min sessions, twice weekly for 4 wks	Average levels during the baseline, 2-wk follow-up and 4-mo follow-up: headache index, 1.7, 0.6, and 0.6; duration 95, 33, 31; frequency, 18, 0.1, 8; medication used, 34, 14, 9; psychosomatic checklist scores, 32, 13, 17	Correlation between reductions in EMG and changes in headache activity: 0.42
Diamond S et al: The value of biofeed-back in the treatment of chronic headache: a 5-year retro-spective study, *Headache* 19:90, 1979.	19 with muscle contraction headaches 265 with combined muscle contrac-tion and vascu-lar headache	Auditory analogue feedback of frontal EMG for 10 min and finger temperature for 20 min, 2-10 times weekly for up to 4 wk	Percent stating that biofeedback helped their headaches: muscle contraction alone, 72; combined muscle contraction and vascular headache, 73	Data unavailable
Fried FE et al: Treatment of tension and migraine head-aches with biofeed-back techniques, *Mo Med* 74:253, 1977.	6 females Age range: 31 to 47; one with tension headaches, two with mixed tension and vas-cular headaches	Home practice of skin temperature raising with a portable trainer twice daily	Number improved by more than 75%: one with tension headache, one with mixed tension and vascular head-ache; number improved little or questionable: one with mixed tension and vascular headache	Data unavailable
Haynes SN et al: Electromyographic biofeedback and relaxation instructions in the treatment of muscle contraction headaches, *Behav Ther* 6:672, 1975.	7 males 14 females Average age 20.9: Average symptom duration, 5.2 yr	Feedback of frontal EMG during 20-min sessions, twice weekly for 3 wk	Average levels during base-line, 1-wk follow-up, 5-7 mo follow-up: frequency, 5.5, 1.5, 1.2; intensity, 3.4, 1.7, 4.1; duration, 4.7, 2.9, 2.3; headache index, 82.1, 20.9, 11.4	Data unavailable
Hutchings DF, Reinking RH: Tension headaches: what form of therapy is most effective? *Biofeedback Self Regul* 1:183, 1976.	14 females 4 males Average age: 23 yr	Auditory analogue feedback of frontal EMG during 10, 15-min sessions	By the end of a 28-day follow-up, 66% improved; composite headache scores (computed by multiplying number of HA hrs times average intensity for that day) were reduced from 10 before treatment to 6 during treatment to 4 after treatment	Average level of EMG in mv/min: 19 before treatment, 8 during treatment, 5 during follow-up

EMG, Electromyogram; *HA,* headache; *mv,* millivolt.

| TABLE 7-1 | Summary of Biofeedback Treatment Studies for Tension Headaches—cont'd |||||

STUDY	PATIENTS	BIOFEEDBACK TREATMENT	SYMPTOMS	BIOLOGICAL FUNCTIONS
Kondo C, Canter A: True and false electromyographic feedback: effect on tension headache, *J Abnorm Psychol* 86:93, 1977.	18 females 2 males Age range: 19-38; Symptom duration: 8-45 mo	Auditory analogue feedback of frontal EMG during 20-min sessions every 1-2 days for 10 sessions	Average number of headaches decreased from approximately 5.3 during the 10 days preceding training to approximately 1.9 during training	Average mv levels of frontal EMG during the first and last 5 min of session #1: 27, 22; during session #10: 15, 10
McKenzie RE, Ehrisman WJ, Montgomery PS, Barnes RH: The treatment of headache by means of electroencephalographic biofeedback, *Headache* 13:164, 1974.	6 females 1 male Average age: 33; Age range: 28-42 yr	Binary visual feedback of EEG activity twice weekly for 5 wk	Average number of headache hours per wk: 41 before treatment 8 during treatment 7 at 1-mo follow-up 2 at 2-mo follow-up	Data unavailable
Phillips C: The modification of tension headache pain using EMG biofeedback, *Behav Res Ther* 15:199, 1977.	15 with headaches at least twice weekly	Auditory feedback of frontal or temporal EMG during 20-min sessions, twice weekly for 6 wk	Average pretreatment, posttreatment, follow-up levels: intensity, 1.1, 0.8, 0.2; frequency, 5.4, 3.8, 2.2; average number of medications used: 6.5, 8.5, 2.6	Average mv levels: pretreatment, 5.6, posttreatment, 2.9, follow-up, 3.6
Wichramaserekera I: Electromyographic feedback training and tension headache: preliminary observations, *Am J Clin Hypn* 15:83, 1972.	5 females with 6-20 yr histories of headache	Feedback of frontal EMG during six 30-min sessions in 6 wk	Average minimum headache intensity: baseline, 4.0; false feedback, 4.3; true feedback, 1.8; average number of hours of headache pain: baseline, 15; false feedback, 15; true feedback, 7.3	Frontal EMG activity averaged 6.2 UV during the baseline and during false feedback and 3.5 during true feedback
Wichramaserekera I: The application of verbal instructions and EMG feedback training to the management of tension headache—preliminary observations, *Headache* 13:74, 1973.	5 females with 6-20 yr histories of headache	Feedback of frontal EMG Feedback of frontal EMG during 10-min sessions, 3 times weekly for 3 weeks; visual feedback was additionally provided during session #1	Average maximum headache intensity: baseline, 4.5; verbal relaxation instructions, 3.8; feedback, 1.9; follow-up, 0.5	Average mv levels of frontal EMG: baseline, 14; relaxation, 14; biofeedback, 6, 0.5; 8-wk follow-up, 5
Bruhn et al: Controlled trial of EMG feedback in muscle contraction headache, *Ann Neurol* 6(1):34, 1979.	28 severe long-standing tension headaches	Experimental group received EMG biofeedback (frontalis placement)	Intensity, duration, and drug intake all reduced	None available
Rokicki LA et al: Change mechanisms associated with combined relaxation/EMG biofeedback training for tension headache, *App Psychophysiol Biofeedback* 22(1):21, 1997.	30 young adults with diagnosed tension headaches compared with 14 controls	EMG relaxation training	51.7% of the experimental group had at least 50% reduction in pain measures compared with none in control	None available

may be detected by monitoring the muscle activity at the most sensitive levels. With continued and constant monitoring, the patient can be taught how to activate and tone these muscles. Theoretically, the patient has identified alternative neurologic routes in the CNS. The method, most of which is performed at an unconscious level, allows many patients to learn how to use their bodies as they did before the loss of function. Bell's Palsy, a paralysis of some facial muscles, is a good example. The use of EMG biofeedback has helped patients who have had strokes regain the use of their tibialis anterior muscles, making the use of splints unnecessary (Table 7-3).

TABLE 7-2 | **Summary of Biofeedback Treatment Studies for Pain Management**

STUDY	PATIENTS	BIOFEEDBACK TREATMENT	SYMPTOMS	BIOLOGICAL FUNCTIONS
Surwit RS et al: Behavioral treatment of Raynaud's disease, *J Behav Med* 1:323, 1978.	32 females Age range: 27-54 yr diagnosed with Raynaud's disease	Visual feedback of changes in finger skin temperature during six 45-min sessions in 11 weeks while performing autogenic relaxation response	Average number of attacks decreased from 2.3 per day during 4 wks preceding training to 1.6 during training; 70 ratings also decreased	Average increase of 3° C while listening to autogenic instructions; no other increases during the session; "patients were able to maintain near normal levels of digital skin temperature after an hour's exposure to ambient temperatures down to 17° C
Ferraccioli G et al: EMG-biofeedback training in fibromyalgia syndrome, *J Rheumatol* 14:4, 820, 1987.	15 patients with fibromyalgia	EMG	56% in long-lasting significant improvement of symptoms of discomfort	
Dohrmann RJ et al: (1978). An evaluation of electromyographic biofeedback in the treatment of myofascial pain-dysfunction syndrome, *J Am Dent Assoc* 96(4):656, 1978.	Myofacial pain	EMG to masseter muscle group	75% total success in reduction of pain, 1 year follow-up	
Cinciripini PM et al: An evaluation of a behavioral program for chronic pain, *J Behav Med* 5(3):375, 1982.	121 patients with pain	EMG in conjunction with total behavioral approaches	Reductions in medications, verbal/nonverbal pain behaviors; Improved physical functioning, employment states	
Kumano H et al: EEG-driven photic stimulation effect on plasma cortisol and beta-endorphine, *Appl Psychophysiol Biofeedback* 22(3):193, 1997.	16 healthy patients	EEG-driven photic stimulation	None	Eight experimental subjects showed significant increases of beta-endorphin and reduction of acute stress compared to eight control subjects
Su XY et al: Application of biofeedback relaxation techniques during chemotherapy, *Chung Hua Hu Li Tsa Chih* 31:11, 627, 1997.	60 patients with cancer during chemotherapy	Thermal	30 experimental subjects less unhealthy psychosomatic reactions to chemotherapy	None available

Incontinence

Fecal incontinency, which is the loss of bowel control, is prevalent in many patients with neurologic disorders, especially those who have experienced cardiovascular events. The original biofeedback methods used with these individuals involved the anal insertion of balloons that measured the pressure of the internal and external sphincters. Although these methods were highly effective in teaching patients to regain control of these muscles, they were difficult to administer. Special EMG instruments monitor muscular activities in relation to both urinary and fecal control.

Thermal Biofeedback

One of the most sensitive correlational physiologic measurements of stress is vasodilation or restriction of blood vessels. Although there are a variety of ways to assess this response, the most efficient and least expensive method is to measure the temperature of the tissue around the area of blood supply. As the vessels are dilated, as occurs with relaxation, the temperature increases. As the vessels restrict, as occurs during stress, the temperature decreases.

Temperature changes can be observed with a simple thermometer. However, thermometers are usually too sluggish to be effective biofeedback monitors to measure the temperature changes in response to subtle stimuli. Special biofeedback temperature instruments are designed to react to a change of temperature in increments of $1/2°$ F in $1/10$ of 1 second, creating an immediacy that allows the patient to learn to affect temperature changes quickly. A skin temperature of $90+°$ F defines a normal, unstressful condition (Figure 7-4).

The administration of temperature biofeedback is relatively easy. It usually requires an electrode attached to the finger, which measures the peripheral temperature of the hand. Occasionally, the therapy requires attachment of the electrode to the toe or another part of the body. The patient monitors the measurements through either a visual cue, such as a meter or graph, or through auditory signals, such as a tone or click pattern. Thermal biofeedback is well researched and recognized as effective treatment for migraine headaches, Raynaud's syndrome, and essential hypertension.

Migraine Headaches

Although migraine headaches can be initiated through muscular tension and treated with EMG, the mechanisms of migraine headaches are cardiovascular. In essence, the pain appears to rebound from vascular restriction, possibly in response to stress of some nature. Stress can also result from external sources such as chemicals or food allergies. Both psychologic and physiologic responses affect the patient's cardiovascular system, inducing headache pain. Successful biofeedback usually helps the patient prevent the onset of headache through the application of relaxation skills, rather than attempting to reduce the pain once the full strength of the syndrome is in process.

The patient is attached to the thermal instrumentation and learns to relax the cardiovascular system by increasing the temperature, as recorded by the finger attachment, while simultaneously reducing the temperature in the temporal area of the head. Patients discover obvious triggers that increase internal stress. Through practicing and "rehearsing" relaxation through imagery techniques, migraine headaches are more easily controlled (Table 7-4).

Case study: Thermal biofeedback

Barbara is a 26-year-old school teacher who has been suffering from migraine headaches for 5 years, ever since graduating from college. Her headaches are inconsistent and come unexpectedly. She has tried to relate the onset of the headaches to diet or work stress. Although there has been an association between her work schedule and headache pain, nothing seemed to help.

Barbara's physician used the standard medication regimen, which seemed to be beneficial in the beginning. Eventually, however, nothing short of total bed rest and major sedatives would help alleviate the pain. This treatment proved unsatisfactory, since she was unable to work or be productive during migraine episodes. Although she

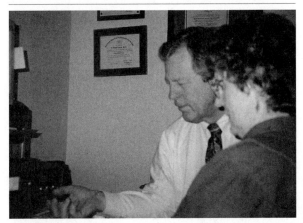

■ **Figure 7-4.** Thermal biofeedback using visual feedback for finger temperature.

TABLE 7-3	Summary of Biofeedback Treatment Studies for Pain Management

STUDY	PATIENTS	BIOFEEDBACK TREATMENT	SYMPTOMS	BIOLOGICAL FUNCTIONS
Andrews JM: Neuro-muscular re-education of the hemiplegic with the aid of the electromyograph, *Arch Phys Med Rehabil* 45:530, 1964.	20 hemiplegics	Feedback of EMG activity from the previously inactive biceps or triceps for 5 min	17 of 20 patients were able to generate EMG activity capable of producing "strong, voluntary, controlled action of the tested muscle"	Data unavailable
Basmajian JV et al: Biofeedback treatment of foot-drop after stroke compared with standard rehabilitation technique: effect on voluntary control and strength, *Arch Phys Med Rehabil* 56:231, 1975.	10 males, 10 females Age range: 30-63 yr	Auditory and visual feedback of EMG activity during 20-min sessions, 3 times weekly for 5 wk	2 of 3 patients were able to walk without their leg braces after training	Dorsiflexion strength increased an average of 2.5 kg; range of motion increased 10.8°
Brudny J et al: Spasmodic torticollis: treatment by feedback display of EMG, *Arch Phys Med Rehabil* 55:403, 1974.	7 males, 3 females with torticollis Age range: 20-58 yr	Visual and auditory feedback of spasmodic and atrophied EMG activity during 30-60 min sessions, 3-5 times weekly for an average of 10 wk	7 became able to maintain a neutral head position with feedback for an indefinite period of time, 1 could do so for hours, 1 could do so for 30 min; following treatment, 7 patients could resume a disturbed normal position without feedback, 1 could do so periodically, and 1 could not	Levels of hypertrophied sternocleidomastoid EMG activity decreased from 95 to 5 (arbitrary) units; ipsilateral activity increased from 31 to 120 units
Brudny J et al: Sensory feedback therapy as a modality of treatment in central nervous system disorders of voluntary movement, *Neurology* 24:925, 1974.	36 patients Age range: 13-68 yr	Feedback of EMG activity from spastic or atrophied muscles during 30-min sessions, 3 times weekly for 8-12 wk	Functional improvement demonstrated by 1 quadriparetic, 10 hemiparetics, 8 patients with torticollis, 2 with hemifacial spasms, and 1 with dystonia	Data unavailable
Brudny J et al: EMG feedback therapy: review of 114 patients, Arch Phys Med Rehabil 57:55, 1976.	114 patients Age range: 13-81 yr	Feedback of EMG activity from spastic or atrophied muscles during 30-45 min sessions, 3 to 5 times weekly for 8-12 wk	23 of 45 hemiparetics partially improved; 19 of 48 with torticollis demonstrated "meaningful" or "major" improvement and decreased medication usage; 2 quadriparetics achieved prehension; 2 of 4 patients with facial spasms improved; 3 with dystonia improved; 2 nonwalking patients with quadriceps muscle atrophy were able to walk	Data unavailable
Carlsson SG et al: Biofeedback in the treatment of long-term temporomandibular joint pain: an outcome study, *Biofeedback Self Regul* 2:161, 1977.	6 males, 5 females with TMJ pain	Visual feedback of masseter muscle activity during 6-18 sessions in 1.5-4 mo	3 patients showed some improvement, 3 showed major improvement; 2 were practically symptom-free, 3 slightly better or totally symptom-free, 1 slightly better, 2 practically unchanged	Lowest UV level of EMG activity at the end of treatment ranged from 4-11

BF, Biofeedback; *CP,* cerebral palsy; *DF,* dorsiflexor; *EMG,* electromylogram; *PT,* physical therapy; *TMJ,* temporomandibular joint; *UV,* ultraviolet.

| TABLE 7-3 | Summary of Biofeedback Treatment Studies for Pain Management—cont'd |

STUDY	PATIENTS	BIOFEEDBACK TREATMENT	SYMPTOMS	BIOLOGICAL FUNCTIONS
Cleeland CS: Behavioral techniques in the modification of spasmodic torticollis, *Neurology* 23:1241, 1973.	4 males, 6 females with torticollis or retrocollis Age range: 15-64 yr	Auditory feedback of sternocleidomastoid activity during six to eight 5-min trials, once or twice daily	Frequency of spasms per 5 min averaged 53.5 and was reduced to 24.8 after treatment; 3 of 10 patients rated as markedly improved, 3 rated moderately improved, 3 showed minimal or no improvement, and 1 lost improvement at follow-up	Data unavailable
Harris FA et al: Electronic sensory aids as treatment for cerebral-palsied children. Inapprop:ioception: part II, *Phys Ther* 54:354, 1974.	18 athetoid cerebral palsied children Age range: 7-18 yr	Auditory and visual feedback of head position, and visual feedback of arm position, during 30-min sessions, 3-7 times weekly for 2-12 months	Children improved ability to maintain neutral head position and normalization of neck muscle tone; decreased tremor in arm and increased smoothness of arm movements; ranges of motion in elbow joints increased; extraneous body movements reduced; drooling decreased; one patient shed crutches and walked independently	Data unavailable
Jacobs A et al: Visual feedback of myoelectric output to facilitate muscle relaxation in normal persons and patients with neck injuries, *Arch Phys Med Rehabil* 50:34, 1969.	14 adults Age range: 21-57 yr	Visual feedback of upper trapezius muscle activity during 10- and 15-min trials	Data unavailable	Trapezius EMG levels were reduced from 5.6-0.79 mm (measured on an oscilloscope)
Johnson HE et al: Muscle re-education in hemiplegia by use of electromyographic device, *Arch Phys Med Rehabil* 54:320, 1973.	6 males, 4 females Age range: 27-73 yr	Auditory and visual feedback of tibialis anterior muscle activity during 30-min sessions, 3 times weekly for 1 wk in the laboratory and twice daily at home	4 patients (40%) became able to walk without a leg brace; 3 demonstrated "fair" improvement, 1 showed minimal improvement, and 2 failed to improve	Data unavailable
Lee K et al: Myofeedback for muscle retraining in hemiplegic patients, *Arch Phys Med Rehabil* 57:588, 1976.	18 adults Age range: 31-79 yr	Auditory and visual analogue feedback of deltoid EMG activity during 20, 5-sec contraction trials, once daily for 3 days	Data unavailable	EMG levels did not change significantly during the trials
Mroczek N et al: Electromyographic feedback and physical therapy for neuromuscular retraining in hemiplegia, *Arch Phys Med Rehabil* 59:258, 1978.	2 females, 7 males with hemiparesis	Auditory and visual feedback of EMG levels in wrist extensors or biceps during twelve 30-min sessions in 4 wk	Data unavailable	In group with sequence biofeedback, then PT: EMG activity increased 23.4 UV during BF, 21.1 during PT; increases in range of motion averaged 14.4% during BF and 18.3% during PT; in group with sequence PT, then biofeedback: EMG activity increased 14.6 UV during PT and 29.6 during BF, increases in range of motion averaged 7.9% during PT and 6.7% during BF

Continued

TABLE 7-3	Summary of Biofeedback Treatment Studies for Pain Management—cont'd			

STUDY	PATIENTS	BIOFEEDBACK TREATMENT	SYMPTOMS	BIOLOGICAL FUNCTIONS
Skrotzky K et al: Effects of electromyographic feedback training on motor control in spastic cerebral palsy, *Phys Ther* 58:547, 1978.	3 males, 1 female with spastic cerebral palsy	Feedback of gastrocnemius EMG activity during 20 sessions in 10 consecutive days	Data unavailable	Range of motion increased by 4.3° to 17°; gastrocnemius EMG activity decreased by 90% to 99% in about 5 seconds for some patients during feedback
Swann D et al: Auditory electromyographic feedback therapy to inhibit undesired motor activity, *Arch Phys Med Rehabil* 55:251, 1974.	4 males 3 females Age range: 17-77 yr	Feedback of EMG activity in the peroneus longus area for 10 min, 3 times weekly for 2 wk	Data unavailable	Increases in range of motion; EMG feedback, 6.3°; PT 2.4°
Wannstedt GT et al: Use of augmented sensory feedback to achieve symmetrical standing, *Phys Ther* 58:553, 1978.	Right and left hemiparetics Age range: 32-75 yr	Auditory feedback of weight placed on affected limb during 20-min sessions, 1 to 28 times daily	During an initial session, 23 of 30 patients achieved symmetric standing; remaining 7 corrected postures somewhat; 16 of 20 continued training for 3-28 sessions and achieved symmetric standing; 4 did not; 14 of 16 maintained symmetric standing at 1-mo follow-up	Data unavailable
Colborne GR et al: Feedback of triceps surae EMG in gain of children with cerebral palsy, *Arch Phys Med Rehabil* 75:(1)40, 1994.	18 children with spastic hemiplegia secondary to cerebral palsy	EMG from the triceps surae group	Stride length and velocity improved/gait symmetry	
Toner LV et al: Improved ankle function in children with cerebral palsy after computer assisted motor learning, *Dev Med Child Neurol* 40(12):829, 1998.	Young children with CP	Auditory and visual feedback of range of motion and ankle DF strength in the laboratory; 3 days a week for 6 wks; at-home component of training using EMG units to train DF muscle recruitment of remaining days	Data unavailable	Tapping ability increased significantly in trained leg posttraining, feel significantly at 6-wk after training test, but remained significantly higher than pretest levels Tapping returned to pretraining levels at 14 mo Active range of motion increased significantly in the trained leg DF strength and active range of motion increased posttraining because of increases in motor-unit recruitment

BF, Biofeedback; *CP,* cerebral palsy; *DF,* dorsiflexor; *EMG,* electromylogram; *PT,* physical therapy; *TMJ,* temporomandibular joint; *UV,* ultraviolet.

had early warning symptoms, such as visional auras and tingling in the base of her skull, she was afraid of committing to social engagements for fear of developing an attack. She was considered by her friends to be a recluse.

Barbara consulted a psychologist in the belief that these attacks may be caused by a neurologic problem related to childhood conflicts with her father. She had read that migraine headaches can

be caused by repressed anger. The psychologist turned out to be certified in biofeedback and integrated some of Barbara's insights about her anger into the biofeedback training.

Thermal biofeedback was administered. The first attempts were very frustrating to her. Finger temperature would drop from 81.2° F to 74.5° F when she attempted to relax. She soon discovered that she was trying to "perform" too much, creat-

TABLE 7-4	Summary of Biofeedback Treatment Studies for Migraine Headaches

STUDY	PATIENTS	BIOFEEDBACK TREATMENT	SYMPTOMS	BIOLOGICAL FUNCTIONS
Andreychuk T et al: Hypnosis and biofeedback in the treatment of migraine headaches, *Int J Clin Exp Hypn* 23:172, 1975.	33 volunteers	Feedback of hand temperature for 45 min, once each week for 10 weeks	Average scores on a headache index for patients scoring high on a hypnotic induction profile: baseline, 156; last 5 weeks of training, 48; average scores for those scoring low on a hypnotic induction profile: baseline, 26; training, 17	Data unavailable
Blanchard EB et al: Temperature biofeedback in the treatment of migraine headaches, *Arch Gen Psychiatry* 35:581, 1978.	25 females, 5 males; average age 39 Age range: 21-77 Average symptom duration 20 yrs, range 5-40	Visual feedback of finger temperature during 30-min sessions, twice weekly for 6 weeks	Average levels per week during the baseline, training, and 1-3 mo follow-up: headache index, 0.74, 0.4, 0.29; frequency, 3.2, 2.2, 1.4; duration, 13.5, 7.6, 2.0; medication index, 13, 7.6, 6.7; intensity, 3.0, 1.9, 1.4	Data unavailable
Friar LR et al: Migraine: management by trained control of vasoconstriction, *J Consult Clin Psychol* 44:46, 1976.	16 females, 3 males Average age: 30	Auditory and visual feedback of skin temperature over the temporal artery during eight 200 heartbeat trials in 3 weeks	Compared with average levels in a 30-day baseline, major attacks reduced 46%, number of episodes reduced 36%, intensity reduced 4%, medication consumption reduced 45%	Average pulse amplitude decreased by 16% during training
Medina JL et al: Biofeedback therapy for migraine, *Headache* 16:115, 1976.	24 females, 3 males Average age: 35; range 10 to 60	Auditory analogue feedback of frontal EMG of 10 min and finger temperature for 20 min, twice weekly for 1 mo	Three markedly improved (76%-100%); 6 moderately improved (51%-75%); 4 mildly improved (30%-50%)	Data unavailable
Reading C et al: Biofeedback control of migraine: a pilot study, *Br J Soc Clin Psychol* 15:429, 1976.	3 females, 3 males Average age: 41; range 26-54 yr	Feedback of finger temperature during sessions of approximately 30 min	Average levels per week during the baseline, training, 1-mo follow-up: frequency, 4.1, 1.9, 1.4, 1.0; duration, 25.3, 10.4, 5.4, 5.1; headache index, 9.0, 5.4, 3.1, 3.0	Subjects able to produce average increases of 1.4° C during final, no feedback baseline, able to produce increases of 7° C at 2-mo follow-up

BPV, Blood-pulse volume; *EMG*, electromylogram.

Continued

ing performance anxiety. She then adopted a more open attitude. She began to focus on nothingness, creating a blank screen in her mind. As she did so, her temperature rose to 90° F! The monitor reading was not as important as the internal pleasure she received from learning to control her body and from experiencing the relaxation response.

During the twelve sessions of biofeedback, Barbara learned to control her temperature with her imagery of openness and began to generalize the technique to her home and work situations. Whenever she experienced signals of an upcoming headache, she would begin her relaxation scheme. If she denied herself this relaxation method, the migraine headache would seize her and nothing would help. Within a short time period, she became adept at avoiding the migraine symptoms with prevention behaviors.

With this new-found sense of control, Barbara began to socialize more and started dating again. Her response to headache symptoms became automatic, and soon headaches were eliminated altogether. The treating psychologist was later invited to her wedding.

Raynaud's Syndrome
Symptoms of Raynaud's syndrome include a sudden onset of severe pain, usually in a limb, and this pain is often associated with physical or thermal shocks to the body. The limb's coloration

TABLE 7-4	Summary of Biofeedback Treatment Studies for Migraine Headaches—cont'd			
STUDY	**PATIENTS**	**BIOFEEDBACK TREATMENT**	**SYMPTOMS**	**BIOLOGICAL FUNCTIONS**
Sargent JD et al: Preliminary report on the use of autogenic feedback training in the treatment of migraine and tension headaches, *Psychosom Med* 35:129, 1973.	74 patients who received at least 270 days of training	Feedback of difference between finger and midforehead skin temperatures	Improvement ratings: 15 very good; 20 good; 16 moderate; 11 slight; 12 no improvement	Data unavailable
Sturgis ET et al: Modification of combined migraine-muscle contraction headaches using BPV and EMG feedback, *J Appl Behav Analysis* 11:215, 1978.	2 females, average age 44	Auditory analogue feedback of blood pulse volume and frontal EMG levels in 20-min sessions	Average duration of headache decreased from 7.4 during baseline, to 1.4 during BPV feedback, to 0.75 during EMG feedback, to 0.75 at follow-up	Data unavailable
Turin A et al: Biofeedback therapy for migraine headaches, *Arch Gen Psychiatry* 33:517, 1976.	3 males 4 females	Feedback of finger temperature for 20 min, twice per week for 6-14 wk	Average levels per week during the baseline and final 4-6 wk of training: frequency, 2.2, 1.3; medication consumption, 4.3, 1.7; duration, 12.4, 5.7	Skin temperature increased during the 10th session by 0.1° C to 1.7° C
Labbé EE et al: Treatment of childhood migraine with autogenic training and skin temperature biofeedback: a component analysis, *Headache* 35(1):10, 1995.	30 children, ages 7-18 yr	Skin temperature biofeedback (finger)	80% of biofeedback group, 50% of autogenics control group, and none of no-treatment group were symptom free	
Sartory G et al: A comparison of psychological and pharmacological treatment of pediatric migraine, *Behav Res Ther* 36(12):1155, 1998.	43 youths (between 8-16 yr) with migraine	Biofeedback cephalic vasomotor feedback with relaxation (compared with metoprolol, beta blocker)	Those treated with cephalic feedback improved significantly in frequency and mood	None reported

BPV, Blood-pulse volume; *EMG,* electromylogram.

grows pale, and intense discomfort is experienced. The cause of this syndrome is unknown, but the reason for the pain is related to a spasm of the cardiovascular system in the particular area of the body in which the pain originates.

A thermal electrode is attached to the finger or digits of other affected limbs, and the patient learns to relax the blood vessels responsible for the pain. Again, situational cues are usually rehearsed for prevention of pain onsets.

Essential Hypertension

Elevated BP, or hypertension, is often a symptom in many disease states; as a result, biofeedback can serve as an integral part of a total health program. In essence, the pressure on the walls of the blood vessels is too great for normal functioning and, when chronic, can cause long-term damage. Hypertension is considered a major factor in incidents of heart attacks and strokes.

Stress has been associated with a wide variety of cardiovascular issues, so it is natural that relaxation biofeedback would affect the total body system and be an effective treatment for hypertension. BP cuffs have been used for monitoring, but because of their sluggish response, these are difficult to use. Because of this, alternative methods of assessing BP are recommended.

The patient is asked to monitor finger temperature after learning how to relax the system by raising the level of peripheral temperature. As the patient learns to raise the temperature consistently, BP readings are taken to substantiate the effect on the total system (i.e., a reduction in BP) (Table 7-5).

Skin Conductance Activity

Sweat gland activity is another physiologic process that is associated with stress and is a component of the "lie detector" test. However, this biological activity is not directly measured through biofeedback instrumentation. What is measured is the correlation of the speed or ease with which electrical impulses travel across the skin. This reaction is called the *galvanic skin response* (GSR). As sweat activity increases, moisture increases the conductivity, thereby reducing the resistance of electrical transmission. Stress is correlated with an increase in recorded conductivity. This is an over-simplified explanation, but the theory supports the use of the instrumentation.

A modicum of electrical current is run across the skin using two electrodes, and the resistance is measured in ohms. (An ohm is a unit of electrical resistance equal to one ampere produced by a potential of one volt crossing the terminals of a conductor.) The GSR is usually converted into an auditory sound for the purposes of biofeedback. However, since the signal of conductivity is the inverse of relaxation, many manufacturers convert the signal to the inverse function (mhos) and refer to the instrumentation as electrodermal response (EDR).

GSR and EDR are difficult parameters to analyze statistically because the measures are not linear and do not have a normal distribution. For example, it appears that a stable measurement—referred to as the tonic state—of a patient is less correlated with stress than a change in the amplitude or strength of resistance—referred to the phasic state. Although biofeedback is useful for training patients with stress syndromes, there is a lack of research for specific disease management.

Electroencephalography

The EEG enjoyed significant interest in the 1970s because research findings based on its use demonstrated definitive states of consciousness related to stress and expansion of creativity. Theorists such as Tart, Krippner, Ornstein, Pelletier and Garfield, Schwartz and Beatty, and Jacobson were among those who made significant contributions and helped mold the fields of humanistic and transpersonal psychology.[7,9,10,11,13,17] However, because of the expense and crude measurements of EEG biofeedback for relaxation, as well as the more reliable applications of EMG and thermal biofeedback, interest waned. A new wave of excitement arose with the development of newer computer-assisted instrumentations and the subsequent discovery of their applications in the treatment of those abusing drugs and those with newly discovered neurologic disorders, such as attention deficient disorders (ADD) (Figure 7-5).

The biofeedback instrumentation is different from the brain diagnostic instrumentation in which various leads across brain areas depict brain mapping of regional neurologic firings, indicative of brain damage. The biofeedback EEG instrumentation consists of measuring brain activity in amplitude and within specified ranges. Although the placement of the electrodes does correlate to certain brain function (e.g., occipital lobes—vision), biofeedback EEG is not referred to as a brain scan. The accepted categories of brain activities for arousal levels are shown in Box 7-1.

It should be noted that research definitions of these ranges vary 1 Hz from article to article. The primary clinical research in biofeedback has been conducted for the alpha, theta, and beta ranges. As indicated previously, alpha state is regarded as the relaxation state. Therefore much of the clinical objectives for clients suffering from stress dis-

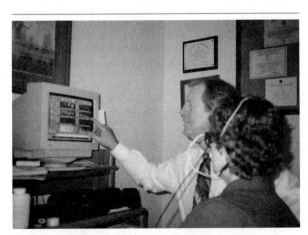

■ *Figure 7-5.* Electroencephalographic therapy using visual feedback of alpha frequency. *(Session conducted by G. Frank Lawlis, PhD.)*

BOX 7-1 Arousal Levels of Brain Activity
0.5 Hz to 3 Hz—delta state (sleep/unconscious)
4.0 Hz to 7.0 Hz—theta state (trance/hypnogogic)
8.0 Hz to 11.0 Hz—alpha state (relaxation)
12.0 Hz to 14.0 Hz—SMR state (calm and focused)
15.1 Hz to beta state (alert/stressed)

TABLE 7-5   **Summary of Biofeedback Treatment Studies for Cardiovascular Disorders**

STUDY	PATIENTS	BIOFEEDBACK TREATMENT	SYMPTOMS	BIOLOGICAL FUNCTIONS
Benson H et al: Decreased blood-pressure in pharmacologically treated hypertensive patients who regularly elicited the relaxation response, *Lancet* 1:289, 1974.	7 hypertensive patients; Age range: 30 to 54 yr	8 to 34 sessions with auditory and visual feedback for decreases in median systolic pressure during 30 trials of 50 heartbeats	Data unavailable	Median systolic pressure averaged 165 mm Hg during the last five baseline sessions and decreased to 148 in the last five training sessions; average in-session decrease 5 mm Hg; heart rate did not change consistently
Blanchard EB et al: A simple feedback system for the treatment of elevated blood pressure, *Behav Ther* 6:241, 1975.	3 males and 1 female with elevated blood pressure Age range: 25-50 yr	Visual feedback of changes in systolic blood pressure and occurrence of Korotkoff sounds during eight 20-min sessions in the first treatment period and during four sessions in the second; sessions generally scheduled each day	Data unavailable	Systolic pressure averaged 154, 128, 137, 122, 127 mm Hg during the first baseline, second feedback, follow-up periods, respectively
Bleecker ER et al: Learned control of cardiac rate and cardiac conduction in the Wolff-Parkinson-White syndrome, *N Engl J Med* 288:560, 1973.	3 males and 3 females with atrial fibrillation Age range: 28-62 yr	Visual feedback for increases and decreases in ventricular rate during 16 to 22 sessions lasting 4-7 min	Data unavailable	Ventricular rates increased average of −0.5-9.5 bpm during speeding, decreased average of 0.8-3.5 bpm during slowing, differed average of 7.2 bpm during alternately speed-slow phase; success rates in sessions averaged 67%, 47%, 86%, respectively
Elder ST et al: Instrumental blood pressure conditioning in out-patient hypertensives, *Behav Res Ther* 13:185, 1975.	14 males and 8 females reporting diagnoses of essential hypertension Age range: 23-80 yr	Visual feedback of relative changes in diastolic blood pressure during either 10 days with feedback sessions once per day (massed practice) or with sessions scheduled in decreasing weekly frequency (spaced practice) for 80 days; sessions included ten 1-min trials	Data unavailable	Baseline pressure of 147/85 mm Hg significantly reduced to 139/82 mm Hg in the last training session; massed practice group reduced diastolic pressure in 88% of sessions; 30-day follow-up of spaced practice group indicated return of systolic pressure to baseline levels, whereas diastolic pressure remained approximately 1% below such values
Elder ST et al: Instrumental conditioning of diastolic blood pressure in essential hypertensive patients, *J Appl Behav Analysis* 6:377, 1973.	18 males with hypertension Age range: 23-59 yr	Visual or visual plus verbal feedback for decreases in systolic blood pressure during 40-min sessions, twice daily for 4 days	Data unavailable	Blood pressure averaged 156/112 mm Hg during baseline and decreased 5/9 mm Hg by follow-up in visual feedback group; visual feedback and verbal reinforcement groups averaged 154/102 mm Hg in baseline and decreased blood pressure levels by 23/19 mm Hg at follow-up
Friedman H et al: A six-month follow-up of the use of hypnosis and biofeedback procedures in essential hypertension, *Am J Clin Hypn* 20:184, 1978.	39 males and 9 females with hypertension Age range: 23-60 yr	Visual feedback of diastolic pressure during seven sessions	Data unavailable	Blood pressure averaged 147/96 mm Hg, 137/94 mm Hg, 140/88 mm Hg during baseline, 1-mo follow-up, 6-mo follow-up periods, respectively

BP, Blood pressure; *EEG,* electroencephalogram; *EMG,* electromyogram; *PVC,* premature ventricular contractions.

| TABLE 7-5 | Summary of Biofeedback Treatment Studies for Cardiovascular Disorders—cont'd |

STUDY	PATIENTS	BIOFEEDBACK TREATMENT	SYMPTOMS	BIOLOGICAL FUNCTIONS
Goldman H et al: Relationship between essential hypertension and cognitive functioning: effects of biofeedback, *Psychophysiology* 12:569, 1975.	7 males with hypertension Age range: 35-68 yr	Auditory and visual feedback of changes of mean systolic blood pressure during 2-hour sessions, once weekly for 3 weeks	Data unavailable	Baseline blood pressure averaged 167/109 mm Hg; reduced to 161/94 mm Hg in last feedback session
Kleinman KM et al: Relationship between essential hypertension and cognitive functioning II: effects of biofeedback training generalize to non-laboratory environment, *Psychophysiology* 14:192, 1977.	8 males with hypertension Age range: 26-63 yr	Auditory and visual feedback of mean systolic pressure during 25 to 30, 30-heartbeat trials during each of 9 sessions	Data unavailable	Laboratory-measured blood pressure averaged 149/95 mm Hg, 152/92 mm Hg, 142/85 mm Hg during the first control session, last control session, last feedback session, respectively; blood pressure determined by patient at home and work averaged 155/97 mm Hg during the control period and 147/89 mm Hg before last two feedback sessions
Kristt DA et al: Learned control of blood pressure in patients with high blood pressure, *Circulation* 51:370, 1975.	4 females and 1 male with hypertension Age range: 46-70 yr	Visual feedback of relative changes in average systolic blood pressure during about 14 sessions per week for 3 weeks	Data unavailable	Pretreatment and posttraining blood pressure: 162/95 mm Hg, 144/87 mm Hg, respectively; no reliable change in heart rate, respiration rate, triceps brachii EMG activity, or alpha EEG activity; systolic blood pressure averaged 141 mm Hg before, and 125 mm Hg after 12-wk home training; 3 patients reduced medication levels while maintaining treatment effect at 12-wk follow-up
Patel C et al: Yoga and biofeedback in the management of hypertension, *Lancet* 2:1053, 1973.	11 females and 9 males with hypertension	Auditory feedback of changes in skin resistance during 30-min sessions, 3 times weekly for 3 months	Data unavailable	Blood pressure averaged 159/100 mm Hg, 139/86 mm Hg, 145/86 mm Hg, 147/88 mm Hg, 144/87 mm Hg in baseline, posttreatment, 3-mo follow-up, 6-mo follow-up, 9-12-mo follow-up periods, respectively
Patel C et al: Randomized controlled trial of yoga and biofeedback in management of hypertension, *Lancet* 2:93, 1975.	13 males and 21 females with hypertension Age range: 34-75 yr	30-min feedback-relaxation sessions twice weekly for 6 weeks	Data unavailable	Blood pressure averaged 168/100 mm Hg during the baseline and decreased to 141/84 mm Hg after treatment; blood pressure in control group, which was later treated averaged 177/104 mm Hg before and 149/89 mm Hg after treatment
Surwit RS et al: Biofeedback and meditation in the treatment of borderline hypertension. In Beatty J, Legewie H, editors: *Biofeedback and behavior,* New York, 1977, Plenum Publishing.	8 hypertensive patients under age 60	Auditory and visual feedback of simultaneous changes in median systolic BP and heart rate during 8-, 60-, to 90-min sessions in 5 weeks; each session included 20 1-min trials alternated with 10 second rests	Data unavailable	No significant change in median systolic pressure across sessions or at follow-up; baseline levels averaged 142 mm Hg systolic and 90 mm Hg diastolic and reduced to 139 mm Hg and 84 mm Hg, respectively at follow-up; heart rate decreased 3 bpm

Continued

TABLE 7-5	Summary of Biofeedback Treatment Studies for Cardiovascular Disorders—cont'd			
STUDY	PATIENTS	BIOFEEDBACK TREATMENT	SYMPTOMS	BIOLOGICAL FUNCTIONS
Surwit RS et al: Comparison of cardiovascular biofeedback, neuromuscular biofeedback, and meditation in the treatment of borderline essential hypertension, *J Consult Clin Psychol* 46:252, 1978.	18 adults with hypertension Age range: 27-59 yr	Auditory and visual feedback of either EMG activity from the frontalis and forearm extensor areas, or integrated (patterned) heart rate and median systolic blood pressure during eight, 60- to 90-min sessions held twice weekly	Data unavailable	Systolic pressure in the cardiovascular group averaged 137 mm Hg during baseline and 139 mm Hg during training sessions; EMG group averaged 137 mm Hg and 140 mm Hg, respectively; within session (first-to-last trial) changes decreased from 139 mm Hg to 128 mm Hg for cardiovascular group and from 142 mm Hg to 139 mm Hg for EMG group
Walsh P et al: Comparison of biofeedback pulse wave velocity and progressive relaxation in essential hypertensives, *Percept Mot Skills* 44(2):839, 1977.	9 females and 15 males with hypertension Age range: 24-69 yr	In phase 1, seven 3-min trials to reduce pulse transit time with auditory and visual feedback once weekly for 5 wks; in phase 2, 90-min sessions once weekly for 5 wk	Data unavailable	Blood pressure averaged 147/94, 133/84, 135/87, 133/86 mm Hg; 135/84 mm Hg during the first session of phase 1, last session of phase 1, last session of phase 2, 3-mo and 12-mo follow-up, respectively; heart and respiration rates did not change significantly across sessions
Weiss T et al: Operant conditioning of heart rate in patients with premature ventricular contractions. In Birk L, editor: *Biofeedback: behavioral medicine*, New York, 1973, Grune and Stratton.	5 males and 3 females with premature ventricular contractions	Visual feedback for heart rate speeding, slowing, alternate speeding and slowing, maintenance in specified limits during approximately 10, 10, 10, 11 sessions, respectively; each session included 34 min of feedback	Some patients became aware of heart beat abnormalities as occurred in environment	Frequency of PVCs averaged 12.9, 11.9, 9.9, 5.1, 4.8, 5.9 per min during pretreatment speeding, slowing, alternate speeding, slowing; maintenance in specified range and follow-up periods, respectively; 5 patients showed decrease in PVCs associated with feedback training
Blanchard EB et al: Controlled evaluation of thermal biofeedback and treatment of elevated blood pressure in unmedicated mild hypertension, *Biofeedback Self Regul* 21(2):167, 1996.	42 unmedicated mild hypertensives	Temperature training (finger)		Significant decrease in DBP for females, not for males
Lal SK et al: Effect of feedback signal and psychological characteristics on blood pressure self-regulated capability, *Psychophysiology* 35(4):405, 1998.	36 normotensives	Visual or auditory continuous systolic feedback	Visual feedback (p=.04), visual plus auditory (p=.03) were significantly better than auditory feedback alone. Increased anger and hostility, state anxiety, and expectation had links to capabilities for control	None available

EEG, Electroencephalogram; *EMG,* electromyogram; *PVC,* premature ventricular contractions.

orders have been directed toward teaching them to achieve alpha states of relaxation with feedback.

The treatment application in EEG biofeedback is the following model: a "normal" individual has at his disposal the brain states of all levels, thereby enabling him to function appropriately in all situations. When rest is needed, the brain can enter the delta state. When creativity and insight are needed, the theta range is available for this purpose, and when relaxation is required, the brain can go into this state. When problem-solving is needed, the brain can gear itself into the beta state. Problems exist when the individual cannot shift into and out of these states as needed or when he or she shifts into these states inappropriately. For example, many people have stress syndromes because they cannot shift into the alpha states appropriately. People with ADD cannot shift out of alpha states easily. By using EEG feedback, they teach themselves these skills and generalize them to life situations.

A great amount of excitement in the clinical field of biofeedback application has been generated for the treatment of drug abuse. Peniston and Kulkosky's landmark studies with alcoholism and other drug abuse disorders established prescribed protocols that proved superior to other treatments.[18] In essence, they used EEG biofeedback to train subjects to generate alpha-theta states, reducing drug abuse behaviors significantly. In theory, many of these individuals were using drugs to shift into relaxation states. Consequently, the need for sedative drugs was reduced or eliminated, and more functional brain patterns allowed the individual to live a more productive life.

As mentioned previously, persons with ADD function in a different manner. Individuals unconsciously seek novel stimulation to satisfy the need for beta excitement, thereby creating hyperactivity as a compensatory outcome. The biofeedback protocol for ADD consists of training the person to generate beta amplitude without the disruptive behaviors, thereby allowing the individual to achieve more focus and less hyperactivity (Figure 7-6).

Case study: **EEG application**

John was a computer engineer who had tremendous aptitude in his vocational field and was considered very successful. However, he had problems focusing on any one project for any period. He became easily distracted, abruptly switching from one thing to another. His long-term projects faltered.

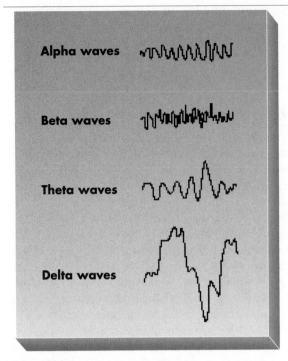

■ **Figure 7-6.** Examples of alpha, beta, theta, and delta waves as seen on an electroencephalogram.

This distraction behavior was obvious in his home life as well. Hundreds of uncompleted projects lay around the house, and his wife was constantly complaining about this trait. John was also unhappy with his constant agitation and inability to complete projects. He took anxiety medications, but these only made him more perturbed. He was afraid that he would eventually have a heart attack or develop an ulcer. He called his condition his "bad nerves."

While viewing a television documentary, John learned of a biofeedback technique called "neurofeedback." He learned that he probably had what was diagnosed as ADD, a condition in which the individual's brain spends too much time in the theta state. In efforts to stimulate the brain into higher states (beta), John attempted novelty-seeking behavior, hence the distraction. Such disorders are often treated with stimulants, such as Ritalin, to balance brain activity; however, there are consequences for long-term usage of these drugs.

Using biofeedback to learn how to shift the brain into beta activity on command, John's distractions decreased and he found himself less agitated. He discovered breathing patterns were related to shifts in consciousness; and, after a period of sensitizing himself to these patterns, a profound change in his overall functionality occurred. His concentration improved dramatically; but, most importantly, John enjoyed life. For the first time, he could honestly say, "I am happy."

■ Frontiers: Old and New

The principles of biofeedback have been used in a wide variety of settings and are usually applied with more than one form of instrumentation. It is exciting to recognize that unlimited applications merely await the appropriate technology. The human capacity for learning to respond within psychophysiologic parameters is unlimited. The following frontiers relate to the treatment of syndromes continually researched with biofeedback:

1. Irritable bowel syndromes (motility of the entire gastrointestinal tract that produces abdominal pain, constipation, or diarrhea)—EMG stress protocol in abdomen area
2. Tinnitus (disturbing noise originating in the ear rather than in the environment)—EMG stress reduction protocol in jaw and head regions
3. Fibromyalgia syndrome (achy pain and stiffness in soft tissues, including muscles, tendons, and ligaments)—temperature-EMG stress reduction protocol in limb area
4. Chronic back pain—thermal stress reduction in hands and feet; EMG stress protocol reduction in lower and upper back areas
5. Constipation—EMG stress reduction protocol in abdomen area
6. Postpoliomyelitis symptoms (progressive muscle weakness, resulting in disability)—EMG stress reduction protocol in affected limbs
7. Schizophrenia (loss of contact with reality, hallucination, and delusions; in some cases, rigid body postures)—EMG stress reduction protocol in arms
8. Phantom-limb pain (pain in area where amputated limb had existed)—EMG stress reduction protocol in stump
9. Asthma (reversible airway narrowing, caused by inflammation or lung hyperreactivity)—temperature stress reduction protocol; EMG stress reduction protocol for respiration
10. Panic attacks—temperature-EMG stress reduction protocol
11. Postural training for idiopathic sclerosis (scarring of skin or joints from unknown causes)—EMG muscle strengthening
12. Oral pharyngeal dysphagia (impairment of speech resulting from pharynx dysfunction)—EMG stress reduction protocol on throat muscles
13. Herpes—EMG stress management protocol on frontalis
14. Sickle cell crisis (sudden worsening of anemia, pain in abdomen or long bones, fever, and shortness of breath)—EMG stress management protocol on frontalis
15. Visual accommodation and oculomotor abnormalities (interference with ability to look upward, downward, and inward effectively)—EMG stress reduction protocol on frontalis and temperature-EMG stress reduction protocol on hands (Tables 7-7 and 7-8)

■ Biofeedback as Research Tool

Biofeedback instruments are used as research tools by a wide variety of scientists who want to assess the effects of stress and relaxation on immune function. The following studies use biofeedback instrumentation for this purpose.

Biofeedback-Assisted Relaxation: Effects on Phagocytic Capacity

The purpose of this study was to investigate whether subjects who self report high levels of stress have lower immunity, and whether low-immunity subjects under high stress could enhance phagocytic activity through biofeedback-assisted relaxation (BAR).[20] During phase 1, the levels of stress and phagocytic immune functioning (determined by nitroblue tetrazolium [NBT] test) were assessed as high or low. Significant chi-square analysis ($\times 2 = 3.8624$, df $= 1$, $p < 0.05$) showed that subjects with high reported stress had low immunity.

Sixteen high stress–low immunity subjects were randomly assigned to BAR and control groups during phase 2. The eight subjects in the BAR treatment were monitored using two EMG and one temperature biofeedback instruments with relaxation instructions. One EMG measurement was taken on the frontalis muscle group, and the second series of measurements was taken on the trapezius muscle group. All subjects showed a clinically significant change in biofeedback readings. The frontalis measurements reduced from 1.88 mv average mean (before treatment) to 1.09 mv average mean (after treatment). The trapezius measurements showed an average decease from 1.86 mv to 1.16 mv, and the average temperature increased from an average of 90.6° F to 95.3° F.

After treatment, NBT testing showed significant increases in the level of phagocytic immune function (F=11.11, p<0.003) for the experimental group as compared with the control group. White blood cell count and differential were unchanged across blood samples for both groups. Experimental subjects reported significant decreases in tension anxiety and increases in overall coping abilities. This research concluded that BAR was improved coping skill ability and phagocytic capacity. BAR affected the quality rather than the quantity of phagocytic neutrophils.

Biofeedback Training as an Adjunctive Therapy for Rheumatoid Arthritis: Study of Relaxation and Temperature

Rheumatoid arthritis (RA) is a painful systemic disease believed to be exacerbated by stress. Relaxation and biofeedback stratagems have demonstrated utility in alleviating both pain and stress-related symptoms; therefore they were tested for efficacy with RA a two-phase study.[1]

First, 24 patients were taught a relaxation technique and then trained with biofeedback to either elevate or reduce temperature. Although EMG studies measured muscle relaxation (frontalis), EMG biofeedback of muscle relaxation was not provided as a component of the training. Second, 15 similarly trained subjects were compared with 8 patients who received traditional physiologic modalities. Psychologic testing and functional and physical evaluations, as well as measurements related to pain, sleep, and other activities, were carried out for all subjects.

In Phase 1, results of the first study where subjects were trained to either elevate or reduce temperature revealed significant and positive changes related to reductions in pain and tension and improved sleep patterns after treatment. No differential effects were noted between temperature elevation and reduced pain and tension. This was attributed to both groups having maintained temperatures above baseline during biofeedback training, confirming the theoretical association of hand warming and relaxation. The temperature enhancement groups raised their temperature from an average of 87.5° F to 91.5° F, whereas the temperature reduction groups also raised their temperature from an average of 84.5° F to 91.0° F. The EMG results also showed reductions of stress for both groups.

The results of Phase 2 consistently favored relaxation and biofeedback over the physiologic group on the physical and functional indices (e.g.,

improvements in sleep, work status, physical activity levels, 50-foot walking time, percentage of time hurting, percentage of body hurting, joint pain, leisure activities, activities of daily living). The psychologic measures tended to remain constant through both phases (tension, depression, anxiety, vigor, fatigue, confusion, and mood changes), leading to the conclusion that the effectiveness of treatment was specific to physical functioning rather than to a psychologic enhancement of well being.

■ Professional Certification

The clinical practice of biofeedback and applied psychophysiology constitutes a multidisciplinary and heterogeneous field of professional disciplines and types of applications. Education and training in this field range from courses in universities and individual workshops to comprehensive biofeedback training programs. The Biofeedback Certification Institute of America (BCIA) provides accreditation for many biofeedback programs. The Association for Applied Psychophysiology and Biofeedback (AAPB) provides much of the standardized training.

In spite of the efforts to certify professionals in this field, expertise is largely determined by the knowledge and experience of a particular field and its applicability. For example, the application of biofeedback to the various syndromes of chronic back pain requires sufficient knowledge of the neurologic and muscular structure of the back and spinal column to accomplish subtle changes for pain relief. Familiarity with orthopedic and neurosurgical procedures are required for the successful application of biofeedback.

To apply biofeedback principles correctly in the field of anxiety management, one must possess a different kind of information, namely an understanding of the psychologic dimensions of biochemistry, psychotropic pharmacology, and psychotherapy related to the syndromes being treated.

In view of the many disciplines involved, some of the following general considerations are essential for health care professionals considering the use of the biofeedback professional:

1. Professional training received
2. Experience of the professional in light of the populations served
3. Reputation of the clinician
4. Research findings for the applicability of biofeedback for the population to be served

An Expert Speaks: Dr. Penelope Montgomery

Penelope Montgomery earned her doctorate in Health and Behavioral Medicine Psychology from North Texas State University. She is a licensed clinical psychologist, certified in biofeedback, and has more than 26 years of experience in her speciality area, the psychology of pain and stress-related diseases. Dr. Montgomery co-authored *Clinical Biofeedback: A Procedural Manual for Behavioral Medicine* (Williams and Wilkins, second edition, 1981) and is author of more than 30 scientific research papers on the management of stress-related disorders. Currently, Dr. Montgomery maintains a private practice in Kansas City, Missouri.

Question. Describe your work in biofeedback.

Answer. My introduction to biofeedback was in 1969 when I met Barbara Brown and began exploring clinical applications of EEG biofeedback. In those days, alpha training was the only EEG frequency used. Fortunately, individual differences are now taken into account, and EEG biofeedback has become neurofeedback.

Throughout these years I have continued to explore clinical applications of biofeedback in a variety of parameters, including EEG, surface EMG, EDR, temperature, borborygmus, and diaphragmatic breathing. This variety takes into account most organ systems that respond to stress appropriately or inappropriately.

The most frequent use of biofeedback over the years has been in the management of stress-related symptoms. Currently, biofeedback and neurofeedback in the management of symptoms of injury or disease are more prevalent than in the management of stress.

I am currently in private practice in Kansas City, Missouri, where I focus on neurofeedback and do some biofeedback. After all of this time, I cannot imagine a more exciting or rewarding professional activity.

Question. What do you see as the future of biofeedback in medicine?

Answer. In the future, I see biofeedback being used more in support of homeostasis; that is, I believe that as science becomes more aware of the mind-body's ability to reinstate balance or health, I believe that biofeedback parameters will be designed more to support and encourage that natural healing.

For example, it is known that more than 90% of the brain's neurons are inhibitory; that means that when the brain needs to correct itself, it does so by inhibiting what should not be there, leaving normal function to prevail. Currently, it is becoming more well known that the safest and most effective method of correcting brain function after injury or illness is to inhibit abnormal patterns, such as spikes in head injury or persistent theta in attention deficit disorders.

Such selected use of inhibition in the brain mimics the brain's natural healing method. I believe that in the future, other biofeedback parameters will also be adjusted to support the homeostatic adaptive process of various organ systems.

I think that more portable devices will be prescribed by physicians and used by patients on a schedule that supports learning.

I see biofeedback used in schools of the future as a regular part of health or biology so that students of the future will measure, regulate, and understand the functional signals of various organ systems. Neurophysiologic baselines will be taken on everyone and stored so that functional signals can be compared on a regular basis as part of a check-up. Brain wave patterns will be stored to determine changes that may result from illness or injury so that specific causes may be determined. This should have implication both in the health and legal arenas.

In short, I see knowledge of the functioning of the body-mind as an integral part of daily experience and understood as part of our usual information system rather than an unorthodox medical technique.

Question. How should these techniques be applied?

Answer. Part of the answer to this question lies in the answer to the former question in that I believe that the most important method of application will be in support of homeostasis, that is, to facilitate the return of the organ system to normal. This may be accomplished by understanding the functional signals emitted by the system and [by understanding] how to measure and feed back the information in a meaningful and accurate manner. It will also require the practitioner to understand and apply the laws of learning. In short, it will require that the clinician know and understand how to use information as therapy.

■ Indications and Contraindications for Biofeedback

Biofeedback has been described as the next frontier in modern medicine. In this new frontier, patients will learn to control their physiologic functions without drugs or surgery. Through biofeedback, we will find the means to modify body function, similar to teaching the body muscular coordination and balance as a means of learning to ride a bicycle. Biofeedback approaches have few negative side effects, and the body is not challenged with the toxicity and potential harm of superficial interventions that do not address the underlying cause of disease. The following metaphor has been used to illustrate this point: To use drugs and surgery to deal with disease is like cutting out the oil pressure meter in a car to solve the problem of poor lubrication in the engine. It eliminates the poor readings, but the engine is still suffering. Applying this metaphor, elevated BP as a measure may be correlated to the real issue or it may only be symptomatic.

The optimistic perspective of past research was that patients, especially those with chronic problems, would storm the doors of biofeedback therapists to embrace the idea of self-control and the possibility of life without disease. Dependence on the over-burdened medical system would therefore be reduced. Medical systems, especially those of the third world, would perceive a new and less-expensive model of health care for managing many of the world's health problems.

In spite of excellent research and many professional advances, these dreams have not been totally realized. There are good bases for the reluctance to accept biofeedback as a new model of health care. (These are listed under the next two sections, "Indications for Biofeedback" and "Contraindications for Biofeedback.")

Indications for Biofeedback

As with any medical or psychologic intervention, some patients will benefit more than others. The primary indications for referral to biofeedback therapy for those individuals most likely to benefit from this treatment are the following:

1. *The patient must be motivated to learn the technique.* Although no studies have been performed, it is estimated that only 20 percent of the population would be motivated to learn biofeedback. The operative tenet in the process of biofeedback is that the patient must have some level of reinforcement, at least a curiosity. In animal studies with operant conditioning, the participants are often deprived of food to develop a reinforcement or reward, which motivates their behaviors. In humans, this practice is not practical. Although there are evaluative instruments, such as the Health Attribution Test,[1] which

purport to identify those most appropriate for biofeedback therapy, the underlying indication is that the person must have the desire to learn to control his or her physiologic functions to benefit from the treatment.

2. Appropriate instrumentation is required to assess disease symptoms and the associated physiologic functions. As indicated, the EEG (temperature or thermal), EMG, and GSR or EDR instruments are excellent measurements for specific syndromes, such as muscular pain, cardiovascular stress, and anxieties. Therefore individuals with symptoms that are particularly sensitive to one of these sources of instrumentations are most likely to benefit from the treatment.

3. *Assessment of substances that may influence the accuracy of measures is required.* Since effective treatment is dependent on accurate and reliable measurements of physiologic parameters, consideration should be given to those patients who are influenced by various substances that influence the accuracy of the measures. For example, the consumption of nicotine and caffeine can affect blood flow and confuse temperature readings. The administration of steroids and sedatives can also be problematic. Therefore patients who are relatively free of these other effects while undergoing biofeedback are most likely to benefit from the treatment.

4. *Patients with stress concerns are good candidates for biofeedback.* Since stress is central to all diseases, either in possible cause or as part of other medical interventions for associated healing processes, those patients with stress concerns are most likely to benefit from biofeedback treatment and the subsequent control of stress.

5. *Highly qualified biofeedback therapists and their skills should be made available to patients.* Experienced, effective biofeedback clinicians can perform psychophysiologic evaluations to alert the patient and health care professional to the potential role of psychologic syndromes in a given problem.

Contraindications for Biofeedback

Biofeedback therapy may be inappropriate for or even place at risk certain populations of patients. Biofeedback is therefore contraindicated in the following situations:

1. *Secondary gains (e.g., perceived benefits) of disease may be too important to surrender.* Secondary gains may include attention from

others or fear of demands if one becomes well. These issues can be generalized to all medical treatments as well.

2. *Chronically depressed patients may react negatively to stress reduction approaches.* Because the lethargic and depressed patient is usually in an already low state of arousal, further lowering often creates anxiety instead of health promotion. However, specific techniques for depressed patients can be effective in the hands of an experienced therapist.

3. *Although stress dimensions have been associated with diabetes and epilepsy, treatment for these patients should be closely integrated with conventional medical supervision.* For patients with epilepsy, the practice of intense stress induction may induce epileptic seizures in susceptible individuals. Most protocols for treatment of seizures strive to help patients achieve specific brain waves (14 Hz to 16 Hz with EEG). Many patients with diabetes have reduced their use of external insulin requirements through stress management. However, at times, the reductions have been abrupt, inducing significant drops in blood sugar and resulting in seizures. An experienced biofeedback clinician is aware of these concerns.

4. *Patients with alexithymia are poor candidates for biofeedback.* Alexithymia is a psychiatric diagnosis for the inability to verbalize one's emotions, which appears to be a neurologic condition from childhood. These patients are poor candidates for biofeedback because of the lack of understanding of emotions themselves, especially the emotions that can be sensed through physiologic means (e.g., anxiety, tension, fear).

5. *An unqualified or overzealous clinician is the primary contraindication for biofeedback.* For practitioners who promise cure from an over-enthusiastic perspective, a cautious eye is advised.

■ Biofeedback Limitations and Some Caveats

Although the research findings discussed in this chapter have many implications for medical care, they are more complex in conclusion. Like so many therapies, the process of learning a biofeedback response is more complicated than the rat learning the rewards of pushing the bar down. For example, learning a stress reduction approach

through raising finger temperature may simply involve a breathing pattern consistent with relaxation. It may also involve the dissolution of the fear of letting go of emotional control. Until such issues are resolved, the effects of biofeedback are often diminished and other relaxation and imagery approaches may be more appropriate.

Although the reviews of research have been positive, biofeedback is consistently recommended as a component in a larger therapeutic approach. In many instances, biofeedback monitoring serves as a catalyst for other therapies or as a validation of certain strategies, such as imagery.

One of the conclusions from metaanalyses of biofeedback research is that, like most therapies, the affect is not determined by the technology or the approach. The success of biofeedback is contingent on the competency of the practitioner. Although it may be true that the social reward of seeing personal change or having personal control is positively reinforcing, imparting the meaningful therapeutic issues to the patient is still an art form. The best outcomes will result from the efforts of an innovative and caring practitioner.

Just as there are therapist variables, patient variables are as important in determining the success of biofeedback as a treatment. Patient agendas that interfere with the success or failure of learning a particular response have been discussed throughout this chapter. One patient once said when he was hooked up to the electrodes of the EMG, "I do not know what you are doing to me, but the healing energy coming from that box sure feels good." (The process had been explained to the patient several times.)

Finally, biofeedback therapy uses a simple approach, measuring one or two parameters at a time. Yet, as any therapist in the mind-body field will explain, the human body is far too complicated to confine disease to only one system. Like magical mirrors, the disease can be reflected in many tissue forms. Is cancer a disease of the immune system, the psychologic systems, the endocrine system, or the circulatory system? Those in different cultures reflect various belief systems and have equivalent research and logic to support their theories. Perhaps all are correct. Further, individuals differ in their constellation of symptoms and interdynamics. Biofeedback is still extremely limited because it monitors the system that may or may not make a difference in the treatment of a specific disease condition. Simply stated, the technology and wisdom necessary to solve the entire "riddle" have not yet arrived.

■ Summary

Biofeedback is a form of therapy for many syndromes. It requires the patient to learn new physiologic and psychologic responses related to the stress dimensions. If immediate feedback of parameters of the disease can be provided, it has been shown that many people can change the related physiologic responses and reduce or eliminate the underlying causes of the disorder.

Although the existing technology and operant learning approaches make these skills available to a majority of the population, these applications are only beneficial for persons motivated to take advantage of them. For example, there are video games available that are "won" by learning to change one's physiologic responses. The success of basketball goals and treasure hunts are connected to the rising of peripheral temperature (thermal) or the lowering of muscle tension (EMG) so that even very young children can learn appropriate responses through the reinforcement of game participation. Future technologic advances will create even more innovative self-regulation opportunities for patients who desire to use them for health management.

The applications are straightforward. They do not require the depth of self-analysis required in psychotherapy, although this can be helpful, the long-term discipline of spiritual training, or unique abilities. The highest benefit to us is a sense of self-destiny, a new understanding, and the capacity to control our personal health and well being.

■ Chapter Review

1. What are the underlying learning concepts on which biofeedback is based?
2. How is thermal biofeedback defined, and how does a patient learn to alter thermal output?
3. What are three medical syndromes that are particularly treatable with thermal biofeedback?
4. How is EMG biofeedback defined, and how does a patient learn to alter the measurements of the feedback system?
5. What are four medical syndromes that are particularly treatable with EMG biofeedback?
6. What is GSR and EDR?
7. What is EEG biofeedback, and how does a patient learn to alter the measurements of the feedback system?
8. What are two medical problems that are especially treatable with EEG biofeedback?
9. What are four indications for biofeedback applications?
10. What are four contraindications for biofeedback application?

SHORT ANSWER ESSAY QUESTIONS

1. What are the underlying learning concepts on which biofeedback is based?
2. What is thermal biofeedback? How does a person learn thermal biofeedback?
3. What are some medical syndromes that are particularly treatable in thermal biofeedback?
4. What is EMG biofeedback? How does a person learn EMG biofeedback?
5. What are some medical syndromes that are particularly treatable with EMG biofeedback?
6. What is GSR or electrodermal biofeedback?
7. What is EEG biofeedback? How does a person learn EEG biofeedback?
8. What are some medical problems that are especially treatable with EEG biofeedback?
9. What are some indications for biofeedback applications?
10. What are some contraindications for biofeedback application?

CRITICAL THINKING AND CLINICAL APPLICATION EXERCISES

1. Most research strongly suggests that regardless of how sophisticated biofeedback technology is, success of the therapy depends largely on the therapist's qualities. How do you explain this conclusion?

2. Nearly all the clinical research has been performed on physical parameters that can be directly measured (e.g., temperature, heart rate). How would you perform biofeedback on physical parameters that are less measurable, such as white blood cell activity or metabolism?

3. If the field of computer technology could make feasible quick measurements of any physical parameter, is there any limitation to the human capacity to learn to modify any system? Provide a cogent analysis of your answer.

4. Consider the development of an Olympics in which the participants participate in internal physical feats, such as lowering BP to the lowest level or racing white blood cells from one hand to another. Would this be a significant event for health care? Provide a critical argument for your response.

References

1. Achterberg J, McGraw P, Lawlis GF: Rheumatoid arthritis: a study of relaxation and temperature biofeedback training as an adjunctive therapy, *Biofeedback Self Regul* 8(2):207, 1981.
2. Basmajian JV: *Biofeedback: principles & practice for clinicians,* ed 3, Baltimore, 1989, Williams & Wilkins.
3. Benson H: *The belief system and health.* Address given to conference entitled, "Spirituality and Health," New York, 1998.
4. Benson H: *The relaxation response,* New York, 1975, Morrow.
5. Benson H, Shapiro D, Tursky B, Schwartz GE: Decreased systolic blood pressure through operant conditioning techniques in patients with essential hypertension, *Science* 173:740, 1971.
6. Brown B: *Stress and the art of biofeedback,* New York, 1977, Harper & Row.
7. Budzynski TH, Stoyva JM, Adler CS, Mullaney DJ: EMG biofeedback and tension headache: a controlled outcome study, *Psychosom Med* 35:484, 1973.
8. Cannon WB: *The wisdom of the body,* New York, 1932, Norton.
9. Chesney MA, Shelton JL: A comparison of muscle relaxation and electromyogram biofeedback treatments for muscle contraction headache, *J Behav Ther Exp Psychiatry* 7:221, 1976.
10. Cox DJ, Freundlich A, Meyer RG: Differential effectiveness of electromyographic feedback, verbal relaxation instructions, and medication placebo with tension headaches, *J Consult Clin Psychol* 43:892, 1975.
11. Dohrmann RJ, Laskin DM: An evaluation of electromyographic biofeedback in the treatment of myofascial pain—dysfunction syndrome, *J Am Dent Assoc* 96(4):656, 1978.
12. Forem J: *Transcendental meditation,* New York, 1974, Dutton.
13. Fried FE, Lamberti J, Sneed P: Treatment of tension and migraine headaches with biofeedback techniques, *Mo Med* 74:253, 1977.
14. Gaarder KR, Montgomery PS: *Clinical biofeedback: a procedural manual for behavioral medicine,* ed 2, Baltimore, 1981, Williams & Wilkins.
15. Green E, Green A: *Beyond biofeedback,* New York, 1977, Delta.
16. Hart JT: Autocontrol of EEG alpha (abstract), *Psychophysiology* 4:506, 1968.

17. Haynes SN, Griffin P, Mooney D, Parise M: Electromyographic biofeedback and relaxation instructions in the treatment of muscle contraction headaches, *Behav Ther* 6:672, 1975.
18. Hutchings D., Reinkin R.H: Tension headaches: what form of therapy is most effective? *Biofeedback Self Regul* 1:183, 1976.
19. Kamiya J: Operant control of the EEG alpha rhythm and some of its reported effects on consciousness. In Tart CT, editor: *Altered states of consciousness,* New York, 1969, Wiley.
20. Kondo C, Canter A: True and false electromyographic feedback: effect on tension headache, *J Abnorm Psychol* 86(1):93, 1977.
21. Mroczek N, Halpern D, McHugh R: Electromyographic feedback and physical therapy for neuromuscular retraining in hemiplegia, *Arch Phys Med Rehab* 59:258, 1978.
22. Nowlis DP, Kamiya J: The control of electroencephalographic alpha rhythms through auditory feedback and the associated mental activity, *Psychophysiol* 6:476, 1970.
23. Ray WJ, Raczynski JM, Rogers T, Kimball WH: *Evaluation of clinical biofeedback,* New York, 1979, Plenum Press.
24. Seifert AR, Lubar JF: Reduction of epileptic seizures through EEG biofeedback training, *Biol Psychol* 3:157, 1975.

Suggested readings

Andrews JM: Neuromuscular re-education of the hemiplegic with the aid of the electromyograph, *Arch Phys Med Rehab* 45:530, 1964.

Andreychuk T, Skriver C: Hypnosis and biofeedback in the treatment of migraine headache, *Int J Clin Exp Hypn* 23:172, 1975.

Basmajian JV, Kukulka CG, Narayan MG, Takebe K: Biofeedback treatment of foot-drop after stroke compared with standard rehabilitation technique: effect on voluntary control and strength, *Arch Phys Med Rehab* 56:231, 1975.

Benson H, Rosner BA, Marzetta BR, Klemchuk HM: Decreased blood-pressure in pharmacologically treated hypertensive patients who regularly elicited the relaxation response, *Lancet* 1:289, 1974.

Blanchard EB, Eilele G, Vollmer A, Payne A, Gordon M, Cornish P, Gilmore L: Controlled evaluation of thermal biofeedback and treatment of elevated blood pressure in unmedicated mild hypertension, *Biofeedback Self Regul* 21(2):167, 1996.

Blanchard EB, Theobald DE, Williamson DA, Silver BV, Brown DA: Temperature biofeedback in the treatment of migraine headaches, *Arch Gen Psychiatry* 35:581, 1978.

Blanchard EB, Young LD, Haynes MR: A simple feedback system for the treatment of elevated blood pressure, *Behav Ther* 6:241, 1975.

Bleecker ER, Engel BT: Learned control of cardiac rate and cardiac conduction in the Wolff-Parkinson-White Syndrome, *N Engl J Med* 288:560, 1973b.

Brudny J, Grynbaum BB, Korein J: Spasmodic torticollis: treatment by feedback display of the EMG, *Arch Phys Med Rehab* 55:403, 1974.

Brudny J, Korein J, Grynbaum BB, Friedmann LW, Weinstein S, Sachs-Frankel G, Belandres PV: EMG feedback therapy: review of 114 patients, *Arch Phys Med Rehab* 57:55, 1976.

Brudny J, Korein J, Levidow L, Grynbaum BB, Lieberman A, Freidmann LW: Sensory feedback therapy as a modality of treatment in central nervous system disorders of voluntary movement, *Neurology* 24:925, 1974.

Budzynski T: Biofeedback in the treatment of muscle-contraction (tension) headache, *Biofeedback Self Regul* 3:409, 1978.

Carlsson SG, Gale EN: Biofeedback in the treatment of long-term temporomandibular joint pain: an outcome study, *Biofeedback Self Regul* 2:161, 1977.

Cinciripini PM, Floreen A: An evaluation of a behavioral program for chronic pain, *J Behav Med* 5(3):375, 1982.

Cleeland CS: Behavioral techniques in the modification of spasmodic torticollis, *Neurology* 23:1241, 1973.

Colborne GR, Wright FV, Naumann S: Feedback of triceps surae EMG in gait of children with cerebral palsy, *Arch Phys Med Rehab* 75(1):40, 1994.

Corr A, Pavloski RP, Black AH: Reducing epileptic seizures through operant conditioning of central nervous system activity: procedural variables, *Science* 203:73, 1979.

Davis MH, Saunders DR, Creer TL, Chai H: Relaxation training facilitated by biofeedback apparatus as a supplemental treatment in bronchial asthma, *J Psychosom Res* 17:121, 1973.

Diamond S, Medina J, Diamond-Falk J, DeVeno T: The value of biofeedback in the treatment of chronic headache: a five-year retrospective study, *Headache* 19:90, 1979.

Eisenberg DM, Delbanco TL, Berkey CS, Kaptchuk TJ, Kupelnick B, Kuhl J, Chalmers TC: Cognitive behavioral techniques for hypertension: are they effective? *Ann Intern Med* 118(12):964, 1993.

Elder ST, Eustis NK: Instrumental blood pressure conditioning in out-patient hypertensives, *Behav Res Ther* 13:185, 1975.

Elder ST, Ruiz ZR, Deabler HL, Dillenkoffer RL: Instrumental conditioning of diastolic blood pressure in essential hypertensive patients, *J Appl Behav Anal* 6:377, 1973.

Engel BT, Nikoomanesh P, Schuster MM: Operant conditioning of rectosphincteric responses in the treatment of fecal incontinence, *N Engl J Med* 290:646, 1974.

Feldman GM: The effect of biofeedback training on respiratory resistance of asthmatic children, *Psychosom Med* 38:27, 1976.

Ferraccioli G, Ghirelli L, Scita F, Nolli M, Mozzani M, Fontana S, Scorsonelli M, Tridenti A, De Risio C: EMG-biofeedback training in fibromyalgia syndrome, *J Rheumatol* 14(4):820, 1987.

Friar LR, Beatty J: Migraine: management by trained control of vasoconstriction, *J Consult Clin Psychol* 44:46, 1976.

Friedman H, Taub HA: The use of hypnosis and biofeedback procedures for essential hypertension, *Int J Clin Exp Hypn* 25:335, 1977.

Friedman H, Taub HA: A six-month follow-up of the use of hypnosis and biofeedback procedures in essential hypertension, *Am J Clin Hypn* 20:184, 1978.

Furman S: Intestinal biofeedback in functional diarrhea: a preliminary report, *J Behav Ther Exp Psychiatry* 4:317, 1973.

Goldman H, Kleinman KM, Snow MY, Bidus DR, Korol B: Relationship between essential hypertension and cognitive functioning: effects of biofeedback, *Psychophysiology* 12:569, 1975.

Harris FA, Spelman FA, Hymer JW: Electronic sensory aids as treatment for cerebral-palsied children. Inapproprioception: part II, *Phys Ther* 54:354, 1974.

Jacobs A, Felton GS: Visual feedback of myoelectric output to facilitate muscle relaxation in normal persons and patients with neck injuries, *Arch Phys Med Rehab* 50:34, 1969.

Jacobson E: *The human mind: a physiological clarification,* Springfield, IL, 1982, Charles C. Thomas.

Johnson HE, Garton WH: Muscle re-education in hemiplegia by use of electromyographic device, *Arch Phys Med Rehab* 54:320, 1973.

Kamiya J: Preface. In Barber T, DiCara L, Kamiya J, Miller N, Shapiro D, Stoyva J, editors: *Biofeedback and self-control,* Chicago, 1971, Aldine-Atherton.

Kaplan BJ: Biofeedback in epileptics: equivocal relationship of reinforced EEG frequency to seizure reduction, *Epilepsia* 16:477, 1975.

Khan AU: Effectiveness of biofeedback and counter-conditioning in the treatment of bronchial asthma, *J Pschosom Res* 21:97, 1977.

Khan AU, Staerk M, Bonk C: Role of counter-conditioning in the treatment of asthma, *J Psychosom Res* 17:389, 1973.

Kleinman KM, Goldman H, Snow MY, Korol B: Relationship between essential hypertension and cognitive functioning II: effects of biofeedback training generalize to non-laboratory environment, *Psychophysiology* 14:192, 1977.

Kotses H, Glaus KD, Bricel SK, Edwards JE, Crawford PL: Operant muscular relaxation and peak expiratory flow rate in asthmatic children, *J Psychosom Res* 22:17, 1978.

Kotses H, Glaus KD, Crawford PL, Edwards JE, Scherr MS: Operant reduction of frontalis EMG activity in the treatment of asthma in children, *J Psychosom Res* 20:453, 1976.

Krippner S: Altered states of consciousness. In White J, editor: *The highest state of consciousness,* Garden City, NY, 1972, Doubleday.

Kristt DA, Engel BT: Learned control of blood pressure in patients with high blood pressure, *Circulation* 51:370, 1975.

Kuhlman WN, Allison T: EEG feedback training in the treatment of epilepsy: some questions and some answers, *Pavlovian J Biolog Sci* 12:112, 1977.

Labbe EE: Treatment of childhood migraine with autogenic training and skin temperature biofeedback: a component analysis, *Headache* 35(1):10, 1995.

Lee K, Hill E, Johnston R, Smiehorowski T: Myofeedback for muscle retraining in hemiplegic patients, *Arch Phys Med Rehab* 57:588, 1976.

Lubar JF, Bahler WW: Behavioral management of epileptic seizures following EEG biofeedback training of the sensorimotor rhythm, *Biofeedback Self Regul* 1:77, 1976.

McKenzie RE, Ehrisman WJ, Montgomery PS, Barnes RH: The treatment of headache by means of electroencephalographic biofeedback, *Headache* 13:164, 1974.

Medina JL, Diamond S, Franklin MA: Biofeedback therapy for migraine, *Headache* 16:115, 1976.

Miller NE: Biofeedback and visceral learning, *Ann Rev Psychol* 29:373, 1978.

Ornstein RE: *The psychology of consciousness,* San Francisco, 1972, Freeman.

Patel C: 12-month follow-up of yoga and biofeedback in the management of hypertension, *Lancet* 1:62, 1975.

Patel C, North WRS: Randomized controlled trial of yoga and biofeedback in management of hypertension, *Lancet* 2:93, 1975.

Patel CH: Yoga and biofeedback in the management of hypertension, *Lancet* 2:1053, 1973.

Peavey B, Lawlis GF, Goven A: Biofeedback-assisted relaxation: effects on phagocytic capacity, *Biofeedback Self Regul* 10(1):33, 1985.

Pelletier KR, Garfield C: *Consciousness: East and West,* New York, 1976, Harper & Row.

Peniston EG, Kulkosky PJ: Alpha-theta brainwave training and endorphin levels of alcoholics, *Alcohol Clin Exp Res* 13(2):271, 1989.

Phillips C: The modification of tension headache pain using EMG biofeedback, *Behav Res Ther* 15:119, 1977b.

Reading C, Mohr PD: Biofeedback control of migraine: a pilot study, *Br J Soc Clin Psychol* 15:429, 1976.

Sargent JD, Green EE, Walters ED: Preliminary report on the use of autogenic feedback training in the treatment of migraine and tension headaches, *Psychosom Med* 35:129, 1973.

Scherr MS, Crawford PL, Sergent CB, Scherr CA: Effect of biofeedback techniques on chronic asthma in a summer camp environment, *Ann Allergy* 35:289, 1975.

Schuster MM: Operant conditioning in gastrointestinal dysfunctions, *Hosp Pract* 9:135, 1974.

Schwartz G, Beatty J: *Biofeedback: theory and research,* New York, 1977, Academic Press.

Skrotzky K, Gallenstein JS, Osternig LR: Effects of electromyographic feedback training on motor control in spastic cerebral palsy, *Phys Ther* 58:547, 1978.

Sterman MB: Neurophysiologic and clinical studies of sensorimotor EEG biofeedback training: some effects on epilepsy. In Birk L, editor: *Biofeedback: behavioral medicine,* New York, 1973, Grune and Stratton.

Sterman MB, MacDonald LR: Effects of central cortical EEG feedback training on incidence of poorly controlled seizures, *Epilepsia* 19:207, 1978.

Sterman MB, MacDonald LR, Stone RK: Biofeedback training of the sensorimotor EEG rhythm in man: effects on epilepsy, *Epilepsia* 15:395, 1974.

Sturgis ET, Tollison CD, Adam HE: Modification of combined migraine-muscle contraction headaches using BVP and EMG feedback, *J Appl Behav Anal* 11:215, 1978.

Surwit RS, Pilon RN, Fenton CH: Behavioral treatment of Raynaud's disease, *J Behav Med* 1:323, 1978.

Surwit RS, Shapiro D: Biofeedback and meditation in the treatment of borderline hypertension. In Beatty J, Legewie H, editors: *Biofeedback and behavior,* New York, 1977, Plenum Publishing.

Surwit RS, Shapiro D, Good MI: Comparison of cardiovascular biofeedback, neuromuscular biofeedback, and meditation in the treatment of borderline essential hypertension, *J Consul Clin Psychol* 46:252, 1978.

Swann D, Van Wieringen PCW, Fokkema SD: Auditory electromyographic feedback therapy to inhibit undesired motor activity, *Arch Phys Med Rehab* 55:251, 1974.

Tart CT: *Altered states of consciousness: a book of readings,* New York, 1969, Wiley.

Turin A, Johnson WG: Biofeedback therapy for migraine headaches, *Arch Gen Psych* 33:517, 1976.

Vachon L, Rich ES Jr: Visceral learning in asthma, *Psychosom Med* 38:122, 1976.

Wannstedt GT, Herman RM: Use of augmented sensory feedback to achieve symmetrical standing, *Phys Ther* 58:553, 1978.

Walsh P, Dale A, Anderson DE: Comparison of biofeedback pulse wave velocity and progressive relaxation in essential hypertensives, *Percept Mot Skills* 44(Pt. 2):839, 1977.

Weiss T, Engel BT: Operant conditioning of heart rate in patients with premature ventricular contractions. In Birk L, editor: *Biofeedback: behavioral medicine,* New York, 1973, Grune and Stratton.

Welgan PR: Biofeedback control of stomach acid secretions and gastrointestinal reactions. In Beatty J, Legewie H, editors: *Biofeedback and behavior,* New York, 1977, Plenum Press.

Wickramasekera I: The application of verbal instructions and EMG feedback training to the management of tension headache—preliminary observations, *Headache* 13:74, 1973a.

Wickramasekera I: Electromyographic feedback training and tension headache: preliminary observations, *Am J Clin Hypn* 15:83, 1972.

8

Hypnosis

Lyn W. Freeman

WHY READ THIS CHAPTER?

Hypnosis presents us with some of the most dramatic examples of the power of the mind to affect the body. When hypnotic procedures are specialized to the needs, personality, and motivations of the individual, hypnosis can be a powerful and effective complementary intervention—one that can succeed where traditional approaches have failed.

Pain, duodenal ulcers, irritable bowel syndrome, and nausea—especially chemotherapy-induced and conditioned nausea—have been effectively treated with hypnosis. Hypnosis is an underused intervention that can, for the appropriate populations, improve the quality of life while reducing health care costs. Health care providers and decision makers need to contemplate the expanded use of hypnosis in hospital settings and as outpatient treatment.

CHAPTER AT A GLANCE

Hypnosis is a state of attentive, focused concentration with suspension of some peripheral awareness. Components of the hypnotic state include absorption, alteration of attention, dissociation, and suggestibility.

The phenomenon of hypnosis has a long history of discovery and rediscovery that predates the written language. Hypnotic phenomena have varied from trance states of mysticism and shamanic practices to the imagery and healing techniques used by the ancient Egyptians and Greeks in their healing temples.

Hypnosis as a clinical discipline was unknown until the eighteenth century when Franz Anton Mesmer defined a discipline he called "animal magnetism." This was the beginning of hypnosis as we know it today. Other individuals soon began to practice hypnotic techniques and made new and interesting discoveries about this unique state of mind. James Esdaile, a surgeon, performed more than 3000 surgical procedures without pain. At that time, the mortality rate after surgery was typically at high 50% and death was mostly caused by neurogenic shock. Esdaile reduced the surgical death rate to 5%.

The best-known hypnotherapist of the twentieth century was Milton Erickson, a psychiatrist who altered the face of hypnosis by his experimental studies of special phenomena encountered in hypnosis. One of the first persons to be certified in psychiatry and neurology, Erickson emphasized the necessity for studying the process, state, and products of hypnosis.

The philosophies used to explain hypnotic effects are from two camps: the neodissociation model and the social psychologic model. The neodissociation model suggests that hypnosis activates subsystems of control; these subsystems have psychologic and physiologic counterparts, which result in an altered state of consciousness. The social psychologic model suggests that hypnosis is not an altered state of consciousness; rather, it is explained by suggestibility, positive attitudes, and expectations.

Some persons are more susceptible to hypnosis than others. Therefore individuals can be categorized as low, moderate, or high hypnotizables. It is hypothesized that this differences can be explained by changes in brain wave patterns, reflected by electroencephalographic (EEG) readings. Both alpha and theta wave changes have been implicated as markers of hypnotizability. One school of thought hypothesizes that there is a hemispheric shift of alpha waves from the left to the right hemisphere in those who are highly hypnotizable. This hypothesis is based on a belief in hemispheric specificity or brain lateralization. Another school of thought claims that a change in wave patterns from the anterior to the posterior brain areas is an indicator of deep hypnosis and high hypnotizability.

Many researchers believe hypnosis is induced most effectively by taking advantage of the "natural waking trance" that occurs during a natural 90-minute ultradian rhythm cycle. There is a 20-minute period during which hormonal and biochemical rhythms make us most susceptible to suggestion and trance.

Hypnosis has been demonstrated to be highly effective in its capacity to alleviate pain. Hypnosis has been successfully used for surgical anesthesia with small, specialized groups of patients, to speed surgical recovery rates, and to reduce cancer, burn, and other forms of pain. Hypnosis has also been used successfully to treat duodenal ulcers, irritable bowel syndrome, anticipatory nausea, pregnancy-induced nausea, and to a lesser degree, anxiety, insomnia, obesity, and smoking cessation.

CHAPTER OBJECTIVES

After completing this chapter, you should be able to:

1. Define hypnosis.
2. List the four major components of the hypnotic state and explain them.
3. Discuss the historical evolution of hypnosis.
4. Define animal magnetism, and explain why the philosophy underlying this belief was faulty.
5. Describe the unique contributions of the psychiatrist, Milton Erickson.
6. Name the two philosophic models of hypnosis, and explain their differences.
7. Define hypnotic susceptibility, and explain how susceptibility is assessed.
8. Explain the hypothesis of hemispheric specificity.
9. Describe the differences in EEG readings between hypnotically susceptible and nonsusceptible subjects, as concluded by researchers.
10. Describe the pain mechanisms related to the effectiveness of hypnosis.
11. Describe the findings of the effects of hypnosis on experimentally induced pain.
12. Explain the findings on the effects of hypnotic pain inhibition at the spinal level.
13. Explain the findings related to hypnosis, endorphins, and adrenocorticotropic hormones.
14. Describe the findings of hypnosis as adjuvant to chemical anesthesia for surgical patients (i.e., surgical recovery findings).
15. Describe the research concerning hypnosis and cancer and burn pain.
16. Describe the outcomes of hypnosis treatment of duodenal ulcers.
17. Describe the research on hypnosis and asthma.
18. Describe the research on hypnosis and irritable bowel syndrome.
19. Describe the research on hypnosis and anticipatory nausea.
20. Describe the research on hypnosis and obesity.
21. Describe the research on hypnosis and smoking cessation and other addictions.

■ Defining Hypnosis

Hypnosis can be defined as a state of attentive, focused concentration with suspension of some peripheral awareness.[128] Major components of the hypnotic state include (1) absorption (capacity to contemplate deeply a selected theme or focal point, Figure 8-1), (2) controlled alteration of one's attention, (3) dissociation (capacity to compartmentalize different aspects of one's experience), and (4) suggestibility (capacity for heightened responsiveness to instructions).[56,101,136] Although suggestibility is an important trait leading to hypnotizability, the therapist does not have "control" of the suggestible client. Client motivation is required for successful induction, and the client will not submit to suggestions that are in opposition to his or her desires.

■ History of Hypnosis

The phenomenon of hypnosis has a long history of discovery and rediscovery. Cultures and individuals have used a variety of rituals and techniques to induce hypnotic, trancelike states. The purposes of these rituals and techniques were to unlock the power of the mind, to experience altered states of consciousness, to participate in spiritual practices, or to heal.

Trance States, Mysticism, and Shamanism

Trance states have been employed as part of mystical and shamanic traditions since the earliest beginnings of the human race. Trance was experienced in the form of meditation, contemplation, and mystical rites during the early formative periods of the major world religions—Buddhism, Taoism, Hinduism, Islam, and Christianity.[53]

Shamanic trance was elicited by a variety of methods, and some of these methods are still practiced today in Siberia, Alaska, Canada, South America, Australia, west Africa, southeast Asia, and numerous other localities[52,98] (Figure 8-2).

Shamanic customs teach that a true shaman travels between and experiences a continuum of many states of consciousness. He or she can bridge the distance between ordinary reality and transpersonal realms, performing many services including healing, prophesying, and retrieving lost souls. Most importantly, the trance experience of the shaman is what allows him or her to perceive a world of total aliveness and to both know and use the energies encountered.[98]

> **Points to Ponder** Historically, hypnotic and imagery techniques were used by the Egyptians and later by the Greeks as part of their healing temple practices. ■

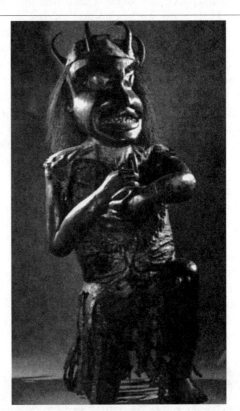

■ Figure 8-2. This wood and leather statue represents a shaman and is from British Columbia, Canada. *From Peterson D, Weise G:* Chiropratic: an illustrated history, *St Louis, 1995, Mosby.*

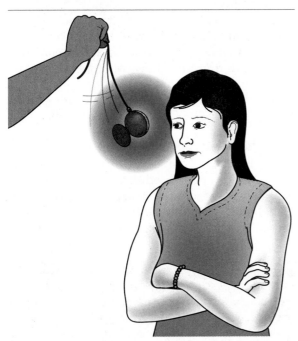

■ Figure 8-1. "You are getting sleepy...VERY sleepy.

Hypnotic Techniques, Imagery, and Healing

Historically, hypnotic and imagery techniques were used by the Egyptians and later the Greeks as part of their healing temple practices. For example, at the time of Alexander the Great (336 BC to 323 BC), there were more than 300 temples dedicated to Askelepios, a physician who was later deified as the god of medicine. Askelepios was considered to be the Greek equivalent of the Egyptian god, Imhotep, who before he was proclaimed a god was a builder of the oldest pyramid in Cairo (2500 BC)[57] One of the rituals practiced in the sleep temples included a type of sleep therapy called *incubation.* Askelepios (probably represented by a priest) visited sick persons while they were in a state of "sleep." This visitation often resulted in a cure. Testimonials of innumerable cures were recorded, and these reports included recovery from paralysis, blindness, and speech disturbances.[143]

Arrival of Clinical Hypnosis

Until the beginning of the eighteenth century, there was no evidence of the establishment of clinical hypnosis as a discipline, as opposed to spiritually based practices. There was little clinical or scientific understanding of the subconscious or of the power of suggestion, and there was no general and consistent body of doctrine to explain the trance state and its effects. Practitioners simply practiced hypnosis in their own way, and that "way" varied from person to person.

In the eighteenth century, the century of enlightenment, a man named Franz Anton Mesmer virtually created a new clinical discipline with a specified context based on what he called "animal magnetism." Animal magnetism was the precursor of modern hypnosis.[60]

Mesmer was a well-educated physician who traveled in the highest circles of Viennese society. He discovered a therapeutic method for treating ailments through the projection of what he believed was a universal but invisible fluid in which all bodies were immersed. He called this substance *animal magnetism* because he believed this substance was transmissible through the human body. He hypothesized that, although all persons possessed animal magnetism, only a few possessed this fluid in sufficient strength to heal others. Mesmer was held up to public ridicule and was eventually discredited professionally because he failed to realize that his cures were because of a psychologic and physiologic phenomenon and not the result of a magnetic fluid. Eventually, the idea of a magnetic fluid was replaced with the concepts of suggestion, visualization, and dissociation (Figure 8-3).

Nonetheless, Mesmer succeeded in stirring sufficient interest in altered states to be followed by a series of individuals who would refine and clarify the real underlying issues of hypnosis and trance.

The Marquis de Puysegur, initially a follower of Mesmer, discovered that the behaviors of individuals in trance were similar to those of sleepwalkers. The sleepwalking condition is called somnambulism. Therefore the Marquis named this induced trance condition *artificial somnambulism.*

The Abbe Faria challenged the ideas of trance as neither animal magnetism nor artificial somnambulism. Instead, he argued that trance was a form of waking sleep that he named *lucid sleep*—not to be confused with lucid dreaming. The Abbe anticipated some of the modern concepts of hypnosis, including the idea that some persons are more susceptible to trance than others and that a good "magnetizer" actually succeeds by exerting his ability to concentrate the power of suggestion onto others.

James Braid discovered that a unique effect of mind could be induced by firmly fixing one's gaze at an inanimate object. He named this condition *hypnotism,* from the Greek word *hypnos,* meaning sleep. He also established that hypnosis was quite different from natural sleep. Other groundbreaking pioneers of hypnosis were to follow.

Early Applications of Hypnosis

James Esdaile, a Scottish surgeon serving in hospitals in India, performed several thousand minor operations and over 300 major surgeries (e.g., amputations of limbs and breasts and removal of scrotal tumors) without pain. Esdaile's use of

---

Points to Ponder   In the eighteenth century, the century of enlightenment, a man named Franz Anton Mesmer virtually created a new clinical discipline with a specified context based on what he called "animal magnetism." Animal magnetism was the precursor of modern hypnosis. ■

Points to Ponder   James Esdaile, a Scottish surgeon serving in hospitals in India, performed several thousand minor operations and over 300 major surgeries (e.g., amputations of limbs and breasts and removal of scrotal tumors) without pain. ■

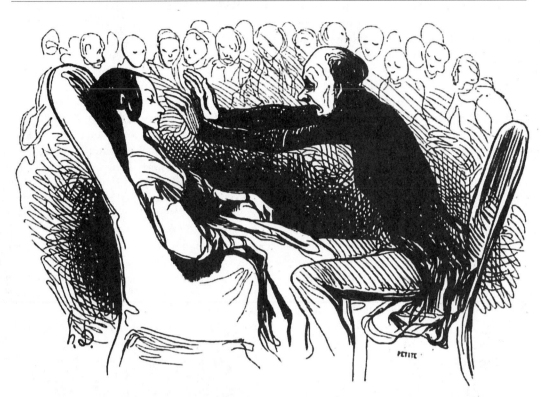

▪ *Figure 8-3.* This was one of the many satirical caricatures of the day representing Mesmer's practice of "animal magnetism." Note how Mesmer's knees are touching the thighs of his female patient—a practice considered sexually suggestive in that day. *Courtesy Bibliotheque Interuniversitaire de Medicine, Paris. From Peterson D, Weise G:* Chiropratic: an illustrated history, *St Louis, 1995, Mosby.*

"mesmeric anesthesia" reduced the surgical mortality rate from 50% to 5%. Improved mortality rates were attributed to a reduction of neurogenic shock after surgical procedures.

Charles Poyen, a Frenchman, introduced mesmerism to America. This led to new advances in psychology, including William James' work on mystical experiences.

Jean-Martin Charcot, a neurologist, hypnotized hysterical and mentally disturbed patients in Paris. His work laid the foundations from which Freud and his followers erected psychoanalysis and psychiatry.[57,61]

Contributions of Milton Erickson

Milton Erickson, a psychiatrist, was the best-known American practitioner of hypnotherapy in the twentieth century. For more than half a century, he altered the face of hypnosis through his experimental studies and publications and his lecturing and teaching. Erickson was a remarkable person who triumphed over two bouts of poliomyelitis that left him badly crippled and in

> **Points to Ponder** Erickson's experimental period, mostly before World War II, opened up the field of hypnosis to investigation. His research bridged the gap between the experimental laboratory experience and clinical experience. ▪

pain. He attributed his survival, in part, to his own hypnotic practices.

While still an undergraduate at the University of Wisconsin, Erickson began his studies of hypnosis with psychologist Clark Hull. He received his Doctor of Medicine degree in 1928, worked at the Colorado Psychopathic Hospital, and eventually became a professor at Wayne State University. In 1949, Erickson severed institutional and academic connections and entered private practice in Phoenix, Arizona, where he remained for the rest of his life.

Erickson's experimental period, mostly before World War II, opened up the field of hypnosis to investigation. His research bridged the gap between the experimental laboratory experience and clinical experience. Innovative experiments covered such topics as special phenomena encountered in hypnosis (e.g., suggested anti-social behavior, negative hallucinations, posthypnotic responses, hypnotic deafness, induced color blindness) and many areas bearing on psychopathology (e.g., induced experimental neuroses, psychosomatic phenomena).[57]

After entering private practice, his publications, mostly descriptive, defined his highly varied and imaginative approaches to hypnosis and psychotherapy. These approaches included indirect suggestion, confusion, puzzlement, and metaphor. He became well known for his utilization and seeding techniques and for his homework assignments. (See Helen Erickson's comments.)

During his years in private practice, his home became a mecca for health care providers, referred patients, and visiting hypnotherapists desiring to learn from the direct experience of his techniques.[61]

An Expert Speaks: Dr. Helen Erickson

Helen Erickson, PhD, RN, HNC, FAAN, emeritus professor at the University of Texas, Austin, is in private practice and also offers training courses in clinical hypnosis. Dr. Erickson is the daughter-in-law of Milton Erickson. She describes her experiences with Milton Erickson and with hypnosis.

Question. How did Milton Erickson's work with hypnosis contribute to health care?

Answer. First of all, I believe that Milton Erickson's work made an enormous contribution to health care by mandating that those who follow him consider mind-body dynamics and the person as a whole entity, not merely a mind or body separate from one another. He helped change what we think about the psychodynamic processes. He emphasized the subconscious and unconscious as reservoirs of important, useful information and knowledge that can heal. This emphasis refocused attention on the nature of these processes. It also provided a basis for the launching of brief therapy and family therapy.

Question. How, in your experience, has hypnosis contributed to health and well being?

Answer. I've carried a private practice since 1976, seen individuals and families, done several federally funded research studies—one working with people with hypertension, another with people who have diabetes, [and] another with people who have Alzheimer's disease. I've found repeatedly that hypnosis—as a way of communi-cating with people, not hypnosis as a set of tricks or techniques—is other-focused communication, designed to bypass conscious resistance and to tap into the "inner being" of individuals. Such communication is the basis for starting the healing process. I'm not talking about curing, although healing sometimes occurs. I'm talking about helping the person live the highest quality of life until he or she takes the last breath. Hypnosis is the basis for such healing.

Question. Can you describe for me one experience with Milton Erickson that, for you, defined him as a hypnotherapist and as a person?

Answer. When I was first married [in 1957], my husband and I visited Phoenix on our way to our new home in Texas. Dad received a phone call from a psychiatrist in New York asking for help. He was caring for a well-to-do woman who had just had her fifth child and was suffering from postpartum psychosis. Several physicians had seen her and decided that the best and only thing to do was hospitalize her. Her husband begged for yet one more consultation, so the doctor called dad and explained the situation as I've described it here. Dad said, "Put her on the phone." He then said to her…this lady with the so-called hallucinations, "What is the matter?" He then told her to let him talk to her husband and he said, " Go buy her a washing machine." He listened intently, then said [to the husband], "You have two choices. Go buy her a washing machine or put her in the hospital." He then hung up. Needless to say, I was astounded, so I asked him to explain. He said that she told him that the problem was that she had a new baby and she couldn't take care of it. Her husband had hired maids, nannies, [and] cooks, and she wasn't even allowed to wash her own baby's diapers. Dad simply said to me, "How many babies does she have to have before she can love one of them?!"

I later talked with the New York doctor. The husband bought the washing machine, the wife "healed miraculously overnight," and every one was in awe. From my view, it was typical Milton Erickson style—treat the symptom and treat it within the context of the individual's view of the world. Don't mess around with all the whys—get straight to the problem. Use whatever the individual brings to the situation—this is known as utilization—and go from there. While many doctors would have charged for such a consultation, dad rarely did. He often took "in-kind" payments or no payments. His intent in life was to help people, not to get rich. While I have observed him using traditional trance induction techniques hundreds of times, I've watched an equal number of times that he has used indirect techniques. His goal was always to help the other person, whether it was a client, a student, or a daughter-in-law! And he did it because he cared about our lives and our learning.

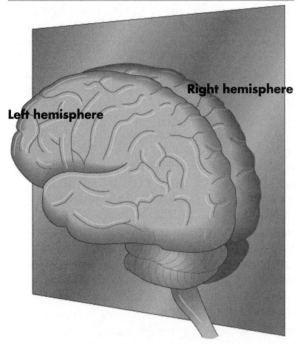

■ **Figure 8-4.** The two hemispheres of the brain. The left hemisphere controls the right side of the body, and the right hemisphere controls the left side of the body. *Adapted from Thibodeau GA, Patton KT:* Anatomy and physiology, *ed 4, St Louis, 1999, Mosby.*

■ Philosophies and Mechanisms Underlying Hypnotic Effects

In their efforts to understand the underlying mechanisms leading to the hypnotic state, researchers assessed the effects of hypnosis on the brain and its electrical activities. The following text offers short definitions of basic brain structure and activity relevant to the understanding of hypnosis research.

Brain: Hemispheres, Lobes, Electrical Activity

The cerebral cortex of the brain is divided into the *left and right hemispheres* with each hemisphere controlling the opposite side of the body (Figure 8-4). The hemispheres are divided into four lobes: frontal, parietal, occipital, and temporal (Figure 8-5).

The *frontal lobe* is primarily involved with motor functions and contains an area called the prefrontal association cortex, which is thought to be involved in higher-level brain processes like problem solving and planning. The *occipital lobe* contains the primary visual areas. The *temporal lobe* controls the primary auditory areas and is involved in the recognition of objects. The *parietal lobe* controls some of our sensory functions, particularly those involving spatial processing.

An EEG is a simple, painless procedure in which 20 wires (leads) are pasted on the scalp to trace and record the brain's electrical activity in the four lobes and/or in the two hemispheres. Recorded wave patterns identify the types of waves and the amplitude of the brain's electrical activity. Frequency spectra of EEG typically range

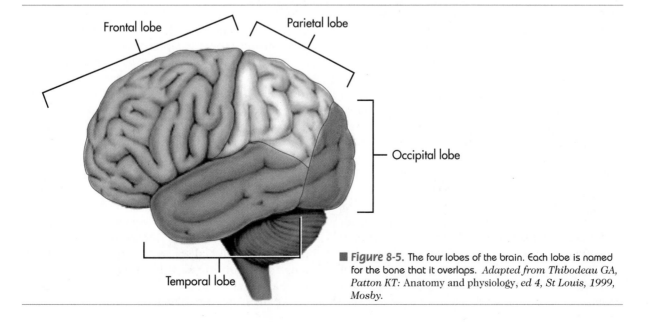

■ **Figure 8-5.** The four lobes of the brain. Each lobe is named for the bone that it overlaps. *Adapted from Thibodeau GA, Patton KT:* Anatomy and physiology, *ed 4, St Louis, 1999, Mosby.*

between 1 Hertz (Hz) to 30 Hz and demonstrate (from fastest to slowest) beta, alpha, theta, and delta waves (see Figures 7-2 and 7-6). *Beta waves* have a frequency of over 13 Hz and a relatively low voltage. *Alpha waves* have a frequency of 8 Hz to 13 Hz and a relatively high voltage. *Theta waves* have both a relatively low frequency, 4 Hz to 7 Hz, and a low voltage. *Delta waves* have the lowest frequency, less than 4 Hz, but a high voltage.

Fast, low-voltage beta waves characterize EEGs recorded from the frontal and central regions of the cerebrum when an individual is awake, alert, attentive, and with eyes open. Beta predominates when the cerebrum is actively processing sensory stimuli or engaged in mental activities and are therefore referred to as "busy waves." Alpha waves are referred to as "relaxed waves" and dominate EEG recordings from the parietal, occipital, and posterior parts of the temporal lobes when the cerebrum is "idling," for example, with eyes closed, relaxed, and in a nonattentive but not sleeping state. Theta waves are called "drowsy waves" because these are registered when we become sleepy. Finally, delta waves are referred to as "deep sleep waves" and characterize a sleep from which one is not easily aroused.[137]

Hypnotically induced states are researched by assessing changes in electrical pathways. In the next section, two philosophies are discussed that attempt to describe how these changes are expressed in consciousness.

Current Philosophies of Hypnosis

The philosophies that attempt to explain hypnotic effects essentially reside in two camps. The *neodissociation model,* also referred to as the *special process view,* suggests that hypnosis activates subsystems of control that are assumed to have psychologic and physiologic counterparts and result in an altered state of consciousness.[54,55] It is assumed that during the hypnotic state, cognitive processing is altered in predictable ways. An example of hypnotic alteration of consciousness is the phenomenon of reversible amnesia, that is, the patient learns and remembers certain information while hypnotized, forgets the information upon awakening, and remembers the information when hypnosis is again induced.

A competing model, called the *social psychologic view,* states that hypnosis is *not* a specialized state of consciousness, but it is more simply explained in terms of the subject's suggestibility, positive attitudes, and expectations. This model supports the idea that hypnosis is no more than social-psychologic interchange.[125] As we will see,

both models have some support in the literature, with the theory of hypnosis as an altered state of consciousness received the most support in subjects who are highly hypnotizable.

Who Is Susceptible to Hypnosis?

An important philosophic issue related to hypnosis is the concept of *hypnotic susceptibility.*[40,109] It has been repeatedly suggested that physiologic changes in electrocortical activity during hypnosis, as reflected by EEG readings, hold the answer to the mystery of hypnotic susceptibility.[67,124,140] The belief that the hypnotic process has a physiologic basis can be traced back as far as the work of James Braid in the 1800s.[13]

Numerous attempts have been made in modern times to define the electrocortical concomitants of hypnosis.[19] Typically, subjects are divided into those who are classified as *high hypnotizables* or *low hypnotizables,* as assessed by validated instruments such as the *Penn State Scale of Hypnotizability* (PSSH) or the *Stanford Hypnotic Susceptibility Scale (SHSS). Measurement of hypnotic susceptibility* has been demonstrated to be as stable a measurement of individual differences as intelligence quotient (IQ) or other personality inventories. EEG readings are then compared and contrasted between low versus high hypnotizables in a restful waking state; during hypnotic induction; during deepening procedures; and while performing tasks suggested under hypnosis. The differences in EEG readings have varied and are often conflicting.

Some authors have found that high-hypnotizable individuals produce more alpha waves in resting conditions (eyes closed but not hypnotized) than low-hypnotizable persons.[24,83,93,99] Other researchers have found no support for a relationship between alpha production and hypnotizability.[29,31,37,104,120] Reviews of the literature by Saborin and by Perline and Spanos have found the literature unproductive, in that it was essentially equivocal or poorly designed and controlled. There were global methodologic problems including inadequate establishment of stable hypnotic susceptibility, limited electrode placement, and inadequate signal-processing technologies.[112]

Another school of thought that associates alpha wave production to hypnosis is based on the hypothesis of *hemispheric specificity.* To test this hypothesis, researchers measured the ratio of right-to-left hemispheric alpha activity during various tasks performed while under hypnosis. An EEG alpha asymmetry ratio is used as an indicator of hemispheric balance, and a relative decrease in alpha activity is assumed to indicate activation of the hemisphere. Some researchers have concluded that high-hypnotizable persons show greater lateralization than low-hypnotizable persons and that hypnosis is, essentially, a right-hemispheric activity.[23,81,82,83,72,91] Others found no such relationship between hemispheric lateralization and hypnotizability, or their research has suggested that high-hypnotizable individuals actually display an increase in either or both hemispheres as compared with low-hypnotizable persons.[19,24,32,93,121]

Susceptibility and Theta Waves

The most solid evidence for a relationship between EEG outcomes and hypnotizability seems to exist for the theta range (4 Hz to 7 Hz).[19] Theta activity has been associated with a variety of processes including hypnagogic imagery, meditation, rapid eye movement sleep, problem solving, focused attention, and cessation of a pleasurable activity.[144] Essentially, theta activity has been associated with continuous concentration of attention and with selective attention. Galbraith and colleagues used stepwise regression methods and found the research literature supported baseline EEG activity in the theta range as most predictive of hypnotic susceptibility.[42] The authors have further suggested that theta activity reflected the high-susceptible person's ability to both focus attention narrowly and specifically and ignore competing stimuli. A variety of studies, including more current literature, continue to report strong relationships between theta activity and hypnotic susceptibility during hypnotic induction.[1,19,42,121,142]

Dynamic Electroencephalgraphic Differences, Chaos Theory, Hypnotizability

Whereas classical EEG activity signal-processing decomposes frequencies (alpha, theta, beta, delta) and thus reflects a one-dimensional view of brain wave activity, newer, more sophisticated methods provide a more dynamic view. This more sophisticated methodology applies measures from nonlinear dynamics—popularly called chaos—such that point-wise or correlation dimensions give important insight into brain

function. It is suggested that the apparently chaotic switching of processes observed in the brain actually contain a mechanism allowing the brain to initiate novel acts perceived as new ideas and bursts of creativity. In chaos language, these ideas and creative modes act as attractors that maintain or reflect a consistency of processing. Therefore a processing time sequence may be used to reflect all the other variables participating in the dynamics of the system.[112]

A well-designed study by Graffin and others used carefully selected subjects and sophisticated signal processing techniques.[45]

They discovered the following:

1. High-susceptible subjects at baseline have greater theta output in the frontal and temporal cortex (the anterior areas of the brain) during resting baseline as compared with low-susceptible subjects. This greater output demonstrates a heightened state of attentional readiness and concentration of attention[121,135] and may be related to the finding that absorption is one of the most consistent correlations of hypnotizability.

2. Although individual differences in EEG before hypnosis appear in the frontal areas of the brain, once the hypnotic induction is underway, state changes are observed more in the posterior locations. As the hypnotic induction proceeds over time, low-hypnotizable individuals increase theta activity in posterior locations as compared with baseline activity, whereas high-hypnotizable persons decrease theta activity as compared with their baseline activity. This observation suggests that the two groups process the hypnotic efforts differently, before and after the hypnotic induction. This finding is consistent with earlier studies.[9,113]

3. During the hypnotic induction and posthypnotic periods, as compared with low-hypnotizable individuals, high-hypnotizable subjects show greater alpha amplitude in all areas of the brain, except for the occipital lobes.

Of additional interest was a similar study by Ray, which found that high-susceptible individuals displayed underlying brain patterns associated with imagery, whereas low-susceptible individuals showed patterns consistent with the performance of cognitive activity (e.g., mental math.)[112]

In terms of localization, the authors have concluded that the anteroposterior issue is more crucial to understanding hypnotic susceptibility than the hemispheric lateralization issue (Figure 8-6). Further, underlying brain patterns associated with the capacity to produce imagery are associated with high-hypnotizable individuals.

These issues (alpha versus theta activity and anteroposterior versus hemispheric lateralization) will continue to be topics of hot debate and ongoing research. Nonetheless, we can conclude that the experience of deep hypnosis will result in an alteration of brain wave function and that some individuals are more hypnotizable than others. The exact "markers" of hypnosis related to imagery production will need further exploration.

Other Theories

Rossi built a theoretical foundation to explain the workings of hypnosis that integrate (1) the findings of mind-body research (see chapters 1 through 4), (2) the works of Milton Erickson, and (3) his own observations of the importance of ultradian rhythms in the use of hypnosis.

Rossi noted that Braid defined hypnotism as a process of dissociation or reversible amnesia giving rise to the "double-conscious state." Modern researchers refer to this process as *state-dependent* memory and learning. State-dependent memory and learning means that what is learned and remembered is dependent on the individual's psychophysiologic state at the time of the experience. The reversibility of amnesia while under hypnosis is one example. Another example is the research of individuals who remember an event that occurred while inebriated only when again becoming inebriated. The biochemical and hormonal condition of the body at the time of experience makes the mind more able to retrieve that memory and emotion when the same biochemical and hormonal conditions occur again. Drugs such as alcohol and the biochemical changes associated with emotional experiences (e.g., Selye's stress syndrome) "set" the ideal recall condition.

Milton Erickson's work has already demonstrated how amnesia caused by psychologic

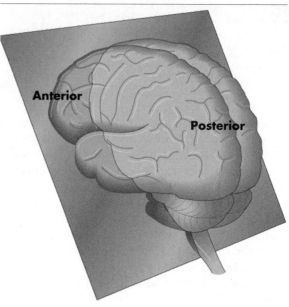

■ *Figure 8-6.* It may be that the changes in brain wave patterns, posterior to anterior, are what are more indicative of hypnotic depth. *Adapted from Thibodeau GA, Patton KT:* Anatomy and physiology, *ed 4, St Louis, 1999, Mosby.*

shocks and traumatic events is, essentially, a psychologic-neurophysiologic dissociation that can be resolved during hypnosis by "inner synthesis." Inner synthesis refers to recreating the biochemical milieu of the event through hypnosis. Once this is accomplished, the inner conflict can be resolved more easily.[33]

Rossi perceived a relationship between hypnosis, state-dependent learning, and the psychobiologic characteristics of *ultradian rhythms.* Ultradian rhythms are 90-minute cycles of psychophysiologic processes involving many parasympathetic and right-hemispheric functions. Erickson had observed and recorded the effects of these cycles in what he called the *common* everyday trance, also a 90-minute cycle.

Based on these combined observations, Rossi developed the hypothesis of *ultradian theory of hypnotherapeutic healing.* His theory proposed that (1) the source of psychosomatic reactions is in stress-induced distortions of the normal periodicity of ultradian cycles, and (2) the naturalistic approach to hypnotherapy facilitates healing by permitting a normalization of these ultradian processes.[117] Rossi noted that new research reports hormones released during periods of stress modulate memory and learning in the limbic system (e.g., amygdala and hippocampus); these are the same hormones of the hypothalamic-pituitary-adrenal (HPA) endocrine system. Further, these are the same hormones as those described by Selye as being related to stress-induced illness[88] (see Selye, Chapter 1). Rossi concluded that the new neurobiologic research on memory and learning and Selye's research are both essentially describing state-dependent memory and learning phenomena.

Hypnosis, Rossi theorized, allows the client to access state-bound information by carefully retrieving the contexts and frames of reference in which it is embedded. Rossi believed that, as Pert suggested (see Chapter 1), memories and emotions are biochemically stored. The state-dependent encoding of life experience is therefore the psychobiologic basis of hypnosis and psychoanalysis. Rossi further hypothesized that this state-dependent encoding of information affects us at the cellular-genetic level and that hypnosis can be used as a process of modulating the effects of this encoded information.[18]

∎ Summary of Hypnosis Mechanisms

In summary, the research and theory on the mechanisms of hypnosis, as we know them, have been presented. In reality, absolute conclusions about these mechanisms have yet to be determined. Future research designs on hypnosis need to address patient motivation carefully, therapist skill level and hypnosis style (naturalistic versus authoritarian), hypnotizability, specifics of imagery used as part of the hypnosis process and the purpose of this imagery, and ultradian effects. A strong grounding in mind-body processes will also result in stronger, more defensible research designs. We now turn our attention to the evolving hypnosis research.

∎ Power of Suggestion: Wart Charming and Other Wonders

Some of the earliest reports of the effectiveness of hypnosis stem from the power of suggestion to eliminate warts. The *charming of warts* was enshrined in American folklore by Mark Twain in his Tom Sawyer stories.[141] Warts are caused by the papillomavirus. Many warts regress spontaneously, but there is no natural history, as occurs in other viral disorders such as the common cold.[119] It is not known why warts locate in a particular area and do not spread with contact to a susceptible person.

Published, controlled studies on the use of hypnosis to cure warts are mostly confined to

Points to Ponder Once warts are removed by hypnosis, they typically "stay" removed. ∎

using directed suggestion, with a reported cure rate between 27% and 55%.[63] Successful hypnotic suggestions for curing warts can vary from "make it cold" and "increase blood supply" to "bring in more antibodies." Each of these suggestions creates a belief in the recipient in their ability to eliminate the warts.

Once warts are removed by hypnosis, they typically "stay" removed. Warts often reoccur after standard medical treatment, but there are no reports of wart recurrence after they are removed by hypnosis. In a study by Bloch, patients who used hypnosis for the treatment of warts had previously experienced as many as 12 recurrences, typically between 1 and 8 weeks after treatment. Bloch employed a single visit using dramatic rituals similar to those used by the original lay "wart charmers".[11] Approximately 55%, or 98 of 179 patients, were "cured."

In a study by Surman, 24 patients with warts were assigned to hypnosis or were assigned to control groups.[132] Treatment patients received hypnosis by eye fixation once a week for 5 weeks. Hypnotic subjects were told the warts on only one side of the body would disappear. At 3 months after the first hypnotic suggestion, 53% of the patients who received hypnosis exhibited significant improvement in size or resolution of warts, but in only one patient did the warts resolve exclusively on the chosen side. The findings suggested that hypnosis may affect the host's response to the causative virus, although side selectivity did not seem to be controlled by hypnosis.

In a more recent study by Ewin, patients unresponsive to standard hypnosis protocols were given direct suggestion, followed by hypnoanalytic techniques that included regressing the patient to the onset of the wart and reframing the context. This technique resulted in 33 of 41 subjects (80%) being "cured" of their warts.[39] The literature supports the hypothesis that directed hypnosis can, in many patients, remove warts, a condition produced by a virus.

Case study: Congenital Ichthyosis

Congenital ichthyosis is a condition where skin progressively thickens with time, reaching a maximum thickness at about the age of 15 years. The condition then remains static throughout life or deteriorates with secondary complications. This condition is resistant to all forms of treatment, including skin grafting.

In a case study, a 16-year-old boy suffering from ichthyosis exhibited a black horny layer that covered his entire body except chest, neck, and face. Papillae projected 2 mm to 6 mm above the surface, with each papillae separated from each other by only a small distance. To the touch, the skin felt as hard as a normal fingernail and was so inelastic that any attempt at bending resulted in a crack in the surface, which then oozed blood-stained serum. In skin flexures, there were fissures that were constantly reopened by movement and were chronically infected and painful. The ichthyosiform layer was numb for a depth of several millimeters. The condition was worst on the hands, feet, thighs, and calves, and least severe on the upper arms, abdomen, and back. The skin on the face, neck, and chest appeared almost normal. The child's education was interrupted because other pupils and teachers objected to his smell. He was shy and lonely but responded well to any teaching and to affection.

The patient was hypnotized and, under hypnosis, the suggestion was made that the left arm would clear. After 5 days, the horny layer softened, became friable, and fell off. From a black casing, the skin on the arm became pink and soft. After 10 days, the arm was completely clear from shoulder to wrist. The right arm was treated in the same way, and 10 days later, the legs and trunk were treated. With time, the palms cleared completely, but the fingers did not improve. However, his arms cleared 95%, his back 90%, his buttocks 60%, his thighs 70%, and his legs and feet, 50%.[87] There was no relapse of improvement 1 year after treatment (Figure 8-7).

■ Hypnosis: Pain Mechanisms

Pain is a complex experience that depends on the stimulation of specific end-organ receptors. Subjectively, however, pain intensity does not necessarily reflect the level of stimulation, the extent of tissue damage, or the danger to the person.[90]

Individual response to pain is mediated by (1) meaning attributed to the pain sensation, (2) past experience, and (3) anxiety and current emotional condition.

Beecher described pain as primary and secondary in nature.[7] The *primary* pain component

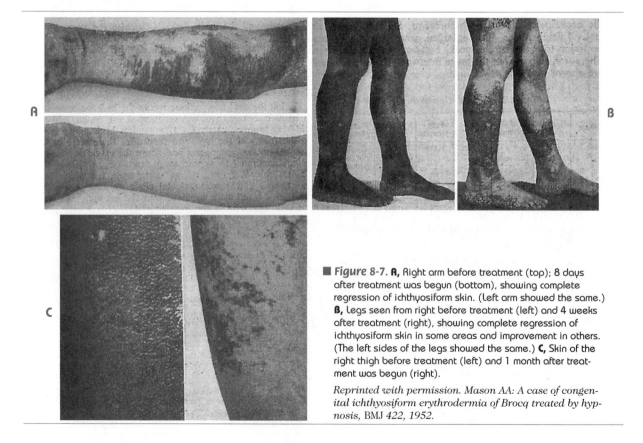

■ *Figure 8-7.* **A,** Right arm before treatment (top); 8 days after treatment was begun (bottom), showing complete regression of ichthyosiform skin. (Left arm showed the same.) **B,** Legs seen from right before treatment (left) and 4 weeks after treatment (right), showing complete regression of ichthyosiform skin in some areas and improvement in others. (The left sides of the legs showed the same.) **C,** Skin of the right thigh before treatment (left) and 1 month after treatment was begun (right).

Reprinted with permission. Mason AA: A case of congenital ichthyosiform erythrodermia of Brocq treated by hypnosis, BMJ 422, 1952.

consists of the pain sensation itself. This includes pain perception and the discrimination and recognition of the noxious stimulus. The *secondary* pain component involves suffering, reactive aspects, anxiety, and emotional responses to pain. The psychologic reaction to pain is considered independent of the primary sensation. It is the primary sensation that may be responsible for many changes in heart rate, blood pressure, and galvanic skin response associated with painful stimulation. In fact, research outcomes often indicate that *hypnotically suggested analgesia* (hypnosis-induced reduction of pain) was generally not associated with a reduction in autonomic response to experimental pain.[6,58]

How Hypnosis Alleviates Pain

How, then, does hypnosis alleviate pain? Shor and others argued that hypnosis relieves pain by reducing anxiety (the secondary pain component) and has little effect on the primary sensation itself.[6,122] Shor, for example, failed to find differences in galvanic skin response when subjects reported that the same level of electric shock that was painful in the waking state was much less painful during hypnotic analgesia. He attributed this outcome to an intentional reduction of anxiety, not the alleviation of the primary pain component.[123] Conceptualized in this manner, hypnotic pain reduction is not unlike the placebo response; both act on the secondary component of pain by reducing anxiety, and both have little effect on primary sensations.

Surgical Pain

Shor's arguments do not fully explain the ability of some patients to experience major surgery without pain. McGlashan and others hypothesized that the mechanism of pain reduction during surgery is one in which the individual's perception of the pain sensation is altered. The altered perception to pain would be analogous to an induced hallucination and would be an additive factor to the relief induced by the placebo aspects of hypnotic treatment.[89]

Experimentally Induced Pain

In an effort to understand how hypnosis affects pain, experiments are often performed to assess how the hypnotic state alters perceived and sensory pain. To accomplish this task, pain is often induced experimentally by the tourniquet technique. In this technique, a tourniquet is applied to the nondominant arm after the arm has been raised toward the ceiling to promote venous drainage. The tourniquet is then inflated, and the arm is lowered. The subject squeezes and releases an exerciser to accelerate the process of ischemic pain. Pain is induced because adequate blood flow is blocked (Figure 8-8).

In the McGlashan and associates study, the effects of hypnotically induced analgesia and response to a placebo—a pill described as a powerful new analgesic drug—were evaluated for the ability to relieve tourniquet-induced ischemic pain. Highly motivated subjects were selected who were known to be either very susceptible or relatively insusceptible to hypnosis. Special procedures were adopted, which establish equal expectation in both groups that both hypnosis and the placebo drug could reduce pain. Hypnosis-insusceptible subjects were convinced they were able to induce hypnotic analgesia by exposing them to a shock test and then significantly reducing the shock after hypnosis with an explanation that the shock was equivalent to that experienced before hypnotic induction.

Experience of pain was similar for susceptible subjects after placebo and for insusceptible subjects after both hypnosis and placebo. Only high-

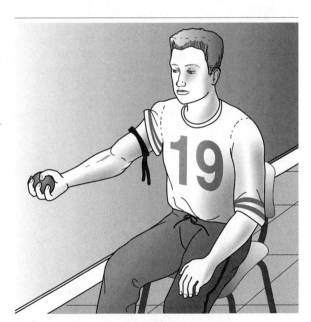

■ *Figure 8-8.* This tourniquet technique accelerates the process of ischemic pain and, before and after hypnosis, allows the researcher to determine how much pain analgesia has been induced.

TABLE 8-1	Effects of Hypnosis on Experimentally Induced Pain

AUTHOR	TYPE OF STUDY	FINDINGS
EXPERIMENTALLY INDUCED PAIN		
McGlashan TH, Evans FJ, Orne MT: The nature of hypnotic analgesia and placebo response to experimental pain, *Psychosom Med* 31(3):227, 1969.	Two groups of subjects (very high and very low hypnotizables, N=24) were assessed for changes in pain threshold and tolerance after hypnosis-induced analgesia and a placebo pill referred to as "a powerful analgesic drug." Pain threshold was tested to induced ischemic muscle pain, elicited by the tourniquet method. Very low hypnotizables were used as an additional placebo check.	For low-hypnotizable subjects, the difference between pain relief for the placebo pill and hypnosis session was nonsignificant. For high-hypnotizables who reached glove-anesthesia depth of hypnosis, difference between placebo pill and hypnosis was highly significant (0.005). Pain threshold increased 63% over baseline with hypnosis and 41% over baseline with placebo pill. The effects of the placebo pill on pain threshold was virtually identical for high and low hypnotizables. Authors concluded that there are two components involved in hypnotic analgesia: the nonspecific placebo effect and the conceptualized distortion of perception specifically induced during deep hypnosis.
Danziger N, Fournier E, Bouhassira D, Michaud D, De Broucker R, Santarcangelo E, Carli G, Chertock L, Willer JC: Different strategies of modulation can be operative during hypnotic analgesia: a neurophysiological study, *Pain* 75:85, 1998.	Nocicepetive electrical stimuli were applied to the sural (calf) nerve of 18 high-susceptible subjects. Pain threshold, nociceptive flexion (RIII) reflex, and late SSEP were investigated with autonomic responses and the spontaneous EEG.	Hypnotic suggestion of analgesia induced a significant increase in pain threshold in all selected subjects. All subjects showed large changes (20% or more) in amplitude of RIII reflexes during hypnotic analgesia as compared with control conditions. Two distinctively different patterns of modulation of the RIII reflex were observed during hypnotic analgesia. Subgroup 1 (N=11) strongly inhibited the reflex, whereas subgroup 2 (N=7) strongly facilitated the reflex. All subjects demonstrated similar decreases in SSEP and no modification in EEG or autonomic parameters were observed. Authors concluded some hypnotic Ns inhibit motor reaction to the stimulus at the spinal level, whereas other hypnotic Ns facilitate that response.
DeBenedittis G, Panerai AA, Villamira MA: Effects of hypnotic analgesia and hypnotizability of experimental ischemic pain, *Int J Clin Exp Hypn* 37(1):55, 1989.	High- and low-hypnotizable patients were administered an ischemic pain test (pain experienced as a result of, in this case, the purposeful blocking of blood flow in the arm) in both wakeful and hypnotic states. Experimentally induced pain was used to assess the efficacy of hypnosis to reduce pain and to determine whether opioids or ACTH activity could be correlated with hypnotically induced pain reductions.	Tolerance for pain and distress were significantly increased during hypnosis as compared with the waking state, with positive correlations between high hypnotizability and relief. A hypnotically induced dissociation between the sensory-discriminative and the affective-motivational dimensions of pain experience was found, but only in high-hypnotizable subjects. Hypnotic analgesia was unrelated to anxiety reduction and was NOT MEDIATED by endorphins or ACTH. When authors subdivided groups by hypnotic performance (e.g., ability to increase, ability not to increase pain tolerance by 50% or more), they found that endorphin levels IN THE WAKING state, but not in the hypnotic state, predicted high-hypnotic performance, independent of hypnotizable scores.

ACTH, Adrenocorticotropic hormone; *EEG,* electroencephalogram; *SSEP,* somatosensory-evoked potentials.

hypnotically susceptible subjects received significant pain relief, exceeding that produced by the placebo effect with hypnotic analgesia. The results supported the hypothesis of two components involved in hypnotic analgesia. One component can be accounted for by the nonspecific or placebo effects of hypnosis; the other can be conceptualized as a distortion of perception (dissociation) specifically induced during deep hypnosis (Table 8-1).

Pain at the Spinal Level

How, exactly, do high-hypnotizable individuals "distort" or block pain? To answer this question, Danziger and others applied pain-inducing electri-

> **Points to Ponder** Only high-hypnotically susceptible subjects received significant pain relief, exceeding that produced by the placebo effect with hypnotic analgesia.

cal stimuli to the *sural nerve*—the nerve in the calf of the leg—of 18 high-hypnotizable subjects while hypnotically suggesting analgesia of the lower left limb.[20] They compared responses with this noxious stimulus before, during, and after hypnotic induction and suggestion. The following indices were evaluated: (1) EEGs, (2) autonomic responses, (3) muscle reflex activity of a knee flexor muscle in response to electrical stimulation of the sural nerve (RIII reflex) assessed by electromyography (EMG), and (4) late *somatosensory-evoked potentials* (SSEP). SSEP is tested in a similar manner as an EEG, but the brain waves are caused, or evoked, by a specific stimulus, in this case, an electrical stimulus.

In subgroup 1, a strong inhibition of the reflex of the knee flexor muscle was observed in 11 subjects, whereas in subgroup 2, there was a strong facilitation of the reflex observed in 7 subjects. The data suggested that different strategies of modulation can operate during effective hypnotic analgesia and that these are subject dependent.

Although all subjects can shift attention away from the painful stimulus, some subjects can, through hypnosis, inhibit their motor reactions to the stimulus at the spinal level. By contrast, this reaction was facilitated in others.

Hypnosis, Endorphins, and Adrenocorticotropic Hormones

Some researchers have hypothesized that the effects of hypnosis result from the release of our "feel good" chemicals, or endorphins. To test this theory, DeBenedittis and others also explored the effects of hypnosis on pain induced by the tourniquet technique.[22] The authors wanted to know how hypnosis affected two distinctive dimensions of pain experience. *Sensory discrimination* is information about the location and intensity of pain, that is, the perceptual quality of pain; *motivational affection,* on the other hand, reflects the aversive affect and the negative emotional resonance of pain, that is, distress or suffering. Pain reduction through hypnotic suggestion has been reported to involve both sensor pain and affective suffering.[58,70]

Although anxiety plays a role in pain tolerance, the authors felt the experimental evidence

suggested that hypnosis for pain reduction acted primarily as an analgesic.[123] They therefore hypothesized that beta-endorphins, or natural opioids, and adrenocorticotropic hormone (ACTH) activity could be altered when hypnosis was successful in increasing pain tolerance. It should be noted that ACTH signals the adrenal cortex to release corticosteroid hormones.

Hypnotic analgesia increased pain and distress tolerance by 63% as compared with waking state. High-hypnotizable individuals increase their tolerance by 113% and low-hypnotizable persons by only 26%. Pain and distress were both reduced by hypnosis, but distress was reduced significantly more than pain, although only for high-hypnotizable individuals. Contrary to the hypothesis, neither beta-endorphin nor ACTH changes were noted for either high- and low-hypnotizable groups.

One interesting finding was discovered. When subjects were considered not by hypnotizable scores but by pain tolerance performance, a significant correlation was found between the ability to induce pain analgesia and the endorphin levels during the waking but not the hypnotic state.

The fact that distress was reduced significantly more than pain, but only for high-hypnotizable subjects, is consistent with the paradox that is often observed when pain is reduced by hypnosis. "Felt pain" (overt response) may be reduced while the involuntary physiologic indicators of pain (covert response) may persist at nearly normal levels.

Although hypnosis affects both pain dimensions, the motivational-affective dimension of stimulation is considered more modifyable.[147] This may explain the dissociative effect induced by hypnosis on the two components of the pain experience (sensory dissociative and motivational affective).

In summary, based on this and other studies, hypnotic analgesia does not appear to be mediated by opiate systems, regardless of hypnotizability,[27,47,100] nor is it induced by stress-induced analgesic mechanisms.[46,95,123]

■ Hypnosis and Surgical Procedures

Hypnosis has been used as an analgesic component of surgery since the first half of the nine-

---

Points to Ponder   Although all subjects can shift attention away from the painful stimulus, some subjects can, through hypnosis, inhibit their motor reactions to the stimulus at the spinal level. ■

Points to Ponder   Contrary to the hypothesis, neither beta-endorphin nor ACTH changes were noted for either high- and low-hypnotizable groups. ■

teenth century. As noted earlier, John Elliotson, an English surgeon, reported using mesmerism as the sole means of analgesia in numerous surgeries of the 1830s. James Esdaile, a Scottish physician working in India, reported more than 300 major surgical cases using mesmerism as the only analgesia.[35]

At the same time Esdaile was reporting his successes, physicians discovered chemical anesthetic agents, beginning with ether in 1846 and chloroform in 1847. Because of the relative safety and effectiveness of these agents, hypnosis fell out of favor as a surgical procedure for pain control. Hypnosis is still used for surgical analgesia for patients for whom chemical anesthesia is contraindicated. It has been clearly demonstrated that hypnosis can serve as a means of surgical anesthesia in a small portion of the population (see Sylvester's case study).

Hypnotic Effects of Anesthesia

There is an interesting hypnotic effect that occurs during the surgical procedure while the patient is anesthetized. Evidence increasingly suggests that the sounds in the operating room register in some areas of the cortex with general anesthesia and that these sounds may influence recovery from surgery.[36]

Although few patients can recall intraoperative events, a more sensitive assessment of learning found significant postoperative recognition of words presented during general anesthesia.[92] Further, patients that are unable to recall instructions made during surgery may still obey them postoperatively. While anesthetized, 11 patients were told to touch their ears during a subsequent interview; they did so significantly more frequently than control patients.[8] This finding was replicated with patients who underwent cardiac surgery.[44] Inappropriate or misinterpreted comments during the surgical procedure may have a harmful effect on recovery, and it has even been suggested that patients' ears should be plugged during surgery.[21,30,59,73]

Hypnosis and Surgical Recovery Rates

Patients may also respond to positive therapeutic suggestions made during surgery. Two uncontrolled studies reported that therapeutic suggestions during anesthesia improved recovery from surgery, a conclusion supported by two double-blind placebo controlled studies.[12,62,103,152]

Evans and Richardson reported significantly shorter periods of hospitalization and fewer instances of elevated temperature when patients received therapeutic suggestions while under anesthesia. Patients who received the instructions also accurately guessed that they had received them; controls guessed no better than chance.[36]

In another study by Bonke and colleagues, 91 patients undergoing bilary tract surgery were randomly assigned to groups who, while under anesthesia, heard (1) positive suggestions for healing; (2) white noise, or (3) noise and conversation as it occurred in the operating room.[12] There were no differences in outcomes for surgical patients under the age of 55 years. For patients 55 years or older, however, positive suggestions provided protection from prolonged hospital stays. The authors concluded that the effects were negligible in the younger population because they seldom had protracted recovery periods.

Blankfield undertook a critical review of eighteen clinical trials that employed hypnosis, suggestion, or relaxation techniques as interventions to facilitate recovery from surgery.[10] Sixteen studies reported that the intervention resulted in improved physical or emotional recovery of patients after the surgical procedure. It appears that hypnosis, suggestion, and relaxation techniques are underused and can result in shorter postoperative hospital stays; they can promote physical recovery of patients and aid in the psychologic and emotional response of patients after surgery.

The type of hypnotic technique, the timing of technique (before anesthesia, after anesthesia, and postoperatively), the study quality, the number of patients, and the type of surgery varied from study to study. There were, nonetheless, positive physical and emotional outcomes postoperatively for 16 of 18 trials.

> **Points to Ponder**   Evidence increasingly suggests that, while under general anesthesia, the sounds in the operating room register in some areas of the cortex and that these sounds may influence recovery from surgery. ■

> **Points to Ponder**   It appears that hypnosis and suggestion and relaxation techniques are underused and can result in shorter postoperative hospital stays; they can promote physical recovery of patients and aid in the psychologic and emotional response of patients after surgery. ■

TABLE 8-2	Effects of Hypnosis on Surgical Recovery Rates	

AUTHOR	TYPE OF STUDY	FINDINGS
SURGICAL RECOVERY		
Evans C, Richardson PH: Improved recovery and reduced postoperative stay after therapeutic suggestions during general anesthesia, *Lancet* 27:491, 1988.	Patients undergoing a hysterectomy were exposed to recorded therapeutic suggestions (treatment group) or a blank tape (control) while under general anesthesia (N=39).	The patients in the suggestion group spent significantly less time in the hospital after surgery, suffered from a significantly shorter period of pyrexia (fever), and were rated by nurses as experiencing better-than-expected recovery. The treatment group experienced significantly less gastrointestinal problems as compared with control subjects. Unlike the control group, those in the treatment group guessed, correctly, that they had been played the therapeutic suggestion tape.
Bonke B, Schmitz PIM, Verhage F, Zwaveling A: Clinical study of so-called unconscious perception during general anesthesia, *Br J Anaesth* 58:957, 1986.	Patients undergoing bilary tract surgery were randomly assigned to (1) positive suggestions played on earphones while under anesthesia; (2) continuous, monotonous low-frequency noise while under anesthesia; or (3) the usual sounds that occur in the operating theatre.	Exposure to positive suggestions during general anesthesia, as compared to noise or operating theatre sounds, protected patients older than 55 years against prolonged postoperative stays in the hospital. Results were not significantly different for younger patients (N=91).

When comparing tape-recorded suggestions with live suggestions from therapists, the results were best for those who used the therapist (e.g., reduced length of hospital stay and analgesic use). Recorded suggestions had the advantages of being efficient and convenient, allowing double blinding and a continued use while under anesthesia. Therapist studies could only be single blinded.

It was also pointed out that positive naturalistic suggestions (e.g., "Your pain will lessen and lessen") were more effective than negative authoritative suggestions (e.g., "You will NOT feel pain").

In summary, there is a small but enticing body of literature that supports the use of hypnotic techniques as adjuvant therapy for patients requiring surgery. The fact that hypnosis offers the possibility of shortened hospital stays and can contribute to the well being of surgical patients makes it certainly worthy of additional study and use (Table 8-2).

Clinical hypnosis is one of the few areas of Western medicine that has always acknowledged the indivisible nature of the body and mind. In the following case study, Sandra Sylvester, PhD, describes how the power of focused attention and deep concentration enabled a 55-year-old woman to undergo an abdominal cholecystectomy during which her gallbladder was removed with little pain or discomfort. Hypnosis was used as the only analgesia. After surgery, she experienced a rapid recovery and was discharged from the hospital 45 hours later. She was gardening 5 days postoperatively.

An Expert Speaks: Dr. Sandra M. Sylvester

Sandra M. Sylvester, Ph.D., is a licensed psychologist who studied with Milton H. Erickson, worked with Erickson's private practice patients and trained professionals in his training seminars. She is author of *Living with Stress,* and has contributed hypnosis chapters entitled "Fear and the Management of Pain," "Preparation for Surgery," "Self-Healing," and "Milton H. Erickson: The Wounded Physician as Healer." She is a faculty member of the Gestalt Institute of Cleveland and is an Approved Consultant of the American Society of Clinical Hypnosis. Dr. Sylvester specializes in presurgical and postsurgical procedures, including using hypnosis as the only anesthesia. In the following text, she describes a case study of hypnosis as anesthesia.

When Lucy learned that she had to have her gallbladder removed surgically, she requested hypnosis as analgesia for surgery rather than a general anesthetic. The reasons she gave for wanting hypnosis in lieu of general anesthesia were: (1) she had negative drug induced psychotic experiences with general anesthesia in the past; and (2) she had two previous successful experiences with clinical hypnosis. Twenty-five years previously, she had a caesarean section with hypnosis supplemented with local anesthesia and 5 years previously, she had a fistula removed with hypnosis supplemented by minimal local anesthesia.

Lucy was highly motivated. She found a surgeon that was willing to do surgery with hypnosis as anesthesia, and then asked if I [Sandra Sylvester] would be willing to do the hypnosis. We decided to proceed with the understanding that standby anesthesia would be available during the surgical procedure, should the need arise.

Through our discussion, Lucy learned that all hypnosis is self-hypnosis and that together we would decide on a method of hypnosis that would build on the concentration skills that Lucy had. The method we arrived at was hypnotic dissociation, a process of concentrating and focusing attention on an activity totally separated from and distant from the operating room procedure and becoming totally absorbed in that other activity. Lucy decided that she would mentally go on a familiar and favorite hike along a mountain stream.

We met for four sessions over a 3-month period. During these sessions, various hypnotic skills were learned, and Lucy was given a cassette tape recording of the session's hypnosis to practice at home for 20 minutes each day.

On the day of surgery, Lucy and I met again in the surgical holding area. Lucy was anxious. I reminded her that she could begin to go to her mountain path along the stream. She could let the sounds in the room and in the hall wash over her, not needing to attend to anything but the sound of my voice; that she would be addressed by name if there was anything that she needed to hear or heed. Otherwise, she need only enjoy her walk along the stream, daydreaming about whatever she wished as she listened to her hypnosis tape. By the time she was taken to the operating room, Lucy was breathing peacefully and was calm.

At 1:10 PM, the patient entered the operating room. Monitors were placed and the patient was prepped and draped. The surgeon and her team were ready. The entire team was trying not to disturb Lucy's concentration. At the moment the surgeon was poised with a scalpel, ready to make the initial incision, I told Lucy that she would have the sensation of the pressure of an eraser end of a pencil being drawn across her body. The surgeon made the initial incision at 1:30 PM, everything remained calm, and we all internally sighed in relief. Approximately 20 minutes into the surgery, Lucy's abdomen had been entered and the liver was lifted to expose the gall bladder. Lucy remarked that she felt like the room was spinning and began to feel nauseous. I asked the anesthesiologist for nasal-prong oxygen and told Lucy to breathe fresh oxygen deeply and the spinning would stop. At this time the anesthesiologist also administered a small amount of a sedative. Lucy's breathing returned to a deep regular rhythm and the surgery continued without further event. Throughout the case, the patient's blood pressure and heart rate remained remarkably stable for an intraabdominal case of this magnitude with only 3 mg Valium, oxygen, and hypnosis for her anesthetic. During the surgery, the patient could answer questions addressed to her by the surgeon. After the wound was closed, the patient asked the surgeon to show her the gallstones. The patient left the operating room at 2:20 PM.

This was the first hypnoanesthesia experience for both the surgeon and the anesthesiologist. The anesthesiologist wheeled Lucy into the recovery room and exclaimed that he didn't know why he was taking her to recovery because she had nothing to recover from! He wrote in his post-surgical note that it was an amazing experience. The surgeon was pleased at Lucy's rapid recovery. Lucy was gardening the fourth day after major abdominal surgery. Lucy had little discomfort or pain during the post-surgical recovery. She was given 10 grains of Tylenol at 6:00 PM the night of surgery, and again at midnight and at 4:00 PM the next morning. She required no further medication for pain. The day after surgery, nursing notes reflect that she was awake and cheerful with no complaints of pain. She showered, walked in the hall, sat up in a chair for meals and had a very stable day with no medication for pain. The following morning she was discharged from the hospital approximately 45 hours after major intraabdominal surgery. Lucy was elated because her experience was personally empowering and noted a tremendous boost in self-confidence.

This is a very unusual case because few patients would choose to have major surgery with clinical hypnosis in lieu of general anesthesia since general anesthesia is so readily available and is the standard of care today. In some cases, however, there are extenuating circumstances or past anesthetic complications which make the administration of a general anesthetic or regional anesthetic very difficult for the patient. In these cases, clinical hypnosis can frequently be used as an adjunct to traditional medical practice by the attending physician or nurse practitioner skilled in its use.

For example, clinical hypnosis can be used for all surgical patients to reduce anxiety and fear. Whenever a physician or nurse practitioner talks to a patient, hypnotic skills can be employed to help the patient focus on a pleasant sensation or event: to experience feelings of warmth, calmness, relaxation. By being observant and discriminating about which patients want to be informed and want to have a certain modicum of control—and which patients want nothing to do with the procedure and would rather be "someplace else"—the physician or nurse practitioner can teach the patient the appropriate hypnotic skills to achieve what the patient wants to achieve. For both types of patients, anxiety is reduced, but by very different means.

In cases where intubation must be achieved while the patient is awake, hypnotic time distortion where long periods of time seem to take only a few moments, can be of great help.

In cases where a regional block has failed or is incomplete, clinical hypnosis can be used to increase the block or spread the field of the block so that the procedure can be completed.

In clinical hypnosis, the power of the mind is used to reinterpret physical sensations, to change the perception of time, to attend to some stimulation and ignore others, and to travel to another space and time. In doing so, the mind empowers an individual and influences his or her health.

■ Hypnosis and Chronic Pain

We have reviewed the mechanisms and effects of hypnosis on acute pain as it occurs during experimentally induced pain and during or after surgery. We now discuss the effectiveness of hypnosis for the treatment of chronic pain (e.g., cancer, burn, and fibromyalgia pain.)

Cancer Pain

Malignant tumors that arise from epithelial tissues are called *carcinomas*. Cells from malignant breast tumors can form secondary tumors in bone, brain, and lung tissues. The cells can then migrate by way of lymphatic or blood vessels. This manner of spreading is called *metastasis*. When cancer spreads in this way, the prognosis is extremely grim. Intense pain often accompanies this form of cancer.

Spiegel and Blo studied 54 women with *metastatic carcinoma* of the breast over the course of a year.[127] In this study, 24 women served

> **Points to Ponder**   The mean pain sensation over time was lowest for the group therapy plus hypnosis group (0.008), higher for the group receiving group therapy without hypnosis (0.05), and the highest for the control group. ■

as controls and 30 women participated in weekly group therapy sessions. Of those in group therapy, 19 persons learned and practiced hypnosis for pain control while 11 attended group therapy but did not learn hypnosis. A significant difference was observed among the three groups for pain sensation. The mean pain sensation over time was lowest for the group therapy plus hypnosis group (0.008), higher for the group receiving group therapy without hypnosis (0.05), and the highest for the control group.

In another study by Syrjala, Cummings, and Donaldson, 67 patients who underwent bone marrow transplant with hematologic malignancies were assigned before transplant to one of four groups: (1) hypnosis training, (2) cognitive behavioral coping skills training, (3) therapist contact control, or (4) control receiving treatment as usual.[134] Patients in the first three groups met with a clinical psychologist for "intervention" twice before transplant surgery and ten times in the hospital after surgery for intervention "boosters." Hypnosis was significantly more effective in reducing reported oral pain, but there was no difference or effect on nausea, vomiting, and opioid use between groups.

Burn Pain

It is well known that a severe burn is one of the most painful experiences possible. Further, the burn care procedure typically creates more pain than the initial trauma. Patients hospitalized with burns endure daily wound care procedures that can last weeks or even months. It is considered too dangerous and too expensive to use general anesthesia on a daily basis for pain control. Opioid drugs, including morphine, are often provided as the main form of pain relief.[105] Unfortunately, opioid drugs almost never control burn pain completely and some patients do not respond well to opioid treatment (i.e., they receive little analgesia from opioid treatment, and side effects of nausea or constipation occur).[106] It is important to control pain for these patients, both for humanitarian reasons and because there is evidence that pain control will improve physical and emotional adjustments.[110]

Even though hypnosis is the most frequently cited nonpharmacologic intervention for burn pain in adults, nearly all published reports of hypnosis for burn pain are anecdotal with few clinically controlled trials. Case studies often fail to document pain measurement, drug dosages, or treatment failures. Even when the poor quality and low number of studies are considered, the number of favorable outcomes and reports of dramatic benefits would suggest that some burn victims benefit from hypnosis interventions.

In a study by Patterson and Ptacek, 61 patients hospitalized for severe burns and averaging 13.95% of total body surface area (TBSA) burned were randomized to hypnosis or a control (sham hypnosis) condition. The control condition consisted of receiving attention, information, and brief relaxation instructions that were described as hypnosis[102] (Figure 8-9). Posttreatment pain scores for the two groups did not differ significantly when all patients were included. However, when a subset of patients who reported the highest levels of baseline pain were compared with the highest baseline controls, hypnosis patients reported less posttreatment pain than control group patients. The sham-hypnotic procedure, especially considering the motivation of patients to avoid pain, may have, in fact, induced a self-hypnotic state. Since no other control group was employed, there is no way to determine whether self-hypnosis actually occurred.

Fibromyalgia Pain

Fibromyalgia syndromes are actually a group of disorders (e.g., myofascial pain syndromes, fibromyositis) characterized by achy pain and stiffness in soft tissue, including muscles, tendons, and ligaments. In a study by Haanen and others, fibromyalgia pain was reduced significantly more by hypnosis than by physical therapy, as were feelings of somatic and psychic discomfort[48] (Table 8-3).

■ Hypnosis and Gastrointestinal Disorders
Duodenal Ulcers

Duodenal ulcers are effectively and rapidly treated with many drugs. However, in the late 1980s, posttreatment relapse was so common that continuous maintenance therapy had been advocated by some physicians.[153] The typical 1-year relapse rate for duodenal ulcers was approximately 85%.[65,86] Data originating from the 1830s and continuing today have chronicled the effects of emotion on the gastric tissues. Stress has since been demonstrated to affect gastric emptying and the secretion of acid and pepsin.[43,138]

In an interesting study, patients with a history of relapsing duodenal ulceration were treated with ranitidine until ulcers were healed and then they were assigned to a hypnosis-preventative group or to regular treatment. Both diagnosis and healing of ulcers were confirmed by endoscopy.[16] Approximately 1 year after treatment, 100% of the control group but only 53% of the hypnosis group relapsed, a statistically significant difference (Table 8-4).

In the 1990s, it was discovered that *H. pylori* (bacteria) was the underlying cause of ulcers. Today, the treatment of choice for duodenal ulcers is antibiotics.[148] This discovery allows us to hypothesize a multifactorial effect of hypnosis for relapse prevention of duodenal ulcers. No doubt, gastric secretions were reduced in this study because of the hypnosis and imagery techniques used with hypnosis. However, relaxation and

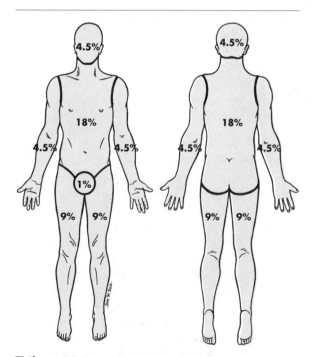

■ *Figure 8-9.* **Rule of Nines.** "Rule of nines" is one method used to estimate the amount of total body surface area burned in an adult. In this population, the average burn size is 13.95%. *Adapted from Thibodeau GA, Patton KT: Anatomy and physiology, ed 4, St Louis, 1999, Mosby.*

Points to Ponder   Approximately 1 year after treatment, 100% of the control group but only 53% of the hypnosis group relapsed, a statistically significant difference.

TABLE 8-3	Effects of Hypnosis on Cancer, Burn, and Fibromyalgia Pain

AUTHOR	TYPE OF STUDY	FINDINGS
PAIN REDUCTION		
Cancer Pain		
Spiegel D, Blo JR: Group therapy and hypnosis reduce metastatic breast carcinoma pain, *Psychosom Med* 45(4):333, 1983.	Women with metastatic carcinoma of the breast were offered weekly group therapy either with or without hypnosis for pain control. The 54 patients were then followed for 1 year.	Both treatment groups demonstrated significantly less self-rated pain sensation (0.02) and suffering (0.03) than a control sample. Those who received group therapy and practiced hypnosis fared better than those who received group therapy alone. They experienced significantly less pain sensation (0.05), although pain frequency and duration were not different from other group therapy. Anxiety, depression, and fatigue subscales were significantly correlated with a reduction in reported pain.
Syrjala KL, Cummings C, Donaldson GW: Hypnosis or cognitive behavioral training for the reduction of pain and nausea during cancer treatment: a controlled clinical trial, *Pain* 48:137, 1992.	Sixty-seven bone marrow transplant patients received (1) hypnosis training; (2) cognitive behavioral coping skills (e.g., relaxation training, cognitive restructuring, information, goal setting, exploration); (3) therapist contact control; or (4) treatment as usual. Patients in groups 1, 2, and 3 received intervention twice before transplant and ten sessions in the hospital.	Hypnosis was effective in reducing reported oral pain for patients undergoing marrow transplantation. Authors concluded that, as hypothesized, hypnosis was effective in reducing persistent pain during cancer treatment. Authors felt that the imagery component of the hypnosis intervention was central to its efficacy; the cognitive behavioral intervention without imagery was not effective; and patients in the cognitive program began, intermittently, to refuse sessions with relaxation alone. Even the patients with hypnosis, when under physical stress, had shortened attention spans and needed briefer inductions and less time spent on relaxation and more time on active, engaging imagery.
Patterson DR, Ptacek JT: Baseline pain as a moderator of hypnotic analgesia for burn injury treatment, *J Consult Clin Psychol* 65(1):60, 1997.	Twenty-seven children enduring bone marrow aspiration and 22 children experiencing lumbar puncture practiced nonhypnotic, distraction techniques or hypnosis for relief of pain and anxiety.	Before intervention, pain during bone marrow aspiration was rated as more painful than lumbar puncture. During bone marrow aspiration, pain was reduced to a large extent by hypnosis (0.001) and to smaller extent by nonhypnotic techniques (0.01). During lumbar puncture, only hypnosis significantly reduced pain (0.001). During bone marrow aspiration, anxiety was reduced only by hypnosis; during lumbar puncture, hypnosis reduced anxiety most (0.001) and, to a lesser degree, by nonhypnotic techniques (0.05).
Burn Pain		
Patterson DR, Ptacek JT: Baseline pain as a moderator of hypnotic analgesia for burn injury treatment, *J Consult Clin Psychol* 65(1):60, 1997.	Sixty-one burn patients were randomly assigned to receive hypnosis or sham hypnosis. Visual imagery of descending a staircase and increasing comfort and relaxation, anchored by touching the patient's shoulder, was used. A shorter version, involving suggestions of descending a staircase, imaging a relaxing place, and anchored with a shoulder touch was used as sham-hypnosis.	Results indicated that the two groups did not differ significantly for their worst pain ratings. However, if highest baseline-pain patients were considered from each group, the hypnosis patients experienced less pain during posttreatment than controls. The possibility that sham-hypnosis served to induce a state of self-hypnosis was a potential flaw in this study.
Fibromyalgia Pain		
Haanen JCM, Hoenderdos HTW, van Romunde LKJ, Hope WCJ, Mallee C, Terwiel JP, Hekster GB: Controlled trial of hypnotherapy in the treatment of refractory fibromyalgia, *J Rheumatol* 18(1):72, 1991.	Forty patients with refractory fibromyalgia were allocated to treatment with hypnotherapy or physical therapy for 12 weeks with follow-up in 24 weeks.	Hypnotherapy patients demonstrated significantly better outcomes in relation to pain experience fatigue on awakening, sleep pattern, and global assessment at 12 and 24 weeks. Somatic and psychic discomfort scores decreased significantly more for hypnosis patients compared with physical therapy patients. Hypnosis may be useful in relieving symptoms in patients with fibromyalgia.

TABLE 8-4	Effects of Hypnosis on Gastric Acid and Duodenal Ulcer Relapse	
AUTHOR	**TYPE OF STUDY**	**FINDINGS**
DUODENAL ULCERS		
Colgan SM, Faragher EB, Whorwell PJ: Controlled trial of hypnotherapy in relapse prevention of duodenal ulceration, *Lancet* 1(8598):1299, 1988.	Thirty patients with rapidly relapsing duodenal ulcers were studied to assess the ability of hypnosis to serve as relapse prevention. Patients were treated with ranitidine until ulcer healing, and another 10 weeks thereafter. Half of patients were taught and practiced hypnosis (i.e., feeling and seeing duodenum warm and acid secretions decrease). Controls received the same medical treatment but no hypnosis.	Both groups were followed for 12 months after completion of treatment. All subjects were confirmed with ulcers by endoscopy, and, similarly, ulcer healing and relapse were confirmed by endoscopy. A direct comparison of 1-year relapse rates for patients demonstrated that 53% of hypnosis patients and 100% of controls relapsed within 1 year.
Klein KB, Spiegel D: Modulation of gastric acid secretion by hypnosis, *Gastroenterology* 96:1383, 1989.	In study one, acid output rose from baseline by 89%. In study two, when compared with the nonhypnotic session, hypnosis produced a 39% reduction in baseline acid output and an 11% reduction in pentagastrin-stimulated peak acid output. Authors concluded that different cognitive states can be induced by hypnosis, which can inhibit or promote gastric acid production—processes clearly controlled by the central nervous system.	In study one, after basal acid secretion was measured, subjects were hypnotized and instructed to imagine all aspects of eating a series of delicious meals. In study two, subjects underwent two sessions of gastric analysis in random order, once with no hypnosis and again with hypnosis to reduce all thoughts of food.

stress reduction techniques also strengthen immune function, most specifically T-cell function. Bacteria in the body are controlled by T-cells. Therefore a strengthening of immune function, leading to the natural destruction of *H. pylori*, may have also been a contributing factor to the differences between groups. It must also be kept in mind that the hypnosis-preventative group was potentially highly motivated to recover and may have practiced the hypnosis techniques more religiously than those in other hypnosis studies.

The early relapse rate in the hypnotherapy subjects in this study was similar to controls, but later the curves demonstrated a much greater separation. The authors concluded that there may have been a subgroup of subjects particularly responsive to therapy. It is possible that the subgroup represented those subjects who were highly hypnotizable.

Irritable Bowel Syndrome

Irritable bowel syndrome (IBS) is defined as the presence of abdominal pain, disordered bowel habit (e.g., diarrhea, constipation or alternating diarrhea and constipation), and abdominal distension. IBS affects about one in seven persons and accounts for up to one half of all outpatient gastroenterologic referrals.[28,50,133,139] Most patients respond to a combination of bulking agents and antispasmodic drugs. Reports of the effects of hypnosis as treatment for IBS have been encour-

> **Points to Ponder** Over time, Whorwell treated 250 patients with hypnosis, with an overall reported improvement rate of 80%. He credits his high success rate with gut-directed imagery—a method whereby the patient directs attention to the inhibition of gastric juice.
> ■

aging.[150,151] A model hypnotherapy intervention with hypnosis includes: (1) patient information of the physiologic model of their disease; (2) hypnosis induced at weekly intervals; (3) therapy targeted at the gut; (4) implementation of daily practice (autohypnosis) and (5) recognition that improvement may take up to 3 months.

Over time, Whorwell treated 250 patients with hypnosis, with an overall reported improvement rate of 80%.[149] He credits his high success rate with gut-directed imagery—a method whereby the patient directs attention to the inhibition of gastric juice. There is clear scientific evidence that gastric secretions can be reduced by hypnosis.[69,131]

A study by Harvey and others of 33 patients with refractory IBS found improvement in 20 of these patients with 11 patients experiencing relief from almost all symptoms[49] (Table 8-5).

Anticipatory and Pregnancy-Induced Nausea

The mechanisms of chemotherapy-induced nausea have been covered in detail in earlier chapters. In essence, when patients undergo chemo-

TABLE 8-5	Effects of Hypnosis on Irritable Bowel Syndrome

AUTHOR	TYPE OF STUDY	FINDINGS
IRRITABLE BOWEL SYMPTOM		
Harvey RF, Hinton RA, Gunay RM, Barry RE: Individual and group hypnotherapy in treatment of refractory irritable bowel syndrome, *Lancet* 25:424, 1989.	Patients with refractory irritable bowel syndrome were treated with four 40-min sessions of hypnotherapy over 7 wks.	Twenty improved, 11 of whom lost almost all symptoms. Short-term improvements were maintained for 3 months without further treatment. Hypnotherapy in groups of up to 8 patients was as effective as individual therapy.
Whorwell PJ, Prior A, Colgan SM: Hypnotherapy in severe irritable bowel syndrome: further experience, *Gut* 28:423, 1987.	Patients with irritable bowel syndrome previously reported as successfully treated with hypnosis were followed for a duration of 18 months (N=15). Another 35 patients were treated and divided into (1) classical cases, (2) atypical cases, and cases exhibiting significant psychologic pathologic conditions.	All 15 patients remained in remission, 2 experienced a single relapse that was overcome by a single session of hypnotherapy. The response rates in the later cases were 95%, 43%, and 60%, respectively. Patients over the age of 50 years responded very poorly (25%), whereas those younger than 50 years with classical irritable bowel syndrome exhibited a 100% response rate. Atypical cases consisted of patients with intractible abdominal pain with little or no abdominal distension or change of bowel habits.
Whorwell PJ, Prior A, Faragher EG: Controlled trial of hypnotherapy in the treatment of severe refractory irritable-bowel syndrome, *Lancet* ii:1232, 1984.	Patients with severe refractory irritable bowel syndrome were randomly allocated to treatment with either hypnotherapy or psychotherapy and placebo.	Psychotherapy patients showed a small but significant improvement in abdominal pain, abdominal distension, and general well being, but no improvement in bowel habit. Hypnotherapy patients showed a dramatic improvement in all features. Differences between groups were highly significant. No relapses were reported at 3-month follow-up in the hypnotherapy group.

therapy as cancer treatment, they experience fatigue, diarrhea, hair loss, and severe nausea and vomiting. After a few months of chemotherapy, some patients develop a conditioned response to their treatments that includes anticipatory nausea; (i.e., they become nauseated in anticipation of treatment).[97] Odors, locations, memories, and persons associated with chemotherapy treatments can all trigger nausea and vomiting. Unfortunately, anticipatory nausea has proven resistant to treatment by antiemetic (nausea-reducing) drugs.[80]

In one study, hypnosis controlled anticipatory nausea and vomiting in six female patients undergoing chemotherapy treatments.[114] Relief provided by hypnosis was replicated across 21 chemotherapy treatments when hypnosis was applied. When three patients trained in hypnosis received one chemotherapy treatment without the aid of hypnosis, the anticipatory nausea and vomiting reappeared.

In another study using hypnosis, 11 of 14 patients experienced less anticipatory nausea and 9 experienced less anticipatory vomiting. Pharmacologic nausea was also reduced in 8 patients, with less vomiting occurring in 5 patients.[146]

Hypnosis also relieves severe nausea and vomiting induced by first-trimester pregnancies. Group hypnosis was found, in one study, to be even more effective than individual hypnotherapy[41] (Table 8-6).

■ Hypnosis and Asthma

A variety of psychosomatic studies have suggested that hypnosis may be useful in the treatment of asthma[3,17,18,26,84,96] (Figure 8-10). Most of these studies lacked a matched control group, or appropriate physiologic or psychologic measurements were not used in the study. None of these earlier studies investigated the effects of hypnosis on bronchial responsiveness. Instead, they may have relied on a decreased awareness of bronchoconstriction—a situation that can jeopardize life if patients delay medical intervention when it is needed.

Treatment of Asthma

Ewer and Stewart, however, did attempt to assess the effects of hypnosis on bronchial hyperresponsiveness with the aid of a methacholine challenge test before and 6 weeks after the learning and practice of hypnosis.[38] Further, two control

TABLE 8-6	Effects of Hypnosis on Chemotherapy-Induced, Anticipatory, and Pregnancy-induced Nausea	
AUTHOR	**TYPE OF STUDY**	**FINDINGS**
CHEMOTHERAPY-INDUCED NAUSEA AND ANTICIPATORY NAUSEA		
Redd WH, Andersen GV, Minagawa RY: Hypnotic control of anticipatory emesis in patients receiving cancer chemotherapy, *J Consult Clin Psychol* 50(1):14, 1982.	Six women suffering from chemotherapy-induced nausea were given two initial training inductions in hypnosis and then patients were hypnotically induced and wheeled into their chemotherapy session. After chemotherapy, patients were wheeled back to the therapist's office and awakened.	Hypnosis suppressed anticipatory vomiting in all patients for all 21 chemotherapy sessions conducted with the aid of hypnosis. Hypnosis was successful regardless of where in the course of chemotherapy hypnosis was introduced. When hypnosis was not used by three patients during one treatment, all three "reverted" and experienced anticipatory vomiting.
Walker LG, Dawson AA, Pollet SM, Ratcliffe MA, Hamilton L: Hypnotherapy for chemotherapy side effects, *Br J Exp Clin Hypn* 5(2):79, 1988.	Fourteen subjects with severe nausea and vomiting after chemotherapy and who also experienced anticipatory nausea and vomiting received hypnosis training and were induced hypnotically before chemotherapy sessions.	Of the 14 patients, 11 reduced anticipatory nausea; 9 reduced anticipatory vomiting; 1 experienced worse anticipatory vomiting, and the remaining patients did not change nor did they worsen with each additional chemotherapy session. After drug administration, 8 patients experienced less nausea, 5 less vomiting, and none worsened. The remaining patients experienced no change of drug-induced nausea and vomiting.
PREGNANCY-INDUCED NAUSEA		
Fuch, K, Paldi E, Abramovici H, Peretz BA: Treatment of hyperemesis gravidarum by hypnosis, *Int J Clin Exp Hypn* 28(4):313, 1980.	Severe nausea and vomiting during the first trimester (hyperemesis gravidarum) were treated with hypnosis; 87 were treated in group sessions and 51 received individual therapy in a hospital setting.	Patients in group therapy improved significantly better than those who received individual treatment. Women in group therapy felt safer and less lonely. The common motivation of those in group sessions appeared to consolidate the psychotherapeutic effect.

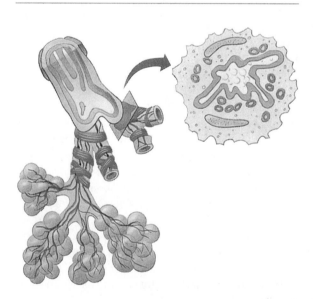

■ *Figure 8-10.* Asthma is an obstructive lung disorder that is characterized by recurring spasms of the smooth muscles in the walls of bronchial air passages. These contractions narrow airways, making breathing difficult. Inflammation is the hallmark of asthma, further obstructing the airways. It is the inflammation component of asthma that is most dangerous. *From Thibodeau GA, Patton KT:* Anatomy and physiology, *ed 4, St Louis, 1999, Mosby.*

groups were used. One control group consisted of low-hypnotizable subjects, and the other control group was made up of persons not receiving hypnosis. The population was mild-to-moderate but not severe asthmatics. Groups were randomized. High-hypnotizable subjects significantly reduced nocturnal symptoms, wheezing, activity limitations, and bronchodilator use, whereas control and low-hypnotizable subjects experienced no change. Further, high-hypnotizable individuals who used hypnosis experienced a 74.9% decrease in bronchial hyperresponsiveness, whereas the two control groups experienced no changes.

Another study, a report to the Research Committee of the British Medical Association, compared hypnosis practice with breathing exercises for relaxation.[115] The hypnosis group significantly reduced wheezing and the use of bronchodilators more than the breathing-relaxation group. Women responded more favorably to hypnosis and less so to the breathing-relaxation exercises. Because there were no differences in forced expiratory volume per second (FEV_1) between groups, it is possible that these differences may have been the result of a reduction in perception of breathing difficulty.

A study by Morrison of 16 patients with chronic asthma compared hospitalization rates and drug usage the year before and after hypnosis treatment.[94] During the year before hypnosis, there were 44 hospital admissions, whereas in the year after, hospitalizations were reduced to 13. For 13 patients, the duration of hospital stays was reduced by 249 days. Prednisolone was withdrawn or reduced in 14 patients, and no patient required a higher prednisolone dose.

In a study by Maher-Loughnan and others, asthmatic patients were assigned to learn hypnosis or to receive a new medi-haler.[84] Although wheezing was reduced by more than 50% for the hypnosis group, no change in eosinophils or any other physical changes were observed. Information was mostly obtained through self-reporting.

Mechanisms Affecting Psychosomatic Response and Cautions

The mechanisms of psychosomatic response in asthma have not been established. One author proposed a model in which a shift in autonomic arousal may induce a change in bronchial sensitivity to local stimuli, such as inhaled allergens or irritants.[108] Anxiety may contribute to this feedback loop, exacerbating asthma bronchoconstriction.[34] Psychosomatic methods may act by decreasing the level of autonomic arousal, deconditioning the primary central stimulus or inhibiting a self-perception feedback loop. Hypnotic suggestion seems to affect large airways, which is consistent with the known distribution of the vagus within the bronchial tree.[116,126] Direct stimulation of the vagus has been shown to induce a heightened response to histamine challenge, whereas atropine and ipratropium both decrease bronchospasm induced by suggestion in patients with mild asthma.

The previous studies address the effects of hypnosis on perceived bronchospasm, but they do not address the inflammatory component of asthma—the critical factor that can mean the difference between life and death. In these studies, neither FEV_1 nor eosinophils were affected by the intervention. Although hypnosis may have affected the inflammatory and bronchospasm components of asthma, it was not demonstrated.

Asthma is an illness that can enter an acute phase with little warning. Patients must respond quickly, and often they must rely on their symptoms as the first signal to respond. Suppressing recognition of those symptoms could be highly dangerous. The use of hypnosis for treatment of asthma must be treated cautiously (Table 8-7). Additional studies assessing the ability of hypnosis to reduce inflammation in asthma are warranted. Although it is probable that targeted imagery used during hypnosis may serve to reduce inflammatory mechanisms, it needs to be clearly demonstrated.

■ Hypnosis and Obesity: Cognitive Behavioral Training

Several studies have been conducted combining hypnosis and behavioral interventions for weight control. In all of these studies the investigators found little if any relationship between hypnotizability and weight loss[25,128,129,145] (Figure 8-11). However, to maximize the hypnotic effects of those persons most likely to benefit from the hypnotic process, one study by Anderson emphasized hypnotic phenomena (e.g., age regression, glove anesthesia, and specialized visualization) accessible primarily to high-hypnotizable individuals.[2] In this intervention, visualization was used in a series of eight suggestions. Subjects lost an average 20.2 pounds. Not surprisingly, high-hypnotizable subjects benefited significantly more from hypnosis (lost more weight) than moderate- and low-hypnotizable subjects. This finding was important because such a relationship supports the specificity of hypnosis as an effective component of weight control.[71]

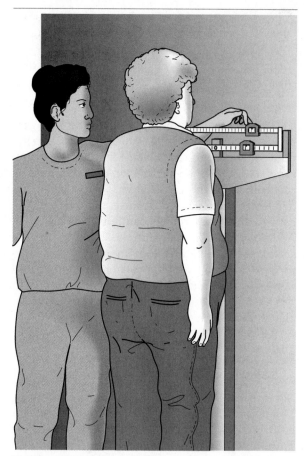

■ **Figure 8-11.** Several studies have been conducted combining hypnosis and behavioral interventions for weight control.

A study by Barabasz and Spiegel attempted to replicate Anderson's findings. This later study added a control group and two comparison hypnosis groups with an improved instrument to identify the higher cognitive levels of trance capacity in those subjects involved in the study.[5] In hypnosis group A, standardized suggestions were used. In hypnosis group B, individualized suggestions, including specific food aversion suggestions for problem foods, were used. Outcomes demonstrated that individualized suggestions appeared to be the most effective method for weight reduction. Further, responsiveness to the therapy was correlated with hypnotizability. The authors hypothesized that hypnosis facilitates the weight loss process by allowing clients to become more absorbed in the broader principle of protecting the body by eating in a healthy pattern.

Another study provided evidence that clients with bulimia were highly hypnotizable, obtaining significantly higher hypnotizable scores than clients with anorexia. This outcome led the authors to conceptualize binge eating as a dissociative process.[4,107]

Points to Ponder   Not surprisingly, high-hypnotizable subjects benefited significantly more from hypnosis (lost more weight) than moderate- and low-hypnotizable subjects. ■

The literature on hypnosis for the treatment of obesity has been fraught with positive reports followed by failed ones. A metaanalysis of six studies using hypnosis for the treatment of obesity concluded that the addition of hypnosis to cognitive behavioral training substantially enhanced treatment outcomes and that the effects were particularly pronounced for treatments of obesity at long-term follow-up. The authors concluded therefore that unlike other weight-loss methods, clients who had used hypnotic inductions continued to lose weight even after treatment ended.[68]

When other authors reassessed the findings of this study and transcription and computational inaccuracies were corrected, the studies yielded a smaller effect size (0.26). The authors concluded that hypnosis as an additive factor to cognitive behavior therapies resulted in a small enhancement of treatment outcomes.

In 1996, Kirsch performed a third metaanalysis of the effect of adding hypnosis to cognitive behavioral treatments for weight reduction, after adding data obtained from the authors of the two studies and after correcting computational inaccuracies of both previous metaanalyses.[66] Averaged mean weight loss was 6.0 pounds without hypnosis and 11.83 pounds with hypnosis. The mean effect size of this difference was 0.66. At the last assessment period, weight loss without hypnosis was 6.03 pounds; weight loss with hypnosis was 14.88 pounds (effect size=0.98). Correlational analyses indicated that the benefits of hypnosis increased substantially with time (r=0.74) and is especially useful for long-term maintenance of weight loss.

One study sought to determine whether client variables (e.g., suggestibility, self-concept, quality of family origin, age of obesity onset, educational level, socioeconomic status, multimodal imagery) would determine the likelihood of successful weight loss.[15] None of the seven variables were significant contributors to weight loss, although individuals practicing hypnosis with or without the aid of audiotapes were significantly more successful than control subjects who did not practice hypnosis (Table 8-8).

Weight loss is a difficult issue to address because food is an ongoing stimulation and because we must eat to maintain life. The temptation to fall back on old habits and the issue of

TABLE 8-7	Effects of Hypnosis on Asthma Symptoms	
AUTHOR	**TYPE OF STUDY**	**FINDINGS**
ASTHMA		
Research Committee of the British Tuberculosis Association: Hypnosis for asthma—a controlled trial, *BMJ* 4(623):71, 1968.	Asthma patients, 10 to 60 years old, with attacks of wheezing and tight chest and capable of relief with bronchodilators. Group 1 was hypnotized monthly and practiced self-hypnosis at home for 1 year. Group 2 practiced breathing exercises for relaxation. N=176 patients from nine chest clinics. Corticosteroid therapy treatment was avoided during the study; 9% of patients were satisfactorily hypnotized.	Both groups showed some improvement of wheezing, need for bronchodilators, and independent clinical assessment. Among men, improvements were similar between groups. However, among women, the hypnosis group showed improvement similar to the men, but those given breathing exercises made much less progress, the difference reaching statistical significance. Independent clinical assessors rated the hypnosis group as "much better" 59% of the time and the control group "much better" 43% of the time. Patients with physicians with previous hypnosis experience did much better than other patients. At year end, hypnosis group used bronchodilators a mean of 17.0 times and controls a mean of 27.7. There were no differences in FEV_1 between groups. Hypnosis group reduced wheezing 52.1% and controls 32.1%, reaching a 0.05 significance difference.
Ewer TC, Stewart DE: Improvement in bronchial hyper-responsiveness in patients with moderate asthma after treatment with a hypnotic technique: a randomized controlled trial, *BMJ* 293:1129, 1986.	Adults with mild to moderate asthma were graded for lower and high susceptibility to hypnosis. Six weeks of hypnosis training and practice followed N=44.	In the 12 high-hypnotizable patients, a 74.9% improvement in degree of bronchial hyperresponsiveness to a standardized methacholine challenge test was observed; nocternal symptoms decreased 62%, peak expiratory flow rates increased 5.5%, wheeze decreased by 53%, and bronchodilator use decreased 26.2%. Controls and patients with low susceptibility to hypnosis had no changes in symptoms or in bronchial hyperresponsiveness.
Morrison JB: Chronic asthma and improvement with relaxation induced by hypnotherapy, *J Royal Soc Med* 81:701, 1988.	Sixteen chronic asthmatic patients inadequately controlled by drugs and suffering from asthma from 2 to 44 years old were hypnotized and given suggestions of reduced wheezing and chest tightening. Patients were asked to practice at home for 5 to 15 minutes, daily.	Approximately 1 year after beginning hypnosis, hospital admission, as compared with the year before, dropped from 44 to 13 days. Duration of stay for 13 patients was reduced by 249 days. Prednisolone was withdrawn in six patients, reduced in eight, and increased in none. Although 62% reported improvement on a visual analogue scale, observations of air flow gave variable results.
Maher-Loughnan GP, MacDonald N, Mason AA, Fry L: Controlled trial of hypnosis in the symptomatic treatment of asthma, *BMJ* ii:371, 1962.	Fifty-seven asthmatics were assigned to hypnosis treatment or control (a new medihaler).	Days with wheezing was reduced for the hypnosis group from 18 to 6 days per month by 6-month follow-up. There was little change in wheezing for controls. No clear-cut physiological changes (eosinophils) were observed from the study.

FEV_1, Forced expiratory volume per second.

the time investment to seek out or prepare appropriate food for weight loss make behavior modification a difficult issue. These studies do suggest, however, that self-monitoring, self-hypnosis with individualized suggestions, and restructuring principles help a client take control of his or her eating habits.

A review of the literature by Cochrane argued that the approach of using hypnosis as the primary therapy of weight reduction is flawed.[14] Obesity is a multifactorial problem. Hypnosis may serve as a valuable adjuvant treatment, but other factors must be included as well. He noted that those persons who succeed in losing weight and keeping it off have a sound knowledge of diet and nutrition, recognize that extreme dieting often fails, and understand the need to exercise regularly and pay attention to diet. One of the most important features of those who succeeded was the sense of personal empowerment, self-worth, and self-esteem. Those who succeeded learned to harness their rebelliousness against the commitment to actions that are necessary to maintain weight successfully.

TABLE 8-8	**Effects of Hypnosis on Weight Loss and Smoking Cessation**	
AUTHOR	**TYPE OF STUDY**	**FINDINGS**

HEALTH BEHAVIOR MANAGEMENT

Weight Loss

AUTHOR	**TYPE OF STUDY**	**FINDINGS**
Barbabasz M, Spiegel D: Hypnotizability and weight loss in obese subjects, *Int J Eat Disord* 8(3):335, 1989.	A controlled study exploring effectiveness of hypnosis in the treatment of obesity. The study also evaluated data methods not previously addressed; e.g., assessment of high cognitive levels of trance capacity as a determinant of hypnotic effectiveness in weight loss management (N=45).	Group 1 simply charted weight loss; group 2 charted and practiced hypnosis with standardized suggestions ("for my body, overeating is poison"), and group 3 practiced hypnosis with individualized suggestions of aversion to problem foods. Group 3 lost significantly more weight than group 1. Group 2 only approached significance as compared with group 1. The differences between groups 2 and 3 were not significant. Group 2 showed only a trend toward a significant correlation between weight loss and hypnotizability, whereas group 3 demonstrated a significant correlation between weight loss and hypnotizability.
Anderson M S: Hypnotizability as a factor in the hypnotic treatment of obesity, *Int J Clin Exp Hypn* 33:150, 1985	This study of hypnosis for weight loss explored the relationships between hypnotizability and weight reduction (N=30). There were eight weekly individual treatment sessions and then 12 weeks of follow-up during which patients practiced hypnosis.	Subjects lost an average of 20.2 pounds. There was a statistically significant positive association between degree of hypnotizability and success at weight reduction. High hypnotizables were significantly more successful at weight loss than medium or low hypnotizables. Note: Eight visualizations were presented, including: (1) See the dinner plate shrink, (2) spontaneously leave food on the plate, (3) regress to a positive effect of physical exercise, (4) glove anesthesia to relieve hunger, and (5) a future picture of thinness.
Cochrane G, Friesen J: Hypnotherapy in weight loss treatment, *J Consult Clin Psychol* 54(4):489, 1986.	Women, ages 20 to 65 and at least 20% overweight were randomized to experimental and control groups. Treatment group 1 consisted of hypnosis plus audiotapes; treatment group 2 practiced hypnosis but had no audiotapes; and the control group received neither hypnosis nor audiotapes (N=60) women.	None of six client variables (suggestibility, self-concept, quality of family origin, age or obesity onset, education level, and socio-economic status) nor one process variable (multimodal imagery) were significant contributors to weight loss. However, both hypnosis groups (with and without audiotape) lost significantly more weight by the 6-month follow-up than the wait-list control group that did not practice hypnosis.

Smoking Cessation

AUTHOR	**TYPE OF STUDY**	**FINDINGS**
Rabkin SW, Boyko E, Shane F, Kaufert J: A randomized trial comparing smoking cessation programs utilizing behavior modification, health education, and hypnosis, *Addict Behav* 9:157, 1984.	140 cigarette smokers were assigned to receive (1) hypnosis, (2) health education, (3) behavior modification, or (4) no treatment.	All three intervention programs significantly reduced smoking as compared with controls. Each program reduced, and equally so, cigarette consumption and serum thiocyanate levels, an indicator of long-term cigarette consumption. Differences were significant as compared with baseline levels and with control group. At 6 months, reported cigarette consumption was not different between the three interventions. Reported cigarette consumption was reduced at least 50% at 3 weeks for the three interventions and 40% at 6 months. Serum thiocyanate fell 30% at the 3-week follow-up.

Problem identification sets the stage for problem resolution, and hypnosis can be beneficial in this area. Hypnotic suggestions related to implementation of the action plan can be helpful. Imagined success; images of a newer, stronger, healthier self; and hypnosis for stress reduction can each play an important part in a comprehensive weight reduction program. Further, high-hypnotizable subjects are better candidates for hypnotic intervention than low-hypnotizable individuals. Assessment of hypnotizability may be a good strategy for persons considering hypnosis for the treatment of obesity.

Hypnosis and Addictive Behaviors: Smoking Cessation

The effectiveness of hypnosis as a treatment to quit smoking has, historically, been difficult to evaluate. Reports are mostly anecdotal, controlled studies are scarce, methodologies are often unsound, information about procedures and results are insufficient for evaluation, and existing reports are often unsystematic and unreplicable. Further, follow-up measures are typically inadequate or lacking altogether.[64]

In 1980, Holroyd reviewed 17 studies of hypnosis (from 1970 to 1979) for smoking cessation. The emphasis of the review was to assess the outcomes of a 6-month program related to total abstinence and to evaluate the variables that contributed to program success or failure. Program success ranged from 4% to 88% reported abstinence at 6 months or longer. Successful programs demonstrating 50% or more success provided the following: (1) several hours of hypnotic treatment; (2) intense interpersonal interaction (e.g., individual sessions, marathon hypnosis, mutual group hypnosis); (3) tailored suggestions to specific motivations of individual patients; and (4) follow-up contact. Tailoring suggestions to specific motivations appeared to be the most critical variable for success. The second most salient variable was the continued supportive contact with phone calls. The studies reviewed were not compared with other forms of smoking cessation interventions. By comparison, a 1976 review of 89 intervention studies comparing hypnosis with other forms of intervention reported that only 30% of persons treated by nonhypnotic interventions remained abstinent after 3 months.[74]

One well-designed program compared and contrasted three separate programs: (1) hypnosis, (2) health education, and (3) behavior modification for efficacy in reducing smoking.[111] Three weeks after program completion, each program showed significant but equal reductions in reported cigarette consumption, as compared with entry data and with a control group. There were no differences among groups in the number of persons who quit smoking, the number of cigarettes smoked, or the change in serum thiocyanate levels. Reported cigarette consumption after 6 months also showed no difference. This study was strengthened by the biomedical assessment of thiocyanate levels, an indicator of cigarette consumption.

One must bear in mind that with few exceptions—monitoring of thiocyanate, for example—research information used to determine success was based purely on self-reporting. Self-report literature has been demonstrated to be highly unreliable, and therefore we must view the studies concluding success with a skeptical eye. Nonetheless, the individual variables that support reported success are worthy of our attention.

Hypnotherapy has been used to treat substance abuse for over a century and is accepted by the American Medical Association (AMA). However, modern practitioners believe that hypnosis alone does not provide a "cure"; rather, it must be used to enhance other modalities.[51,130]

Hypnosis and Treatment of Anxiety and Phobias

Twenty-eight outpatients diagnosed with phobias were treated with hypnosis or systematic desensitization.[85] The patients received one weekly session for 12 weeks. After a 6-week delay, unimproved patients then received twelve sessions of the alternative procedure in a crossover design. In all, 23 patients had desensitization and 18 patients received hypnosis. The patients were rated for symptoms and social adjustment before, during, and after treatment and at 1-year follow-up. Both treatments produced significant improvement in phobias, with desensitization producing a slightly greater improvement in phobias than hypnosis, but only for one set of ratings. Suggestibility correlated only slightly with improvement during hypnosis and insignificantly with desensitization.

Autogenic Training: Form of Hypnosis

Autogenic training is categorized as a self-hypnotic procedure. The role of the instructor is to teach the technique by following a set of six formulas that are repeated and suggest specific autonomic sensations.[76,79] The formulas are as follows:

1. My arm is very heavy (muscular relaxation).
2. My arm is very warm (vascular dilation).
3. My heartbeat is very regular (stabilization of heart function).
4. It breathes me (regulation of breath).
5. Warmth is radiating over my stomach (regulation of visceral organs).
6. There is a cool breeze across my forehead (regulation of blood flow in the head).

Each autogenic formula suggests a somatic function. The images and sensations accompanying each function are those commonly reported by patients in deep relaxation and hypnotic trances. Research has demonstrated that measurable physiologic changes accompany the practice of these imagery exercises.[75,77]

In a review of 24 controlled trials, the authors found that autogenic training was helpful in childbirth, in the treatment of infertility, angina, eczema, headache, and in the rehabilitation from myocardial infarction.[78] They noted that the small number of studies for each condition called for caution. The authors found that autogenic training was associated with medium effect sizes for biological indices of change ($d = 0.43$) and for psychologic and behavioral indices ($d = 0.58$). These effect sizes approximate the effects of biofeedback and muscular relaxation. Length of treatment did not affect clinical outcome.

An Expert Speaks: Dr. Arthur Hastings

Arthur Hastings, PhD, is a faculty member at the Institute of Transpersonal Psychology, a graduate psychology school in Palo Alto, California. He is professor and co-director of the William James Center for Consciousness Studies where he teaches research training, transpersonal theory, and the psychology of hypnosis. He has published works on the relationship of hypnotism to transpersonal psychology and has conducted research on the use of hypnosis to create non–drug altered states and transpersonal experiences. Dr. Hastings' publications include one of the first books on holistic approaches to medicine, *Health for the Whole Person.* Other books include *Argumentation and Advocacy* and *With Tongues of Men and Angels: A Study of Channeling,* a work that reviewers have called the "standard" on this controversial topic. He has written articles on health, communication, semantics, and parapsychology. Dr. Hastings is a former president of the Association for Transpersonal Psychology and has also been dean and President of the Institute of Transpersonal Psychology. Dr. Hastings' personal acquaintance with Charles T. Tart, G.R. Anderson, Milton H. Erickson, and David Cheek has contributed to his knowledge and approach to hypnosis. He and his family live in Mountain View, California.

Question. How did you become interested in the practice of hypnosis?

Answer. From high school days, I was always interested in hypnosis, and I began by reading books such as George Estabrooks' *Hypnotism.* I remember his great story of the hallucinated bear that would not go away. There were no courses in college or graduate school on hypnosis, so I had to learn from the literature and talented hypnotists. At Northwestern University, [I met] Gary Anderson, and later I learned much from Charles T. Tart (Stanford University and UC Davis), who also introduced psychology and the concept of altered states of consciousness as a way of studying hypnosis and other mind-body states. The altered states of consciousness approach developed into one of my specializations in transpersonal psychology. Later, I visited Milton H. Erickson several times, even before he was a "cult" figure. I was there once when he was asked about persons saying that they were doing Ericksonian hypnosis. "I know it," he said, "I can't do anything about it." I would not presume to say I practice Ericksonian hypnosis, but I certainly learned much from him, consciously and, I am sure, unconsciously. I also came to know Dr. David B. Cheek of San Francisco, one of the pioneers in using hypnosis for birth preparation and childbirth and in mind-body medicine. Now, there are more conferences, courses, and workshops in hypnosis, as well as private programs that offer certification and training. Two societies, American Society for Clinical Hypnosis and the International Society for Experimental and Clinical Hypnosis, and many local organizations now make it more possible for professionals to learn hypnosis theory and practice.

Question. Can you describe your current hypnosis practice?

Answer. I consider myself an educator and researcher in hypnosis, and I also have a small private practice. At the Institute of Transpersonal Psychology, I teach courses on the subject and have conducted research using hypnosis to evoke experiential states similar to drug-induced states, but without the drug. In classes, I occasionally include hypnotic mini-sessions to assist students in their preparation of papers and dissertations. My work with individuals covers three areas. One is using hypnosis as an adjuvant for minor and major operations and dental procedures. Patient and doctor reports indicate less anxiety, reduced bleeding during surgery, and more comfortable healing. A second area is using hypnosis with applicants for licensing examinations in psychology, medicine, nursing, law, counseling, and other professions. Here, the intention is to get the person's conscious and unconscious resources to work together, as well as relieve the almost inevitable anxiety. A third area of application is in transpersonal and personal issues, such as performance, exploring personal goals, negative habits, stress, career decisions, and emotional reactions. I find that hypnosis often gives access to the deeper self in terms of purposes, values, insights, and transcendent experiences.

Question. What do you think will be the future of hypnosis as a medical intervention?

Answer. I cannot predict what will emerge, but I can suggest some potential uses of hypnosis that would be beneficial for physicians and for medical treatment. The first is for physicians to learn the basics of hypnotic suggestion and communication. Since patients are often in semitrance states during appointments, doctors can use informal hypnotic communication with patients to influence healing, reassure, improve compliance, and enhance the effects of medication. Nurses can learn hypnotic approaches for use during inpatient care, as well as outpatient treatment. Also, I hope that schools of medicine and hospital in-service courses will offer training in hypnosis for internists and also specializations. This is not everyone's cup of tea as a technique, but basic knowledge of hypnosis also enables referrals for specific treatment. I am sure that anesthesiologists can enhance and direct the effects of anesthetics by using hypnotic instructions in conjunction with regular procedures. Hypnosis can sometimes be used in place of anesthetics when called for because of allergic reactions, but I consider that it is almost always helpful to use it to assist anesthesia and also to facilitate the body's elimination of the anesthetic at the end of the procedure. Surgeons can give hypnotic suggestions during operations that will reduce shock, decrease blood loss, and improve recovery. Psychiatrists will benefit from recognizing hypnotic reactions in patients and from being able to use hypnosis for therapeutic motivation and change. A third area of potential use for hypnosis can be for the physician's personal development. In medical school, hypnotic instructions can facilitate memory, study habits, and focus of attention. In school and in medical practice, doctors can use hypnosis to reduce their stress, to mentally review decisions on diagnosis and treatment, and to protect their own health.

■ Indications and Contraindications

As with any therapy, hypnosis is indicated for some subpopulations and not for others. Hypnosis is most likely to be indicated for:

- Patients motivated to learn and practice hypnosis

- Persons who are moderately to highly hypnotizable
- Patients who have illnesses exacerbated by stress and anxiety
- Patients who are not frightened by the idea of hypnosis and not obsessively concerned with loss of control

Hypnosis may be contraindicated in patients with epileptic seizure disorders and patients with some forms of depression. If these conditions exist, caution must be exercised; specialized skill in the use of hypnosis as therapy for these conditions is required.

■ Chapter Review

In a metaanalysis of 18 studies in which a cognitive behavioral therapy was compared with the same therapy supplemented with hypnosis, results indicated that the addition of hypnosis substantially enhanced treatment outcome.[68] Studies evaluated were for the treatment of pain, insomnia, hypertension, anxiety, obesity, phobias, and ulcers. Clients receiving cognitive behavioral hypnotherapy showed greater improvement than at least 70% of clients receiving nonhypnotic treatment alone.

Based on the review of the literature presented in this chapter, it can be concluded that hypnosis can be a valuable adjuvant therapy for the treatment of pain (e.g., cancer pain, burn pain, surgical pain), for anticipatory nausea, IBS, and duodenal ulcers. The effectiveness of hypnosis for the treatment of obesity and smoking cessation depends on the patient's motivation, hypnotic susceptibility, and the inclusion of hypnosis as a component of a comprehensive cognitive behavioral training program.

To be most effective, hypnotic procedures should be tailored to the needs, personality, and motivations of the individual. Hypnosis is an underused intervention that can, for the appropriate populations, improve quality of life while reducing health care costs. Health care providers and decision makers need to contemplate the expanded use of hypnosis in hospital settings and in outpatient treatment.

> **Points to Ponder**   Based on the review of the literature presented in this chapter, it can be concluded that hypnosis can be a valuable adjuvant therapy for the treatment of pain (e.g., cancer pain, burn pain, surgical pain), for anticipatory nausea, IBS, and duodenal ulcers.   ■

Matching Terms and Definitions

Match each numbered definition with the correct term. Place the corresponding letter in the space provided.

a. Brain lateralization
b. Alpha
c. Beta
d. Theta
e. Delta
f. EEG
g. Frontal lobe
h. Occipital lobe
i. Temporal lobe
j. Parietal lobe
k. Hypnotic susceptibility
l. Congenital ichthyosis
m. Sensory discrimination
n. Motivational-affection
o. Autogenic training

_____ 1. Primary auditory areas
_____ 2. 8 Hz to 13 Hz
_____ 3. Related to capacity to benefit from hypnosis
_____ 4. Sensory areas
_____ 5. 1 Hz to 3 Hz
_____ 6. Primary visual areas
_____ 7. Skin progressively thickens with time
_____ 8. Shift of alpha waves from the left to right hemisphere
_____ 9. Involved in higher-level brain processes like problem solving and planning
_____10. Set of six formulas that are repeated and suggest specific sensations
_____11. Information about the location and intensity of pain
_____12. 4 Hz to 7 Hz
_____13. Aversive affect and negative emotional resonance of pain
_____14. Higher than 13 Hz
_____15. Simple, painless procedure in which 20 wire leads are pasted on the scalp to trace and record the brain's electrical activity

SHORT ANSWER ESSAY QUESTIONS

1. Write a comprehensive review of the historical evolution of hypnosis. Discuss Askelopios, Mesmer, the Marquis de Puysegur, the Abbe Faria, James Braid, James Esdaile, Charles Poyen, Jean-Martin Charcot, and Milton Erickson.
2. Compare and contrast the neodissociation model and the social psychologic model.
3. Describe the pain mechanisms related to hypnosis analgesia.

CRITICAL THINKING AND CLINICAL APPLICATION EXERCISES

1. Discuss the research related to the pain-alleviating effects of hypnosis—spinal effects, endorphin and ACTH findings, and EEG findings of the high-hypnotizable individual. Trace what you believe to be the major pathways from the brain–spinal chord to pain receptors. How do you believe these pathways are fueled, if not by endorphin–natural opiate mechanisms?
2. Hypnosis has been shown to alleviate viral and bacterial-driven conditions, such as warts and duodenal ulcers. Explain how and why you think this occurs.
3. Consider the findings related to relaxation, meditation, and biofeedback. What does hypnosis have in common with these other forms of intervention:
   a. In relation to shared pathways?
   b. In relation to medical research findings?

References

1. Akpinar S, Ulett GA, Itil TM: Hypnotizability predicted by digital computer-analyzed EEG pattern, *Biol Psychol* 3:387, 1971.

2. Anderson M S: Hypnotizability as a factor in the hypnotic treatment of obesity, *Int J Clin Exp Hypn* 33:150, 1985.

3. Aronoff GM, Arooff S, Peck LW: Hypnotherapy in the treatment of bronchial asthma, *Ann Allergy* 34:356, 1975.

4. Barbabasz M: *Bulimia, hypnotizability, and dissociative capacity,* The Hague, The Netherlands, 1988, Paper presented at the 10th International Congress of Hypnosis and Psychosomatic Medicine.

5. Barbabasz M, Spiegel D: Hypnotizability and weight loss in obese subjects, *Int J Eat Disord* 8(3):335, 1989.

6. Barber TX: The effects of hypnosis on pain, a critical review of experimental and clinical findings, *Psychosom Med* 25:303, 1963.

7. Beecher HK: *Measurement of subjective responses: quantitative effects of drugs,* New York, 1959, Oxford University Press.

8. Bennett HL, Davis HS, Gianii JA: Non-verbal response to intra-operative conversation, *Br J Anaesth* 57:174, 1985.

9. Berfield KA, Ray WJ, Newcombe N: Sex role and spatial ability: an EEG study, *Neuropsychology* 24:731, 1986.

10. Blankfield RP: Suggestion, relaxation, and hypnosis as adjuncts in the care of surgery patients: a review of the literature, *Am J Clin Hypn* 33(3):172, 1991.

11. Bloch B: Uber die heilung der warzen durch suggestion, *Klinische Wochenschrift* 6:2271, 1927.

12. Bonke B, Schmitz PIM, Verhage F, Zwaveling A: Clinical study of so-called unconscious perception during general anesthesia, *Br J Anaesth* 58:957, 1986.

13. Braid J: *Braid on hypnotism: the beginnings of modern hypnosis,* New York, 1960, Julian.

14. Cochrane G: Hypnosis and weight reduction: which is the cart and which is the horse? *Am J Clin Hypn* 35(2):109, 1992.

15. Cochrane G, Friesen J: Hypnotherapy in weight loss treatment, *J Consult Clin Psychol* 54(4):489, 1986.

16. Colgan SM, Faragher EB, Whorwell PJ: Controlled trial of hypnotherapy in relapse prevention of duodenal ulceration, *Lancet* 1(8598):1299, 1988.

17. Collison DR: Hypnotherapy in the management of asthma, *Am J Clin Hypn* 11:6, 1968.

18. Cooper AJ: A case of bronchial asthma treated by behavioral therapy, *Int J Psychoanal* 1:351, 1964.

19. Crawford H, Gruzelier J: A midstream view of the neuropsychophysiology of hypnosis: recent research and future direction. In Fromm E, Nash M, editors: *Contemporary hypnosis research,* New York, 1992, Guilford Press.

20. Danziger N, Fournier E, Bouhassira D, Michaud D, De Broucker R, Santarcangelo E, Carli G, Chertock L, Willer JC: Different strategies of modulation can be operative during hypnotic analgesia: a neurophysiological study, *Pain* 75:85, 1998.

21. Davis R: Anesthesia, amnesia, dreams, and awareness, *Med J Aust* 146:4, 1987.

22. DeBenedittis G, Panerai AA, Villamira MA: Effects of hypnotic analgesia and hypnotizability of experimental ischemic pain, *Int J Clin Exp Hypn* 37(1):55, 1989.

23. De Pascalis V, Penna PM: 40-Hz EEG activity during hypnotic induction and hypnotic testing, *Int J Clin Exp Hypn* 38(2):125, 1990.

24. DePascalis V, Silveri A, Palumbo G: EEG asymmetry during covert mental activity and its relationship with hypnotizability, *Int J Clin Exp Hypn* 36:38, 1988.

25. Deyoub PL, Wilkie R: Suggestions with and without hypnotic induction in a weight reduction program, *Int J Clin Exp Hypn* 28:333, 1980.

26. Diamond HH: Hypnosis in children: complete cure of 40 cases of asthma, *Am J Hypn* 1:124, 1959.

27. Domangue BB, Margolis CG, Lieberman D, Haji H: Biochemical correlates of hypnoanalgesia in arthritic pain patients, *J Clin Psychiatry* 46:235, 1985.

28. Drossman DA, Sandler RS, McKee DC, Lovitz AJ: Bowel dysfunction among subjects not seeking health care, *Gastroenterology* 83:529, 1982.

29. Duman RA: EEG alpha-hypnotizability correlations: a review, *Psychophysiology* 14:431, 1977.

30. Editorial: Is your anesthetized patient listening? *JAMA* 206:1004, 1968.

31. Edmondston WE Jr, Grotevant WR: Hypnosis and alpha density, *Am J Clin Hypn* 17:221, 1975.

32. Edmondston WE Jr, Moscovitz HC: Hypnosis and lateralized brain functions, *Inter J Clin Exp Hypn* 38(1):70, 1990.

33. Erickson M, Rossi E: Varieties of hypnotic amnesia. In Rossi E, editor: *The collected papers of Milton H. Erickson on hypnosis. III. Hypnotic investigations of psychodynamic processes,* New York, 1974/1980, Irvington.

34. Erskine-Milliss J, Schonell M: Relaxation therapy in asthma: a critical review, *Psychosom Med* 43:365, 1981.

35. Esdaile J: *Hypnosis in medicine and surgery,* New York, 1946/1957, Julian Press. (Original work published in 1846.)

36. Evans C, Richardson PH: Improved recovery and reduced postoperative stay after therapeutic suggestions during general anesthesia, *Lancet* 27:491, 1988.

37. Evans FJ: Hypnosis and sleep: techniques for exploring cognitive activity during sleep. In Fromm E, Shor RE, editors: *Hypnosis: research developments and perspectives,* London, 1973, Scientific Books.

38. Ewer TC, Stewart DE: Improvement in bronchial hyperresponsiveness in patients with moderate asthma after treatment with a hypnotic technique: a randomized controlled trial, *BMJ* 293:1129, 1986.

39. Ewin DM: Hypnotherapy for warts (Veruca Vulgaris): 41 consecutive cases with 33 cures, *Am J Clin Hypn* 35(1):1, 1992.

40. Fromm E, Nash M: *Contemporary hypnosis research,* New York, 1992, Guilford Press.

41. Fuch, K, Paldi E, Abramovici H, Peretz BA: Treatment of hyperemesis gravidarum by hypnosis, *Int J Clin Exp Hypn* 28(4):313, 1980.

42. Galbraith GC, London P, Leibovitz MP, Cooper LM, Hart JT: Electroencephalography and hypnotic susceptibility, *J Comp Physiol Psychol* 72:125, 1970.

43. Goldman MC: Gastric secretion during a medical interview, *Psychosom Med* 25:351, 1963.

44. Goldmann L, Shah MV, Hebden MW: Memory of cardiac anesthesia. Psychological sequelae in cardiac patients of intra-operative suggestion and operating room conversation, *Anesthesia* 42:596, 1987.

45. Graffin NF, Ray WJ, Lundy R: EEG concomitants of hypnosis and hypnotic susceptibility, *J Abnorm Psychol* 104(1):123, 1995.

46. Green RJ, Reyher J: Pain tolerance in hypnotic analgesic and imagination states, *J Abnorm Psychol* 79:29, 1972.

47. Guerra, G, Guantieri G, Tagliaro F: Hypnosis and plasmatic beta-endorphins. In Waxman D, Misra PC, Gibson M, Basker MA, editors: *Modern trends in hypnosis,* New York, 1985, Plenum.

48. Haanen JCM, Hoenderdos HTW, van Romunde LKJ, Hope WCJ, Mallee C, Terwiel JP, Hekster GB: Controlled trial of hypnotherapy in the treatment of refractory fibromyalgia, *J Rheumatol* 18(1):72, 1991.

49. Harvey RF, Hinton RA, Gunay RM, Barry RE: Individual and group hypnotherapy in treatment of refractory irritable bowel syndrome, *Lancet* 25:424, 1989.

50. Harvey RF, Salih SY, Read AE: Organic and functional disorders in 2000 gastroenterology outpatients, *Lancet* 1:963, 1983.

51. Haxby D: Treatment of nicotine dependence, *Am J Health Sys Pharm* 52(3):265, 1995.

52. Heinze R-I: *Shamans of the 20th Century,* Falls Villages, Conn, 1991, Bramble.
53. Heinze R-I: *Trance and healing in Southeast Asia today,* Berkeley, CA, 1988, White Lotus.
54. Hilgard ER: Dissociation and theories of hypnosis. In Fromm E, Nash M, editors: *Contemporary hypnosis research,* New York, 1992, Guilford Press.
55. Hilgard ER: *Divided consciousness: multiple controls in human thought and action,* New York, 1986, Wiley.
56. Hilgard ER: *Hypnotic susceptibility,* New York, 1965, Harcourt, Brace and World.
57. Hilgard ER: *Psychology in America: a historical survey,* New York, 1987, Harcourt Brace Jovanovich.
58. Hilgard ER, Hilgard JR: *Hypnosis in the relief of pain,* Los Altos, CA, 1975, Kaufman.
59. Howard JF: Incidents of auditory perception during anesthesia with traumatic sequelae, *Med J Aust* 146:44, 1987.
60. Hughes JC, Rothovius AE: *The world's greatest hypnotists,* New York, 1996, University Press of America.
61. Hughes JC, Rothovius AE: *The world's greatest hypnotists,* New York, 1996, University Press of America.
62. Hutchings DD: The value of suggestion given under anesthesia: a report and evaluation of 200 cases, *Am J Clin Hypn* 4:26, 1961.
63. Johnson RF, Barber TX: Hypnosis, suggestions and warts: an experimental investigation implicating the importance of "believed-in efficacy," *Am J Clin Hypn* 20:165, 1978.
64. Johnston E, Donoghue JR: Hypnosis and smoking: a review of the literature, *J Clin Psychol* 13:431, 1971.
65. Kang JY, Piper DW: Cimetidine and colloidal bismuth in treatment of chronic duodenal ulcer, *Digestion* 23:73, 1982.
66. Kirsch I: Hypnotic enhancement of cognitive-behavioral weight loss treatments—another meta-reanalysis, *J Consult Clin Psychol* 64(3):517, 1996.
67. Kirsch I, Council J: Situational and personality correlates of hypnotic responsiveness. In Fromm E, Nash M, editors: *Contemporary hypnosis research,* New York, 1992, Guilford Press.
68. Kirsch I, Montgomery G, Sapirstein G: Hypnosis as an adjunct to cognitive-behavioral psychotherapy: a meta-analysis, *J Consult Clin Psychol* 63:214, 1995.
69. Klein KB, Spiegel D: Modulation of gastric acid secretion by hypnosis, *Gastroenterology* 96:1383, 1989.
70. Knox VJ, Morgan AH, Hilgard ER: Pain and suffering in ischemia: the paradox of hypnotically suggested anesthesia as contradicted by report from the "hidden observer," *Arch Gen Psychiatry* 30:840, 1974.
71. Kroger WS: Comprehensive management of obesity, *Am J Clin Hypn* 12:165, 1970.
72. La Briola F, Karlin R, Goldstein L: EEG laterality changes from prehypnotic to hypnotic periods: preliminary results, *Adv Biolog Psych* 16:1, 1987.
73. Levinson BW: States of awareness during general anesthesia, *Br J Anaesth* 37:544, 1965.
74. Lichtenstein E, Danaher BG: Modification of smoking behavior: a critical analysis of theory, research and practice. In Hersen M, Eisler RM, Miller PM, editors: *Progress in Behavior Modification,* New York, 1976, Academic Press.
75. Lichtenstein KL: *Clinical relaxation strategies,* New York, 1988, Wiley.
76. Linden W: *Psychological perspectives of essential hypertension,* Basel, Switzerland, 1984, S. Karger.
77. Linden W: *Autogenic training: a clinical guide,* New York, 1990, Guilford.
78. Linden W: Autogenic training: a narrative and quantitative review of clinical outcome, *Biofeedback Self Regul* 19(3):227, 1994.
79. Linden W: Self-regulation theory in behavioral medicine. In Linden W, editor: *Biological barriers in behavioral medicine,* New York, 1988, Plenum.
80. Lucas VS, Laszlo J: Tetrahyrocannabinol for refractory vomiting induced by cancer chemotherapy, *JAMA* 243:1241, 1980.
81. MacLeod-Morgan C: EEG lateralization in hypnosis: a preliminary report, *Aust J Clin Exp Hypn* 10:99, 1982.
82. MacLeod-Morgan C: Hemispheric specificity and hypnotizability: an overview of ongoing EEG research in South Australia. In Waxman D, Misra PC, Gibson MC, Basker MA, editors: *Modern trends in hypnosis,* New York, 1985, Plenum.
83. MacLeod-Morgan C: Hypnotic susceptibility, EEG theta and alpha waves, and hemispheric specificity. In Burrows GD, Collinson DR, Dennerstein L, editors: *Hypnosis,* Amsterdam, 1979, Elsevier/North-Holland.
84. Maher-Loughnan GP, MacDonald N, Mason AA, Fry L: Controlled trial of hypnosis in the symptomatic treatment of asthma, *BMJ* ii:371, 1962.
85. Marks IM, Gelder MG, Edwards G: Hypnosis and desensitization for phobias: a controlled prospective trial, *Br J Psychiatry* 114:1263, 1968.
86. Martin DG, Hollanders D, May .J, Ravencroft MM, Tweedle DEF, Miller JP: Difference in relapse rates of duodenal ulcer after healing with cimetidine or tripotassium dicitratobismuthate, *Lancet* I:7, 1981.
87. Mason AA: A case of congenital ichthyosiform erythrodermia of Brocq treated by hypnosis, *BMJ* 422, 1952.
88. McGaugh J: Preserving the presence of the past: hormonal influences on memory storage, *Am Psychol* 38(2):161, 1983.
89. McGlashan TH, Evans FJ, Orne MT: The nature of hypnotic analgesia and placebo response to experimental pain, *Psychosom Med* 31(3):227, 1969.
90. McGlashan TH, Evans FJ, Orne MT: The nature of hypnotic analgesia and placebo response to experimental pain, *Psychosom Med* 31(3):227, 1969.
91. Meszaros I, Banyai E, Greguss AC: *Enhanced right hemisphere activation during hypnosis: EEG and behavioural task performance evidence.* Paper presented at the Third International Conference of the International Organization of Psychophysiology, Vienna, Austria, 1986.
92. Miller K, Watkinson N: Recognition of words presented during general anesthesia, *Ergonomics* 26:585, 1983.
93. Morgan AH, MacDonald H, Hilgard ER: EEG alpha: lateral asymmetry related to task and hypnotizability, *Psychophysiology* 11:275, 1974.
94. Morrison JB: Chronic asthma and improvement with relaxation induced by hypnotherapy, *J Royal Soc Med* 81:701, 1988.
95. Nasrallah HA, Holley T, Janowsky DS: Opiate antagonism fails to reverse hypnotic-induced analgesia, *Lancet* 1(8130):1355, 1979.
96. Neinstein LS, Dash J: Hypnosis as an adjunct for asthma, *J Adolesc Health* 3:45, 1982.
97. Nesse RM, Carli T, Curtis GC, Kleinman PD: Pretreatment nausea in cancer chemotherapy, *Psychosom Med* 42:33, 1980.
98. Nicholson S: *Shamanism,* London, 1987, Theosophical Publishing House.
99. Nowlis DP, Rhead JC: Relation of eyes-closed resting EEG alpha activity to hypnotic susceptibility, *Percept Mot Skills* 27:1047, 1968.
100. Olness K, Wain HJ, Lorenz NG: A pilot study of blood endorphin levels in children using self-hypnosis to control pain, *J Dev Behav Pediatr* 4:187, 1980.
101. Orne MT: The nature of hypnosis: artifact and essence, *J Abnorm Child Psychol* 58:277, 1959.
102. Patterson DR, Ptacek JT: Baseline pain as a moderator of hypnotic analgesia for burn injury treatment, *J Consult Clin Psychol* 65(1):60, 1997.
103. Pearson RE: Response to suggestions given under general anesthesia, *Am J Clin Hypn* 4:106, 1961.

104. Perlini A, Spanos N: EEG alpha methodologies and hypnotizability: a critical review, *Psychophyology* 28:511, 1991.
105. Perry S, Heidrich G: Management of pain during débridement: a survey of U.S. burn units, *Pain* 12:26, 1982.
106. Perry S, Heidrich G, Ramon E: Assessment of pain in burn patients, *J Burn Care Rehabil* 2:322, 1981.
107. Pettenati HM, Horne RL, Staats JM: Hypnotizability in patients with anorexia nervosa and bulimia, *Arch Gen Psychiatry* 42:1014, 1985.
108. Phillip RL, Wilde GJS, Day JH: Suggestion and relaxation in asthmatics, *J Psychosom Res* 16:193, 1972.
109. Piccione C, Hilgard E, Zimbardo P: On the degree of stability of measured hypnotizability over a 25-year period, *J Pers Soc Psychol* 56:289, 1989.
110. Ptacek JT, Everett JE, Patterson DR, Montgomery BM, Heimbach DR: Pain, coping and adjustment in patients with burns: preliminary summary findings from a prospective study, *J Pain Symptom Manage* 10:446, 1995.
111. Rabkin SW, Boyko E, Shane F, Kaufert J: A randomized trial comparing smoking cessation programs utilizing behavior modification, health education, and hypnosis, *Addict Behav* 9:157, 1984.
112. Ray WJ: EEG concomitants of hypnotic susceptibility, *Int J Clin Exp Hypn* XLV(3):301, 1997.
113. Ray WJ, Cole HC: EEG alpha activity reflects attentional demands, and beta activity reflects emotional and cognitive processes, *Science* 228:750, 1985.
114. Redd WH, Andersen GV, Minagawa RY: Hypnotic control of anticipatory emesis in patients receiving cancer chemotherapy, *J Consult Clin Psychol* 50(1):14, 1982.
115. Research Committee of the British Tuberculosis Association: Hypnosis for asthma—a controlled trial, *BMJ* 4(623):71, 1968.
116. Richardson JB: Innervation of the lung, *Eur J Resp Dis* 117:237, 1981.
117. Rossi EL: Hypnosis and ultradian cycles. A new state(s) theory of hypnosis? *Am J Clin Hypn* 25:21, 1982.
118. Rossi EL: *The psychobiology of mind-body healing: new concepts of therapeutic hypnosis,* New York, 1993, Norton.
119. Rulison RH: Warts: a statistical study of nine hundred and twenty-one cases, *Arch Dermatol Syphilol* 46:66, 1942.
120. Sabourin M: Hypnosis and brain function: EEG correlates of state-trait differences, *Res Commun Psychol Psych Behav* 7:149, 1982.
121. Sabourin M, Cutcomb SD, Crawford HJ, Pribham K: EEG correlates of hypnotic susceptibility and hypnotic trance: spectral analysis and coherence, *Int J Psychophysiol* 10:125, 1990.
122. Shor RE: On the physiological effects of painful stimulation during hypnotic analgesia: basic issues for further research. In Estabrooks GH, editor: *Hypnosis: current problems,* New York, 1962, Harper.
123. Shor RE: Physiological effects of painful stimulation during hypnotic analgesia under conditions designed to minimize anxiety, *Int J Clin Exp Hypn* 10:183, 1962.
124. Silva C, Kirsch I: Interpretive sets, expectancy, fantasy proneness, and dissociation as predictors of hypnotic response, *J Pers Soc Psychol* 63:847, 1992.
125. Spanos N, Cow W: A social psychological approach to hypnosis. In Fromm E, Nash M, editors: *Contemporary hypnosis research,* New York, 1992, Guilford Press.
126. Spector S, Luparello TJ, Kopetzky MT, Souhrada J, Kinsman RA: Response of asthmatics to methacholine and suggestion, *Am Rev Resp Dis* 113:43, 1976.
127. Spiegel D, Blo JR: Group therapy and hypnosis reduce metastatic breast carcinoma pain, *Psychosom Med* 45(4):333, 1983.
128. Spiegel H, Spiegel D: *Trance and treatment: clinical uses of hypnosis,* New York, 1978, asic Books.
129. Stanton HE: Weight loss through hypnosis, *Am J Clin Hypn* 18:94, 1975.
130. Stoil M: Problems in the evaluation of hypnosis in the treatment of alcoholism, *J Subst Abuse* 6:31, 1989.
131. Stratcher G, Berner P, Naske R et al: Effect of hypnotic suggestion of relaxation on basal and betazole-stimulated gastric acid secretion, *Gastroenterology* 68:656, 1975.
132. Surman OS, Gottlieb SK, Hackett TP, Silverberg EL: Hypnosis in the treatment of warts, *Arch Gen Psychiatry* 28:439, 1973.
133. Switz DM: What the gastroenterologist does all day, *Gastroenterology* 70:1048, 1976.
134. Syrjala KL, Cummings C, Donaldson GW: Hypnosis or cognitive behavioral training for the reduction of pain and nausea during cancer treatment: a controlled clinical trial, *Pain* 48:137, 1992.
135. Tebecis AK, Provins KA, Farnbach RW, Pentany: Hypnosis and the EEGA: a quantitative investigation, *J Nerv Ment Dis* 161:1, 1975.
136. Tellegen A, Atkinson G: Openness to absorbing and self-altering experiences ("absorption"), a trait related to hypnotic susceptibility, *J Abnorm Psychol* 83:268, 1974.
137. Thibodeau GA, Patton KT: *Anatomy and physiology,* ed 3, St Louis, 1996, Mosby.
138. Thompson DG, Richelson E, Malagelada JR: Pertubation of upper gastrointestinal function by cold stress, *Gut* 24:277, 1983.
139. Thompson WG, Heaton KW: Functional bowel disorders in apparently healthy people, *Gastroenterology* 79:283, 1980.
140. Tomarken A, Davidson R, Henriques J: Resting frontal brain asymmetry predicts affective responses to films, *J Pers Soc Psychol* 59:791, 1990.
141. Twain M: *The Adventures of Tom Sawyer,* New York, 1936, Heritage Press.
142. Ulett GA, Akpinar S, Itel TM: Hypnosis: physiological, pharmacological reality, *Am J Psychiatry* 128:799, 1972.
143. Veith I: *Hysteria: the history of a disease,* Chicago, 1965, University of Chicago Press.
144. Vogel W, Broverman DM, Klaiber EL: EEG and mental abilities, *Electroencephalogr Clin Neurophysiol* 24:166, 1968.
145. Wadden T.A, Flaxman J: Hypnosis and weight loss: a preliminary study, *Int J Clin Exp Hypn* 29:162, 1981.
146. Walker LG, Dawson AA, Pollet SM, Ratcliffe MA, Hamilton L: Hypnotherapy for chemotherapy side effects, *Br J Exp Clin Hypn* 5(2):79, 1988.
147. Wall PD: The physiology of controls on sensory pathways with special reference to pain. In Chertok L, editor: *Psychophysiological mechanisms of hypnosis,* Berlin-Heidelberg, 1969, Springer-Verlag.
148. White R: *Personal communication,* 1998.
149. Whorwell PJ: Use of hypnotherapy in gastrointestinal disease, *Br J Hosp Med* 45:27, 1991.
150. Whorwell PJ, Prior A, Colgan SM: Hypnotherapy in severe irritable bowel syndrome: further experience, *Gut* 28:423, 1987.
151. Whorwell PJ, Prior A, Faragher EG: Controlled trial of hypnotherapy in the treatment of severe refractory irritable-bowel syndrome, *Lancet* ii:1232, 1984.
152. Wolfe LS, Millett JB: Control of post-operative pain by suggestions under general anesthesia, *Am J Clin Hypn* 3:109, 1960.
153. Wormsley KG: Relapse of duodenal ulcers, *BMJ* 293:1501, 1986.

9

Imagery

Lyn W. Freeman

WHY READ THIS CHAPTER?

Imagery is the foundation of mind-body medicine. It is the essential and activating element in the clinical use of relaxation therapy, meditation, biofeedback, and hypnosis. Imagery, in the forms of placebo and event-interpretation, also affects quality of life and health outcomes every day.

The effective incorporation of imagery into any intervention requires that the clinician have a thorough understanding of the way the body functions in relation to the health condition being addressed. He or she must also understand the types of imagery used in interventions, how these varying types affect the body biochemically and hormonally, and how to facilitate imagery sessions that are biologically accurate yet represent the individual's personal expressiveness. The effects of imagery are subtle but powerful. This chapter gives the health professional an overview of what must be considered in the effective use of imagery as intervention.

CHAPTER AT A GLANCE

Imagery is the thought process that invokes and uses the senses. These include vision, sound, smell, and taste, and the senses of movement, position, and touch. Virtually nothing exists in our experience that we do not image in some way, and those images can produce physiologic, biochemical, and immunologic changes in the body that affect health outcomes.

Most typically, when imagery procedures are used for clinical or experimental purposes, they fall into one of three categories: diagnostic imagery, mental rehearsal imagery, and end-state imagery. These forms and their combined clinical uses are described in this chapter.

Imagery has been found beneficial in the treatment of eczema, acne, diabetes, breast cancer, arthritis, migraine and tension headaches, and severe burns. Imagery has also been used as treatment to improve lactation in mothers of premature infants, to increase coping skills with birth pain, and as intervention with anticipatory grief.

Research strongly suggests that imagery is capable of altering specific immune parameters, hormonal responses, and immune cell migration. Further, imagery assessment tools have been used to assess treatment for cancer, spinal pain, and diabetes and have been proven highly accurate as predictors of treatment outcomes. Imagery is the foundation of mind-body medicine. It is a powerful tool that, when used effectively, can assist in healing the mind, body, and spirit.

The image is more than an idea. It is a vortex or cluster of fused ideas and is endowed with energy.

EZRA POUND. SELECTED PROSE, 1909-1965, "AFFIRMATIONS—AS FOR IMAGISME" (WILLIAM COOKSON, EDITOR, 1973)

CHAPTER OBJECTIVES

After completing this chapter, you should be able to:

1. Define imagery.
2. Define, compare, and contrast diagnostic imagery, mental rehearsal imagery, and end-state imagery.
3. Explain how and why imagery is a critical factor in the practices of relaxation therapy, meditation, biofeedback, and hypnosis.
4. Summarize the findings concerning the biochemical and hormonal effects of imagery.
5. Summarize the findings of the beneficial effects of imagery as treatment for disease and illness.
6. Describe how a clinician and patient can prepare for the effective use of imagery.

■ What Is Imagery and What Does It Do?

Imagery is the thought process that invokes and uses the senses. These include vision, sound, smell, and taste, and the senses of movement, position, and touch.[1] Based on neurologic and psychologic models and on research, imagery can be considered a doorway to conscious reality[33] (Figure 9-1). In fact, imagery representations are stored as memories so that each person can tap into related emotions at any time and experience them all over again.

Imagery can powerfully affect a person in emotional and physical ways. For victims of crime, continually reliving—imaging—a traumatic event can lead to chronic depression and anxiety. The recalled events elicit imagery that evokes the same responses—emotional, mental, physiologic, and biochemical—that were experienced during the originating events.

■ History of Imagery

As discussed in earlier chapters, healing practices have existed throughout history that use the mind and imagination to heal the body. Even though dreams and visions were universally the most common methods for inquiring into the cause and cure of disease, these practices were most systematically incorporated into standard medical practices during the Grecian era.[1] In the Asclepian temples of Greece, imagery was evoked in a state of consciousness that occurred in a lucid state just before sleep (Figure 9-2). During this phase, images flow forth with great ease. This lucid sleep phase is referred to as *hypnogogic sleep*. There is some evidence that even major surgery was occasionally performed while patients were in this state of consciousness. This was, perhaps, the precursor to what is known today as hypnotic imagery. The blind, lame, and deaf, and

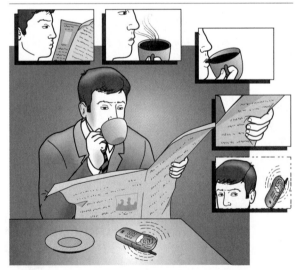

■ *Figure 9-1.* Imagery is much more than visualization. Imagery uses the senses of vision, sound, smell, and taste, and the senses of movement, position, and touch. Imagery is a doorway to conscious reality. What we image can be translated into changes in individual biochemistry, physiology, immunology and health outcomes.

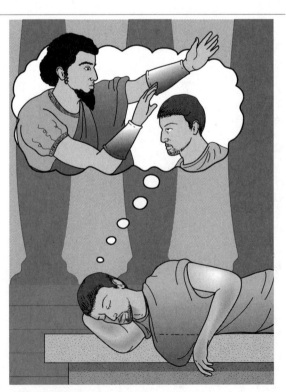

■ *Figure 9-2.* The Asclepian dream state.

those who were ill left written descriptions of their temple cures.[1]

Aristotle, Hippocrates, and Galen were trained in the Asclepian method of imagery and all could articulate its role in healing. Aristotle stated that physicians of his day paid diligent attention to the dreams of their patients. Galen believed that the content of a patient's dreams offered clinically important diagnostic information.

Dream images and imagery in general are important components of modern-day psychotherapy. Imagery is, quite simply, the conveyor of the messages that result in physiologic, biochemical, and emotional change in the body. The history of imagery can also be traced throughout the histories of meditation, relaxation practices, hypnosis, and biofeedback (see previous chapters).

■ Physiology and Mechanisms of Imagery

It will come as no surprise to the discerning reader that the first eight chapters of the book have already introduced the majority of the physiology, mechanisms, and research outcomes related to imagery.

Chapter 1 reviews the physiology of how our interpretation of events (our imagery) affects the hypothalamic-pituitary-adrenal (HPA) cortex pathway and the sympathetic-adrenal medullary (SAM) pathway, resulting in biochemical and hormonal changes. These changes have powerful implications for health outcomes.

Chapter 2 reviews the four lines of evidence— observational, physiologic, epidemiologic, and clinical—of the mind's influence on the body. These influences are produced by our interpretation of and reaction to internal imagery.

Chapter 3 introduces the reader to the field of psychoneuroimmunology (PNI) and the conditioning of immune function. Conditioning of immunity is often elicited by the pairing of an emotional or a mental event with a biochemical or physiologic event. Imagery is often the evocative factor— the catalyst—in these conditioning events.

Chapter 4 describes how relationships and life events affect our health or, more accurately, how our interpretation and experience of these events alter health status. For example, in the case of divorce, the effect on immune function can depend on which person chose to leave and which one did not. Divorce may result in immune enhancement for the person initiating the separation, whereas it can result in immune suppression for the person interpreting this event as abandonment and loss.

Chapters 5 through 8—relaxation, meditation, biofeedback, and hypnosis—describe the clinical techniques used to invoke purposefully the physiologic and biochemical changes in the body. Without imagery, these clinical techniques would be ineffectual.

Because the research studies and clinical outcomes of imagery used during relaxation, meditation, biofeedback, and hypnosis were reviewed previously, these findings will not be repeated here. Rather, the emphasis will be on studies that deepen our understanding of how different types of imagery, offered in specific ways, modify bodily processes. This chapter also emphasizes the critical importance of applying this understanding to all mind-body interventions.

■ Pervasiveness of Imagery

It has been stated by researchers, as well as clinicians who use imagery in their practices, that virtually nothing exists in our experience that we do not image in some way (Figure 9-3). It has been argued that every voluntary behavior is preceded by an image of what will occur. Our emotions are also preceded and accompanied by images. In fact, the field of sports psychology is built on the premise that the body-mind does not know the difference between an actual event and an imaged one.[13]

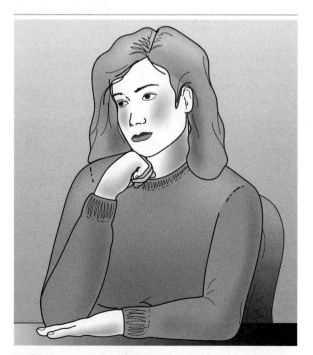

■ **Figure 9-3.** Virtually nothing exists in our experiences that we do not image in some way.

Imagery is acknowledged as the critical factor in biofeedback that allows subjects to learn to alter physical responses.[24] Green and Green refer to biofeedback as an "imagery trainer." One study found that individuals who were unable to fantasize, could not remember dreams, or were not particularly creative had the most difficulty learning to elicit a biofeedback response.[6]

■ Imagery in Current Day Health Practices

Imagery is the very foundation of all mind-body interactions and effects. In fact, imagery plays a critical role in all health care, even the most orthodox Western medical practices. The diagnosis and communication between patient and physician and the images invoked by these interactions have powerful effects on health outcomes. For example, a patient with asthma experienced exacerbations of her asthma every time she visited her physician. On one occasion, she experienced a severe attack within hours of leaving the physician's office, which resulted in hospitalization. When questioned about this, she stated that her physician was often unresponsive or critical of her during their visits. On the visit that resulted in hospitalization, the physician lectured her harshly, accusing her of failing to follow orders diligently. Even though this patient could think of no way in which she failed to follow instructions, she blamed herself for her worsening condition and began to cry in the car on the way home. Within hours, her asthma condition had deteriorated in spite of all attempts to control the attack with medication. This client was older and believed that she should never question a physician; rather, she thought she should simply comply with medical instructions. After some counseling, this patient reviewed the effects of her physician's attitudes on her health and decided to seek another specialist. Her asthma condition improved and became more manageable over the following months.

■ Imagery and Placebo Effect

Positive imagery, often in the form of the placebo effect, can also heal. The placebo effect refers to actual biochemical, physiologic, and symptom changes that occur in the body because the person believes a substance, an event, or a person can produce healing effects. For example, belief in the power of a tribal healer to heal can improve health outcomes. Belief can produce physiologic changes in response to a sugar pill presented to the patient as a potent medication.

The placebo effect has been reported to account for healing in 30% to 70% of all drug and surgical interventions. Repair of injured tissues has also been enhanced by placebo. The active properties of drugs can actually be altered by the placebo effect.[59] A pregnant woman, suffering from morning sickness, was given ipecac, a strong and well-known emetic that is used to induce vomiting in those who have swallowed poison. She was told the "medication" would eliminate her morning sickness. The woman experienced the elimination of her nausea and vomiting symptoms in response to ipecac, even though this drug typically induces severe vomiting and nausea when ingested.

■ How Imagery Effects Can Differ

Imagery has been found beneficial in the treatment of eczema, acne, birth pain, diabetes, breast cancer, arthritis, migraine and tension headaches, and severe burns.[3,4,6,17,23,26,29,36] A few of these studies are reviewed in this chapter, but, most importantly, we explore the more subtle nature of imagery. For example, imagery that reduces anxiety and imagery that reinforces coping skills can produce different hormonal changes.

Targeted imagery—imagery in which the patient is taught the actual processes by which the body produces a physiologic change and then images that exact process—can produce extremely exacting outcomes. For example, a person can be taught to increase the output of a particular immunoglobulin, to speed up wound healing, or to teach the brain to fire specific neurons. Targeted imagery requires the patient to understand fully what outcome is desired and to craft imagery that will produce the desired outcome.

Although eloquent and accurate imagery can produce desired results, inaccurate or misleading

Points to Ponder   Imagery is the very foundation of all mind-body interactions and effects. In fact, imagery plays a critical role in all health care, even the most orthodox Western medical practices. ■

Points to Ponder   Imagery has been found beneficial in the treatment of eczema, acne, birth pain, diabetes, breast cancer, arthritis, migraine and tension headaches, and severe burns. ■

Points to Ponder   Although eloquent and accurate imagery can produce desired results, inaccurate or misleading imagery can produce the exact opposite of what is desired.   ■

imagery can produce the exact opposite of what is desired. Therefore an understanding of imagery and its relationship to physiologic change is an absolute necessity for its proper use in relaxation, meditation, biofeedback, or hypnosis interventions.

■ Types of Imagery Used for Clinical Intervention

Imagery has been classified in a variety of ways. It has been categorized as cellular imagery (i.e., imagery used for strengthening the immune system); physiologic imagery (i.e., imagery intended to affect the cardiovascular system); psychologic imagery (i.e., imagery for maintaining emotional resiliency); and relationship imagery (i.e., imagery for healing personal associations).[41] Lawlis emphasizes what is known as vision quest imagery, that is, imagery related to the person's life story and personal myth of empowerment. This type of imagery strengthens the person's journey to wholeness in an integrated, meaningful, and personal manner.[33]

Most typically, when imagery procedures are used for clinical or experimental purposes, they fall into one of three categories:
1. Diagnostic imagery
2. Mental rehearsal imagery
3. End-state imagery[1]

Diagnostic Imagery

Diagnostic imagery is valuable because it provides the information needed to design individualized and meaningful imagery sessions for each client. The client is asked to describe how he or she feels in sensory and emotional terms. This information is then used to design mental rehearsal or other therapeutic interventions that are specific to the person and to his or her condition.

Mental Rehearsal Imagery

Mental rehearsal is an imagery technique often used to prepare the patient for medical procedures (Figure 9-4). Mental rehearsal imagery is used to relieve anxiety, pain, and side effects that are exacerbated by heightened emotional reactions. For example, surgical procedures, burn débridement, or childbirth may be rehearsed

before the event so the patient is emotionally and mentally prepared for what is to come.

Typically, a relaxation strategy is taught, then the treatment and recovery period are described in sensory terms while the patient takes a "guided imagery trip." Care is taken to be factual, to avoid emotionally laden or fear-provoking words, and to reframe the medical procedure in a realistic but positive light. Other coping techniques such as distraction, mental dissociation, muscle relaxation, and abdominal breathing may be practiced as part of the imagery application.

Published outcomes from research on mental rehearsal imagery are almost uniformly positive and include significant reductions in pain and anxiety, length of hospital stays, pain medication use, and reported side effects.

End-State Imagery

End-state imagery is a technique intended to produce a specific physiologic or biological change in the body (Figure 9-5). For example, imagery may be used to reduce sympathetic nervous system arousal; to enhance immune function; or to calm a hyperreactive immune response. In these situations, a healthier functioning of a physiologic or biological process is "targeted."

Physiologic and biochemical end-state imagery has been used successfully to alleviate nausea induced by chemotherapy or pregnancy; to facilitate weight gain in patients with cancer; to control surgical, chronic, and acute pain; and as an adjuvant therapy for a variety of diseases, including diabetes. End-state imagery has also been found to enhance immunity in the geriatric population and, in combination with other behavioral programs, has been found to mobilize immune function in

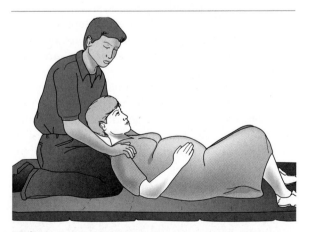

■ **Figure 9-4.** Childbirth preparation is one way in which mental rehearsal is used to reduce anxiety, increase perceived coping, and reduce pain.

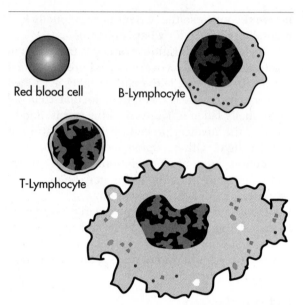

■ *Figure 9-5.* End-state imagery is often used to target changes in immune function, as occurs with cancer and asthma patients.

Points to Ponder   To affect change in a particular body system, we must intervene somewhere inside that system. Points of entry are our perceptions, our emotions, our cognitions, and our experience of sensation—in other words, our images.

patients with cancer. It has also been used as part of a cardiac rehabilitation program. (This research is reviewed in earlier chapters as part of research interventions using relaxation, meditation, hypnosis, and biofeedback.)

Imagery is the driving mechanism that allows these various interventions to work. To affect change in a particular body system, we must intervene somewhere inside that system. Points of entry are our perceptions, our emotions, our cognitions, and our experience of sensation—in other words, our images.

Many of the concepts of imagery were lost to medicine in the nineteenth and twentieth century because imagery was considered unscientific. However, the scientific study of the placebo effect (i.e., actual biochemical and physiologic changes and symptom changes occurring because of belief) led to recognition of the power of the mind and of imagery.

Finally, the explosion of the field of PNI, beginning with Ader and Cohen's 1981 text and the scientific studies of the pathways of mind-body communication, has brought imagery to the

forefront again (see Chapter 3). Today, the working hypothesis of imagery and its research component, PNI, is that for every change of the mind, emotion, and body, there is a preceding or concomitant image, whether conscious or unconscious. As a result, emotions, thoughts, behaviors, bodily reactions, and autonomic physiologic functions are accompanied or preceded by imagery.

■ Effects of Imagery on Physiology and Biochemistry

In previous chapters, we describe the effects of imagery on specific health outcomes. In this chapter, we review studies that describe some of the biochemical changes imagery is capable of producing, based on the nature of the imagery. Imagery has been demonstrated to alter certain immune parameters. These include salivary immunoglobulin in both adults and children and T-cell responses. Imagery has been demonstrated to alter cortisol (an immunosuppressant agent) and corticosteroid levels in response to stressful events, such as surgery and night-shift work. Imagery has even been found capable of altering cellular migration patterns.

You will notice in these studies that the more directed or targeted the imagery, the more specific the effects. In addition, you will observe how imagery that alters mood state or perception—an increase in perceived control or attempts to decrease anxiety, for example—produce differing biochemical effects. The preparation of imagery for different populations must also be carefully crafted. You will notice the different imagery strategies used for children as compared with adults. The image IS the message. In the following text, we review varying imagery strategies used for different populations and outcomes.

Salivary Immunoglobulin A in Children

In one case, 57 healthy children were selected to determine whether 6- to 12-year-old children could increase salivary immunoglobulin A (IgA) by practicing biologically targeted imagery. In this case, the specific imagery used reflected how the body actually produces salivary IgA.

The children were first shown a videotape entitled, "The Toymaker's Magic Microscope." This videotape used puppets to explain bacteria, viruses, and basic immune system components. The children were then introduced to the use of generalized relaxation and imagery audiotapes. Saliva samples were taken at baseline and before relaxation and imagery to assess normal levels of IgA.

At a session 2 weeks later, saliva samples and peripheral temperatures were taken at baseline. The children were then randomized into one of three groups. The children in group A listened to a relaxation tape and were given nonspecific imagery instructions, but they were told these instructions would increase immune substances. The children in group B listened to the same relaxation tape, but they were given very specific imagery instructions about how the body would increase salivary IgA. The children in Control group C engaged in conversation for the same 25-minute period that the other children practiced relaxation and imagery.

Specimens of saliva were taken again at the end of the imagery sessions. Baseline levels of IgA remained stable between the introductory session and the later session.

At the second session, IgA concentrations before and after relaxation and imagery practice were significantly different for group B only (the specific imagery group). There were no significant differences between baseline and before-imagery IgA levels for group A (the nonspecific imagery group) or group C (the control group). The results indicated that biologically targeted imagery alone resulted in significant increases in the specific immune component of salivary IgA (p<0.01).

Salivary Immunoglobulin A in Adults

In a similar but longer-term study, 45 college students were assigned to one of three groups. Group 1 received educational training on how secretory IgA was produced.[45] Photographs and drawings of B-cells migrating out of bone marrow and plasma cells producing and secreting hundreds of thousands of antibody molecules were used in the training sessions. The double Y–shape of the salivary IgA molecule was strongly emphasized (Figures 9-6 and 9-7).

Group 1 then listened to a 17-minute audiotape of specific imagery instructions with specially composed background entrainment music designed to enhance imagery. Group 2 listened to the same music, but those in this group received nondirected imagery, (i.e., they focused on non–immune-related imagery generated without direction). Group 3, a control group, experienced 17

minutes of no activity. All three groups were tested for salivary IgA before and after the 25-minute exercise. Groups 1 and 2 were then given audiotapes of their relaxation and imagery process and asked to listen to the tapes every other day for 6 weeks.

At the initial trial, groups 1 and 2 produced significantly more salivary IgA than the control group, but neither group produced significantly more than the other. In trial 2 (3 weeks into the practice sessions), both groups 1 and 2 again increased salivary IgA significantly more than the control group, but this time group 1 (the specific imagery group) also increased salivary IgA significantly more than group 2 (the nonspecific imagery, [p<0.008]). At trial 3 (6 weeks into the practice sessions), groups 1 and 2 again produced significantly more salivary IgA than group 3, and group 1 once again increased salivary IgA significantly more than group 2 (p<0.03).

The authors concluded that, in adults, 3 weeks of imagery training is needed before significant differences in salivary IgA emerge between relaxation and nonspecific imagery practice and relaxation and targeted imagery practice.

The differences in salivary IgA concentrations were apparently not affected by skin temperature, since there were no group differences on this physiologic measure. Since temperature changes reflect physiologic relaxation, relaxation alone was not responsible for changes in salivary IgA in groups 1 and 2. The imagery produced the differing effects, which is an important point since relaxation alone has also been demonstrated to enhance immune function.

Conclusions From Salivary Immunoglobulin A Studies

These studies suggest that children are more immediately susceptible to imagery as a method for altering certain parameters of immune function, but adults can also be "trained" to modulate immune function when more practice is provided. These types of outcomes are not surprising, since children are more open, imaginative, and responsive to their beliefs than adults.

Points to Ponder   The results indicated that biologically targeted imagery alone resulted in significant increases in the specific immune component of salivary IgA.

Points to Ponder   These studies suggest that children are more immediately susceptible to imagery as a method for altering certain parameters of immune function, but adults can also be "trained" to modulate immune function when more practice is provided.

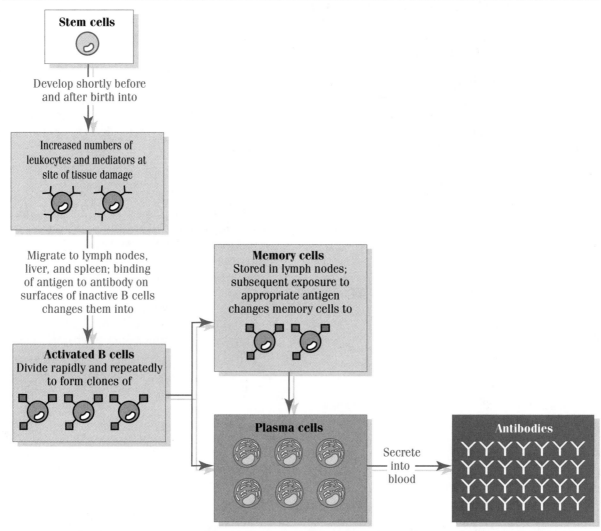

■ *Figure 9-6.* Antibodies are proteins of the family called **immunoglobulins,** which are formed by B cells. This figure shows how stem cells, developed both before and after birth, become inactive B cells that migrate to various parts of the body. Antigen then binds to inactive B cells, causing them to divide and form plasma cells that secrete antibodies. Memory cells stored in lymph nodes can also form plasma cells when reexposed to antigens. *Modified from Thibodeau GA, Patton KT:* Anatomy and physiology, *ed 4, St Louis, 1996, Mosby.*

Hormonal Responses to Stress

Surgical Stress

Although the evidence suggesting that endocrine responses influence clinical outcome is not absolute, anesthetic techniques are widely used for reducing such responses. It is accepted medical belief that elevated cortisol and adrenaline responses promote muscle wasting, immune suppression, and postoperative fatigue.[7,19] Because of this fact, psychologic interventions have been created that attempt to reduce the cortisol and norepinephrine increases that accompany surgical stress.

Although counterintuitive, evidence strongly suggests that preoperative psychologic preparation designed to reduce anxiety may, in fact, result in an elevation of the cortisol and adrenaline responses to surgery.[38,47,58] In these studies, postoperative preparation used to reduce anxiety was associated with increased cortisol and adrenaline responses, even though the patients reported a reduction in stress. Other studies have reported that cortisol responses to stress are reduced when individuals feel able to "cope" with a stressful challenge and when they are not subjected to demands for additional adaptation.[9,12,54]

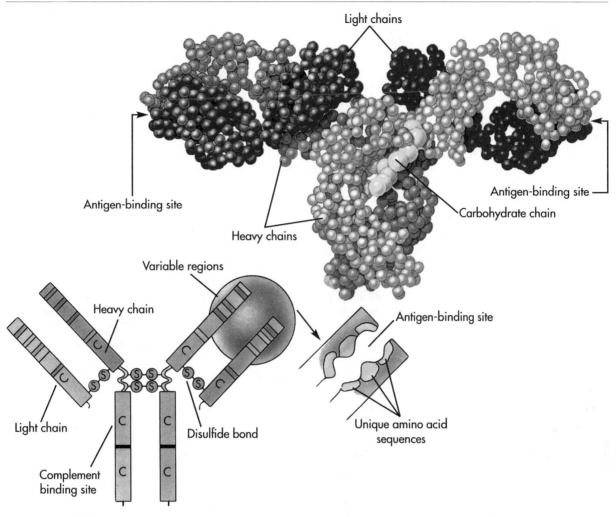

■ **Figure 9-7.** Notice how IgA is composed of two basic antibody units, forming a double-ended Y shape. *Modified from Thibodeau GA, Patton KT:* Anatomy and physiology, *ed 4, St Louis, 1996, Mosby.*

Janis has hypothesized surgical stress can be reduced when patients "work through" impending events, a process he terms the "work of worry." [30] Based on these findings, Manyande and others designed an experiment in which patients who underwent abdominal surgery were preoperatively prepared for surgery using guided imagery. This preparation was not designed to reduce anxiety; rather, it was intended to increase the patients' feelings of being able to cope with surgical stress.[37]

In this mental rehearsal form of imagery, 26 patients first imagined different aspects of the preoperative and postoperative discomforts (e.g., hunger and thirst, dry mouth, pain, nausea, and weakness) and the experiences surrounding surgery. They then rehearsed scenarios of successful postsurgical coping with these discomforts. Serving as a control group, 25 patients listened to a brief audiotape that gave general information about the hospital.

Hormone levels did not differ between groups on the afternoon of admission or before intervention. Outcomes demonstrated that cortisol levels were lower in imagery patients than control patients immediately before and after surgery (p<0.01). However, norepinephrine levels were greater in imagery patients than in the control group on these two occasions (p<0.001), suggesting that norepinephrine was stimulated as part of the coping process.

Imagery patients reported less pain intensity, less pain distress, and better pain coping skills than those in the control group; they also requested less analgesia (pain medication). Compared with the control group, patients who practiced imagery had lower heart rates during surgery and in recovery. Imagery did not affect reported anxiety, indicating that imagery procedures had not only relaxed or reassured patients but had induced a coping response.

These findings are supported by other studies that suggest that cortisol response to stress is reduced by coping imagery. By contrast, images of active coping have been associated with increased norepinephrine responses, particularly when the coping strategy is perceived as difficult.[22,50] Duration of postoperative stays did not differ between groups.

A study was undertaken to determine the effects of relaxation and guided imagery on surgical stress response and wound healing[27] (Figure 9-8).

After gallbladder surgery, 24 patients either observed 20 minutes of quiet time daily for 5 days, beginning the day before surgery (group 1), or they practiced a series of audiotapes consisting of 20 minutes of relaxation and guided imagery for the same 5-day period (group 2).

For group 2, an introductory audiotape introduced the concept of relaxation and planted the notion of positive surgical recovery and successful wound healing in general. Three additional tapes focused on relaxation and normal wound healing. A mental journey was taken through the body, and a picture of the normal phases of successful wound healing was suggested in imagery. Tape 2 focused on the inflammatory phase of wound healing, tape 3 targeted the proliferative phase, and tape 4 was directed toward the maturation phase.

> **Points to Ponder** These findings are supported by other studies that suggest that cortisol response to stress is reduced by coping imagery. ■

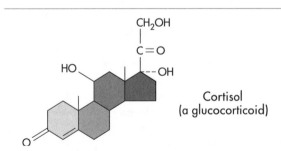

■ **Figure 9-8.** Cortisol, a glucocorticoid, is a steroid hormone manufactured by endocrine cells from cholesterol. Effects of cortisol include increased catabolism of tissue proteins, hyperglycemia, decreased lymphocyte and immune response, and decreased eosinophil and allergic response. *Modified from Thibodeau GA, Patton KT:* Anatomy and physiology, *ed 4, St Louis, 1996, Mosby.*

The relaxation and guided-imagery group (group 2) demonstrated a steady downward linear trend in anxiety levels after surgery, whereas those in the control group exhibited their highest anxiety levels after surgery. For those in the imagery group, cortisol levels were lower than those in the control group the first day after surgery, with other levels being equivocal. Thereafter, cortisol levels rose strikingly for both groups after surgery, increasing 12.5 times over preoperative levels in the control group and 4.7 times over preoperative levels in the relaxation and imagery group. Compared with those in the control group, significantly less surgical wound erythema (redness of skin) was observed at wound margins in patients who practiced imagery.

The results of the study indicated that the relaxation and imagery group demonstrated a smoother postoperative recovery than the control group. The primary findings of the study were that (1) patients who listened to relaxation and imagery audiotapes before and after surgery showed significant reductions in state anxiety levels as compared with those in the control group, and (2) this reduction in anxiety was, for this study, associated with lower postoperative levels of cortisol.

It is possible that the imagery used in this study served to reduce anxiety and elicit a sense of effective coping. Suggestions were given for both relaxation (anxiety reduction) and effective but self-directed wound healing. This approach may explain the differences in outcomes for this study as compared with other anxiety-reduction studies.

Hormonal Responses During Depressed Mood State

The Bonnie Method of Guided Imagery and Music (GIM) uses music to serve as a catalyst to evoke free-flowing imagery for accessing and working through emotional processes. While listening to the music, a therapist encourages active, ongoing dialogue with the client. The client is encouraged to stay with uncomfortable emotions while accessing imagery that is open ended and symbolic. Sessions can also include intense experiences of positive emotion and imagery. Progress is assessed by the spontaneous transformation of the images and a broader range of behavioral, affective, and interpersonal changes.[10,11]

In this study, 28 healthy adults were randomized to 13 weeks of GIM intervention or wait-list control conditions. The Profile of Mood States (POMS) was used to assess emotional status; and blood was taken before the intervention, at the end of the 13-week intervention, and at a 6-week follow-up.[39] Compared with wait-list control adults, GIM participants reported significant preintervention to postintervention decreases in depression, fatigue, and total mood disturbance, as well as significant decreases in cortisol level by the 6-week follow-up. Decreases in cortisol from pretest to follow-up were significantly associated with a decrease in mood disturbance.

The reader should keep in mind that emotion is often driven by our interpretation of events (our images) and that the release of negative emotion has been demonstrated to decrease the likelihood of viral and other illnesses, as noted in Chapter 4. In this study, releasing the images of emotion led to a reduction in cortisol.

In this study, imagery was used in a different but no less significant manner than in studies previously reviewed. Instead of targeting specific images in advance, this method allowed whatever emotions that were troubling to the individual to be identified and expressed as they surfaced.

Imagery and Circadian Rhythm Retraining

The physical stress of shift work and its effects on mental acuity and on health are well-known. In the next study, Rider and others wanted to determine whether they could more quickly "retrain" circadian rhythm effects in shift workers, thereby reducing the corticosteroids produced in response to this naturally occurring stressor.

This study sought to determine whether music and guided imagery could retrain circadian rhythms and reduce stress hormones (corticosteroids) in nurses who worked rotating shifts or night shifts[46] (Figure 9-9). Six of the nurses rotated every 10 to 14 days between morning and evening shifts, and six worked permanent night shifts.

Imagery sessions consisted first of Jacobson's muscle-group relaxation technique followed by the imagery of turning themselves into clouds and observing a problem area from their elevated vantage point. They then conceptualized possible solutions to the problems. (You will note that this form of imagery would serve to increase perceived coping skills.)

Urine was collected and body temperatures recorded simultaneously, four times each measurement day, and at 4- to 5-day intervals over the period of 1 month. The authors compared data collected before beginning imagery practice with the data collected during the 3 weeks of practice. Outcomes demonstrated that circadian amplitude effects decreased significantly (p=0.007), and corticosteroid and temperature rhythms were significantly more entrained (p<0.01) during the taped conditions. Mean corticosteroid levels also declined during tape listening, but not significantly (p=0.15). The small sample size in this study may have served to mask a corticosteroid effect, as observed in previous studies.

Immune Cell Migration

Can we actually succeed in "commanding" our cells via imagery to increase surveillant vigilance in the body? This study suggests that this may be the case.

Neutrophils and lymphocytes are the two most prolific subsets of leukocytes, making up approximately 85% to 90% of the total leukocyte count (Figure 9-10). Because activation and life span of leukocytes involve considerable time, short-term effects of imagery would affect leuko-

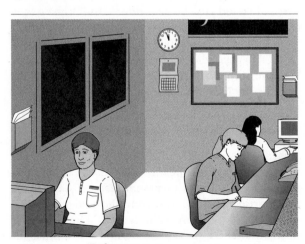

■ *Figure 9-9.* Nurses at work.

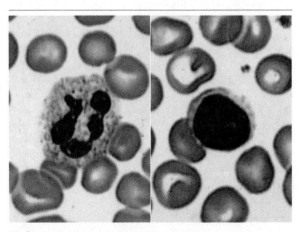

■ *Figure 9-10.* Neutrophils (left) and lymphocytes (right) are the two most prolific subsets of leukocytes, comprising approximately 85% to 90% of the total leukocyte count. *Modified from Thibodeau GA, Patton KT:* Anatomy and physiology, *ed 4, St Louis, 1996, Mosby.*

cyte count (e.g., differential white blood cell counts) through their migration patterns rather than through cell maturation or proliferation.[32]

When neutrophils and lymphocytes are activated, they migrate out of the bloodstream to perform their mission of surveillance in lymphatic and body tissues. Therefore the count in the peripheral bloodstream will drop when these cells are activated or called into action. In the following study, imagery was used to activate these cells.

For a 6-week imagery intervention, 30 music students were randomly assigned to one of two groups.[44] Group 1 focused on images of morphology, location, and movement of neutrophils; group 2 focused on the same types of images of lymphocytes. Photographs and drawings of the neutrophils or lymphocytes were used, and the students drew these images and discussed them to enhance the imagery effect. Cassette audiotapes of the imagery, prepared in consultation with an immunologist, were practiced at home. Entrainment music was used to enhance imagery. To be included in the study, the subjects had to have a minimum of ten imagery sessions in 6 weeks and have an experience of positive shift in imagery— vividness, movement, color, symbolism, and other dimensions. In other words, the subjects had to succeed in imaging the cells effectively. Cells not imaged by each group served as a control factor; no additional control group was included.

Peripheral white blood cell and differential counts were determined before and after a 20-minute imagery session at the end of the 6-week intervention. Neutrophils decreased significantly ($p < 0.04$) for the neutrophil imaging group, whereas lymphocytes did not. The reverse occurred for the lymphocyte group, with a significant decrease of lymphocytes ($p > 0.03$).

It should be noted that positive emotional states have been found to increase certain subpopulations of lymphocytes, in contrast to the decrease shown in this study. The authors hypothesized that imagery mechanisms may trigger the immune response into action (migration) in the short term, whereas more positive emotional states over a longer term may benefit the immune response by making more cells available in the bloodstream.

In another study by Jasnoski, 30 Harvard undergraduate students, identified as high in absorption ability (i.e., the ability to concentrate intently and respond intensely to experiences and imagination), were randomly assigned to one of three groups.[31]

Group 1 practiced progressive muscle relaxation and focused breathing; group 2 practiced progressive muscle relaxation, focused breathing, and potent imagery depicting the immune system; and group 3 participated in a vigilance task control exercise where subjects discriminated between two tones after variable intervals. The subjects participated in a single, 1-hour trial.

At the completion of the trial, the two relaxation groups produced identical increases in salivary IgA, whereas the vigilance task group demonstrated significant reductions in salivary IgA. When cortisol was controlled, the relaxation-only group appeared to produce more salivary IgA than the relaxation group with immune imagery.

The authors were not specific in their descriptions of the type of imagery used. Consequently, it is impossible to know whether specific imagery of IgA was used. They stated that the imagery was "power imagery" that combined an arousing psychologic state with a relaxed physiologic one. Since the type of imagery must be specific, if a single immune component is targeted for change, this lack of specificity may explain why the imagery group did not produce more of a specific immune component than the relaxation-only group. The imagery in this study may not have been precise enough to elicit the proposed difference between the relaxation-only group and the immune imagery group. This is an example of the critical need to both understand the exact imagery needed and consider carefully the emotional effect of the imagery type used for "delivery." The psychologic state evoked in the imagery session may not have been the most appropriate one for the intended outcome.

■ Summary of Imagery Effects

Research strongly suggests the potential for imagery to alter specific immune parameters (immunoglobulins), hormonal responses (cortisol and corticosteroid), and immune cell migration (neutrophils and lymphocytes). The imagery used to affect a particular outcome (1) must be specific and biologically accurate, and (2) the

> **Points to Ponder**   The authors hypothesized that imagery mechanisms may trigger the immune response into action (migration) in the short term, whereas more positive emotional states over a longer term may benefit the immune response by making more cells available in the bloodstream. ■

effect of imagery "delivery" on mood state must be carefully considered. Outcomes differ or are affected by the elicitation of mood factors such as anxiety-reduction, perceived control, or reduction of depression. Finally, each person's interpretation of images and each person's dominant images are unique to that person. In using guided imagery, the facilitator must be careful to allow the individual to form images that, while being accurate, are meaningful and appropriate for that person.

One method for facilitating beneficial imagery for the individual is to use imagery assessment tools. Such tools can assist in the selection and therapeutic use of imagery and can, in some instances, even predict health outcomes.

■ Imagery Assessment Tools

Perhaps the finest imagery assessment instruments for use in clinical and rehabilitation settings are those developed by Achterberg and Lawlis. Their instruments have been used to assess treatment for cancer (Image CA), spinal pain (Image SP), and diabetes (Image DB) and have proven to be highly accurate predictors of treatment outcomes.[4] For example, the total scores on the Image CA were found to predict with 100% certainty those who would die or show significant deterioration within 2 months and with 93% accuracy those who would go into remission within that same time frame.

The following brief summary of how imagery is used for diagnosis is provided. However, for a more comprehensive understanding of how diagnostic imagery is used, the reader should consult the textbook provided by Achterberg and Lawlis.

■ Imagery for Diagnosis: An Overview

When using imagery for diagnosis, the first step is to use a technique that induces relaxation without being too wordy. Excessive verbal content activates the left brain in a manner that interferes with free-flowing imagery.

The second step is to ensure that the setting used during the diagnosis protocol is appropriate and conducive to imagery. The setting and the imagery ritual should support belief in the efficacy of imagery and should reduce patient anxiety. For this reason, personal ritual is often helpful. Some patients find that candles, scents, or personal objects create an atmosphere conducive to imagery. Others find music, drums, or chimes beneficial.

The therapist's next goal is to encourage the patient to create a picture expressive of his or her intimate knowledge of the disease—a picture unencumbered by the suggested images of others. These images must flow naturally from the patient.

Patients are asked to draw three imagery components: the disease, the treatment, and the defenses. The disease imagery is later examined and evaluated for vividness, including its strength or weakness and its ability to persist. The treatment imagery is examined for vividness and effectiveness of the mechanism for cure. The personal defense imagery is examined for vividness of the patient's description and the effectiveness of the imagery's action to defend the body from the disease state. The coherence of the three components, along with how well the "story" is integrated and the degree of symbolism, are all considered. Most importantly, the symbolic images, rather than the realistic and anatomically correct ones, are the best predictors of health outcomes.

■ Imagery as Therapy

Diagnostic imagery not only provides information concerning the likelihood of recovery, but it also provides valuable information for the therapeutic procedure. For example, images of treatment may be inaccurate or blurry. Our perceived personal defenses may be lacking, and education about these defenses may increase our understanding of disease and provide data for healing imagery.

Those serious about using imagery for healing must invest time everyday to the effort. This effort may involve continued drawings of the images, but it must be composed of a relaxation process followed by imagery practice. Typically, 30 minutes or more are required, always preceded by relaxation. Many persons experience sensation in the affected part when they image; most experience spontaneous changes in their imagery as their condition changes.

The following text reviews various types of imagery used for pain management and surgical recovery. We also discuss research outcomes of imagery used as treatment for cancer.

■ Imagery for Treatment of Pain

Imagery for the treatment of pain is either (1) pain-transforming imagery or (2) pain-incompatible imagery. Pain-transforming imagery concentrates on changing specific aspects of the pain experience (e.g., a contextual change by mentally rehearsing to prepare for an upcoming

Pain-transforming imagery concentrates on changing specific aspects of the pain experience (e.g., a contextual change by mentally rehearsing to prepare oneself for a coming débridement experience), whereas pain-incompatible imagery consists of imaginations of events or feelings and sensations that are not compatible with pain.

débridement experience). Pain-incompatible imagery consists of imaging events or feelings and sensations that are not compatible with pain. The incompatible images can be further divided into emotive images or sensory images. For example, imaging a sense of relaxation, tranquility, and joy (emotive) and analgesic numbness (sensory) are images incompatible with burn pain.[20,49,57]

A study by Neumann and others sought to determine whether imagery could influence tolerance for pain. Specifically, they wanted to determine whether subjects trained in pain-incompatible imagery differed in heart rate and skin resistance from subjects not trained in this manner.[42]

In the study, 39 subjects were randomly assigned to pain-incompatible imagery or to a control group. For the imagery group, pain tolerance and the psychophysiologic reaction to pain were assessed with a pressure algometer before and after imagery training and in response to two pain-induction sessions. (A pain algometer is a metal cylinder placed on the middle phalanx of the ring finger that applies constant pressure using an electrical motor. Pressure is applied until the subject reaches a pain threshold [i.e., the pain is no longer bearable, and the subject then pushes a button to release the pressure]).

At the end of the first pain assessment, imagery subjects designed imagery that, to them, was incompatible with the pain induced by the algometer. Their individual imagery and imagery taught by the instructor were combined and used in the second pain tolerance session.

Those in the control group also received two pain tolerance assessments but without benefit of imagery.

Pain tolerance was significantly increased in the group that used pain-incompatible imagery, as compared with those in the control group and with the subject's pain tolerance scores before imagery. Subjects trained in pain-incompatible imagery also demonstrated lower heart rates than control subjects during the second pain induction. The groups did not differ with regard to skin resistance.

Outcomes demonstrated that not only was pain tolerance extended, but one psychophysiologic reaction to pain was also altered. The authors concluded that pain-incompatible imagery may be the best form of imagery for the treatment of acute pain, such as occurs in dental procedures, endoscopy, or lumbar puncture, whereas pain-transforming imagery may be more appropriate for chronic forms of pain.

Imagery for Pain of Severe Burn Injury

There is no more debilitating or painful trauma than the pain experienced during the treatment for severe burn injury. In fact, patients regard the treatment as more horrific than the experience of the burn itself.[8]

As part of burn treatment, patients endure having dead skin removed by scrubbing, a process called débridement. Because this process is performed regularly over the course of weeks or months, patients cannot be anesthetized for these treatments. The procedural pain experienced during débridement is excruciating and uncontrollable even with high doses of opioid drugs. To make matters worse, because of concerns of narcotic addiction and possible narcotic inhibition of the immune response, patients must endure this excruciatingly painful process with limited pain medication. Behavioral interventions that can blunt the anxiety and pain of débridement are, therefore, potentially very valuable for humanitarian reasons and to support the healing process. (You will recall from earlier chapters that stress can also impair wound healing) (Figure 9-11).

Using a mental rehearsal form of imagery, Achterberg and others tested three audiotape procedures to determine which would be most valuable as an intervention for burn pain. Burn victims received training in relaxation, relaxation with imagery, or relaxation, imagery, and biofeedback. Other patients with burns received no training, but they served as a control group. The audiotaped procedure consisted of relaxation instructions followed by an imagery trip through the wound care procedure. The imagery tapes were designed to address specifically patient experience of treatment. Anxiety, discomfort, and cold and shivering after the tub treatments were included as sensory components that were mentally rehearsed but done so in a state of deep calm.

This research took place under extremely demanding conditions of a hospital burn care unit. Patient schedules could be changed with no notice; or infections on the unit could result in

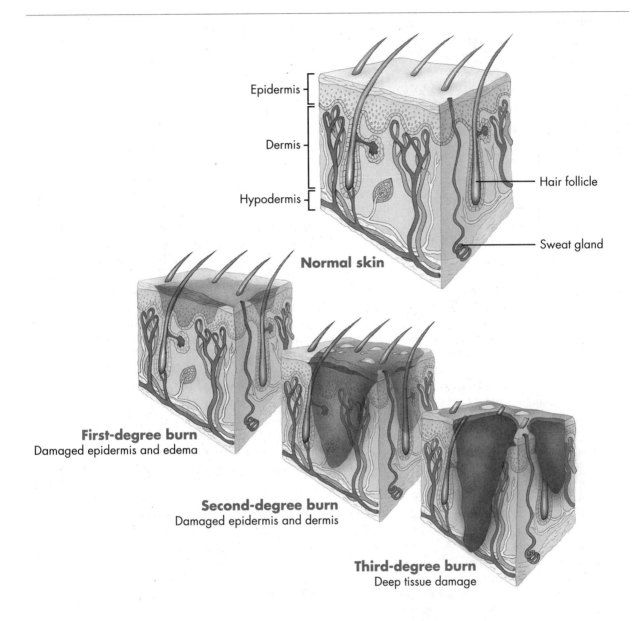

■ *Figure* 9-11. **First-degree burns** (typical sunburn) will cause minor discomfort and some reddening of the skin. Although surface layers may peel in 1 to 2 days, no blistering occurs and skin damage is minimal. **Second-degree burns** involve deep epidermal layers and always cause injury to the upper level of the dermis. In deep second-degree burns, damage to the sweat glands, hair follicles, and sebaceous glands may occur, but tissue death is not complete. Blisters, severe pain, swelling, edema, and scarring typically occur. **Third-degree burns** are characterized by destruction of both the epidermis and dermis. Tissue death extends below the hair follicles and sweat glands and may involve underlying muscles, fasciae, and even bone. The third-degree burn is insensitive to pain immediately after surgery because of destruction of nerve endings. Scarring is serious. *Modified from Thibodeau GA, Patton KT: Anatomy and physiology, ed 4, St Louis, 1996, Mosby.*

patient setbacks. The authors learned that six uninterrupted imagery sessions were the most they could hope for in a burn unit setting. However, part of what they wanted to determine was not only what would be effective—but also what could be reasonably applied in such a hectic and challenging environment.

The control group demonstrated no improvement, pretreatment to posttreatment, for any measurement of pain or anxiety. Compared with control subjects, all three behavioral protocols demonstrated improvements in pain and anxiety reduction. Relaxation/imagery and relaxation/imagery/biofeedback produced the best and essentially equivocal outcomes. Because imagery without biofeedback is more easily administered in a busy hospital setting, the relaxation/imagery intervention was recommended as the treatment of choice for severe burn injury. One point to be learned from this study is that imagery must not only be affective for its intended purpose, but the facilitator must also develop an imagery protocol that can be inserted into the intended hospital or health care setting.

■ Imagery and Surgical Recovery

A study by Tusek and others was designed to determine whether guided imagery in the preoperative and postoperative periods could improve the outcomes of colorectal surgery patients (N=130). Patients were assigned to (1) receive standard care (e.g., control group) or (2) listen to a guided imagery tape 3 days preoperatively; a music-only tape during induction, during surgery, and postoperatively in the recovery room; and a guided imagery tape during each of the first 6 postoperative days (e.g., treatment group).

The imagery tape instructed patients to go "to a special place" in their mind that was safe, secure, protected, and relaxed. The imagery story encouraged patients to work through feelings of fear, anxiety, and negativity. Patients listened to the tape twice daily, in the morning and evening.

Before surgery, anxiety increased in the control group, but it decreased in the guided imagery group. Postoperatively, pain scores were significantly lower for the imagery group as compared with the control subjects. Total opioid use and time to first bowel movement were also lower for the imagery group. The authors concluded that guided imagery significantly reduced postoperative anxiety, pain, and narcotic requirements and that patient satisfaction increased with treatment.

■ Imagery in the Treatment of Cancer

Cancer intrudes on the patient's life, pulling the rug out from under him or her. Cancer invokes fear and anxiety, alters the lifestyle of the patient and family, and forces the endurance of a variety of unpleasant or painful side effects brought about by chemotherapy, radiation, surgical procedures, or other treatment protocols. Imagery can help

alleviate some of these intrusions. It can help alleviate the nausea and vomiting caused by chemotherapy; reduce perceived pain, fear, and anxiety; and address the spiritual distress experienced as part of this life-threatening disease.[14-16,21,52]

Imagery has also been shown to improve immune function, specifically natural killer (NK) cell functioning—a critical component of the body's ability to fight cancer.[28,60] A variety of studies using imagery for the treatment of cancer or cancer-treatment side effects are reviewed in the chapters on hypnosis and relaxation. The reader is referred to these chapters for additional data beyond what is covered in this chapter.

When patients hear the diagnosis of cancer, their imagery is often powerful and, more often than not, negative. Guided imagery can be used to reacquaint patients with their healthy side, to give them a sense of control over side effects and pain, and to reduce the stress and anxiety that may work against optimal immune functioning.

Cancer Pain

Wallace reviewed controlled trials of imagery for the relief of cancer pain published between 1982 and 1995. He located nine clinical studies. He found that imagery used in the treatment of cancer appeared to (1) significantly reduce the sensory experience of pain; (2) significantly improve affective (depression, anxiety) status; and (3) have no effect on functional status (activities of daily living, movement, and posture).[56] Most studies reviewed by Wallace had such small sample sizes that identifying significant effects was impossible. Intervention methods and length of interventions were highly variable, and several studies had no control groups. Some studies were part of more comprehensive packages, and subjects were limited to adults.

A more recent study with more research subjects conducted by Syrjala and others compared oral mucositis pain levels in four groups of patients with cancer receiving bone marrow transplants.[51] Oral mucositis refers to mouth inflammation and its accompanying pain caused by immunosuppressive drugs. These drugs are required to prevent rejection of transplanted tissue and fluids.

In this study, 94 patients received (1) relaxation and imagery training; (2) training in a package of cognitive behavioral coping skills (self-statements, distraction, and short-term goals) that also included relaxation and imagery training and practice; (3) therapist support; or (4) treatment as usual (control group).

Imagery consisted of deep breathing followed by progressive muscle relaxation (session 1), abbreviated autogenic relaxation (session 2), deepening imagery using descending a staircase or a counting method (session 3), and imagery of a place the patient had chosen (session 4). Images of cold as a form of sensory transformation for pain control, as well as references to patient well-being, strength, competence, and comfort, were included in all imagery sessions. Patients practiced audiotapes of guided imagery sessions twice daily between regular sessions. Intervention included two on-site training sessions before treatment and two weekly booster sessions during the first 5 weeks of treatment.

Patients in the relaxation/imagery group and in the relaxation/imagery/cognitive coping skills group experienced significant reduction in pain. The cognitive coping skills addition did not significantly add to pain reduction nor did therapist support significantly reduce pain more than regular treatment. The authors concluded that relaxation/imagery alone was the most efficient method for oral pain management in this group of patients with cancer.

Immunologic Responses of Patients With Breast Cancer

Thirteen patients, each recovering from a modified radical mastectomy who had not undergone chemotherapy or radiation and who were lymph node–negative (cancer free), were randomly assigned to either full treatment or a delayed treatment control group.[25] The treatment group was given a 9-week sequence of relaxation training, guided imagery, and EMG biofeedback training.

The treatment group learned about the immune system and was given Jacobsonian relaxation training during the first week. They then received a relaxation audiotape to practice at home. Week 2 was used to deepen relaxation. At week 3, guided imagery was introduced and added to the home-practice audiotape. General guidelines were given to the patients regarding the immune system and the development of health-promoting processes in the body. No specific imagery was suggested to patients; imagery was selected individually. EMG biofeedback training was implemented in week 4. Throughout training and follow-up, the patients were instructed to practice relaxation and guided imagery twice daily. Each month over the 15 months of the project, monthly brush-up sessions were held during which relaxation practice and help with imagery were provided. Patients made drawings of their imagery, and it was scored

> **Points to Ponder** Relaxation, imagery, and biofeedback training produced statistically significant effects primarily on T-cell populations. Several weeks to several months were required for changes to reach statistical significance. ■

according to the standardized Image CA forms.[5] After 6 months into the study, group 2 controls were trained in relaxation and imagery the same as group 1.

Relaxation, imagery, and biofeedback training produced statistically significant effects primarily on T-cell populations. As compared with the control group and with outcomes before and after intervention, significant effects of intervention were found for NK cell activity ($p<0.017$), mixed lymphocyte responsiveness ($p<0.001$), concanavalin A (Con A) responsiveness ($p>0.001$), and the number of peripheral blood lymphocytes ($p>0.01$). Antibodies were minimally affected. Several weeks to several months were required for changes to reach statistical significance.

■ Imagery for Other Medical Conditions

Imagery has been used as treatment to improve lactation in mothers of premature infants and as intervention with anticipatory grief. The following text reviews these studies.

Improved Lactation in Mothers of Premature Infants

Many women with premature infants find that emotional stress inhibits lactation. This is a critical problem since expressed breast milk aids the survival of the premature infant. A study of 55 mothers of premature infants found that the 30 who listened to a 20-minute imagery audiotape produced 63% more breast milk than the 25 who did not. A subgroup of mothers with ventilator-dependent babies increased milk flow 121% (Figure 9-12).

Intervention With Anticipatory Grief

In this day of chronic disease and protracted death, many patients and their families live with the knowledge that death is inevitable but that its occurrence is weeks, months, or even years in the future. These types of experiences are typical with the conditions of acquired immunodeficiency syndrome (AIDS), Alzheimer's disease, or a variety of conditions where life-extending medical technology prolongs the dying process. Long-term anticipatory grief can often lead to pathologic anxiety, disruption of family and support net-

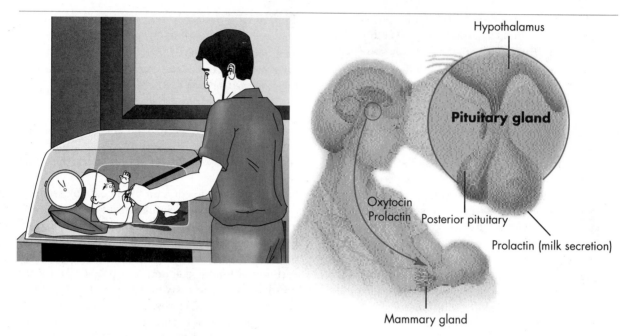

■ *Figure 9-12.* Nursing provides a rich source of proteins, fat, calcium, vitamins, and other nutrients in proportions to the need of the infant. It also provides passive immunity in the form of maternal antibodies and strengthens the bonding process. Nursing increases the likelihood of survival in premature infants. *Figure at right modified from Thibodeau GA, Patton KT:* Anatomy and physiology, *ed 4, St Louis, 1996, Mosby.*

works, displaced anger, and even abandonment of the patient. Lebow defined anticipatory grief as a phenomenon with an identifiable pattern of cognitive, affective, cultural, and social reactions to an anticipated death.[35] The process work of anticipatory grief involves the constant recognition and acceptance of a future loss and the process of gradual, continual, and incremental detachment for the patient and family.[43]

Characteristics of normal anticipatory grief include verbal expressions of distress at anticipated loss; anger, sorrow, crying, and choked feelings; changes in eating and sleeping habits; altered dream patterns; modified activity level and libido; and altered ability to concentrate.[53] When these characteristics become extreme, they can include disruption of communication between a patient and loved ones, abandonment of the patient, pathologic hopelessness, isolation and withdrawal, delusions and hallucinations, dysfunctional denial, and inability to participate in decision making. Further, anticipatory loss can trigger physical as well as emotional illness in family members. As we have discussed previously, Alzheimer's caregivers can often suffer excessive short- and long-term illnesses and even shortened life spans (see Chapter 4).

Even though little research exists in this area, a variety of researchers have argued that imagery is a potent intervention for anticipatory grief.[18,34,48,55] Imagery is beneficial for the patient and involved family members, often improving lines of communication and providing a process for preparation of loss and for closure. The following is an abbreviated case study of the use of guided imagery for this purpose.

Case study: **Cancer and Imagery**

Mr. Bee, a 76-year-old retired salesperson, had a diagnosis of terminal lung cancer and esophageal cancer. He was unable to eat or retain food and suffered from increasing pain. Because nothing further could be done in a hospital setting, he was released to his home to die, but in-home nursing care was provided. Mr. Bee acknowledged his terminal state by such comments as, "You girls will have to look after my wife when I am gone." However, when he tried to discuss his impending death with his wife, she would change the subject or respond, "Now, honey, you mustn't talk that way. Everything will be alright, just as soon as we get you stronger." Mr. Bee soon succumbed to his wife's wishes by meeting her denial. The nurses noted that when his wife was in the room for long periods, his need for pain medication doubled. He was increasingly strained by her visits and became uneasy when she was with him. He became less and less communicative to his wife and to his caregivers.

Mrs. Bee constantly pushed her husband to eat, and when he responded by choking or vomiting, she would run from the room and demand to know why this was happening. She became argumentative and demanding with caregivers and became angry with any family member who tried to talk to her about his impending death. Soon, her children became frustrated with her and ceased efforts to communicate with her. At this point, a gerontologic home care specialist suggested the use of guided imagery and the family and patient agreed, although Mrs. Bee was reluctant. It was explained that the goal of imagery was to reduce pain for Mr. Bee and reduce stress and tension for the rest of the family.

The therapist began sessions by encouraging Mr. Bee to visualize a happy time in his life when he had no discomfort or pain and to describe the scene in detail. Mr. Bee began to describe a scene of his wife and him in a canoe, with gentle lapping water, sunshine, the sounds of loons, and the smell of pine trees. Mrs. Bee joined in by describing how pleasant the water felt when she trailed her hand in it and how they shed their worries in this environment. After the first session, Mr. Bee fell into a peaceful sleep, and he breathed easier. Mrs. Bee noticed an improvement, commenting that he looked "younger" than before the session. Subsequent sessions followed, emphasizing the canoe trip. Mr. Bee was encouraged to recall how his breathing was relaxed as he glided along in the canoe and how at peace he was. Eventually, Mrs. Bee began visualizing herself alone with her children, discussing happy and humorous memories of Mr. Bee. She visualized herself preparing the family's favorite foods for a birthday party and talking to her grandchildren about memories of Mr. Bee.

With the help of imagery, Mr. Bee had less pain and slept with less distress. He experienced less pain when he had trouble breathing, and he regained his sense of humor. Mrs. Bee was less anxious about his food intake and became more accepting of the nurses. Family gatherings took on a new tone. They were often full of laughter, less stressed, and full of anecdotes like, "Remember when...." Mr. Bee was able to talk to his children about taking care of Mrs. Bee after he died, even with her present. The family's shared prayers were no longer for recovery but for help to meet future challenges.

On Mr. Bee's last day, Mrs. Bee sat by his bedside, talking to him. "Just picture our canoe, honey, the sun is shining on the water, and we can hear the kids playing on shore. Do you hear that loon over there? He's telling us night is almost here...."[53]

■ Preparation for Using Imagery in Medical Practices

Selecting the appropriate imagery for any intervention cannot be overemphasized. In her text "Imagery in Healing," Achterberg offers specific advice for individuals interested in incorporating imagery as a healing tool.[1]

Both the therapist and patient must develop a solid understanding of the way the body functions in relation to the health condition being addressed and the treatments and physical limitations imposed by the illness. Further, the therapist should clearly and fully identify the goal of imagery. Exploring diagnostic imagery is an excellent way to ensure that the goals are clear and accurate. Without a clear "picture" of what the problem or disease is, the individual cannot create accurate imagery. The cancer patient faces unique symptoms, treatment, and living experiences that are different from the patient who experiences, for example, myocardial infarction. To be beneficial, imagery must be both realistic and accurate in relation to the medical condition.

Patients have different life experiences and imagery preferences that must be considered when creating therapeutic imagery that will be effective and acceptable to the patient. For example, the therapeutic imagery of sharks attacking cancer cells was used in earlier research, but this imagery was not found to be the best or even acceptable for all cancer patients. The most useful information on imagery for the treatment of disease has come from patients who have been diagnosed with the specific condition and who can articulate how they mastered the illness and learned to live a full life in spite of it. Patients can also provide specific imagery details, such as what the actual healing felt like; and what sensations, thoughts, or behaviors accompanied or preceded the healing process.

The patient must relax before practicing imagery so the mind can become receptive to the inner dialogue. Further, the patient must end the session with images of the desired state of wellness—the representation of health for the specific condition (end-state imagery). Imagery must be practiced often if beneficial outcomes are to occur.

■ Indications and Contraindications for the Clinical Application of Imagery

Indications for using imagery in any of its forms (e.g., relaxation, meditation, biofeedback, hypnosis, targeted imagery) are the following:

- The patient exhibits interest in assuming personal responsibility for health management.
- Secondary gains from the disease state under treatment are not a significant confounding factor. In other words, is the condition to be treated providing certain benefits to the patient? For example, one patient with chronic asthma believed that her husband stayed in their marriage only because she was ill. She believed he only stayed in the marriage because he did not want to upset her and potentially induce a fatal asthma attack. To be restored to health meant, to her, the potential loss of her marriage. In such a situation, the underlying issues must be dealt with before imagery interventions are likely to be effective.
- The patient believes that mind-body effects can be altered by imagery and that altering these underlying dimensions of illness (e.g., stress, lifestyle, information deficit) can result in improved health.

Contraindications for the use of imagery as clinical intervention in any of its forms include the following:

- Imagery practices alter brain wave activity and, in patients susceptible to uncontrolled epileptic episodes, can induce seizures. Specialists in the treatment of epileptic seizures who also use biofeedback techniques have used imagery techniques to teach their patients to control their seizures. However, such attempts should be undertaken only by persons trained and experienced in the use of this type of intervention.
- Patients with unstable diabetes may be inappropriate candidates for imagery techniques. Even for persons with stable diabetes, sugar levels need to be monitored carefully when they embark on the consistent use of imagery techniques. Many patients with diabetes require less insulin when altering physiology with relaxation and imagery.
- Patients with chronic severe depression, unless anxiety is the underlying feature, may be inappropriate candidates for clinical intervention with imagery techniques. Such patients may be too unstable to cope effectively with the surfacing of images, memories, and emotions that accompany certain types of imagery interventions. However, a psychologist or psychiatrist who is well-trained in imagery effects may be able to use imagery interventions safely and effectively with the clinically depressed.

An Expert Speaks: Dr. Jeanne Achterberg

Jeanne Achterberg, PhD, is author or co-author of more than 100 journal articles related to imagery and/or mind-body healing and has written several books including Rituals in Healing: Creating Health through Imagery; Woman as Healer; Imagery in Healing; Imagery and Disease; and Bridges of the Bodymind. She has created or co-created several health assessment instruments including the Health Attribution Test, the Trauma Impact Survey, and the Image CA, Image SP, and Image DB assessment tools. Dr. Achterberg, a member of the Executive Faculty of Saybrook Institute and Graduate School in San Francisco, CA, is also Senior Editor of the peer-reviewed journal Alternative Therapies in Health and Medicine. Here, she shares her experiences and view of imagery as a healing modality.

Question. How did you become interested in imagery?

Answer. About 25 years ago, I was serving as the Research Director for Carol Simonton's cancer center in Ft. Worth, Texas. Imagery was (and is) a very important part of the mind-body therapy for those groups. I made the decision to focus a research career on the subject because it seemed to be a correlate as well as a predictor of response to treatment, side effects, rehabilitation potential, and, in many cases, life expectancy, as well. The same results held true for the indigent patients being treated at the medical school where I was a faculty member for many years. In addition, I had the opportunity to study the role of imagery with many chronic diseases, as well as with acute conditions such as orthopedic trauma and burn injury. Unfortunately, the word "imagery" is a little word that does not adequately convey the whole story. Essentially, imagery relates to larger issues of consciousness: belief, hope, trust, and the inner phenomenology of health and disease.

Question. For what conditions is imagery most appropriate?

Answer. People use imagery all the time—it is simply thought with a sensory quality. Every time someone walks into a doctor's office or a nurse nods or gestures, images are created in the patient's mind. We create images with every communication with another sentient being—a fact that would be helpful to keep in mind! However, we also speak of imagery as a meditation practice or a formal protocol that is done on a regular basis. The most practical and noncontroversial uses of imagery are for stress management [and the] preparation for surgical or other medical procedures—examinations, cast removal, spinal taps. Imagery is very helpful for anticipatory nausea for chemotherapy and is generally associated with a reduction in side effects from cancer and other treatments. Problems such as autoimmune disorders that have a known relationship to stress—either at onset or before exacerbations—are good candidates for imagery. There is some basic research showing an isomorphic effect on various physical components—such as the immune system—because of imagery training. Whether imagery is a useful adjunct or a "cure" for disease remains a matter of conjecture. Anecdotal evidence abounds for its curative value, but controlled research is lacking.

Question. What are the past, present, and future of imagery?

Answer. Imagery is the most ancient of the healing modalities. It probably dates back to the time when humans were first capable of reflecting on their own mortality. Ancient art, as well as living tribal traditions, suggests that images were used for both power and healing. I believe it sustains itself in medicine quite naturally because it is the way that the mind and body communicate—the bridge between what we consider psyche and soma. Imagery is the final common ground in many psychotherapies as well—hypnosis, psychosynthesis, the creative [and] expressive therapies (art, music, dance), Gestalt [psychology], and so on. The database is fairly extensive compared with many of the so-called alternative and complementary therapies.[2] The continued future of imagery as a therapy is bright, provided it is not oversold and that practitioners have a broad understanding of the pathology, course, and treatment of the problems that they face in working in a medical setting.

■ Chapter Review

Imagery is the foundation of mind-body medicine. It is a powerful tool that, when used effectively, can assist in healing the mind, body, and spirit. When used ineptly, it can accomplish little and, in a worst-case scenario, produce results in opposition to the desired outcome. Those interested in using imagery for clinical intervention are encouraged to invest the time and effort necessary to guarantee that the use of patient-directed imagery will be appropriate and beneficial. It is important to recall that imagery is the underlying catalyst in the uses of relaxation, meditation, biofeedback, and hypnosis. Therefore it would benefit practitioners to review the research on specific imagery effects so that the potency of their own practices may be improved. The appendix offers the reader a list of organizations and individuals competent to train clinicians in the effective use of imagery.

Matching Terms and Definitions

Match each numbered definition with the correct term. Place the corresponding letter in the space provided.

a. Imagery
b. Targeted imagery
c. Vision quest imagery
d. Diagnostic imagery
e. Mental rehearsal imagery
f. End-state imagery
g. Imagery assessment instruments

_____ 1. Image CA, Image SP, and Image DB

_____ 2. Imagery technique often used to prepare the patient for medical procedures

_____ 3. Provides the information needed to design individualized and meaningful imagery sessions for a client and can often predict health outcomes

_____ 4. Imagery intended to produce a specific physiologic or biological change in the body

_____ 5. Imagery related to the person's life story and personal myth of empowerment

_____ 6. Thought process that invokes and uses the senses including vision, sound, smell, taste, and the senses of movement, position, and touch

_____ 7. Imagery where the patient is taught actual processes by which the body produces a physiologic change and then images that exact process, a technique that can produce extremely exacting outcomes

CRITICAL THINKING AND CLINICAL APPLICATION EXERCISES

1. Select the type of imagery that you would use to assist a patient with chronic arthritic pain. Describe what steps you would take to develop an imagery scenario with patient participation.
2. Create an imagery scenario for improving NK cellular response in a patient with cancer. Review Chapter 2 (immune function) for assistance in creating biologically targeted imagery. Describe how you would combine biologically targeted imagery with the individualized imagery of the patient.

References

1. Achterberg J: *Imagery in healing: shamanism and modern medicine,* Boston, 1985, Shambhala.
2. Achterberg J, Dossey L, Gordon J et al: Mind-body interventions. In *Alternative medicine, expanding medical horizons. A report to the National Institutes of Health on Alternative Medical Systems and practices in the United States,* Washington, 1994, Government Printing Office.
3. Achterberg J, Kenner L, Lawlis GF: Severe burn injury: a comparison of relaxation, imagery and biofeedback for pain management, *J Ment Imagery* 12(1):33, 1988.
4. Achterberg J, Lawlis GF: *Imagery and disease,* Champaign, Ill, 1984, Institute of Personality and Ability Testing.
5. Achterberg J, Lawlis GF: *Imagery of cancer,* Champaign, Ill, 1978, Institute for Personality and Ability testing.
6. Achterberg J, McGraw P, Lawlis GF: Rheumatoid arthritis: a study of relaxation and temperature biofeedback as an adjunctive therapy, *Biofeedback Self Regul* 6(2):207, 1981.
7. Anand KJS: The stress response to surgical trauma: from physiological basis to therapeutic implications, *Prog Food Nutr Sci* 10:67, 1986.
8. Anderson NJC, Noyes R, Hartford CE: Factors influencing adjustment of burn patients during hospitalization, *Psychosom Med* 34:785, 1972.
9. Bohnen N, Nicolson N, Sulon J et al: Coping style, trait anxiety, and cortisol reactivity during mental stress, *J Psychosom Res* 35:141, 1991.
10. Bonny HL: *Facilitating guided imagery and music sessions,* Salina, KS, 1978, Bonnie Foundation.
11. Bonny HL: Twenty-five years later: a GIM update, *Music Ther Perspect* 12:70, 1995.
12. Brandtstadter J, Baltes-Gotz G, Kirschbaum C et al: Developmental and personality correlates of adrenocortical activity indexed by salivary cortisol: observations in the age range of 35-65 years, *J Psychosom Res* 35:173, 1991.
13. Brigham DD: Imagery for getting well. Clinical applications of behavioral medicine, New York, 1994, Norton.
14. Brown-Saltzman K: Replenishing the spirit by meditative prayer and guided imagery, *Semin Oncol Nurs* 13(4):255, 1997.
15. Carey MP, Burish TG: Etiology and treatment of the psychological side effects associated with cancer chemotherapy: a critical review and discussion, *Psychol Bull* 104:307, 1988.
16. Caudel KA: Psychoneuroimmunology and innovative behavioral interventions in patients with leukemia, *Oncol Nurs Forum* 23:493, 1996.
17. Cott A, Parkison W, Fitch W, Bedard M, Marlin R: Long term efficacy of combined relaxation and biofeedback treatment for chronic headache, *Pain* 5(1):49, 1992.
18. Dossey R, Keegan L, Guzzeta C, Kilkmeier L: *Holistic nursing: a handbook for practice,* ed 2, Gaithersburg, MD, 1995, Aspen Publishers.
19. Ellis RF, Humphrey DE: Clinical aspects of endocrine and metabolic changes relating to anesthesia and surgery. In Watkins J, Salo M, editors: *Trauma stress and immunity in anesthesia and surgery,* London, 1982, Butterworth.
20. Fernandez E: A classification system of cognitive coping strategies for pain, *Pain* 6:141, 1986.
21. Fessele KS: Managing the multiple causes of nausea and vomiting in the patient with cancer, *Oncol Nurs Forum* 9:1409, 1996.
22. Frankenhaueser M: Psychobiological aspects of life stress. In Levine S, Ursin H, editors: *Coping and health,* New York, 1980, Academic Press.
23. Gray S, Lawlis GF: A case study of pruritic eczema treated by relaxation and imagery, *Psychol Rep* 51(3):23, 1982.
24. Green E, Green A: *Beyond biofeedback,* New York, 1977, Delta.
25. Gruber BL, Hersh SP, Hall NRS, Waletzky LR, Kunz JF, Carpenter JK, Kverno KS, Weiss SM: Immunological responses of breast cancer patients to behavioral interventions, *Biofeedback Self Regul* 18(1):1, 1993.
26. Gruber E, Hall N, Hersh E, Dubois T: Immune system and psychological changes in metastatic cancer patients using relaxation and guided imagery, *Scand J Behav Ther* 17:25, 1988.
27. Holden-Lund C: Effects of relaxation with guided imagery on surgical stress and wound healing, *Res Nurs Health* 11:235, 1988.
28. Houldin A, Lev E, Prystowsk, M et al: Review of psycho-immunological literature, *Holistic Nurs Pract* 5:10, 1991.
29. Hughes H, Brown B, Lawlis GF: Biofeedback-assisted relaxation and imagery for acne vulgaris, *J Psychosom Res* 27(4):16, 1983.
30. Janis IL: Psychological stress, New York, 1958, Wiley.
31. Jasnoski ML: Relaxation, imagery, and neuroimmunomodulation, *Ann N Y Acad Sci* 496:723, 1987.
32. Klein J: *Immunology: the science of self-nonself discrimination,* New York, 1982, Wiley.
33. Lawlis GF: *Imagery and consciousness development,* unpublished manuscript.
34. LeBaron S: The role of imagery in the treatment of a patient with malignant melanoma, *Hospice J* 5(2):13, 1989.
35. Lebow G: Facilitating adaptation in anticipatory mourning, *Soc Casework* 57:458, 1976.
36. Lindberg C, Lawlis GF: The effectiveness of imagery as a childbirth preparatory technique, *J Ment Imagery* 12(1):31, 1988.
37. Manyande A, Berg S, Gettins D, Stanford SC, Mazhero S, Marks DF, Salmon P: Preoperative rehearsal of active coping imagery influences subjective and hormonal responses to abdominal surgery, *Psychosom Med* 57:177, 1995.
38. Manyande A, Chayen S, Priyakumar P et al: Anxiety and endocrine responses to surgery: paradoxical effects of preoperative relaxation training, *Psychosom Med* 54:275, 1992.
39. McKinney CH, Antoni MH, Kumar M, Tims FC, McCabe PM: Effects of guided imagery and music (GIM) therapy on mood and cortisol in healthy adults, *Health Psychol* 16(4):390, 1997.

40. Turkoski B, Lance B: The use of guided imagery with anticipatory grief, *Home Healthcare Nurs* 14(11):884, 1996.

41. Naperstek B: *Staying well with guided imagery*, New York, 1994, Time Warner.

42. Neumann W, Kugler J, Pfand-Neumann P, Schmitz N, Seelbach H, Kruskemper GM: Effects of pain-incompatible imagery on tolerance of pain, heart rate, and skin resistance, *Percept Mot Skills* 84:939, 1997.

43. Rando T: *Grief, dying, and death: clinical interactions for caregivers*, Champaign, IL, 1984, Research Press.

44. Rider MS, Achterberg J: Effect of music-assisted imagery on neutrophils and lymphocytes, *Biofeedback Self Regul* 14(3):247, 1989.

45. Rider MS, Achterberg J, Lawlis GF, Goven A, Toledo R, Butler JR: Effect of immune system imagery on secretory IgA, *Biofeedback Self Regul* 15(4):317, 1990.

46. Rider MS, Floyd JW, Kirkpatrick J: The effect of music, imagery, and relaxation on adrenal corticosteroids and the re-entrainment of circadian rhythms, *J Music Ther* XXII(1):46, 1985.

47. Salmon P, Evans R, Humphrey D: Anxiety and endocrine changes in surgical patients, *Br J Clin Psychol* 25:135, 1986.

48. Simonton OC, Matthews-Simonton S, Creighton J: *Getting well again*, Los Angeles, 1978, JP Tarcher.

49. Spanos N, Horton C, Chaves J: The effects of two cognitive strategies on pain threshold, *J Abnorm Psychol* 84:165, 1975.

50. Steptoe A: Stress, helplessness, and control: the implications of laboratory studies, *J Psychosom Res* 27:361, 1983.

51. Syrjala KL, Donaldson GW, David MW, Kippes ME, Carr JE: Relaxation and imagery and cognitive-behavioral training reduce pain during cancer treatment: a controlled clinical trial, *Pain* 63:189, 1995.

52. Troesch LM, Rodeher CB, Delaney EA, Yanes B: The influence of guided imagery on chemotherapy-related nausea and vomiting, *Oncol Nurs Forum* 20(8):1179, 1993.

53. Turkoski B, Lance B: The use of guided imagery with anticipatory grief, *Home Healthcare Nurs* 14(11):878, 1996.

54. Vickers RR Jr: Effectiveness of defenses: a significant predictor of cortisol excretion under stress, *J Psychosom Res* 32:21, 1988.

55. Vines SW: The therapeutics of guided imagery, *Holistic Nurs Prac* 8(2):34, 1988.

56. Wallace KG: Analysis of recent literature concerning relaxation and imagery interventions for cancer pain, *Cancer Nurs* 20(2):79, 1997.

57. Wescott JB, Hogan JJ: The effects of anger and relaxation forms of "in vivo" emotive imagery on pain tolerance, *Can J Behav Sci* 9:216, 1977.

58. Wilson HF: Behavioral preparation for surgery: benefit or harm? *J Behav Med* 4:79, 1981.

59. Wolf S: Effects of suggestion and conditioning on the action of chemical agents in human subjects: the pharmacology of placebos. *J Clin Invest* 29:100, 1950.

60. Zachariae R, Kirstense JS, Hokland P et al: Effect of psychological intervention in the form of relaxation and guided imagery on cellular immune function in normal health subjects: an overview, *Psychother Psychosom* 54:32, 1990.

UNIT *three*

Alternative Professionals

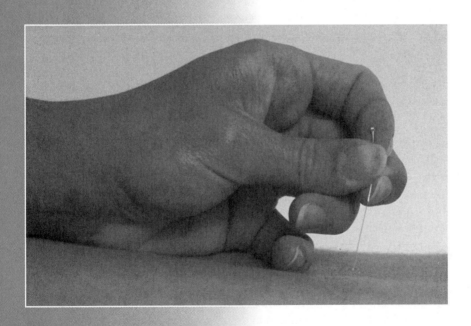

10

Chiropractic

Lyn W. Freeman

WHY READ THIS CHAPTER?

After physicians, chiropractors are the second largest group of primary care providers in the United States. Chiropractic is the most widely disseminated indigenous American system of healing and, today, is the most frequently used alternative health care profession in the United States. Yet, few understand the history, philosophy, or mechanisms underlying chiropractic practice. Consumers of chiropractic care and health care professionals who must advise patients concerning complementary medicine should inform themselves of how chiropractic is most beneficial and understand its limitations and its indications and contraindications. Chiropractic has a rich and intriguing history, a history that explains much about the tensions between conventional medicine and alternative therapies in general. It is always wise to be an informed consumer of any medical intervention—conventional or alternative. The reader can become more informed by reading this chapter.

CHAPTER OVERVIEW

Chiropractic is a profession that works on the musculoskeletal system of the body. Manipulation as a form of treatment is an ancient healing art. No single origin of the practice of manipulation can be identified, although many of the concepts of basic manipulation appear to be shared across time and by various cultures. Daniel David Palmer (known as D.D. Palmer), a self-styled magnetic healer, founded chiropractic in 1895. D.D. Palmer's son, B.J. Palmer, became known as "the developer" of the chiropractic movement and was initially responsible for its continuing success and survival.

Historically, the main emphasis of chiropractic has been and still is on the spine and its effects on the nervous system. The original chiropractic theory suggested that misaligned spinal vertebrae interfered with nerve function, ultimately resulting in an altered physiologic condition that contributed to pain and disease. It was believed that if a nerve was impinged because of a misalignment in the spine, a condition called subluxation occurred. Although the main symptom of a subluxation was pain, chiropractors also believed that spinal misalignment impaired the body's defenses.

Today, chiropractors still believe and emphasize that adjusting the spinal joints and resolving subluxations will restore normal nerve function and optimal health. However, the meaning of subluxation has been expanded. Improved joint mobility and the alleviation of spinal fixation or restricted movement is a focus of chiropractic today.[58]

In recent decades, chiropractic theories concerning how mechanical spinal joint dysfunction may influence neurophysiology have also undergone significant modification and now reflect a more contemporary view of physiology.[29] This modification of theory has continued to expand the meaning of subluxation.

The Intelligent Life-Force of Creation is God. It is individualized in each of us...God—the Universal Intelligence—the Life-Force of Creation—has been struggling for countless ages to improve upon itself—to express itself intellectually and physically higher in the scale of evolution.[58]

D. D. PALMER

The effects of manipulation are currently categorized as mechanical and neurologic. The mechanical effects are defined in terms of the subluxation, characterized as a spinal joint strain or sprain with associated local and referred pain and muscle spasm. Relieving subluxations is proposed to induce mechanical issues that result in the reduction of pain and restoration of mobility. The neurologic effects originally revolved around the "pinched nerve" hypothesis, but this classical theory has given way to a model that includes both direct and indirect effects on the function of the peripheral and central nervous systems because of spinal dysfunction.

Chiropractic research has demonstrated some effects on physiologic, biochemical, and immunologic parameters, although the clinical significance of these findings is currently unknown.

Chiropractic research has demonstrated short-term benefits in the treatment of acute low back pain, as well as neck and headache pain. Its effects on other musculoskeletal conditions are mixed, and its effects on nonmusculoskeletal conditions have not been adequately researched to demonstrate benefit. More clinically controlled trials with specified variables are needed.

CHAPTER OBJECTIVES

After completing this chapter, you should be able to:

1. Define chiropractic.
2. Describe and discuss the history and evolution of chiropractic.
3. Define and explain subluxation. Explain how its definition has expanded with time.
4. Describe and discuss the physiology underlying the chiropractic philosophy.
5. Explain the differences among adjustment, manipulation, and mobilization.
6. Define and explain the difference between physiologic and paraphysiologic joint space.
7. Summarize the findings of chiropractic treatment for low back pain.
8. Summarize the findings of chiropractic treatment for other musculoskeletal conditions, such as neck pain and migraine headaches.
9. Summarize the findings of chiropractic treatment for nonmusculoskeletal conditions, such as menstrual pain, asthma, and colic.
10. Describe the indications and contraindications for chiropractic treatment.

■ Chiropractic Defined

The word chiropractic is derived from the Greek words *cheir,* meaning hand, and *praktikos,* meaning done by. Chiropractic is essentially a profession that works on the musculoskeletal system of the body (i.e., bones, joints, muscles, ligaments, and tendons that give the body its form). A chiropractor may adjust the joints of the hand and wrist to relieve pain associated with carpel tunnel syndrome, or ankle pain may be alleviated by an adjustment to the joints of the ankle. The focus of chiropractic, however, is on the spine and its effects on the nervous system. This focus is described in detail when we discuss chiropractic philosophy and mechanisms. First, we review the history of manipulation and how chiropractic evolved in relation to that history.

■ History of Manipulation

Manipulation as a form of therapy is an ancient healing art. No single origin of the practice of manipulation can be identified, although many of the concepts of basic manipulation appear to be shared across time and by various cultures. The ancient cultures of China, Japan, Polynesia, India, Egypt, and Tibet all practiced a manipulative form of therapy. Therapeutic manipulation has been practiced by a variety of Indian cultures, such as the Aztec, Toltec, Tarascan, Inca, Maya, Sioux, and Winnebago.[65]

Well into the seventeen century, Greek, Roman, Byzantine, Cretan, Arabic, Spanish, Turkish, Italian, French, and German authors reported the use of traction applied to the head and feet while pressure was exerted on a specific spinal area.[51]

Hippocrates and Manipulation Practices

Hippocrates, the father of medicine (460-370 BC), was also a practitioner of manipulation (Figure 10-1). Two chapters in his monumental work, *Corpus Hippocrateum,* were dedicated to manipulative procedures. These chapters were entitled *Peri Arthron* (about joints) and *Moch-likon* (the lever); they described spinal manipulation with traction (extension).[51,64] Hippocrates wrote:

"Such extension would not do great harm, if well arranged, unless one deliberately wanted to do harm. The physician, or an assistant who is strong and not untrained, should put the palm of his hand on the hump, and the palm of the other on that, to reduce it forcibly, taking into consideration whether the reduction should naturally be made straight downwards, or towards the head, or towards the hip."[36]

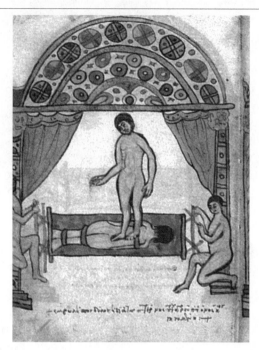

■ *Figure 10-1.* The Hippocratic method of manipulation relied on combined traction applied with a thrust or sustained pressure. Traction was applied with cloths pulled by helpers. The thrust would come from a person sitting or standing on the back of the patient or by means of a board acting as a lever (Apollonius of Cyprus). *From Peterson D, Wiese G:* Chiropractic: an illustrated history, *St Louis, 1994, Mosby.*

Hippocrates went on to describe using the physician's foot to apply full body weight in the manipulative process. He also suggested using the end of a stout board placed in a cleft in a wall as a lever for applying pressure to the "hump" (misaligned spinous process).

The physician, Galen (130-202 AD), was known as the "prince of physicians" and was strongly influenced by Hippocrates' teachings of manipulation. Galen reportedly relieved the paralysis of the right hand of Eudemas, a prominent Roman scholar, by manipulating the cervical vertebrae.[65]

Bonesetters

During the middle ages and Renaissance, manipulation was performed by a group of practitioners known as *bonesetters* (Figure 10-2). The art of bonesetting was practiced in Europe, North Africa, and Asia where bonesetters honed their skills through apprenticeships.[64] Some bonesetters, such as Sarah Mapp and Sir Herbert Barker, became famous for their skills. Mrs. Mapp's success medically and financially is credited with encouraging many bonesetters to set up permanent practices. Sir Herbert Barker's patients

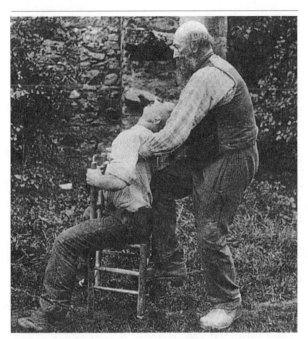

■ *Figure 10-2.* This French postcard, circa 1880, shows a bone-setter treating a lumbago or acute low back pain. This picture was shot in Brittany, France. *Courtesy of Musee des Artset Traditions Populaires, Paris. From Peterson D, Wiese G:* Chiropractic: an illustrated history, *St Louis, 1994, Mosby.*

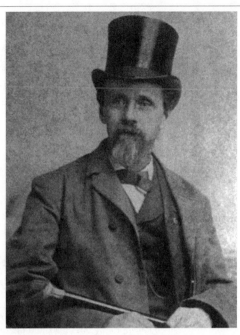

■ *Figure 10-3.* A portrait of A.T. Still, the founder of osteopathy, circa 1900. *Courtesy: Kirksville College of Osteopathy, A.T. Still Memorial Library, Archives Department, Kirksville, Missouri. From Peterson D, Wiese G:* Chiropractic: an illustrated history, *St Louis, 1994, Mosby.*

included English royalty, nobles, members of Parliament, and even H. G. Wells. In 1936, Sir Herbert was asked to demonstrate his skills for over 100 orthopedic surgeons. The August 1936 edition of the *British Medical Journal* reported that he presented a most interesting demonstration. In spite of the fact that Sir Herbert had been knighted in 1922 for his service to the public health, his manipulative practice was still considered unorthodox and was never accepted by organized medicine.

Osteopathy and Manipulation

Andrew Taylor Still (1828-1917) founded osteopathy, a therapeutic manipulation practice[64] (Figure 10-3). After losing three of his children to cerebrospinal meningitis, Still became convinced that physicians of his day did more harm than good. He became convinced that the body had to heal itself essentially, but the body had to be structurally sound to accomplish this healing. A structurally sound body would be able to access successfully its *life force*, a term he used to describe the body's innate healing abilities. Still believed that manipulation of the spine could relieve mechanical pressure on blood vessels and nerves. Pressure on the nerves led, he believed, to ischemia (i.e., reduced blood flow to tissue, often

resulting in pain), eventual necrosis (i.e., death of cells or tissues), and impingement of the healing life force. In 1892 he opened a school of osteopathy at Kirksville, Missouri. By 1958 there were more than 1300 practicing osteopaths. By 1968 the American Medical Association (AMA) began the amalgamation of medicine and osteopathy. Today, osteopathic practitioners receive full medical licensure in most states, and many no longer employ manipulation as part of their practice. Through specialization, most osteopaths have become indistinguishable from allopathic medical physicians.

■ Founding of Chiropractic

Daniel David Palmer (1845-1913), an emigrant from Canada, founded chiropractic (Figure 10-4). Initially, Palmer made a living as a schoolteacher, a farmer, and, finally, a grocer. In 1886, Palmer undertook a career as a magnetic healer. With the help of a creative advertising campaign, Palmer's practice grew quickly. He wrote and distributed a publication called the *Educator* that argued for the benefits of magnetic healing and against the "wickedness" of vaccinations and other conventional medical practices. Patients flooded his office, some from cities many miles away.[60]

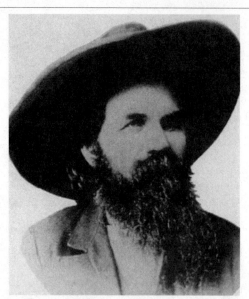

■ *Figure 10-4.* D.D. Palmer, circa 1870. *Courtesy of Palmer College of Chiropractic Archives, Davenport, Iowa. From Peterson D, Wiese G:* Chiropractic: an illustrated history, *St Louis, 1994, Mosby.*

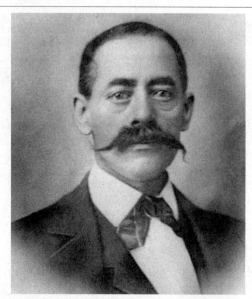

■ *Figure 10-5.* Harvey Lillard, a black American who operated a janitorial service in the building where D.D. Palmer maintained his offices, was the first chiropractic patient. *Courtesy of Palmer College of Chiropractic Archives, Davenport, Iowa. From Peterson D, Wiese G:* Chiropractic: an illustrated history, *St Louis, 1994, Mosby.*

■ Birth of Chiropractic

Palmer performed his first chiropractic adjustment on a janitor named Harvey Lillard on September 18, 1895, a time before the advent of licensing laws for physicians and at a time when many physicians had no medical education. Palmer was, however, a self-taught student of anatomy and physiology. Palmer describes what happened on that day.

> Harvey Lillard, a janitor in the Ryan Block, where I had my office, had been so deaf for 17 years that he could not hear the racket of a wagon on the street or the ticking of a watch. I made inquiry as to the cause of his deafness and was informed that when he was exerting himself in a cramped, stooping position, he felt something give in his back and immediately became deaf. An examination showed a vertebra racked from its normal position. I reasoned that if that vertebra was replaced, the man's hearing should be restored. With this object in view, a half-hour talk persuaded Mr. Lillard to allow me to replace it. I racked it into position by using the spinous process as a lever and soon the man could hear as before. There was nothing "accidental" about this, as it was accomplished with an object in view, and the result expected was obtained. There was nothing "crude" about this adjustment; it was specific, so much so that no chiropractor has equaled it.[58]

Convinced he had made a profound discovery related to health care, D.D. Palmer became very

secretive about his methods, making it impossible for patients or others to observe his palpations and adjustments (Figures 10-5 and 10-6).

Some persons believed that Palmer had gleaned information on manipulation from A.T. Still, the founder of osteopathy. Palmer and Still had much in common. Both had been magnetic healers and both practiced manipulative procedures. Palmer had once traveled from Davenport, Iowa, to observe Still's practice, but it is debatable how influenced he was by the principles of osteopathy.[30,32] Palmer claimed to have first learned the art of manipulation from a person named Dr. Atkinson, who also resided in Davenport.[58] Palmer was also quick to point out that manipulation had existed for a very long time.[58]

> I have, both in print and by word of mouth, repeatedly stated and now most emphatically repeat the statement, that I am not the first person to replace subluxated vertebrae, for this art has been practiced for thousands of years. I do, however, claim to be the first to replace displaced vertebrae by using the spinous and transverse processes as levers wherewith to rack subluxated vertebrae into normal position, and from this basic fact, to create a science which is destined to revolutionize the theory and practice of the healing art.[58]

In January, 1898, D.D. Palmer accepted his first chiropractic student. On January 6, 1902,

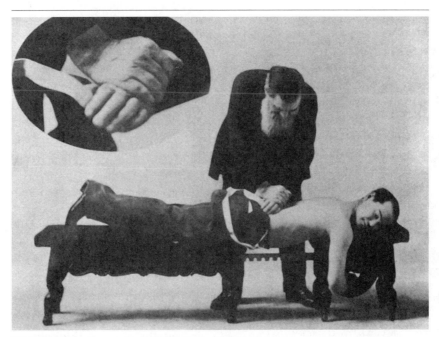

■ Figure 10-6. One of the few photographs of D.D. Palmer giving an adjustment. *From Palmer DD, Palmer BJ: The science of chiropractic: its principles and adjustments.* In Peterson D, Wiese G: Chiropractic: an illustrated history, *St Louis, 1994, Mosby.*

D.D. graduated four Doctors of Chiropractic, among them Bartlett Joshua, known as B.J., D.D. Palmer's son.

In 1906, D.D. Palmer was convicted of practicing medicine without a license. He was jailed for a short time because he initially refused to pay the fine that would free him. After his release, Palmer sold his interest in his chiropractic school to his son, B.J. Although he began or was involved with other chiropractic schools between 1908 and 1910, the elder Palmer's involvement in them did not continue for long. He did, however, continue to lecture and teach at the Ratledge College of Chiropractic. On October 20, 1913, D.D. Palmer died of typhoid fever after an illness of 28 days.

■ Developer of Chiropractic

Just as D.D. Palmer has been called "the founder," so B.J. became known as "the developer" of the chiropractic movement (Figure 10-7). After purchasing the school from his father, B.J. expanded the school and many of its related activities. He advertised, set up a correspondence program, and published two magazines, *Fountain Head News* and *The Chiropractor.* B.J. also brought the first x-ray machine to Davenport and eventually offered a course leading to a special diploma for the use of x-ray technology. Under the influence

of B.J., the student body grew by leaps and bounds. By 1920 the Palmer School boasted over 1000 future chiropractors in training.

■ Continuing Battle for Acceptance

Just as B.J. inherited the responsibility for developing the future of chiropractic, a new and significant challenge to the profession was being born. At the turn of the nineteenth century, there were numerous competing medical practitioners—magnetic healers, herbologists, hydro healers, bonesetters, and homeopathic practitioners. Scientific research methods and adequate medical training were sorely lacking during this period, as evidenced by the condemnation of traditional medical colleges in the Flexner Report.[27] Medical education's foremost critic, Abraham Flexner, although not a physician, was commissioned by the Carnegie Foundation to survey all medical schools during 1909 and 1910. The resulting study, the *Flexner Report,* led to the reformation of medical education in the United States. In the wake of this report, organized medicine promoted licensing regulations, believing that the inferior education of chiropractics and other alternative practitioners would prevent them from passing state board licensing examinations.[75] In the coming years, chiropractors would be arrested repeat-

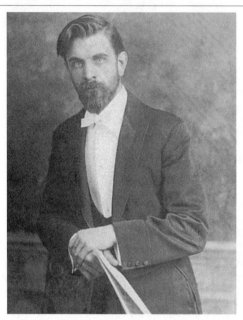

■ *Figure 10-7.* A photograph of B.J. Palmer, circa 1910. *(Courtesy: Palmer College of Chiropractic Archives, Davenport, Iowa. From Peterson D, Wiese G:* Chiropractic: an illustrated history, *St Louis, 1994, Mosby.)*

edly and prosecuted for practicing medicine without a license. The prosecutions continued in states where chiropractic legislation was not enacted and was especially vehement in California and Texas.[60] Introduction of the Basic Science Board in 1925 created a further obstacle for chiropractors who were under trained in these areas. Applicants of all "healing" professions—medicine, osteopathy, chiropractic, and naturopathy—were required to pass tests in physiology, pathology, chemistry, and, in some cases, bacteriology, toxicology, and diagnosis. The requirement to pass the Basic Science Board proved to be a devastating blow for the chiropractic movement. Chiropractic leaders argued against the basic science requirements, stating that chiropractic and allopathic medical approaches differed in philosophy, rationale, and approach. This argument went unheeded.[42]

The 1930s served as a crucible for chiropractic. The economic depression, coupled with legal attacks, resulted in a drastic reduction of chiropractic schools and students. In Nebraska, one of the first states to license chiropractors (1915), the right to practice was virtually eliminated for 4 decades. Between 1929 and 1950, not a single chiropractor was able to pass the licensing examinations, and the state board could only record 70 licensed chiropractors in 1945. Nationwide, the Federation of Medical Licensing Boards reported that between 1927 and 1944, 87% of medical stu-dents, or 17,400 physicians, passed the basic sciences examination. By contrast, only 28% of chiropractors passed these boards (93 total).[60]

In November, 1963, with increased numbers of ex-servicemen becoming chiropractors, the AMA began a renewed campaign to "contain and eliminate" chiropractic. The AMA formed a Committee on Quackery, and AMA members were forbidden to associate professionally with chiropractors. Physicians could not teach in chiropractic schools, lecture at chiropractic conventions, or accept patient referrals from a chiropractor.

Aggressive action on the part of conventional medicine usually backfired, however. For example, in 1916, Tullius Ratledge, a California chiropractor, was sentenced to 90 days in jail for practicing medicine without a license. The charge arose not from patient complaints but from medically instigated entrapment. California chiropractors adopted the slogan, "Go to jail for chiropractic"; at the apex of the controversy, 450 chiropractors were jailed in a single year. In defiance, chiropractors continued to set up portable tables to treat fellow prisoners and even treated visiting patients. By the time a woman chiropractor collapsed from a 10-day hunger strike, public sympathy for chiropractors had reached a fevered pitch and the medical lobby was routed. In 1922, Californians voted overwhelmingly to license the profession, and all chiropractors still in jail were pardoned on the grounds that they had been unjustly accused.[75] Repeatedly through the years, the heavy-handed tactics of the conventional medical lobby has only resulted in continual "wins" for chiropractic.

Chiropractic continued to make inroads. Between 1913 and 1937, forty of the fifty states passed licensing laws for chiropractors. By 1974, chiropractic education received federally recognized accreditation, and doctors of chiropractic were licensed in all 50 states.[18] Finally, in 1976, Chester Wilks and four other chiropractors filed a federal lawsuit against the AMA, the American Hospital Association, and six other medical associations. Wilks and others charged these organizations with antitrust violations of conspiring to eliminate chiropractic and refusal to associate with chiropractors. In 1987 the U.S. District court of Illinois found the AMA and its associates, including the American College of Radiology and the American College of Surgeons, guilty of conspiracy against chiropractors and in violation of the federal antitrust laws. The permanent injunction against the AMA required *The Journal of the American Medical Association* to publish the court's judgment.[31] In 1990 the U.S. Supreme Court let this decision stand without comment. Chiropractic's historic enemy, the AMA, was ordered to cease and desist—a phenomenal win for the chiropractic profession.

■ Chiropractic Education Today

In 1996, there were 16 colleges of Chiropractic in the United States accredited by the Council of Chiropractic Education (CCE).[2] Admission to a college of chiropractic requires at least 2 years of undergraduate study with course work in biology and chemistry.[63] The chiropractic curriculum requires 4 years of full-time education and a minimum of 4200 hours of course work. A typical chiropractic curriculum includes but is not limited to anatomy; biochemistry; physiology; microbiology; pathology; public health; physical, clinical, and laboratory diagnosis; gynecology; obstetrics; pediatrics; geriatrics; dermatology; roentgenology (x-ray); psychology; dietetics; orthopedics; physical therapy; first aid and emergency medicine; spinal analysis; principles and practice of chiropractic; adjustive techniques; and research methods and procedures.

There are also specialization areas available to chiropractors, some of which require an additional 3 years of study. Postgraduate educational programs are available in family practice, applied chiropractic sciences, clinical neurology, orthopedics, sports injuries, pediatrics, nutrition, rehabilitation, and industrial consulting.[50] Residency programs include radiology, orthopedics, family practice, and clinical sciences.[18]

■ Chiropractic Philosophy and Mechanisms

As mentioned previously, the main emphasis of chiropractic is the spine and its effects on the nervous system. The original chiropractic theory suggested that misaligned spinal vertebrae interfered with nerve function, ultimately resulting in physiologic alterations that contributed to pain and disease. It was believed that if a nerve was impinged because of a misalignment in the spine, a condition called *subluxation* occurred. Although the main symptom of a subluxation is pain, chiropractors also believed that spinal subluxation impaired the body's defenses.

Today, chiropractors still believe and emphasize that by adjusting the spinal joints and resolving subluxations, normal nerve function and optimal health are restored. However, the meaning of subluxation has expanded with time, first to

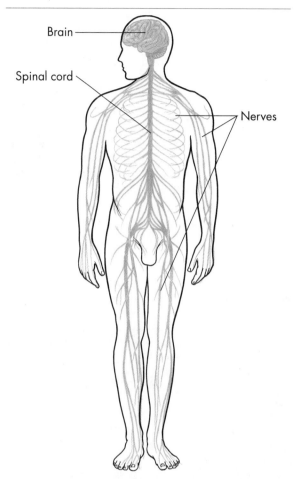

■ **Figure 10-8.** The nervous system. The brain and spinal cord constitute the **central nervous system** and the nerves make up the **peripheral nervous system.** *Modified from Thibodeau GA, Patton KT:* The human body in health & disease, *St Louis, 1996, Mosby.*

include the issues of joint mobility and then to make spinal fixation, or restricted movement, the focus of chiropractic manipulation.[26,33]

In recent decades, chiropractic theories about how mechanical spinal joint dysfunction may influence neurophysiologic conditions have undergone significant modification and reflect more contemporary views of physiology.[29] These contemporary views are discussed in detail in the section entitled "Mechanisms of Chiropractic."

Physiology Underlying Chiropractic Care

The *nervous system* is composed of three overlapping systems: the *central nervous system* (CNS), the *autonomic nervous system* (ANS), and the *peripheral nervous system* (PNS). The two main structures of the CNS are the brain and the spinal cord (Figure 10-8). Whereas the brain is protected by the cranial cavity of the skull, the spinal cord is protected by the *vertebral column,* also referred to as the *spinal column.* The spinal column—the bony structure that surrounds the spinal cord—is composed of 24 bones, or *vertebrae.* Between each individual vertebra, pairs of spinal nerves exit and extend to every body part including muscles, bones, organs, and glands. The spinal nerves, in turn, send and receive messages to all the other nerves in the body, referred to as the PNS. The ANS consists of certain motor neurons that conduct impulses from the spinal cord and brainstem to cardiac, smooth muscle, and glandular tissues. The ANS therefore consists of the parts of the nervous system that regulate what are considered involuntary functions (e.g., heartbeat, contractions of the stomach and intestines, secretions of the glands) (Figure 10-9).

For health to be maintained, balance and equilibrium of function must exist between these three systems. Chiropractors emphasize that this balance can be disturbed by spinal injury, spinal subluxation, certain illnesses, and even stress. Damage, disease, or structural change to the spine can affect the health of the rest of the body.

Chiropractic Mechanisms and Practices

Chiropractic treatments, as well as diagnostic practices, vary by geographic region because of

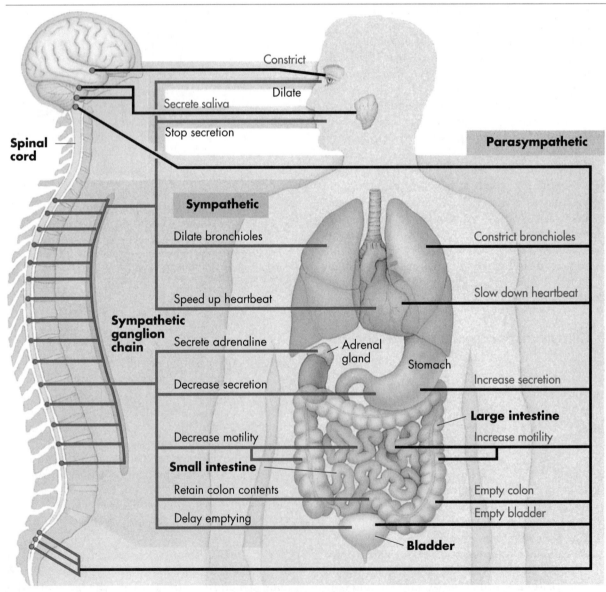

■ **Figure 10-9.** Innervation of the major target organs by the autonomic nervous system. *Modified from Thibodeau GA, Patton KT:* The human body in health & disease, *St Louis, 1996, Mosby.*

the differences in state laws governing scope of practice and practitioner philosophy. The therapeutic procedure most closely associated with chiropractic is spinal manipulation. However, chiropractic patient management often includes lifestyle counseling, nutritional management, rehabilitation, various physiotherapeutic modalities, and a variety of other interventions.[29,35]

Chiropractors examine the spine and then apply specialized manipulative techniques designed to return the spine to optimal function. In this manner, chiropractors diagnose and treat numerous disorders ranging from headache to back pain.

In chiropractic, *spinal adjustments* are made to bring the spinal column into proper function, thereby protecting the function and integrity of the CNS and PNS (Figure 10-10). Chiropractors diagnose problems by observation, x-ray films, and hands-on examination called *palpation*. The spine is then *manipulated* by applying force to the spinous processes, joints, and other tissues of the body (Figure 10-11). Other techniques such as *mobilization* may also be applied. (These terms are defined in the following text.)

Techniques of Care

Almost from its inception, chiropractors were repeatedly prosecuted for practicing medicine without a license. As a means of defense, and to clarify the differences between chiropractic and other medical treatments, a specialized terminology was developed for chiropractic. This new terminology emphasized that chiropractors do not treat disease, as do physicians; rather, they promote the healing of the body by focusing on the body's "innate intelligence," or the homeostasis of the body to heal itself.

Chiropractic Adjustment

Chiropractic adjustment, the mainstay of chiropractic treatment, refers to a wide variety of manual and mechanical interventions that may be delivered with (1) high or low velocity (speed); (2) short or long lever (direct application to spinous processes versus using arms and legs as fulcrums); (3) high or low amplitude (force); and (4) with or without recoil. Procedures are usually directed at specific joints or anatomic regions and may or may not involve cavitation or gapping of a joint, which produces the "pop" or "click" sound.[35] The common denominator of all of these interventions is the purpose for their delivery (e.g., the removal of a subluxation, that is, the structural dysfunction of joints and muscles associated with neurologic alterations.)

However, the adjustment procedure that is the hallmark and defining technique of chiropractic treatment is the delivery of the short-lever, high-velocity, low-amplitude thrust to the bony

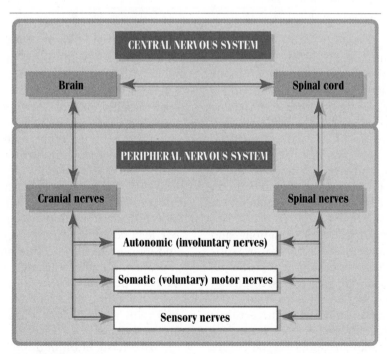

■ **Figure 10-10.** Divisions of the nervous system. *Modified from Thibodeau GA, Patton KT:* The human body in health & disease, *St Louis, 1996, Mosby.*

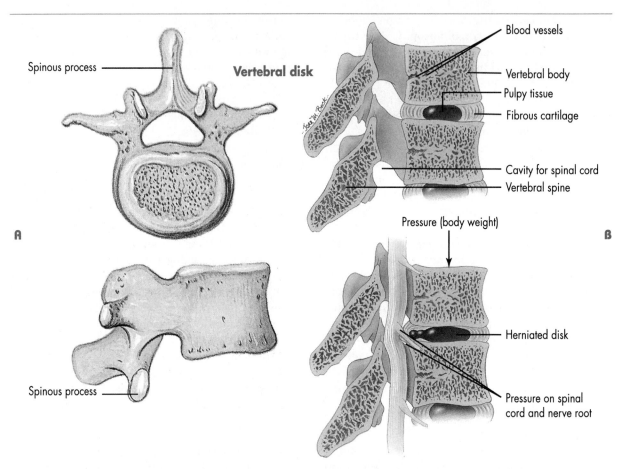

Spinous process

Vertebral disk

Blood vessels

Vertebral body

Pulpy tissue

Fibrous cartilage

Cavity for spinal cord

Vertebral spine

R

B

Pressure (body weight)

Spinous process

Herniated disk

Pressure on spinal cord and nerve root

■ *Figure* 10-11. **R,** The spinous process. **B,** Sagittal section of vertebrae showing normal and abnormal disk alignment. *Parts A and B modified from Thibodeau GA, Patton KT:* The human body in health & disease, *St Louis, 1996, Mosby.*

processes of the spine. This adjustment procedure often results in cavitation or gapping of a joint and produces an audible popping sound.[49] Another description to explain this type of adjustment is a very fast but highly controlled thrust of specific force that is applied directly to the bony processes. The length of the lever arm used to adjust the spinous process is what makes this technique "short lever." A chiropractor is trained to thrust into a spinal joint with a specific and exact amount of force and speed, resulting in a correct realignment of the spine.

The terms adjustment, manipulation, and mobilization are often confusing to persons reviewing the literature on chiropractic, osteopathy, physiotherapy, and massage. This confusion occurs because often these terms are given multiple definitions. To understand what these terms mean in relation to chiropractic and how they relate to this entire body of literature, the reader needs to place them in the context of joint movement, as explained in the following text.

Terminology of Joint Movement

There are three end-range barriers to joint movement. The first is the *active end range,* which refers to how far the patient can, with his or her own muscular effort, move a joint in a particular direction. Once a patient has reached the end of this first active end range, a clinician can still passively move the joint further without injury or pain. This extra "stretch" provided by the clinician enters the second barrier called the *passive end range.* Movement to the passive end range is also termed *physiologic joint space.* The third barrier encountered is the *anatomic end range,* and movement **beyond** this range would result in rupture of the joint's ligaments. If joint movement exceeds the physiologic joint space (passive end range) but not the anatomic end range barrier, this joint movement is termed the *paraphysiologic joint space.*[35]

The term *manipulation* refers to a passive movement of low amplitude and high velocity, which moves the joint into the paraphysiologic range, often resulting in joint cavitation accompanied by the popping sound.

Mobilization refers to the clinician-assisted passive movement within the third barrier, physiologic joint space, resulting in an increased overall range-of-joint motion.

Although chiropractors rely most heavily on their hallmark manipulation technique of short-lever, low-amplitude, high-velocity thrusts to the spinous processes, they may also employ manipulation of joints other than the spine or may use mobilization techniques. There are currently more than 150 chiropractic techniques. We explore three of the most basic forms.

Direct Thrust Technique

Chiropractors will use different parts of the hand to direct the thrust, depending on the joint being adjusted. For example, the middle or base of the index finger may be used to adjust the neck, whereas an area of the wrist bone may be used to adjust the lumbar spine.

Indirect Thrust Techniques

If, because of the nature of an injury, the direct thrust technique of adjustment would be too uncomfortable for a patient, an indirect thrust technique may be used. The joint to be manipulated may be gently stretched over a pad or wedge-shaped block until realignment is accomplished.

Soft-Tissue Techniques

Soft-tissue techniques are methods used before an adjustment to relax the joint or reduce muscle tension. These methods are often used to release "trigger points (e.g., tender or reflex points where tension is stored in the musculature).

Other Tools of Chiropractic

X-ray studies, a major diagnostic tool for chiropractors, are often used during the first evaluation. Other supportive measures include the use of electrical stimulation, ice, heat, ultrasound, and traction. Electrical stimulation involves placing a pad onto the body and introducing a mild electric current into the body. This can be used as a form of deep-tissue massage or to move body fluids away from swollen tissues.[30] Ice is used for pain control, and heat is used for sedation. Ultrasound (i.e., the use of sound vibrations) stimulates circulation and removes toxins and swelling around an injured area. Traction may be imposed to lengthen the spine and/or to relieve the pressure of a deranged disk or spinal nerve.

■ Mechanisms of Chiropractic

Chiropractic philosophy holds that subluxation of the spinal vertebrae interferes with nerve function, alters physiology, and contributes to pain and disease. If chiropractic reduces pain and disease, by what mechanisms do these results occur?

The effects of manipulation are currently categorized as *mechanical* and *neurologic*. In mechanical terms, a manipulable spinal disorder, traditionally termed *subluxation,* is characterized as a spinal joint strain or sprain with associated and referred pain and muscle spasm. The spinal joint's function is deranged by virtue of static misalignment and reduction of motion.

The second category, neurologic effects, revolved around the classical theory of the "pinched nerve" hypothesis. This theory has now given way to a model that includes both direct and indirect effects on the function of the PNS and CNS resulting from spinal dysfunction. Direct effects involve compression or irritation of the neural structures in and around the intervertebral foramen; indirect effects involve persistent spinal pain and hypomobility of the reflex activities of the associated spinal cord levels.[71]

Support for the original ideas of subluxation was undermined when published research suggested that vertebral displacement could not impinge on a spinal nerve at the intervertebral foramen.[21] Today, many scientists no longer refer to simply subluxation; rather, they use the terminology "vertebral subluxation complex," meaning mechanical impediments beyond bone displacement that can include mobility, posture, blood flow, muscle tone, and condition of the nerves themselves.[48] Some researchers suggest abandoning the term altogether, whereas others refer to manipulable spinal lesions or vertebral blockage.[34,39-41]

Various studies have also attempted to assess the physiologic, biochemical, and immunologic effects that explain chiropractic's effectiveness. Some of these studies are discussed in the following text.

Chiropractic, Applied Force, and Immunologic Changes

Triano, Brennan, and their associates quantified the applied forces of manipulation and correlated them to changes in leukocyte function. At 500 N or more applied force, neutrophil and mononuclear cells were primed for enhanced endotoxin-stimulated tumor necrosis factor production, demonstrating a slight but significant elevation in substance P. The authors determined that a threshold of approximately 500 N was required to produce these effects and that less than this threshold resulted in no effect on this variable.[12,70] An elevated respiratory burst in vitro when challenged with opsonized zymosan was also demonstrated.[12] (Note: Respiratory burst is a bacterial killing process in which oxygen is metabolized to produce potent germ-killing, oxidizing substances, such as bleach and hydrogen peroxide.)

Beta-Endorphin Levels and Chiropractic

In three studies of the effects of manipulation on plasma beta-endorphin levels, one study found a statistically significant increase in endorphins, whereas the other two studies did not.[19,62,73]

Brennen recently reviewed the hypothesized mechanisms used to explain the effects of chiropractic. She concluded that nearly all the theories of the effects and mechanisms of action of spinal manipulation still lacked adequate research.[11] Further, the clinical significance of the observed physiologic and biochemical effects are unknown.

■ Use of Chiropractic Care

Back pain is the most frequently reported ailment for which alternative treatments are sought.[25] It is not surprising therefore that after physicians, chiropractors are the second largest group of primary care providers in the United States.[67] Chiropractic is the most widely disseminated indigenous American system of healing and, today, is the most frequently used alternative health care profession in the United States.[25]

In 1970 there were an estimated 13,000 licensed chiropractors in the United States. By 1994 there are more than 50,000 chiropractors in the United States.[20] More than two thirds of all health care treatment for back pain are provided by chiropractors. In excess of $3.5 billion per year is spent on chiropractic care, with 32% to 45% of visits for the treatment of low back pain.[1,54,68] In the United States, chiropractors deliver 94% of manipulative therapies, with the rate of use of chiropractic services approximating 50 visits per 100 person years.[68] Overall, chiropractic services are used by approximately 11% of the total population annually, with a mean of 9.8 visits per client, per year.[24] Even though the relative cost-effectiveness of chiropractic care has not been convincingly established, patients with back pain typically report being more satisfied with chiropractic treatment than those patients receiving conventional medical care.[4,14,17,52]

■ Chiropractic Research Outcomes: An Overview

Patient Response to Chiropractic Care

In spite of the fact that there is no experimentally validated biological mechanism for the effectiveness of chiropractic, in the past 18 years, chiropractic has consistently assumed an increasing role in the health care industry.[69,74] For example, an analysis of the RAND Health Insurance Experiment (HIE), a community-based study of the use of health services, found that 7.5% of the population used chiropractic care, and 42% of all visits were for back pain.

Patients have consistently reported high levels of satisfaction with chiropractic care.[14,16,38] Kane and others identified workmen's compensation records for treatment of back or spinal problems. In this study, physicians treated 110 patients and chiropractors treated 122. In terms of the patient perception of improvement in functional status and patient satisfaction, chiropractors were reported to be as effective with the patients they treated as were those treated by physicians.

A Cherkin survey found chiropractic patients with back pain more satisfied with all aspects of their care than patients with back pain treated by physicians. It is not known whether these results are due to self-selection of patients with strong beliefs and expectations in chiropractic care.

Chiropractic Treatment of Low Back Pain

Acute back pain is defined as pain of less than 3 weeks' duration. Subacute low back pain is pain of 3 to 13 weeks' duration, whereas chronic low back pain is pain that lasts longer than 13 weeks. Most patients with acute low back pain without sciatic nerve root irritation have been reported to recover spontaneously within a few weeks.[23,28] (Note: Sciatic nerve root irritation is defined by shooting pain in the posterior thigh or calf and pain upon straight-leg raising.) (Table 10-1)

There have been more than 36 randomized clinical trials of spinal manipulation for patients with low back pain.[45] Studies have been of variable quality. Three of the better reviews reached differing conclusions. The first review, conducted by Koes, noted heterogeneity in treatments and did not attempt statistical combinations of individual studies.

Koes: Review of Low Back Pain Studies

Koes and others evaluated 35 randomized clinical trials of patient back and neck pain that compared spinal manipulation with other treatments. Most studies were found to be of poor quality.

TABLE 10-1	Manipulation Treatment for Low Back Pain and Back and Neck Pain

AUTHOR(S)	TREATMENT	COMPARISON TREATMENT	SAMPLE SIZE	RESULTS AND OUTCOMES
Hadler NM et al: A benefit of spinal manipulation as adjunctive therapy for acute lowback pain: a stratified controlled trial, *Spine* 12(7):703, 1987.	Single long-lever; high-velocity; thrust to lower spine while stabilizing the thorax	Spinal mobilization without rotational forces and leverage required to move facet joints	54	No difference for patients with pain of less than 2 wks; however, if pain was of 2-4 wks duration, manipulation achieved 50% reduction in pain more quickly; differences emerged at day 3 of treatment
Mathews JA et al: Back pain and sciatica: controlled trials of manipulation, traction, sclerosant and epidural injections, *Br J Rheumatol* 26:416, 1987.	Manipulation, defined as overpressure at the extremes of range, including a straight thrust	Infrared heat	260	In groups with low back and dorsal pain, in the group with limited straight-leg raising (n=207), significantly more persons recovered in 2 wks; in group without limited straight-leg raising, only a trend for greater improvement was found (n=53)
Coyer AB, Curwen IHM: Low back pain treated by manipulation, *BMJ* 705, 1955.	Manipulation of lumbar spine	Bed rest, lumbar pillow, and analgesics	136	Significant benefit of manipulation found at 1 wk (50% vs 27%) No significant difference at 6 wks
Hoehler FK et al: Spinal manipulation for low back pain, *JAMA* 245(18):1835, 1981.	Short, high-velocity thrusts to the pelvis	Soft-tissue massage	95	Significantly greater benefit to chiropractic patients for sitting in chair and bed, reaching, dressing, amount of pain, improvement in straight-leg raising to pain level Manipulation provided immediate subjective alleviation of pain
MacDonald RS, Bell J: An open controlled assessment of osteopathic manipulation in nonspecific low-back pain, *Spine* 15(5):364, 1990.	Low-velocity, high amplitude movements to hypermobile joints and high-velocity, low-amplitude thrust techniques	Control group-received advice on posture, exercise, and avoidance of stress	95	Subjects with pain duration of 14-28 days improved; no response to shorter episodes of presenting pain Maximal benefit was during the first 2 wks of treatment, with no difference at 4 wks
Meade TW et al: Low back pain of mechanical origin: randomized comparison of chiropractic and hospital outpatient treatment, *BMJ* 300:1431, 1990.	Chiropractic treatment at discretion of chiropractor, maximum of ten treatments; high-velocity, low-amplitude thrusts	Hospital outpatient treatment	741	Chiropractic care was most effective for patients with a history of chronic or severe pain Reduction in pain over time was significantly greater for the chiropractic group; changes in straight-leg raising and lumbar flexion were significantly more improved for the chiropractic group
Cherkin DC: A comparison of physical therapy, chiropractic manipulation, and provision of an educational booklet for the treatment of patients with low back pain, *N Engl J Med* 339:1021, 1998.	Chiropractic	McKenzie method of physical therapy and an educational booklet	321	McKenzie method and chiropractic had similar effects and costs and produced marginally better outcomes than the booklet group Over 2 yrs, costs were $437 for physical therapy, $429 for chiropractic, $153 for booklet group

Continued

| | **TABLE** 10-1 | **Manipulation Treatment for Low Back Pain and Back and Neck Pain—cont'd** | | | |

AUTHOR(S)	TREATMENT	COMPARISON TREATMENT	SAMPLE SIZE	RESULTS AND OUTCOMES
BACK AND NECK STUDIES				
Skargren EI: Cost and effectiveness analysis of chiropractic and physiotherapy treatment for low back pain: six month follow-up, *Spine* 22(18):2167. 1997.	Chiropractic treatment at therapist discretion	Physiotherapy	323	No difference in outcome or direct/indirect costs between groups; no difference in subgroups defined as duration, history, or severity There was a highly significant improvement in pain, function, and general health for both groups immediately after treatment and at 6-mo follow-up
Jordan A et al: Intensive training, physiotherapy, or manipulation for patients with chronic neck pain, *Spine* 23(3):311, 1998.	Chiropractic treatment for chronic neck pain	Intensive training of musculature; physiotherapy	119	No difference between the three treatments All three treatments demonstrated meaningful improvements in all primary effective parameters Improvements were maintained at 4 and 12 mos
Skargren EI: Cost and effectiveness analysis of chiropractic and physiotherapy treatment for low back and neck pain: six month follow-up, *Spine* 22(18):2167, 1997.	Chiropractic care at discretion of chiropractor	Physiotherapy at discretion of physiotherapist	323	Effectiveness and total costs of chiropractic and physiotherapy as primary treatment were similar to reach the same result at completion of treatment and at 6-mo follow-up No differences were found in subgroups defined as duration, history, or severity

Approximately 51% showed favorable results for manipulation, whereas 14% of the studies reported positive results in one or more subgroups. Although results were promising, the efficacy of manipulation was not convincingly demonstrated because of poor study quality.[44]

As often occurs in traditional medical journals, this review combined manipulation forms, rather than evaluate chiropractic practice exclusively. Seven studies were clearly defined "chiropractic," whereas other manipulation studies evaluated a variety of methods including osteopathy, Maitland, rotational, and Cyriax. Although it is valuable to determine whether manipulation, in its general sense, is efficacious, one has to be careful not to confuse chiropractic outcomes with other forms of manipulation and mobilization that are not delivered by chiropractors and do not use the hallmark chiropractic technique of short-lever, high-velocity, low-amplitude thrusts to spinous processes.

Anderson: Metaanalysis of Back Pain Studies
In a more thoughtful metaanalysis performed by Anderson and others, 23 randomized, controlled trials were assessed for their efficacy to manage back pain.[3] Care was taken to include the *Chiropractic Research Archives Collection* and to hand search professional chiropractic journals. Because one trial can include more than one comparison

of treatment, these trials produced 34 mutually exclusive, discrete samples. Effect sizes were calculated for nine outcome variables at eight time points after treatment initiation. Of the 44 effect sizes, 38 indicated that spinal manipulation was more effective than comparison treatments (i.e., manipulation was found to be more effective than mobilization).

Shekelle: Metaanalysis of Low Back Pain Studies
Shekelle and others performed a metaanalysis of nine studies of patients with acute or subacute low back pain, uncomplicated by sciatica. The authors tested the effect of manipulation against other conservative treatments or sham manipulation.[68] Variables assessed included relief of pain, time to relief of pain, improvement in functional status, and days lost from work. For patients with uncomplicated, acute low back pain, the difference in probability of recovery at 3 weeks favored treatment with spinal manipulation (0.17, an increase in recovery from 50% to 67%). The authors also reviewed three studies of patients further complicated with sciatic nerve irritation. Differences in probability of recovery at 4 weeks were not statistically significant (0.098). The authors concluded that spinal manipulation has short-term benefit in some patients, especially those with uncomplicated acute low back pain. At that time, data were insufficient to determine

efficacy of spinal manipulation for chronic low back pain.

The combined manipulative treatments in this review were described as (1) long-lever manipulation; (2) osteopathic manipulation; (3) combined physiotherapy including manipulation; (4) manipulation and physical therapy; (5) Maitland manipulation and mobilization; (6) rotational manipulation and mobilization; and (7) Cyriax manipulation. It quickly becomes apparent that although this review evaluated methods described as "manipulation," this review did not reflect outcomes from chiropractic practice alone. Only four of the nine studies of uncomplicated back pain appeared to have been delivered by chiropractors or to offer (as occurred in the osteopathic study) clearly defined techniques typically used by chiropractors. Manipulation, as defined in most review articles (if clearly defined at all), did not represent the hallmark chiropractic method of manipulation (i.e., low amplitude and high velocity, which moves the joint into the paraphysiologic range, resulting in joint cavitation accompanied by the "popping" sound.)

Review of Mixed Studies of Low Back Pain

After an exhaustive review of the literature, a recent systematic review assessed the effectiveness of chiropractic treatment for patients with low back pain.[6] Eight controlled trials were found, four for the treatment of chronic pain and four for combined acute and chronic pain. Outcomes were mixed. All studies had serious design flaws with differing outcome measures and follow-up periods, making statistical combination impossible. The authors concluded that the number of studies and their poor quality provided no convincing evidence for or against the effectiveness of chiropractic for acute and chronic low back pain. The authors concluded higher quality studies are needed before the efficacy of chiropractic for low back pain can be demonstrated or refuted.

These findings should not come as a total surprise. For the issue of back pain, seriously flawed studies with inconclusive outcomes are common in the conventional medical literature. An evidence-based review of conservative and surgical interventions for acute back pain failed to identify any conventional medical interventions supported by multiple high-quality scientific studies.[8] In spite of the low number and poor quality of chiropractic studies, there is as much or more evidence for the efficacy of spinal manipulation and chiropractic as for other nonsurgical treatments for back pain.

It should not be assumed that research conclusions find no benefit for manipulation. In the *Journal of the American Medical Association*, Assendelft and others literally assessed 51 reviews of spinal manipulation for low back pain. Of the 51 reviews, 17 found neutral results and 34 found positive results. For spinal manipulation, 9 of the 10 highest quality reviews found positive results. The authors, nonetheless, pointed to the need for improvement in the overall quality of all manipulative studies.[5] In the *New England Journal of Medicine,* the bastion journal of conventional and conservative allopathic medicine, an article evaluating the role of chiropractic in health care states: "That spinal manipulation is a somewhat effective symptomatic therapy for some patients is, I believe, no longer in dispute."[66] Although this may seem to be damning with faint praise, this statement is actually remarkable, considering the history between conventional medicine and chiropractic. This article goes on to point out that it is the use of chiropractic for other than spinal pain and the cost effectiveness of chiropractic that is still in question. Recent guidelines published by the federal Agency for Health Care Policy and Research (AHCPR) concluded that spinal manipulation was one of only three treatments for acute low back pain for which there was at least moderate research-based evidence of effectiveness.[8] Other commonly accepted treatments for back pain (e.g., muscle relaxants, physical therapy) lack even moderate amounts of evidence because of the paucity of research.

■ Chiropractic and Musculoskeletal Conditions

Neck Pain

In a randomized controlled trial to determine the immediate results of manipulation, 100 consecutive outpatients suffering from unilateral neck pain with referral into the trapezius muscle were randomized to receive manipulation or mobilization. Manipulation subjects received a single rotational manipulation (high-velocity, low-amplitude thrust); mobilization subjects were mobilized with a muscle energy technique. Both treatments increased range of motion, but manipulation had a significantly greater effect on pain intensity; 85% of manipulated patients and 69% of mobilized patients reported immediate pain relief, with the decrease of pain for manipulated subjects more than 1.5 times greater than mobilized subjects ($p=0.05$).[15]

In another study, 119 patients with neck pain received chiropractic care, intensive training of the cervical musculature, or a physiotherapy regimen. No clinically significant differences between groups were found, although all three groups significantly reduced pain and disability.[37] In a smaller study with only 20 patients, half received six sessions of high-velocity, low-amplitude manipulation over a 3- to 4-week period, or they practiced stretching exercises twice a day for the same period. Manipulation patients reduced pain 44%, whereas stretching only reduced pain 9%.[61] Studies of manipulation for neck pain are few, and outcomes are mixed; it can be stated that research outcomes suggest manipulation may be beneficial for neck pain, but more trials of consistent design are needed (Table 10-2).

Headache Pain

Studies of manipulation for headache have focused on migraine headache, tension headache, or cervicogenic headache pain. Headaches of cervical origin are referred to as cervicogenic headaches, that is, pain rising from neck dysfunction.[72] The following text examines the studies of these three forms of headache pain.

Migraine Headaches

In a 6-month trial, 85 volunteers suffering from migraine headache pain were randomly assigned to manipulation by a physiotherapist, manipulation by a chiropractor, or mobilization by a medical practitioner. For all persons, migraine symptoms were significantly reduced. Chiropractic did not reduce frequency, duration, or severity of migraine pain compared with the other two groups; however, chiropractic patients experienced less pain when they had attacks.[59] Another study compared outcomes of 218 migraine sufferers receiving 4 weeks of spinal manipulation, amitriptyline (a serotonin agonist), or amitriptyline plus spinal manipulation. Manipulation was as effective as amitriptyline; no advantage to combining the two was found.[53]

Tension Headaches

Another randomized controlled trial compared spinal manipulation with amitriptyline for the treatment of chronic tension headache pain in 102 patients. During the treatment period, both groups improved at similar rates. Ten weeks after beginning treatment, the manipulation group demonstrated significantly greater improvements (e.g., intensity, frequency, and over-the-counter medication use [$p < 0.001$] and functional status [$p < 0.008$]) than the medication group. The authors concluded that manipulation was as effective as amitriptyline therapy in the treatment of tension headaches with fewer reported side effects and a lower need for over-the-counter medications.[9]

Bove and others compared soft-tissue therapy and manipulation with soft-tissue therapy and

TABLE 10-2	Treatment for Neck Disorders			
AUTHOR(S)	**TREATMENT**	**COMPARISON TREATMENT**	**SAMPLE SIZE**	**RESULTS AND OUTCOMES**
Jordan A et al: Intensive training, physiotherapy, or manipulation for patients with chronic neck pain. A prospective, single-blinded, randomized clinical trial, *Spine* 23(3):311, 1998.	Chiropractic care	(1) Intensive training of cervical musculature (2) Physiotherapy regimen	119	Patients from all three groups demonstrate significant improvements in self-report of pain and disability at study completion Improvements were maintained throughout the 4- and 12-mo follow-up period There were no significant differences between groups at any pretreatment point Intensive training resulted in greater endurance than did chiropractic care.
Rogers RG: The effects of spinal manipulation on cervical kinesthesia in patients with chronic neck pain: a pilot study, *J Manip Physiol Ther* 20(2):80, 1997.	Six sessions of high-velocity, low-amplitude manipulation (chiropractic) over 3- to 4-wk period	Stretching exercises to be performed twice daily for 3- to 4-wk period	20	Pain levels were assessed at baseline and at six follow-up sessions using a 100-mm visual analogue scale Manipulation patients reduced pain 44%, with a 41% improvement in head repositioning skills Stretching patients reduced pain by 9% and head repositioning by 12% ($p < 0.05$)

placebo laser treatments for episodic tension headache pain. Both groups experienced significant reductions in the number of daily headache hours and analgesic use, but the differences between groups were not significant.[10]

Cervicogenic Headaches

Nilsson and others applied high-velocity, low-amplitude cervical manipulation (the hallmark technique of chiropractic) for treatment of cervicogenic headache pain. The manipulation group experienced significant reductions in the number of headache hours, pain intensity, and use of analgesics as compared with the control group that received low-level, laser treatment.[56] In an earlier study, Nilsson had compared high-velocity, low-amplitude spinal manipulation with treatment of low-level laser with deep friction massage and trigger point therapy. Although the manipulation group experienced significant reductions in analgesic use, headache intensity, and number of headache hours per day, differences between groups failed to reach statistical significance.[57]

Outcomes for manipulation as treatment for headache pain are mixed. Some of the comparison groups clearly provided some pain relief, masking some of the benefits of chiropractic manipulation for headache pain. The literature suggests that manipulation may be therapeutically beneficial for the treatment of headache pain; some of the comparison treatments (e.g., soft-tissue therapy, deep friction massage, and trigger point treatment) were also beneficial.

Most impressive were the benefits of spinal manipulation as compared with drug therapy (e.g., amitriptyline) during treatment and 4 weeks after treatment completion. The literature strongly suggests that manipulation can be an effective treatment for reducing headache pain, at least as effective as treatment with some forms of drug therapy, massage with trigger point therapy, and soft-tissue therapy (Table 10-3).

■ Chiropractic and Nonmusculoskeletal Conditions

Based on their personal experience, many chiropractors believe that spinal manipulation is beneficial as a treatment for many conditions in addition to neuromusculoskeletal pain. There is a small body of studies examining the effects of chiropractic manipulative care on nonmusculoskeletal conditions. The following text reviews some of these studies.

Menstrual Pain

In one study, 45 women with a history of primary dysmenorrhea were randomly assigned to receive manipulation or sham manipulation. In the manipulation group, short-lever, high-velocity, low-amplitude thrusts (a chiropractic hallmark technique) were applied to relevant vertebrae. Sham treatment consisted of a gentle thrust to the sacrum with the patient's knees and hips flexed. Immediately after treatment, perception of pain and level of menstrual distress was significantly reduced by manipulation. Manipulation was significantly more effective in relieving reported abdominal and back pain and menstrual distress. This decrease was associated with a significant reduction in plasma prostaglandins, a chemical related to menstrual cramping. However, a significant and similar reduction in plasma prostaglandin levels occurred in the sham group as well, suggesting that a biochemical placebo effect was associated with a single manipulation.[46]

Asthma

In another study, 31 patients, aged 18 to 44, who were suffering from asthma controlled by bronchodilators and/or inhaled steroids, were randomized to receive active or sham chiropractic manipulation twice weekly for 4 weeks. No clinically important differences were found between the chiropractic and sham treatments, although nonspecific bronchial hyperreactivity and patient symptom severity were significantly reduced for both groups compared with baseline.[55] Another randomized controlled trial of 80 symptomatic children with asthma also found no difference between chiropractic treatment and sham treatment.[7]

Colic and Carpal Tunnel Syndrome

In an uncontrolled study of 316 infants suffering from infantile colic and selected by well-defined criteria, the infants significantly improved within 2 weeks and after an average of three treatments.[43]

In another study, carpel tunnel syndrome was treated by chiropractic and conservative medical care (e.g., ibuprofen and wrist supports). Both groups demonstrated improvement, but no difference in efficacy between groups was found.[22]

Nonmusculoskeletal Conditions: Review

A recent systematic review of the literature of the efficacy of spinal manipulation for nonmusculoskeletal conditions concluded that spinal manipulation was nonefficacious for the treatment of

TABLE 10-3	**Manipulation in the Treatment of Headache**			

AUTHOR(S)	TREATMENT	COMPARISON TREATMENT	SAMPLE SIZE	RESULTS AND OUTCOMES
Boline PD et al: Spinal manipulation vs amitriptyline for the treatment of chronic tension-type headaches: a randomized clinical trial, *J Manip Physiol Ther* 18(3):148, 1995.	6 weeks of chiropractic manipulation and treatment	6 weeks of amitriptyline treatment provided by medical physician	125	During treatment, both groups completed improved at similar rates 4 wks after treatment ended, manipulation group reduced headache intensity by 32%; headache frequency reduced by 42%; OTC medications dropped by 30%; functional health improved 16% For amitriptyline group, all variables showed no improvement or degraded slightly Group differences 4 wks after cessation for all categories were both clinically and statistically significant 82.1% of amitriptyline subjects had side effects; 4.3% of manipulation group had side effects of **chronic tension headache**
Bove G, Nilsson N: Spinal manipulation in the treatment of episodic tension-type headache, *JAMA* 280(18):1576, 1998.	Soft tissue therapy and spinal manipulation (manipulation group)	Soft tissue therapy and placebo laser treatment (control group)	76	Eight treatments over 4 wks were delivered by chiropractor Based on intent to treat analysis, no significant differences were found between groups for three outcome measures: (1) daily hrs of headache, (2) pain intensity per episode, (3) daily analgesic use By wk 7, both groups experienced significant reductions in daily headache hrs (2.8 to 1.5 hrs in manipulation group, and 3.4 to 1.9 hrs in control groups); mean analgesics per day (0.66 to 0.38 for manipulation group, 0.82 and 0.59 for control groups) Headache pain intensity was unchanged during trial conclusions: as an isolated intervention, spinal manipulation does not seem to affect positively **episodic tension-type headache pain**

hypertension and chronic moderately severe asthma in adults.[13] The same review concluded that because of the small number and poor quality of the existing studies, there is insufficient evidence to advise, for or against, the use of spinal manipulation for the treatment of vertigo, nocturnal childhood enuresis, dysmenorrhea, chronic obstructive pulmonary disease, duodenal ulcer, or infantile colic.

An Expert Speaks: Dr. Dana Lawrence

Dana Lawrence, DC, FICC, has more than 19 years teaching and administrative experience in chiropractic education, with an emphasis on teaching spinal and extravertebral chiropractic techniques and orthopedics. Dr. Lawrence is a biomedical editor, writer, and textbook consult-

ant and has served as editor of the *Journal of Manipulative and Physiological Therapeutics* since 1987. He is also editor of the *Journal of Sports Chiropractic and Rehabilitation*. In 1998, Dr. Lawrence was named "Researcher of the Year" by the Foundation for Chiropractic Education and Research. In the following interview, he shares his thoughts on the benefits, challenges, and future of chiropractic.

Question. How did you become involved in the chiropractic profession and chiropractic research?

Answer. I am afraid that my answer to this is rather mundane. I had always wanted to work in one of three fields: high-energy physics; English, humanities, teaching; or health care. After graduating from Michigan State University with a bachelor's degree in biology, I had applied to both

TABLE 10-3	Manipulation in the Treatment of Headache—cont'd			
AUTHOR(S)	**TREATMENT**	**COMPARISON TREATMENT**	**SAMPLE SIZE**	**RESULTS AND OUTCOMES**
Nilsson N, Christensen HW, Hartvigsen J: The effect of spinal manipulation in the treatment of cervicogenic headache, *J Manip Physiol Ther* 20(5):326, 1997.	High-velocity, low-amplitude cervical manipulation twice a wk for 3 wks	Low-level laser in the upper cervical region for 3 wks	53	**Patients were cervicogenic headache sufferers** From 1 to 5, analgesic use decreased 36% in the manipulation group, but was unchanged in control group; (p=0.04); headache hrs per day decreased 69% for manipulation group, 37% in control patients (p=0.03); headache intensity per episode decreased 36% with manipulation and 17% in control groups (p=0.04) Conclusion: spinal manipulation has a significant positive effect on cervicogenic headache
Nelson CF et al: The efficacy of spinal manipulation, amitriptyline and the combination of both therapies for the prophylaxis of migraine headache, *J Manip Physiol Ther* 21(8):511, 1998.	Spinal manipulation for 4 wks with 4-wk follow-up	Amitriptyline or amitriptyline plus spinal manipulation	218	Patients were **migraine sufferers** Pre to post treatment, headache index scores improved 49% with amitriptyline, 40% with manipulation, 41% with combined treatment (p=0.66) During the 4-wk after follow-up period, improvement from baseline was 24% with amitriptyline, 42% for spinal manipulation, 25% for combined treatment (p=0.05) Conclusion: there was no advantage to combining drug with manipulation for treatment of migraine; manipulation was as effective as amitriptyline with fewer side effects
Nilsson N: A randomized controlled trial of the effect of spinal manipulation in the treatment of cervicogenic headache, *J Manip Physiol Ther* 18(7):435, 1995.	High-elocity, low-amplitude spinal manipulation, twice a week for 3 wks	Low-level laser of upper cervical region and deep friction massage (including trigger points) of lower cervical and upper thoracic region, twice a wk for 3 wks	39	Change from wk 2 to 6: Despite a significant reduction in manipulation group on outcomes of analgesic use, headache intensity per episode, and number of headache hours per day, differences between groups failed to reach statistical significance Patients had **cervicogenic headache**

dental school and to [the] master's program in biology. My initial interest in chiropractic came about by serendipity, when my father brought me material from a friend of his for whom he was developing a radio ad. The material was from the National College of Chiropractic and laid out its full program in chiropractic. I then investigated the profession and found that there was something that appealed to my idiosyncratic feelings. I was drawn by the essentially conservative nature of the profession. Once in the college, I thrived and did quite well and began, even as a student, to work in the college as a physiology lab assistant. After graduation, I was able to merge two of my interests, teaching and health care, by becoming a faculty member. I rose through the ranks and was asked to help out a colleague who was working with the college's journal. By that time, I had become involved in my own research projects, which had grown out of a desire by the then president, Dr. Joseph Janse, to increase our research productivity. My own work was on the short leg phenomenon.

Question. As editor of the *Journal of Manipulative and Physiological Therapeutics,* you have had a unique opportunity to review the research on chiropractic thoroughly. From your viewpoint, what benefits from chiropractic have been most strongly documented with clinically controlled trials?

Answer. There is little question that the greatest benefits of chiropractic care have been shown in low back pain, headache [pain], and neck pain. Indeed, a number of comprehensive reviews have concluded that manipulative care confers good benefit to patients suffering from low back pain in particular. Given the pervasive nature of low back pain, this has significant policy and health care implications. Indeed, health economist Pran Manga has recommended, based upon his review of the literature, that the government of the province of Ontario include chiropractic coverage in its health policies. Similar recommendations have been made in the United States, Canada, and Australia as the result of consensus conferences. In addition to the conditions I noted, there is also research to show benefit for childhood asthma, for otitis media, and for dysmenorrhea. I must also note that there are significant numbers of case reports, low on the evidence hierarchy, of course, which show the full gamut of the involvement of chiropractic care.

Question. There are always clashes of politics among the health care research communities, and chiropractic has had to deal with more than its equal share of those political issues. Can you describe your observations of the political challenges chiropractic has faced from a research perspective?

Answer. The most significant problem the profession has faced with regard to research is lack of funding. For a long time, the single major funding agency for chiropractic research was the Foundation for Chiropractic Education and Research. One single source is insufficient. Federal funds were virtually nonexistent. As a result, we had to bootstrap ourselves in research. We also lack a large-scale research infrastructure, though much has happened to assuage this problem. The establishment of the Consortial Center for Chiropractic Research at the Palmer College of Chiropractic, with funds from the Government, has opened new vistas for chiropractic research. Also, recognition of the public interest in CAM [complementary and alternative medicine] therapies has made possible for the Office of Alternative Medicine to become a national center. There is growing interest by the public in receiving "alternative" health care. I must also note a small amount of antiscientific attitudes within the chiropractic profession, from those who believe that "chiropractic works" and therefore needs no scientific documentation.

Question. What do you see as the future of chiropractic and health care?

Answer. The future will see greater cooperation between medical, chiropractic, and osteopathic professionals. There are a growing number of chiropractors serving in hospital settings and greater amounts of collaboration both for research and in the clinical setting. Chiropractors will provide greater amounts of primary care in the future, while maintaining their traditional strength in musculoskeletal management.

■ Recommendations for Future Research

The literature to date most strongly supports the efficacy of chiropractic in the treatment of low back pain. Therefore a chiropractic research strategy could be implemented that targets the treatment of low back pain with the following considerations:

1. Treatment is provided by licensed chiropractors only.
2. Study uses a black-box design, which allows chiropractors to treat as they deem most appropriate, but which incorporates the use of the short-lever, low-amplitude, high-velocity treatment technique.
3. Patients are matched and then randomized by age, gender, and duration of pain to receive chiropractic treatment or no treatment (control group).
4. Treatment time period is set, including a maximum number of adjustments.
5. Study assesses both short- and long-term (1 year or more) outcomes.

Once such a design is created, chiropractic researchers in other parts of the country could repeatedly replicate the study. Chronic, acute, and subacute trials should not be mixed. Other conditions (e.g., neck pain, headache pain) could be similarly investigated. Future reviews and meta-analyses of multiple replications could then more accurately depict the benefits of chiropractic care than the "mixed" reviews currently available.

More long-term research evaluating the preventive role of chiropractic also needs to be performed. The cost effectiveness of chiropractic care needs to be determined, as well as the necessary number of treatments for subcategories of pain and other conditions.

■ Indications and Contraindications

Spinal manipulation is indicated for treatment of the following conditions:

1. Back pain, especially treatment of low back pain of short duration
2. Neck pain

3. Headache pain (migraine, cervicogenic, and tension)

Some evidence suggests efficacy of chiropractic for treatment of:

1. Menstrual pain
2. Colic
3. Carpel tunnel syndrome

Spinal manipulation to the indicated pathologic site is contraindicated for the following conditions:

1. Vascular complications, such as compromise of the vertebral arteries that cause interruption of the flow of blood into the basilar area of the brain (vertebral-basilar insufficiency)
2. Arteriosclerosis of major blood vessels
3. Aneurysm
4. Tumors of the lung, thyroid, prostate, breast, or bone
5. Bone infections, such as tuberculosis or bacterial infection
6. Traumatic injuries, such as fractures, joint instability or hypermobility, severe sprains or strains, or unstable spondylolisthesis
7. Arthritis
8. Psychologic considerations, including malingering, hysteria, hypochondriacs, and pain intolerance
9. Metabolic disorders, such as clotting disorders and osteopenia
10. Neurologic complications, such as sacral nerve root involvement from disk protrusion, disk lesions, and space-occupying lesions[30]

■ Complications From Manipulation

Serious complications of manipulation, including paraplegia and death, have been reported. Although the incidence of these complications is unknown, it is probably very low.[68] A review of the world's literature between 1950 and 1980 found 135 case reports of serious complications, including 18 deaths caused by manipulation.[47] The development of cauda equina syndrome, a serious complication of lumbar spinal manipulation, is estimated to occur in less than 1 case per 100 million manipulations.

■ Chapter Review

Chiropractic has been demonstrated efficacious in the treatment of low back pain, and the data suggest its efficacy in the treatment of neck pain and headache syndromes. More research is needed to confirm its benefits for other conditions, such as vertigo, nocturnal childhood enuresis, dysmenorrhea, chronic obstructive pulmonary disease, duodenal ulcer, or infantile colic. In the past few years, research in the area of chiropractic has increased significantly, bolstering the scientific credibility of chiropractic care. Chiropractic will no doubt continue to maintain and improve its status as an efficacious health profession as more research is forthcoming.

CRITICAL THINKING AND CLINICAL APPLICATION EXERCISES

1. Compare and contrast the differences between manipulation, mobilization, and classical chiropractic adjustment. What do you think are the benefits and limitations of each procedure?
2. Define and explain the two categories of the effects of manipulation. Then describe the research that supports each of these categories. What are the limitations and implications of this research?
3. In spite of limitations to chiropractic research, chiropractic care is an extremely popular form of complementary medicine. Describe the literature on patient response to chiropractic care. Explain why and how chiropractic has such a loyal following.
4. Compare and contrast the findings on the benefits of chiropractic for the treatment of low back pain.
5. Compare and contrast the findings of the benefits of chiropractic for the treatment of other musculoskeletal methods. What are the limitations and strengths of this research?
6. Design a replicable chiropractic research protocol intended to address the weaknesses in the current research.
7. Compare the research of chiropractic care to the research of more conventional medical treatments for back pain.
8. Clearly define the indications and contraindications for chiropractic treatment. Considering the complications resulting from manipulation, argue for the safety or dangers in administering chiropractic care.

Matching Terms and Definitions

Match each numbered definition with the correct term. Place the corresponding letter in the space provided.

a. Chiropractic
b. Chester Wilks
c. Hallmark adjustment of chiropractic
d. Bonesetters
e. Flexner Report
f. Subluxation
g. Basic science requirements
h. Passive end range
i. B.J. Palmer
j. American Medical Association
k. Palpation
l. Anatomic end range
m. Paraphysiologic joint space
n. Harvey Lillard
o. Hippocrates
p. D.D. Palmer
q. Active end range
r. Andrew Taylor Still

_____ 1. Founder of chiropractic
_____ 2. Developer of chiropractic
_____ 3. Father of osteopathy
_____ 4. Means done by hand
_____ 5. Father of modern medicine; wrote some of the first texts on manipulation
_____ 6. Fist professional manipulators, trained by apprenticeship
_____ 7. Boundary beyond which movement results in rupture of joint ligaments
_____ 8. First chiropractic patient, cured of his deafness by chiropractic adjustment
_____ 9. Study commissioned by the Carnegie Foundation to survey the quality of all medical schools
_____ 10. Criteria that prevented licensure for most chiropractors
_____ 11. Began a campaign to "contain and eliminate" chiropractic
_____ 12. Won an antitrust lawsuit based on a conspiracy to eliminate chiropractic
_____ 13. Nerve impingement by misalignment of spine
_____ 14. Extra "stretch" provided by clinician to the physiologic joint space
_____ 15. On-hands chiropractic examinations
_____ 16. Short-lever, high-velocity, low-amplitude thrust to the spinous processes
_____ 17. Point to which a patient can move a joint with his or her own muscular effort
_____ 18. Joint exceeds the passive end range but not the anatomic end range

References

1. A study of chiropractic worldwide: *FACTS Bull* 3:32, 1989.
2. Agency for Health Care Policy and Research: *Chiropractic in the United States: training, practice, and research*, 98-N002, 1997, AHCPR.
3. Anderson R, Meeker WC, Wirick B, Mootz RD, Kirk DH, Adams A: A meta-analysis of clinical trials of spinal manipulation, *J Manipulative Physiol Ther* 15(3):181, 1992.
4. Assendelft WWJ, Bouter LM: Does the goose really lay golden eggs? A methodological review of workmen's compensation studies, *J Manipulative Physiol Ther* 16:161, 1993.
5. Assendelft WJJ, Koes BW, Knipschild PG, Bouter LM: The relationship between methodological quality and conclusions in reviews of spinal manipulation, *JAMA* 274:1942, 1995.
6. Assendelft WJJ, Koes BW, van der Heijden GJMG, Bouter LM: The effectiveness of chiropractic for treatment of low back pain: an update and attempt at statistical pooling, *J Manipulative Physiol Ther* 19:499, 1996.
7. Balon J, Aker PD, Crowther ER, Danielson C, Cox PG, O'Shaughnessy D, Walker C, Goldsmith CH, Duku E, Sears MR: A comparison of active and simulated chiropractic manipulation as adjunctive treatment for childhood asthma, *N Engl J Med* 339(15):1013, 1998.
8. Bigos S, Bowyer O, Braen G et al: *Acute low back problems in adults*, (clinical practice guidelines no 14. AHCPR publication No 95-0642), Rockville, MD, 1994, Agency for Health Care Policy and Research.
9. Boline PD, Kassak K et al: Spinal manipulation vs. amitriptyline for the treatment of chronic tension-type headaches: a randomized clinical trial, *J Manipulative Physiol Ther* 18(3):148, 1995.
10. Bove G, Nilsson N: Spinal manipulation in the treatment of episodic tension-type headaches, *JAMA* 280(18):1576, 1998.
11. Brennen PC, Cramer GD, Kirstukas SJ, Cullum ME: Basic science research in chiropractic: state-of-the-art and recommendations for a research agenda, *J Manipulative Physiol Ther* 20(3):150, 1997.
12. Brennen PC, Triano JJ, McGregor M, Kokjohn K, Hondras MA, Brennan DT: Enhanced neutrophil respiratory burst as a biological marker for manipulation forces: duration of the effect and association with substance P and tumor necrosis factor, *J Manipulative Physiol Ther* 15:83, 1992.
13. Bronfort G, Assendelft WJJ, Bounter, LM: *Efficacy of spinal manipulation for conditions other than neck and back pain: a systematic review and best evidence synthesis*, Bournemouth, Engl, 1996, International Conference on Spinal Manipulation.

14. Carey TS, Garrett J, Jackman A, McLaughlin C, Fryer J, Smucker D: The outcomes and costs of care for acute low back pain among patients seen by primary care practitioners, chiropractors, and orthopedic surgeons, *N Engl J Med* 333(14):913, 1995.

15. Cassidy JD, Lopes AA, Yong-Hing K: The immediate effect of manipulation versus mobilization on pain and range of motion in the cervical spine: a randomized controlled trial, *J Manipulative Physiol Ther* 15(9):570, 1992.

16. Cherkin DC, MacCornack FA: Patient evaluations of low back pain care from family physicians and chiropractors, *West J Med* 150:351, 1989.

17. Cherkin DC, MacCornack FA, Berg AO: The management of low back pain: a comparison of the beliefs and behaviors of family physicians and chiropractors, *West J Med* 15:351, 1988.

18. Christensen M, Morgan D, editors: *Job analysis of chiropractic: a project report, survey analysis, and summary of the practice of chiropractic within the United States,* Greeley, CO, 1993, National Board of Chiropractic Examiners.

19. Christian GH, Stanton GJ, Sissons D, How HY, Jamison J, Alder B, Fullerton M, Funder JW: Immunoreactive ACTH, beta-endorphin and cortisol levels in plasma following spinal manipulative therapy, *Spine* 13:1411, 1988.

20. Cooper RA, Stoflet SJ: Trends in the education and practice of alternative medicine clinicians, *Health Aff* 15:226, 1996.

21. Crelin ES: A scientific test of the chiropractic theory, *Am Sci* 61:574, 1973.

22. Davis PT, Hulbert JR, Kassak KM, Meyer JJ: Comparative efficacy of conservative medical and chiropractic treatments for carpel tunnel syndrome: a randomized clinical trial, *J Manipulative Physiol Ther* 21(5):317, 1998.

23. Deyo RS: Conservative therapy for low back pain. Distinguishing useful from useless therapy, *JAMA* 250:1057, 1983.

24. Eisenberg DM et al: Trends in alternative medicine use in the United States, 1990-1997: results of a follow-up national survey, *JAMA* 280(18):1569, 1998.

25. Eisenberg DM, Kessler RC, Foster C, Norlock FE, Calkins DR, Delbanco TL: Unconventional medicine in the United States: prevalence, costs, and patterns of use, *N Engl J Med* 328(4):246, 1993.

26. Faye LJ, Wiles MR: Manual examination of the spine. In Haldeman S, editor: *Principles and practice of chiropractic,* Norfolk, CN, 1992, Appleton & Lange.

27. Flexner A: *Medical education in the United States and Canada,* New York, 1910, Carnegie Foundation for the Advancement of Teaching.

28. Frymoyer JW: Back pain and sciatica, *N Engl J Med* 318:291, 1988.

29. Gatterman MI, editor: *Foundations of chiropractic: subluxation,* St Louis, 1995, Mosby.

30. Gatterman MI: *Chiropractic management of spinal disorders,* Baltimore, 1990, Williams & Wilkins.

31. Getzendanner S: Permanent injunction order against the AMA (special communication), *JAMA* 259:81, 1988.

32. Gibbins RW: The evaluation of chiropractic: medical and social protest in America. In Haldeman S, editor: *Modern principles and practice of chiropractic,* East Norwalk, CN, 1979, Appleton-Century-Crofts.

33. Gillet H: The history of motion palpation, *Eur J Chiropractic* 31:196, 1983.

34. Haldeman S: Spinal manipulation therapy: a status report, *Clin Orthopedic Related Res* 179:62, 1983.

35. Haldeman S, Chapman-Smith D, Petersen D, editors: *Guidelines for chiropractic quality assurance and practice parameters,* Gaithersburg, MD, 1993, Aspen Publishers.

36. Hippocrates: *Hippocrates with an English translation by ET Withington,* ed 3, Cambridge, 1959, Howard University Press.

37. Jordan A, Bendix T et al: Intensive training, physiotherapy, or manipulation for patients with chronic neck pain. A prospective, single-blinded randomized clinical trial. *Spine* 23(3):311, 1998.

38. Kane RL, Olsen D, Leymaster C, Woolley FR, Fisher FD: Manipulating the patient: a comparison of the effectiveness of physician and chiropractor care, *Lancet* 1:1333, 1974.

39. Kaptchuk TJ, Eisenberg DM: Chiropractic: origins, controversies, and contributions, *Arch Intern Med* 158:2215, 1998.

40. Keating JC Jr: Science and politics and the subluxation, *Am J Chiropractic Med* 113:109, 1988.

41. Keating JC Jr: Shades of straight: diversity among the purists, *J Manipulative Physiol Ther* 15:203, 1992.

42. Keating JC, Mootz RD: The influence of political medicine on chiropractic dogma: implications for scientific development, *J Manipulative Physiol Ther* 12(5):393, 1989.

43. Klougart N, Nilsson N, Jacobsen J: Infantile colic treated by chiropractors: a prospective study of 316 cases, *J Manipulative Physiol Ther* 12(4):281, 1989.

44. Koes BW, Assendelft WJJ, van der Heijden GJMG, Bouter LM, Knipschild PG: Spinal manipulation and mobilisation for back and neck pain: a blinded review, *BMJ* 303:1298, 1991.

45. Koes BW, Assendelft WJJ, van der Heijden GJMG, Bouter LM: Spinal manipulation for low back pain: an updated systematic review of randomized clinical trials, *Spine* 2:2860, 1996.

46. Kokjohn K, Schmid DM, Triano JJ, Brennan PC: The effect of spinal manipulation on pain and prostaglandin levels in women with primary dysmenorrhea, *J Manipulative Physiol Ther* 15(5):279, 1992.

47. Ladermann JP: Accidents of spinal manipulations, *Ann Swiss Chiropractors Assoc* 7:161, 1981.

48. Lantz CA: The vertebral subluxation complex. Introduction to the model and the kinesiological component, *Chiropractic Res J* 13:23, 1989.

49. Leach RA: *The chiropractic theories: a symposium of scientific research,* Mississippi, 1980, Mid-South Scientific Publishers.

50. Liebensen C: Rehabilitation and chiropractic practice, (commentary), *J Manipulative Physiol Ther* 19:134, 1996.

51. Ligeros KA: *How ancient healing governs modern therapeutics: the contribution of hellenic science to modern medicine and scientific progress,* New York, 1937, Putnam.

52. Manga P, Angus D, Swan WR: Findings and recommendations from an independent review of chiropractic management of low back pain, *J Neuromusculoskeletal Syst* 2(3):157, 1994.

53. Nelson CF, Bronford G et al: The efficacy of spinal manipulation, amitriptyline and the combination of both therapies for the prophylaxis of migraine headache, *J Manipulative Physiol Ther* 21(8):511, 1998.

54. Nichols LM: *Nonphysician health care providers: use of ambulatory services, expenditures, and sources of payment* (National Medical Expenditure Survey Research Findings 27), Rockville, MD, 1966, AHCPR.

55. Nielsen NH, Bronfort G, Bendix T, Madsen F, Weeke B: Chronic asthma and chiropractic spinal manipulation: a randomized clinical trial, *Clin Exp Allergy* 25:80, 1995.

56. Nilsson N, Christensen HW, Hartvigsen J: The effect of spinal manipulation in the treatment of cervicogenic headache, *J Manipulative Physiol Ther* 20(5):326, 1997.

57. Nilsson N: A randomized controlled trial of the effect of spinal manipulation in the treatment of cervicogenic headache, *J Manipulative Physiol Ther* 18(7):435, 1995.

58. Palmer DD: *The chiropractic adjuster: the science, art and philosophy of chiropractic,* Portland, 1910, Portland Printing House.

59. Parker GB, Tupling H, Pryor DS: A controlled trial of cervical manipulation for migraine, *Australian N Z J Med* 8:589, 1978.

60. Peterson D, Wiese G: *Chiropractic: an illustrated history,* St Louis, 1995, Mosby.

61. Rogers RG: The effects of spinal manipulation on cervical kinesthesia in patients with chronic neck pain: a pilot study, *J Manipulative Physiol Ther* 20(2):80, 1997.

62. Sanders GE, Reinnert O, Tepe R, Maloney P: Chiropractic adjustive manipulation on subjects with acute low back pain: visual analog scores and plasma beta-endorphin levels, *J Manipulative Physiol Ther* 13:39, 1990.

63. Schafer RC, Sportelli L: *Opportunities in chiropractic health care careers,* Lincolnwood, IL, 1987, American Chiropractic Association and VGM Career Horizons.

64. Schoitz EH, Cyriax J: *Manipulation past and present,* London, 1975, William Heinemann Medical Books.

65. Shafer RC: *Chiropractic health care,* Des Moines, 1976, FCER.

66. Shekelle PG: What role for chiropractic in health care? *N Engl J Med* 339(15):1074, 1998.

67. Shekelle PG et al: *The appropriateness of spinal manipulation for low-back pain, project overview and literature review,* Santa Monica, VA, 1991, Rand.

68. Shekelle PG, Adams AH, Chassin MR, Hurwitz EL, Brooks RH: Spinal manipulation for low-back pain, *Ann Intern Med* 117(7):590, 1992.

69. Shekelle PG, Brook RH: A community based study of the use of chiropractic services, *Am J Public Health* 81:439, 1991.

70. Triano JJ: Studies of the biomechanical effects of a spinal adjustment, *J Manipulative Physiol Ther* 15:71, 1992.

71. Vernon HT: Biological rationale for possible benefits of spinal manipulation. In *Chiropractic in the United States: training, practice, and research,* 1997, US Dept of Commerce, Group Health Cooperative of Puget Sound.

72. Vernon HT: Spinal manipulation and headaches of cervical origin, *J Manipulative Physiol Ther* 12(6):455, 1989.

73. Vernon HT, Dhami MS, Howl TP, Annett R: Spinal manipulation and beta-endorphin: a controlled study of the effect of a spinal manipulation on plasma beta-endorphin levels in normal males, *J Manipulative Physiol Ther* 9:115, 1986.

74. Von Kuster T: *Chiropractic health care: a national study of cost of education, service, utilization, number of practicing doctors of chiropractic, and other key policy issues,* Washington, DC, 1980, The Foundation for the Advancement of Chiropractic Tenets and Science.

75. Wardwell WI: *Chiropractic: history and evolution of a new profession,* St Louis, 1992, Mosby.

11

Acupuncture

Lyn W. Freeman

WHY READ THIS CHAPTER?

Acupuncture is one of the most researched forms of complementary medicine in the world today; because of this, it is becoming more accepted by traditional medicine. One of the reasons for its acceptance is that its underlying mechanisms are defined, (i.e., its effects on the nervous system and on the endogenous opioids can be used to explain pain-relieving, biochemical, and systemic changes).

Much of the research on acupuncture is methodologically flawed; nonetheless, findings suggest that it is a potent intervention with few side effects for pain and nausea, symptoms of drug detoxification, and other issues inadequately addressed by traditional medical approaches.

The history, philosophy, mechanisms, and outcomes related to acupuncture are fascinating topics of study, shedding light on one of the oldest systems of healing in the world today. The reader is encouraged to acquaint him or herself with the fruits of this ancient discipline.

CHAPTER AT A GLANCE

Acupuncture involves stimulating specific anatomic points in the body for therapeutic purposes. It is believed that acupuncture works by correcting the balance of qi in the body. Qi flows through the 12 major energy pathways called meridians, each linked to specific internal organs or organ systems and 365 to 2000 acupoints.

Historically, acupuncture evolved as one component of the complex tradition known as Chinese medicine. Widespread awareness of acupuncture came to North America in 1971 when James Reston described how his postoperative pain from an emergency appendectomy was alleviated by acupuncture. His description was published in the New York Times.

Bioelectrical properties of acupuncture were identified when low resistance points on the body were found to correlate with the traditional acupuncture channels. Later, research revealed that radioactive tracers injected into classical acupuncture points were diffused along the pathways of the classical acupuncture channels.

Acupuncture has been researched and demonstrated (to varying degrees) to alleviate low back pain, headache, pain from osteoarthritis, neck pain, musculoskeletal and myofascial pain, organic pain, and pain before and after surgery. Acupuncture has also been used for the treatment of postoperative and chemotherapy-induced nausea, neurologic dysfunction, gynecologic and obstetric conditions, asthma, and substance abuse.

It's supposed to be a professional secret, but I'll tell you anyway.
We doctors do nothing.
We only help and encourage the doctor within.

ALBERT SCHWEITZER

CHAPTER OBJECTIVES

After completing this chapter, you should be able to:

1. Define acupuncture.
2. Describe Tao, the yin-yang theory, the eight principles, the three treasures, and the five elements.
3. Explain the historical evolution of acupuncture.
4. Discuss the bioelectrical properties of acupuncture.
5. Describe how acupuncture activates the autonomic nervous system.
6. Explain the theory of diffuse noxious inhibitory control.
7. Discuss the challenges to and failings of acupuncture research.
8. Describe the outcomes from acupuncture as treatment for low back pain.
9. Explain the outcomes of acupuncture for relief of headache pain.
10. Evaluate the effects of acupuncture on osteoarthritic pain.
11. Review the findings of acupuncture for treatment of neck, musculoskeletal, and myofascial pain.
12. Discuss the benefits and limitations of acupuncture for procedural, surgical, and postoperative pain.
13. Explain the findings of acupuncture as treatment for postoperative and chemotherapy-induced nausea.
14. Describe the acupuncture outcomes for treatment of neurologic dysfunction and gynecologic and obstetric conditions.
15. Define the benefits and limitations of acupuncture for the treatment of asthma.
16. Evaluate the findings of acupuncture treatment for substance abuse.
17. Explain the indications and contraindications for acupuncture.

Acupuncture Defined

Acupuncture involves stimulating specific anatomic points in the body for therapeutic purposes. Puncturing the skin with a needle is the usual method of application, but practitioners may also apply heat, pressure, friction, or suction. They may also apply impulses of electromagnetic stimulation directly to the needle points.[5] Needles are inserted into acupoints identified as in need of stimulation to treat the condition in question. The angle and depth of insertion at each point is critical; the needles may be twirled. Smoldering cones of herbs may also be applied at acupoints.[115,175]

It is believed that acupuncture works by correcting the balance of *qi* (pronounced chee) in the body. *Qi*, the vital energy or the life force, is believed to flow through 12 major energy pathways called meridians, each linked to specific internal organs or organ systems and to 365 to 2000 acupuncture points.

Philosophy Underlying Acupuncture

The philosophy of acupuncture is based on the principles of *Tao* (Dao); *yin-yang* theory, the *eight principles;* the *three treasures;* and the *five elements.*

Principle of Tao

The Tao can best be interpreted as the "path" or "way of life." However, it is difficult to interpret in English terms, and even its definition in Chinese frustrates attempts to classify or describe it. It is said, "The Tao that can be told of is not the Tao." Therefore the Chinese have developed ways of alluding to Tao in aphorisms, parables, and tales that are like poetry of thought. Tao can be comprehended only by recognizing that everything takes place within a context of flux, interconnectedness, and dynamism. This principle is applied in Chinese medicine by accepting that a patient may have many signs and symptoms, but to comprehend the true condition and treat it, one must seek the pattern within those signs and symptoms. Each sign means nothing by itself and acquires meaning only in relationship to other signs.[20]

This emphasis on perception of patterns is based on Taoist thought, which altogether lacks the idea of a creator and whose concern is insight into the "web" of phenomena, not a comprehension of the "weaver." One way of contrasting the difference between Western and Eastern medicine is to recognize that in Taoist thought, the web has no weaver, no creator. By contrast, in Western thought the ultimate concern is always the creator or **cause**—as in cause and effect—and the phenomena (symptoms) is merely its reflection.

In Chinese medicine, a person who is well or "in harmony" has no distressing symptoms and expresses mental, physical, and spiritual balance. The purpose of Chinese medicine is to return a patient who is expressing disharmony in mind, body, emotion, or behavior to a state of harmony, balance, and well-being.

Yin-Yang Theory

In Chinese medical theory, the logic that explains relationships, patterns, and change is called *yin-yang*. The *yin-yang* theory is based on the philosophic construct of two polar complements, called *yin* and *yang*. *Yin* and *yang* are labels used to describe how things function in relation to each other and to the universe; they are used to explain the continuous process of natural change. *Yin* and *yang,* when properly understood, also represent a way of thinking. In this system of thought, all things are seen as parts of the whole. No entity can ever be isolated from its relationship to other entities, and no thing can exist in and of itself. Therefore *yin* and *yang* contain within themselves the possibility of opposition and change.

Yin originally meant the shady side of the mountain. It is associated with qualities such as cold, rest, responsiveness, passivity, darkness, interiority, downwardness, inwardness, and decrease.

Yang originally meant the sunny side of the mountain. It is associated with qualities such as heat, stimulation, movement, activity, excitement, vigor, light, exteriority, upwardness, outwardness, and increase.[84]

Yin and *yang* are represented by the tai chi symbol; a little yin always existing in the yang, and vice versa (Figure 11-1). When the two forces are in balance, the patient feels good, but if one force dominates the other, it brings about imbalance and poor health. One of the main aims of acupuncture is to maintain the balance between yin and yang and therefore prevent illness and restore health.

Eight Principles

In Chinese medicine, the pattern within the patient's symptoms must always be comprehended and addressed if the patient is to be made healthy and balanced. Essentially, there are *eight principle patterns* that can be ascertained. One of the essential tasks of the Chinese physician is to discern the eight principal patterns within the signs and symptoms of a patient. The eight principle patterns are composed of four pairs of polar

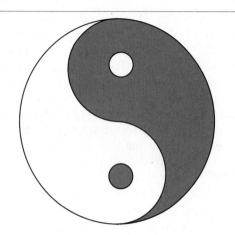

■ **Figure 11-1.** Yin and yang are represented by the tai chi symbol, with a little yin always existing in the yang and vice versa.

opposites: *yin* and *yang, interior* and *exterior, deficiency* and *excess,* and *cold* and *hot.* These eight principle patterns actually subdivide *yin* and *yang* into six subcategories.

Each patient is defined by a unique relationship between his or her own bodily signs and the overall movement of *yin* and *yang.* The eight principle patterns are a model for mediating between these two realms. The physician uses them to build a conceptual matrix that delineates an organized relationship between particular clinical signs and *yin* and *yang,* leading to a medical diagnosis and treatment plan. For example, an illness could be described as *internal deficient cold,* meaning the illness is internal, one of weakness, and has a cold nature.

In Chinese medicine the essential principles of Tao are further delineated by the three treasures: *shen, jing,* and *qi.*

Three Treasures

Shen: Spirit

Shen is best represented as the spirit; it is the treasure that brings light and joy to life. It is an elusive concept because, in the medical tradition, it is the substance unique to human life. Shen is responsible for consciousness and is associated with the force of human personality and the abilities to think, discriminate, and choose appropriately. It is said that, "Shen is the awareness that shines out of our eyes when we are truly awake."[84]

Jing: Substance of Organic Life

Jing is the essence of our being, the substance that underlies all organic life and the source of organic change. *Jing* is supportive and nutritive

and is the basis of reproduction and development. It is believed that each person is born with a set quota of *jing,* and that once this quota is gone, it cannot be restored. *Jing* is preserved by temperate living and by acupuncture. Reckless living depletes *jing.* Thus the job of the acupuncturist is to restore health and help the patient live by the principles of the Tao. Extreme sexual excess, more than any other source, depletes *jing,* which results in premature death.

Qi: Vital Energy In a State of Transformation

The idea of *qi* is fundamental to Chinese medical thinking, yet no English word can adequately capture its meaning. Everything in the universe, organic and inorganic, is composed of and defined by *qi.* One can think of *qi* as matter on the verge of becoming energy or energy at the point of materializing.[9]

Physical, emotional, and mental harmony rely on the unobstructed flow of *qi,* believed to be the vital energy or life force that drives every cell in the body. However, *qi* is more than just the "vital energy." It is also defined functionally by what it does.

1. *Qi* is the source of all movement in the body and accompanies all movement.
2. *Qi* protects the body; it resists the entry into the body of pathologic agents called *external pernicious influences.*
3. *Qi* is the source of harmonious transformation in the body. When food is ingested, it is transformed into other substances such as blood and *qi,* itself, as well as tears, sweat, and urine. These changes cannot occur without the transformation function of *qi.*
4. *Qi* governs retention of the body's substances and organs; *qi* "keeps everything in." It holds the organs in their proper places, keeps blood in its pathways, and prevents excessive loss of bodily fluid.
5. *Qi* warms the body. Maintenance of normal heat in the body depends on the warming effect of the *qi.*

If *qi* is in a state of disharmony, the patterns of disharmony are designated as one or more of the following:

1. *Deficient. Qi* is insufficient and therefore unable to perform the five *qi* functions previously listed.
2. *Collapsed.* A subcategory of deficient that implies the *qi* is insufficient to the extent that it can no longer hold organs in place.
3. *Stagnant.* Normal movement of *qi* is impaired.
4. *Rebellious. Qi* is going in the wrong direction.

Qi, Meridian System, and Acupoints

Clinical researchers describe *qi* in electromagnetic terms. It flows through 12 channels known as meridians; six are *yin* channels and six are *yang* channels. Each meridian is related to and named for an organ or function (Figure 11-2), which are the lung (LU), large intestine (LI), spleen (SP), stomach (ST), heart (HT), small intestine (SI), urinary bladder (BL), kidney (KI), pericardium (PC [heart protector or sex meridian]), san jiao (TE [three heater]), gallbladder (GB), and liver (LR). Along these meridians lie 361 acupoints.

When *qi* flows freely, the person is healthy and well-balanced; if *qi* is blocked, the person may become mentally, emotionally, or physically ill. Inappropriate expressions of anger, excitement, self-pity, grief, and fear often signal an imbalance of *qi*.

To restore health, the acupuncturist stimulates the points that will produce balance. For example, if *qi* is stagnant (blocked), points are stimulated that will increase its flow; if *qi* is cold, points will be stimulated to produce warmth. If *qi* is weak, points will be stimulated to increase it.

The five elements is one additional concept related to the Tao.

Five Elements: Categories of Functions and Qualities

The principles of *yin* and *yang* also subdivide into a system called the *five elements*. The elements are *wood, fire, earth, metal,* and *water*. Each element denotes a category of related functions and qualities and allow additional tools for diagnosis. For example, the element *wood* is associated with active functions that are in a growing phase, whereas *fire* designates functions that have reached a maximal activity level and are now headed toward a declining state or a resting period. *Metal* represents functions in a declining state, whereas *water* represents a maximal state of rest, heading toward the direction of activity. *Earth* designates balance or neutrality; it is essentially a buffer between the other elements. The elements therefore allow distinctions concerning the direction of change of the *yin* and *yang*.

In concrete terms, the elements can also be used to describe other cyclical change issues including the annual cycle in terms of biological growth, development, and even seasonal changes. For example, *wood* represents spring; *fire* represents summer; *metal* represents autumn; and *water* represents winter. *Earth* represents the transition between each season.

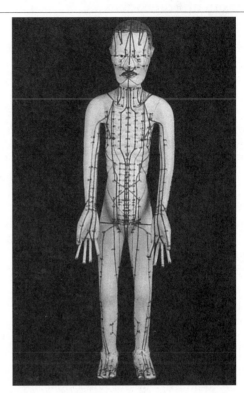

■ **Figure 11-2. Meridian system.** This important Chinese therapeutic modality has been continually used for thousands of years to treat various organs, often quite distant from each other. *From Peterson, Weiss:* Chiropractic: an illustrated history, *St Louis, 1995, Mosby.*

Each element is further associated with a color, emotion, sound, smell, taste, climate, body part, and function. Correlations are also made between the elements and various organs and anatomic regions, which is how the connection between the elements and medicine came about.[84] This system is based on the belief that life is an ever-changing, cyclical process, with each element flowing into the next, just as each season flows into the next. For example, summer is connected to *fire,* which contains the heart, small intestines, pericardium, and the *three heater* (i.e., the body's physical and emotional thermostat).

These principles, Tao (Dao); *yin* and *yang;* the eight principles; the three treasures; and the five elements, are all used as diagnostic tools in Chinese medicine to comprehend the web of phenomena as it relates to health and well-being. These interrelated principles can be considered analogous to the anatomy, physiology, biochemistry, and electrical principles studied as part of conventional Western medicine. The difference is that in Western medicine, the body is considered in relationship to its parts; in Chinese medicine, the body is considered only in relationship to the whole.

■ History of Acupuncture

China and Acupuncture's Beginnings

Acupuncture evolved as one component of the complex tradition known as Chinese medicine.[165] One of the earliest sources of information on acupuncture is found in a text known as the *Yellow Emperor's Inner Classic (Huang Di Nei Jing),* a collection of 81 treatises. The nucleus of the book was compiled between 206 BC and 220 AD.[107] The philosophic context of these teachings are that the human body should be regarded as a microcosmic reflection of the universe. Medicine and the healing arts should therefore be directed toward maintaining the body's balance, both internally and as one relates to the external world.[112]

The *Comprehensive Manual of Acupuncture and Moxibustion (Zhen Jiu Jia Yi Jing)* is the oldest existing classical text devoted entirely to acupuncture and moxibustion and was written around 282 AD by Huang-Fu Mi. This text is based on the combined classical concepts concerning the theories and teachings of acupuncture points, channels, and the cause of illness, diagnosis, and therapeutic needling.[166,183]

In 618 AD, education in acupuncture reached its apex in China with the founding of the Imperial Medical College; other similar colleges were then founded in each province. Dissemination of acupuncture teachings to Korea, Japan, and Southeast Asia occurred quickly. Buddhist missionaries transported Chinese medical texts, including the *Jia Yi Jing,* to Korea and Japan, resulting in the *Jia Yi Jing* becoming the fundamental text of acupuncture for both countries.[74]

Acupuncture reached its greatest refinement at the end of the sixteenth century. Research, education, clinical refinements, and compilation and commentary on previous classics flourished. The *Great Compendium of Acupuncture and Moxibustion (Zhen Jui Da Cheng)* was published in 1601 and remained the most influential medical text for generations. Dabry de Thiersant used this text as a method of transmitting information on acupuncture to Europe in the nineteenth century, as did Soulie de Morant in the twentieth century.[184] George Soulie de Morant was a French diplomat to China and an accomplished acupuncturist who systematically introduced acupuncture to the French and European medical communities.[185]

China in the Nineteenth and Twentieth Centuries

As early as 1822, the Qing emperor ordered that acupuncture no longer be taught at the Imperial Medical College. During this and later periods, China became exposed to Western medicine. Western medicine was demonstrated to be highly successful in the fields of drugs, surgery, and public hygiene. These successes undermined the status of acupuncture and traditional Chinese medicine.[71,167] However, during the 1940s, many parts of China suffered from infectious epidemics. In an effort to provide inexpensive medical treatment, the corps of "barefoot doctors" was created. These barefoot doctors were members of the rural communities who were trained to treat medical emergencies by using basic Chinese medicine, as well as some Western medical interventions. By the 1960s, 70% to 80% of all illnesses were treated by the "barefoot doctors" using acupuncture or herbs.[1,54]

Acupuncture in the West

The first documented practice and research of acupuncture in the United States was the 1825 publication of Morand's *Memoir on Acupuncturation,* a document translated from French by Franklin Bache, the grandson of Benjamin Franklin.[122] In 1826, Bache reported his own experiments with acupuncture for the treatment of rheumatism and neuralgia in Pennsylvania prisoners.[7]

Then, for nearly 140 years, there were few published references to acupuncture. A brief reference in an American Civil War surgeon's manual and descriptions of acupuncture's efficacy in treating cases of lumbago and sciatica in Sir William Osler's *The Principles and Practice of Medicine* were the only references during that time.[132,174] Osler's book was first published in 1892 and republished sixteen times with the final edition published in 1947.[110] His text recommended acupuncture treatment for low back pain and other conditions.

Widespread awareness of acupuncture came to North America in 1971 when James Reston described how his postoperative pain from an emergency appendectomy was alleviated by acupuncture. His description was published in a front-page article in the *New York Times.*[141] Approximately 3 months later, a team of U.S. physicians traveled to China and observed acupuncture used for surgical analgesia. Physician observations were reported in the *Journal of the American Medical Association.*[41] In 1972, President Nixon traveled to China with his personal physician and witnessed several surgeries where acupuncture was used as the only form of analgesia.[163] The National Institutes of Health (NIH) then sponsored a team of physicians to study the health care system in China. Soon after, research grants were offered to evaluate acupuncture's mechanisms and its clinical efficacy.[22]

U.S. schools of acupuncture began to incorporate traditional Chinese medicine, European acupuncture, and traditional elements from Japan, Korea, and Vietnam.[23] Acupuncture in the United States was often modeled more on a "mixed bag" approach rather than on traditional Chinese practices of acupuncture.

Acupuncture soon gained unprecedented popularity in the United States. Asian practitioners were overwhelmed with patients seeking their help; teachers were sought to train physicians; tours of China were organized; and individuals traveled to China, Japan, Korea, England, France, and Germany to gain clinical experience.[71] Soon, training programs were created around North America, fundamental textbooks were imported and translated, and the tenets of Chinese medicine and acupuncture were presented and reworked in the English language.

Acupuncture analgesia was soon linked to the central nervous system and to the activities of endogenous opioid peptides.[116] With clinical acupuncture experimentally linked to neurotransmitter mechanisms, scientific skepticism among medical professionals diminished and many sought professional training in the use of acupuncture. By 1991, approximately 1500 physicians and 8000 nonphysicians were practicing acupuncture in the United States.[110]

■ Hypothesized Mechanisms of Acupuncture

Bioelectrical Properties of Acupuncture

Niboyet, a French researcher, believed that a correlation existed between acupuncture points and skin points of lowered electrical resistance. In the 1940s and 1950s, he scanned skin surfaces with a galvanometer and then stimulated points of low resistance with direct and alternating currents. His research suggested that electrical conductance at acupuncture points is different from that at other skin sites, and that stimulating acupuncture points results in physiologic responses that will not be elicited from other skin sites similarly stimulated.[130] Niboyet's work supported the assertion that points of lowered electrical resistance are usually found in the acupuncture zones illustrated on Chinese charts. Grall verified Niboyet's work in 1962 and asserted that points of low resistance on the face and forearms corresponded to acupuncture points.[65] As research continued, it was found that resistance values varied from subject to subject and from anatomic zone to zone, ranging from 5 to 50 kilo ohms at acupuncture points, whereas neutral nonacupuncture points ranged between 0.5 and 3 mega ohms. When the low resistance points were delineated with overlaying paper, the classical acupuncture channels were revealed.[78,142]

Tracing Acupuncture Channels

One method of identifying acupuncture channels involved injecting a radioactive tracer, Technetium 99, into classical acupuncture points and into locations that were neutral (e.g., nonacupuncture points). Pathways were then compared by following the tracer with a scintillation camera. The pathways of the radioisotope diffusion from the acupuncture points corresponded to the classically described acupuncture channels. However, neutral points displayed a diffusion pattern without linear tracings.[35] Other researchers concluded that transportation away from acupuncture and control points occurred through the vein and lymphatic systems, not acupuncture networks.[145] Darras, an investigator using nuclear tracers, rejected this argument with the observation that the scanned pathway moved beyond a tourniquet blocking surface peripheral blood circulation. Further, he observed that the tracer injected into the lymphatic vessels demonstrated these vessels to be distinct from acupuncture channels. Stimulation of the injected points with a needle, electricity, or helium-neon laser increased the migration rate along the channels. Since these rates did not correspond to vascular or lymphatic circulation rates, the authors concluded that the observed isotopic migration demonstrates the pathways of acupuncture channels.[33,34] In another study, the French researcher, De Vernejoul, injected radioactive isotopes into the acupoints of human beings and tracked their movement with a gamma imaging camera. Within 4 to 6 minutes, the isotopes traveled approximately 30 cm along previously identified acupuncture meridian tracks. To challenge his work, he then injected isotopes into blood vessels at random points. Isotopes injected into the blood vessels did not travel in any manner similar to how they traveled at acupoints, suggesting that meridians make up a separate pathway system within the body.[38]

Electrical Current Along Acupuncture Channels

Resistance to a current passed between acupuncture points on the **same** classical channel has been consistently shown to be less than the resistance between two nearby control points.[140] The French researcher Mussat determined that electrodes placed on the surface of two unstimulated acupuncture points along the same channel did not register a significant current. However, when needles were inserted into these points, a current resulted of 10 to 30 nanoamperes between the two points; this current diminished exponentially with the passage of time. A 9-volt battery was then connected to the needles inserted into two acupuncture points along the same channel. When the battery was disconnected, a discharge current of 15 to 25 microamperes took place between the two points. When the same measurements were made between needled neutral points not connected by a muscle cleavage plane, no current was measured.[123]

It has been postulated that the fascia and interstitial fluid are the most likely vehicles to transmit electromagnetic bioinformation and that the continuum of electron-rich fascia acts as a semiconductor of electrical impulses. Cleavage planes between fascial sheaths surrounding muscles allow unencumbered flow of the ionic fluid from the interior to the surface (Figure 11-3).[71]

Mussat found that the charge carried in the acupuncture channel was measurable and was independent of the surrounding tissue. Mussat continued experimentation with the intensity of electrical current, the time of propagation of current along the channel, and the electrical potential differences linked vertically along acupuncture channels. He concluded that the current passing between acupuncture points follows the organization of traditional acupuncture channels and that this circulation is not random.[123]

Acupuncture Points

Acupuncture points have a surface area of 1 to 5 square millimeters; most points are situated in surface depressions along the cleavage between muscles. The depressions can be identified by palpation and are typically hypersensitive.[13] Acupuncture points are located in a vertical column of loose connective tissue, surrounded by the thick, dense connective tissue of the skin, itself not a good electrical conductor (Figure 11-4). Dissection of over three hundred sites on cadavers demonstrated acupuncture points to correspond to peripheral endings of cranial and spinal nerves, with their terminals dispersed in the area of the surface point.[76] Another study found nerve-vessel bundles present at the sites corresponding to acupuncture points.[70]

The nature of sensitivity at acupuncture points is not fully understood, although the points appear to be specific regions of hyperalgesia arising spontaneously from local irritation or from excitation of somatic or visceral structures distant from the painful point.[131] The number and sensitivity of classical acupuncture points increase with the duration and intensity of pain, and the diameter of a sensitive acupuncture point expands with increasing pain intensity. Diseased viscera combine with the noxious sensation of active acupuncture point stimulation to produce referred pain to a larger surface around the sensi-

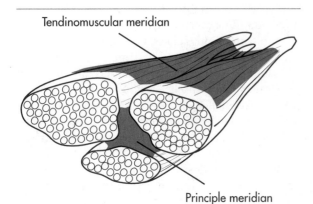

Tendinomuscular meridian

Principle meridian

■ *Figure 11-3.* Most acupuncture points are situated in surface depressions along the cleavage between muscles. The depressions can be identified by palpation and are typically hypersensitive.

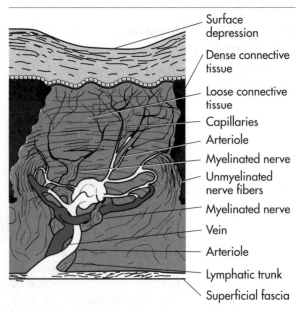

Surface depression

Dense connective tissue

Loose connective tissue

Capillaries

Arteriole

Myelinated nerve

Unmyelinated nerve fibers

Myelinated nerve

Vein

Arteriole

Lymphatic trunk

Superficial fascia

■ *Figure 11-4.* Acupuncture points are located in a vertical column of loose connective tissue, surrounded by the thick, dense connective tissue of the skin, itself not a good electrical conductor.

tive point. Points become tender in orderly progression and disappear in reverse order when disease progression is arrested or when healing occurs.[48]

Acupuncture Analgesia

The most researched area of acupuncture relates to acupuncture analgesia (numbing of pain sensation).[96] By 1980, connections had been established between the endogenous opioid peptide system and analgesic events observed with electrical acupuncture stimulation. This connection has also been demonstrated in a variety of experimental animal studies, suggesting that acupuncture analgesia is a general phenomenon in the mammalian world.[29,116,138]

Peripheral and Autonomic Nervous Systems Pathways

Acupuncture needles inserted into the skin, tissue, and deeper structures of fascia, muscle, tendon, and periosteum appear to stimulate primarily small myelinated A-∂ (fast pain) *afferent* (traveling toward the central nervous system [CNS]) nerve fibers and small *myelinated* (covering contributing to high speed conductance) group II and group III nerve fibers in muscles.[154] The autonomic nervous system (ANS) appears to be activated both centrally and locally by acupuncture stimulation. Inserting a needle at the myotome segmental level associated with muscular pain, whether the problem is located on the trunk or an extremity, stimulates the somatic nerve endings in the muscle.[173] (Note: a myotome is a region of skeletal muscle innervated by motor fibers of a given spinal nerve.)

Theories of Pain Control: Diffuse Noxious Inhibitory Control

Some of the best known and documented effects of acupuncture are related to acute and chronic pain control and surgical anesthesia. One neuroanatomically based model used to explain acupuncture's ability to produce pain relief is *diffuse noxious inhibitory control* (DNIC). DNIC can be described as an inhibition of pain by counter-irritation stimulation. DNIC can be triggered by a noxious stimulus produced from any part of the body, at the site of pain or at a location unrelated to the painful area.[94] In the DNIC model, inhibition is directly related to the intensity of the noxious stimulus.[62] Interestingly, the distance between the painful site and the site of application of inhibitory noxious stimulation is

not a critical factor in determining the strength of pain inhibition, and effective stimulation is not limited to acupuncture points.[121] Further, inhibition of pain persists after acupuncture stimulation is discontinued.

The mechanism of DNIC involves a complex loop ascending from and descending to the spinal cord. There is both endorphin and serotonin activity involved in the mechanism.[71] DNIC depends on intense stimulation of a large population of A-∂, C, and group IV fibers. These fibers converge at multiple segments of the spinal cord. DNIC involves a complex mechanism of nerve impulses and neurotransmitter responses in all levels of the nervous system.

Enduring analgesic effects of acupuncture stimulation for chronic pain depend on a cumulative effect of sequential acupuncture treatments. Acupuncture-induced inhibition of pain builds up slowly, reaching a peak 30 minutes after beginning treatment. If low-frequency electrostimulation is applied, inhibition of pain can be maintained for several hours after stimulation is discontinued. If a second acupuncture treatment is given 90 minutes after an initial 15-minute treatment, the effects of the first treatment are potentiated. This suggests that the first endorphin effect modulates synapses so that the second effect, which may not be endorphinergic, is more powerful.[139] It has been suggested that duration of acupuncture analgesia can be explained by (1) the potentiation of the effect for a second treatment after the first, and (2) the cumulative effect of sequential treatments that (3) use the synthesis of endorphin precursors. Maximum elevation for pain relief is reached within 24 hours and can last up to 96 hours.

Challenges to Acupuncture Research

Because of the nature of acupuncture (its historical traditions and application), it is often difficult to perform acupuncture research that meets the gold standard double-blind, placebo-controlled trial of Western medicine. Criteria for traditional acupuncture diagnoses and needling sites are not standardized; indeed, traditionally, acupuncture sites (often multiple sites) were selected based on individual symptoms and history, as well as traditional needling sites for the complaint at hand. As symptoms changed, so did the treatment.

Because of a lack of funding for research, subject numbers in acupuncture studies were typically small, leaving studies statistically under powered. Blinding was another issue; the acupuncturist had to know the intended goal. Reviews of the literature were often difficult to summarize, as acupuncture methods, research designs, and group sizes varied.[100,101,134,143,171]

■ Clinical Research on the Effects of Acupuncture

This section begins by reiterating that Chinese medicine uses acupuncture to treat the whole person and that patient symptoms are meaningless if considered in isolation from the entire identified pattern of health. However, since this text is targeted to the Western reader, we review the clinically controlled trials of the efficacy of acupuncture—trials that do, in fact, consider only individual signs or symptoms related to patient care. The reader should remember that acupuncture and Chinese medicine is used to treat the patient for a broad spectrum of conditions, as defined by Chinese diagnosis. However, in the West, acupuncture has been evaluated clinically for its efficacy in limited ways. In this chapter, we review these trials.

In discussing the randomized, controlled trials on acupuncture, there are three major acupuncture categories worthy of attention: (1) chronic and acute pain management, including surgical analgesia, (2) substance abuse control, and (3) postoperative and chemotherapy-induced nausea. Other uses of acupuncture less tested by clinically controlled trials are also reviewed.

Acupuncture and Pain Management

Acupuncture for the treatment of pain has been researched for its efficacy to relieve low back pain, headache pain, procedural and preoperative and postoperative pain, osteoarthritic pain, cervical pain, musculoskeletal pain, pain associated with organic lesions, and cancer pain. It has also been assessed for its capacity to provide surgical analgesia. The following text reviews some the studies of acupuncture and pain management.

Low Back Pain

In the studies of low back pain, acupuncture has been compared with wait-list controls; sham acupuncture (i.e., needles inserted into nonacupuncture points); transcutaneous electrical stimulation (TENS); sham TENS (i.e., current was not on); and placebo acupuncture (i.e., numbing of nonacupuncture points followed by shallow insertion of needles). All of these techniques, with the exception of wait-list or no treatment, have been criticized for methodologic reasons. Sham TENS

does not produce the skin pricking sensation of acupuncture; nor does it "feel" like "real" TENS. It has been suggested that superficial needle insertion is the best form of placebo treatment; however, some researchers argue that DNIC effects may release endorphins in response to needling, providing some pain relief.[104] Determining what is a "real" placebo in acupuncture and what is a less effective form of treatment has been hotly debated. Nonetheless, we review examples of each type of research and their outcomes.

Thirteen controlled studies of acupuncture for the treatment of low back pain are illustrated in Table 11-1. Gunn and associates (1983), Lehmann and colleagues (1983 and 1986), MacDonald and others (1983), and Garvey and associates (1989) all concluded that acupuncture was superior to no treatment, sham acupuncture, or control interventions such as TENS, sham TENS, or trigger point injections.[57,66,98,99,111] Ghia and colleagues found acupuncture equally effective whether using the technique of tender area needling or the technique of classical meridian loci needling.[63] Coan and others (1978), Laitinen (1976), Mendelson and associates (1983), and Fox and Melzack (1976) reported improvements with the administration of acupuncture, but these results were not statistically significant nor statistically analyzed.[31,53,91,118,119] Emery and Lythgoe and Edelist and others concluded that acupuncture was not clinically effective.[49,51]

In evaluating these studies, we can say that acupuncture:

1. Performed slightly better than TENS in three studies (Laitinen, Fox and Melzack, and Lehmann and others);
2. Enhanced the effectiveness of standard treatment relative to standard treatment alone (Gunn); and
3. Performed better than mock TENS or no treatment (MacDonald and others and Coan and associates).

When a broad range of controlled trials, reviews, and metaanalyses are considered, we can conclude that a majority of patients with back pain will derive some clinically significant short-term benefits from acupuncture. The figures in individual studies are highly variable, with reported improvements ranging from 26% to 79%.[31,120] This conclusion is not surprising based on the methodologic flaws and differences in research designs.

The longer-term effects are harder to assess. In the Fox and Melzack study, acupuncture benefits lasted only 40 hours, whereas the Laitinen study reported the continuation of gains 6 months after treatment.

It is troubling that a majority of literature reports no significant differences between TENS and sham (no point) needling, although acupuncture often demonstrated a trend for greater improvement. One possible explanation for the differences in study outcomes is that formularized or standardized methods of needling are most typically used, rather than the individualized treatments of traditional Chinese medicine; the Coan study was an exception.

The methodologic issues related to acupuncture and low back pain continue to be a problem; more studies addressing these methodologic shortfalls are needed.

Headache Pain

Acupuncture studies for the treatment of headache pain are usually categorized as migraine,

TABLE 11-1	Acupuncture for Treatment of Low Back Pain		
STUDY	**NUMBER**	**GROUPS**	**RESULTS**
Coan R et al: The acupuncture treatment of low back pain: a randomized controlled treatment, *Am J Chin Med* 8:181, 1980.	50	(1) Immediate acupuncture (2) Waiting list for acupuncture later	Acupuncture was manual with some electro-acupuncture Differences between immediate and wait-list groups at 15 wks revealed 32% reduction in pain vs 0% for wait-list; mean pain score, 51% vs 2% decrease; increase of activity 19% vs 0%; reportedly improved, 83% vs 31% Of those patients who completed "adequate" treatment, 79% showed significant improvement and at final follow-up, (30 wks) 58% were still significantly improved
Edelist G et al: Treatment of low back pain with acupuncture, *Can Anaesthesiol Soc J* 23:303, 1976.	30	(1) "True" acupuncture (2) Sham acupuncture	Both groups got manual and electrical stimulation of points (real or sham) Authors were unable to demonstrate any benefit of acupuncture vs sham treatment
Emery P, Lythgoe S: The effect of acupuncture on ankylosing spondylitis, *Br J Rheumatol* 25:132, 1986.	10	Cross-over design; all patients received active and sham needling at different times	Neither sham nor real acupuncture was found to be beneficial for ankylosing spondylitis Note: Ankylosing spondylitis is a severe condition; long-term treatment would probably be necessary to identify improvement from acupuncture, if it were to be effective
Fox E, Malzack R: Transcutaneous electrical stimulation and acupuncture: comparison of treatment for low-back pain, *Pain* 2:141, 1976.	12	(1) Acupuncture (2) TENS	Cross-over design; all patients received both at different times Following each course of treatment, patients reporting 33% or better pain relief were 75% and 66% for acupuncture and 57% and 46% for TENS Mean duration of pain relief was 40 hours for acupuncture vs 23 hours for TENS Numbers were too small to reach statistical significance
Garvey TA et al: A prospective, randomized, double-blind evaluation of trigger-point injection therapy for low-back pain, *Spine* 14:962, 1989.	63	(1) Lidocaine injection (2) Lidocaine with a steroid (3) Acupuncture (4) Vapocoolant spray with acupressure	Therapy without injected medication (63% improvement rate) was at least as effective as therapy with drug injection (42% improvement rate, difference p>0.09) Trigger point is a useful treatment for low back pain; injection of the substance is not the critical factor
Ghia JN et al: Acupuncture and chronic pain mechanisms, *Pain* 2:285, 1976. Ghia JN et al: Acupuncture and chronic pain mechanisms, *Pain* 2(3):285, 1976.	40	(1) Meridian loci acupuncture (2) Tender area needling	Groups were not significantly different in reported improvement Comparing group 1 vs group 2, 4 vs 5 reported excellent results; 0 vs 3 good; 4 vs 1 fair; 11 vs 10 reported failure

TENS, Transcutaneous electrical stimulation.

Continued

TABLE 11-1	Acupuncture for Treatment of Low Back Pain—cont'd		
STUDY	**NUMBER**	**GROUPS**	**RESULTS**
Gunn CC et al: Dry needling of muscle motor points for chronic low back pain, *Spine* 5(3):279, 1980.	56	(1) Physical therapy, remedial exercises and occupational therapy AND acupuncture (2) Above therapies without acupuncture	Acupuncture patients had significant improvement of symptoms (p<0.005); of the 29 in the acupuncture group, 18 returned to original or equivalent jobs and 10 to lighter duty; in control group, only 4 returned to original jobs at 27 wks
Laitinen J: Acupuncture and TENS in the treatment of chronic sacrolumbalgia and ishialgia, *Am J Chin Med* 4:169, 1976.	100	(1) Acupuncture (2) TENS	Complete and moderate improvement ratings were compared for acupuncture vs TENS Acupuncture performed better (but not statistically so) compared with TENS; it is essentially as useful as TENS
Lehmann TR et al: The impact of patients with nonorganic physical findings on a controlled trial of transcutaneous electrical nerve stimulation and electroacupuncture, *Spine* 8(6):625, 1983.	54	(1) Electroacupuncture (2) TENS (3) Sham TENS	Acupuncture group gained significantly more relief of peak pain and pain on average day at 3-mo follow-up
Lehmann TR et al: Efficacy of electroacupuncture and TENS in the rehabilitation of chronic low back pain patients, *Pain* 26:277, 1986.	53	(1) Electroacupuncture (2) TENS (3) Sham TENS	Without regard for treatment group, mean scores for all 10 outcome measures were significantly (and highly) improved (p ranged from 0.0117 to 0.0001) between admission and discharge Over time (6 mos), sham TENS improved during admission (p=0.03) and then had a nonsignificant loss discharge to 6 mos; during admiting, acupuncture group improved (p=0.005) and had significant gain during 6 months TENS and sham TENS did not demonstrate significant long-term gains (p=0.50 and 0.23) compared with acupuncture (p=0.0008)
MacDonald AJR et al: Superficial acupuncture in the relief of chronic low back pain: a placebo-controlled randomized trial, *Ann Royal Coll Surg Engl* 65:44, 1983.	17	(1) Manual and electro-acupuncture (2) Sham TENS	When comparing acupuncture vs sham, pain relief was 77.35% vs 30.13% (p<0.01); pain score reduction 57.15% vs 22.74%; activity pain reduction 52.04% vs 5.83% (p<0.05); and physical signs reduction 96.78% vs 29.17% (p<0.01); and combined average reduction 71.41% vs 21.35% (p<0.01)
Mendelson G et al: Acupuncture analgesia for chronic low back pain, *Clin Exp Neurol* 15:182, 1978. Mendelson G et al: Acupuncture treatment of chronic back pain: a double-blind, placebo-controlled trial, *Am J Med* 74:49, 1983.	77	(1) Real acupuncture (2) Placebo acupuncture of a subcutaneous injection of lidocaine into nonpoints, then shallowing inserting needles into numb spots	Patients received both treatments, in a crossover design There were no significant differences between the two treatments, leading authors to conclude that the placebo-component was more clinically important than its physiologic effects

tension, or mixed disorder. Ten controlled trials on the effects of acupuncture for tension or migraine headache pain are summarized in Table 11-2. Two studies found that acupuncture reduced headache pain, but it was not significantly more effective than physical therapy control. Further, physical therapy relieved muscle tension more than acupuncture.[18,19] Three studies found acupuncture as effective for pain relief as physical therapy or sham needling.[3,164,170] Four studies concluded that acupuncture was significantly more effective for pain relief than control (no treatment).[68,79,103,169] Two studies found acupuncture significantly more effective than sham acupuncture.[12,82] One study produced no statistically significant improvements between mock TENS and classical acupuncture.[42]

Patients are often referred to acupuncture trials only after traditional medical treatment has failed. Therefore these subjects are particularly

TABLE 11-2	Acupuncture and Headache Pain				
AUTHOR	**TYPE HEADACHE**	**NUMBER**	**CONTROL**	**TYPE**	**RESULTS**
Ahon E et al: Acupuncture and physiotherapy for the treatment of myogenic headache patients: pain relief and EMG activity, *Adv Pain Res Ther* 5:571, 1983.	Tension (myogenic)	22	Physiotherapy plus ultrasound	Classical 4 sessions	Both groups had significant changes in pain and frequency; 4 acupuncture sessions and 8 physiotherapy sessions were equivalent
Borglum-Jensen et al: Effect of acupuncture on myogenic headache, *Scand J Dent Res* 87:373, 1979.	Not stated	29	Sham acupuncture	Classical, single session	Acupuncture group had significant reduction in frequency of headache and medication use; placebo group also reduced medication use
Carlsson J et al: Muscle tenderness in tension headache treated with acupuncture or physiotherapy, *Cephalalgia* 10:131, 1990.	Tension headache	62	Physiotherapy	Classical	Intensity of pain improved for both groups ($p<0.05$ acupuncture and $p<0.001$ physiotherapy) Muscle tension reduced in 6 muscles for physiotherapy group ($p<0.01$) and 3 muscles for acupuncture group Authors concluded both were highly successful for reducing headache pain, but acupuncture was not superior to physiotherapy
Carlsson J, Rosenthal U: Oculomotor disturbances in patients with tension headache treated with acupuncture or physiotherapy, *Cephalalgia* 10:123, 1990.	Tension headache	48	Physiotherapy	Classical	Headache intensity was reduced for both groups; trapezius muscle tension reduced by physiotherapy but not acupuncture; acupuncture was not found superior to physiotherapy
Dowson D et al: The effects of acupuncture versus placebo in the treatment of headache, *Pain* 21:35, 1985.	Migraine	48	Mock TENS	Classical 6 sessions	Acupuncture group experienced 56% and 44% improvement in severity and frequency compared with 30% and 57% for placebo Differences not significant between groups
Hansen PE, Hansen JH: Acupuncture treatment of chronic tension headache: a controlled cross-over trial, *Cephalalgia* 5:137, 1985.	Chronic tension	18	Sham acupuncture	Classical	Acupuncture found to relieve significantly more pain than sham Pain reduction=31% This was a cross-over design
Jensen LB et al: Effect of acupuncture of headache measured by reduction in number of attacks and use of drugs, *Scand J Dent Res* 87:373, 1979.	Mixed	29	Sham acupuncture	Classical	Placebo resulted in nonsignificant reduction of headache attacks; acupuncture produced a significant reduction in attacks A reduction in the use of drugs after acupuncture was also noted
Johansson et al: Effect of acupuncture in tension headache and brainstem reflexes, *Adv Pain Res Ther* 839, 1976.	Tension	33	Sham acupuncture	Classical	Acupuncture group reported significant improvement as compared with sham group

Continued

TABLE 11-2	Acupuncture and Headache Pain—cont'd				
AUTHOR	**TYPE HEADACHE**	**NUMBER**	**CONTROL**	**TYPE**	**RESULTS**
Loh L et al: Acupuncture versus medical treatment for migraine and muscle tension headaches, *J Neurol Neurosurg Psychiatry* 47:333, 1984.	Migraine and tension	48	Standard drug/medical care	Classical and EA (crossover)	59% of acupuncture improved, with 39% showing marked improvement for standard treatment group 25% showed a benefit with 11% markedly improved
Tavola T et al: Traditional Chinese acupuncture in tension-type headache: a controlled study, *Pain* 48:325, 1992.	Tension headache	30	Sham needling	Classical	No significant differences between groups for frequency, medication use, headache index Authors found no difference in treatment effects between sham and classical acupuncture
Vincent CA: A controlled trial of the treatment of migraine by acupuncture, *Clin J Pain* 5:305, 1989.	Chronic migraine	30	Sham needling at "nonpoints"	Classical	For classical vs sham, pain was reduced 43% and 14%, respectively; medication use 38% vs 28%, respectively At 1 year, pain was reduced 71% and 8%, respectively; medication use 71% and 21%, respectively Author found acupuncture significantly more effective at reducing pain than sham
Vincent CA: The treatment of tension headache by acupuncture: a controlled single case design with time series analysis, *J Psychosom Res* 34(5):553, 1990.	Tension headache	14	Sham needling (crossover)	Classical (crossover)	Single case design; sham and classical delivered in random order Medication use reduced 52% in group and pain reduced 54% Medication reduction $p<0.02$; pain $p<0.001$ Classical and sham did not differ significantly

difficult to treat. In spite of this fact, results from the literature at large have generally been encouraging with moderate (54%) to marked (92%) improvements in subjective pain.[24,90]

Pain from Osteoarthritis

In studies of acupuncture as treatment for osteoarthritis pain, Junnila (1982), Thomas and colleagues (1992), and Christensen and others (1993) found acupuncture significantly more effective in reducing pain than control and comparison treatments including wait-list controls, pain medication (e.g., piroxicam and diazepam), sham acupuncture, and placebo medication[25,26,83,162] (Table 11-3). Dickens and Lewith found acupuncture more effective than TENS.[40] Gaw and others and Takeda and Wessel found acupuncture effective but not significantly more effective than sham acupuncture (nonpoint needling).[15,58] The authors therefore concluded that "sham" acupuncture may act as a pain relieving treatment.

A thorough and systematic review of the literature found outcomes from the previously discussed studies and other trials contradictory. Most trials had serious methodologic flaws, and sham acupuncture seemed to produce effects equal to acupuncture. Almost all studies employed formula acupuncture (i.e., needling of a predefined set of points) as opposed to traditional acupuncture (i.e., needling individualized sets of points according to traditional Chinese diagnosis). This failure to "individualize" treatment may have masked stronger outcomes. Ernst stated that, based on current existing clinical trials, one cannot draw the conclusion that acupuncture is superior to sham needling in pain associated with osteoarthritis. Better designed and controlled trials that test traditional acupuncture need to be conducted.[52]

Cervical Neck Pain

In studies of acupuncture for the treatment of neck pain, controlled trials by Petrie and Langley

TABLE 11-3	Acupuncture for Treatment of Osteoarthritis			
STUDY	**NUMBER**	**GROUPS**	**TYPE**	**RESULTS**
Christensen BV et al: Acupuncture treatment of severe knee osteoarthritis: a long-term study, *Acta Anaesthesiologica Scandinavica* 36:519, 1992.	29	(1) Received immediately after knee surgery (2) Received 9 wks after surgery	Knee	Group treated immediately had significantly better knee function scores, time to walk, and stair climbing than did delayed treatment (p<0.0001) At wk 12, both groups had significant improvements in objective scores and pain levels (p<0.02) At wk 16, 80% experienced pain relief; 56% improvements in objective findings NSAIDS and other medications were reduced (p<0.01 and p<0.002) 7 patients in wait-group avoided surgery, a savings of $63,000 Authors found acupuncture highly effective as treatment
Christensen et al: Acupuncture treatment of knee arthrosis. A long-term study (abstract), *Ugeskrift for Laeger* (Copenhagen), 155(49):4007, 1993.	17	Follow-up of Christensen	Knee	17 patients (and 29 knees) continued to receive treatment Treatment resulted in significant reduction in pain, analgesic consumption and in most objective measures This demonstrated that acupuncture treatment can result in a maintenance of its original gains
Dickens W, Lewith GT: A single-blind, controlled and randomized clinical trial to evaluate the effect of acupuncture for the treatment of trapezio-metacarpal osteoarthritis, *Complementary Med Res* 3(2):5, 1989.	12	(1) Acupuncture (2) Mock TENS	Trapezio-meta-carpel	Acupuncture patients experienced significant thumb pain relief (p=0.02) and retained gains at follow-up (p=0.04) compared with pretreatment scores; TENS produced nonsignificant improvements
Gaw AC et al: Efficacy of acupuncture on osteoarthritic pain, *N Engl J Med* 293(8):375, 1975.	40	(1) Acupuncture at standard points (2) Needling at nonpoints		Improvement was found in joint tenderness, subjective pain, and joint activity (p=0.05) No significant differences were found among groups Both interventions may have acted as a treatment (i.e., nonpoint needling may have produced some beneficial effects as a less-effective form of true acupuncture)
Junnila SYT: Acupuncture superior to Piroxicam for the treatment of osteoarthritis, *Am J Acupunct* 10(4):341, 1982.	32	(1) Acupuncture (2) Piroxicam	Hip, knee humeroscapular	Improvements at 2 wks were equal (30%); after that, acupuncture was superior Acupuncture group improved pain scores from13.9 to 4.9; the piroxicam group improved from 11.7 to 7.8
Takeda W, Wessel J: Acupuncture for the treatment of pain of osteoarthritic knees, *Arthritis Care Res* 7(3):118, 1994.	40	(1) Acupuncture (2) Sham acupuncture	Knee	Both groups significantly reduced pain, stiffness, and physical disability of knee There were no differences found between the two groups Authors concluded acupuncture is not more effective than sham for treatment of osteoarthritis
Thomas M et al: A comparative study of Diazepam and acupuncture in patients with osteoarthritis pain: a placebo controlled study, *Am J Chin Med* 19(2):95, 1991.	44	(1) Acupuncture (2) Sham acupuncture (3) Diazepam (4) Placebo diazepam	Cervical	Diazepam reduced affective and sensory pain (p<0.01 and 0.05) Placebo reduced affective pain only (p<0.05) Acupuncture significantly removed affective (p<0.0001) and sensory pain (p<0.005) Sham acupuncture reduced affective & sensory pain as well (p<0.05) Acupuncture was the most effective treatment

TENS, Transcutaneous electrical stimulation.

and Petrie and Hazelman found that acupuncture is no more effective than placebo TENS.[136,137] Loy found electroacupuncture more effective than physical therapy for cervical pain, although both treatments were effective. Electroacupuncture produced earlier symptomatic improvement with increased neck movement, especially in patients with mild degenerative changes of the cervical spine.[105]

In a study by Coan and others, 15 sufferers with chronic neck pain (mean of 8 years) were treated with acupuncture. At 12 weeks, 12 (80%) of the treated subjects improved, some dramatically. A 40% reduction of pain score, 54% reduction of pain pills, 68% reduction of pain hours per day, and 32% less limitation were demonstrated. Only 2 of 15 (13%) treated subjects reported improvement after 12 weeks of treatment.[32]

Musculoskeletal and Myofascial Pain

The earliest study of musculoskeletal pain was published in 1978 by Godfrey and Morgan. It concluded that acupuncture reduced musculoskeletal pain, but no more effectively than sham acupuncture.[64] By contrast, Deluze and others found acupuncture superior to sham acupuncture in the relief of fibromyalgia pain.[36] Lundenberg found acupuncture equally as effective as TENS or vibratory stimulation for the treatment of chronic myalgia; this study also found that acupuncture, TENS, and vibratory stimulation all produced superior pain relief to placebo oral analgesics[106] (Table 11-4).

Organic Pain

Co and colleagues demonstrated that pain from sickle cell anemia crisis was effectively relieved by needling at both "real" acupuncture sites and at sham locations.[30] Lee and associates also found acupuncture as effective as intramuscular analgesics in the treatment of renal colic pain.[97] In a study by Ballegard and Christophersen, chronic pancreatitis pain was relieved equally by "real" and sham acupuncture; however, both acupuncture and TENS were judged not to be of significant clinical value for the treatment of pancreatitis pain.[8]

Surgical Analgesia

No doubt, the most dramatic use of acupuncture has been in the area of surgical analgesia. The use of acupuncture as a surgical analgesia brought this therapy prominently to the attention of Western medicine. In 1973, it was reported that 15% to 25% of all surgical procedures in Chinese hospitals were performed using acupuncture analgesia, and that its success rate for surgical analgesia was 90%. This report was later questioned, however; outside observers reported only 6% to 7% of Chinese surgeries using acupuncture as an analgesia.[41,127]

TABLE 11-4	**Acupuncture for Treatment of Musculoskeletal Pain**		
STUDY	**NUMBER**	**GROUPS**	**RESULTS**
Deluze C et al: Electroacupuncture in fibromyalgia: results of controlled trial, *BMJ* 305:1249, 1993.	70	(1) Electroacupuncture (2) Sham (shallow needling at nonpoints)	Compared with sham, electroacupuncture group improved significantly more, ranging from p<0.001 to 0.0627 (71% on pain threshhold; 34% for number of tablets used; 39% for regional pain scores; 30% for VAS pain; 45% for sleep quality; 29% for morning stiffness; patient and physical evaluation 34%)
Godfrey CM, Morgan P: A controlled trial of the theory of acupuncture in musculoskeletal pain, *J Rheumatol* 2:121, 1978.		(1) Correct-site acupuncture (2) Noncorrect site acupuncture	Although 60% had reduced pain after only 3 treatments There were no significant differences between treatments Although not disproving acupuncture, findings do not support the theory that certain specific points must be needled to relieve specific areas of pain
Lundenberg T: A comparative study of the pain alleviating effect of vibratory stimulation, TENS, electroacupuncture, and placebo, *Am J Chin Med* 12:1, 1984.	36	(1) Vibrostimulation (2) TENS (3) Electroacupuncture (4) Placebo(sugar pill)	All subjects (chronic myalgia patients) received random order treatment for 3 weeks No significant difference was found in pain relief between treatments, although vibrostimulation and electroacupuncture produced analgesia for longer periods of time than TENS and placebo

TENS, Transcutaneous electrical stimulation.

In spite of dramatic reports of its effectiveness, acupuncture for surgical analgesia has seldom been used in Western countries, with the exceptions of oral surgery and dental extractions. The failure of acupuncture analgesia to be more accepted and used in Western countries may be because of its mechanisms. Although pain is modified by acupuncture, the sensations of touch, pressure, stretch, vibration, and temperature are still experienced by the patient, sensations unacceptable to Western clients accustomed to a lack of sensation of any kind during surgery[69,95,128] (Table 11-5).

Procedural Analgesia

Endoscopy is an examination of the body's internal organs and structures using a fiberoptic viewing tube called an endoscope. The endoscopic procedure that examines the rectum and lower

TABLE 11-5	**Acupuncture for Examination, Surgical Analgesia, Postoperative Analgesia**					
AUTHOR	**TYPE HEADACHE**	**NUMBER**	**CONTROL**	**TYPE**	**RESULTS**
EXAMINATION PROCEDURES					
Cahn AM et al: Acupuncture in gastroscopy, *Lancet* 1(8057):182, 1978.	Gastroscopy	90	Sham acupuncture 12-needle placement 1 cm away from "real" acupoints	12-needle placement at acupoints	Electrical stimulation used for both groups Acupuncture group had significantly less belching, agitation, and vomiting attempts ($p<0.001$); and number of attempts to insertion ($p<0.05$) There was less pain in pharynx ($p<0.01$); and less bloating ($p<0.05$)
Wang HH et al: A study in the effectiveness of acupuncture analgesia for colonoscopic examination compared with conventional premedication, *A J Acupunct* 20(3):217, 1992.	Colonoscopic examination	200	Analgesic medication buscopan and pethidine	Acupuncture	88 of 100 acupuncture patients reported good to excellent pain relief while 96 of 100 in the medication group rated pain relief good to excellent Pain was not significantly different between groups although acpuncture group had significantly fewer side effects ($p<0.001$)
SURGICAL ANALGESIA					
Lee MHM et al: Acupuncture anesthesia in dentistry, *N Y State Dent J* 39:299, 1973.	Anesthetic, dental procedures	20	No control group—need for analgesia served as control	Extraction, cavity, curettage	16 or 20 (80%) used acupuncture as the only anesthetic; 4 required other analgesia medications
POST-OPERATIVE ANALGESIA					
Chen et al: The effect of location of transcutaneous electrical nerve stimulation on postoperative opioid analgesic requirement: acupoint versus nonacupoint stimulation, *Anesth Analg* 87(5):1129, 1998.	Total hysterectomy or myomectomy	100W	(1) Sham TENS (no current) (2) Nonacupoint and TENS at shoulder (3) TENS at surgical incision	"Real" acupuncture and TENS	At 24 hours, opioid use in 3 and 4 decreased 37% and 39%, respectively, compared with sham; 35% and 38% compared with group 2 Analgesia use, nausea and dizziness also reduced in groups 3 and 4 compared with 1 and 2 Authors found that TENS applied at incision was as effective as acupuncture and both were more effective than nonacupoint stimulation

TENS, Transcutaneous electrical stimulation.

Continued

TABLE 11-5	Acupuncture for Examination, Surgical Analgesia, Postoperative Analgesia—cont'd				
AUTHOR	**TYPE HEADACHE**	**NUMBER**	**CONTROL**	**TYPE**	**RESULTS**
Christensen PA et al: Electroacupuncture and postoperative pain, *Br J Anaesth* 62:258, 1989.	Postoperative pain control after abdominal surgery	20	No further treatment	Electroacupuncture after wound closure	Acupuncture group consumed half the quantity of pethidine of controls; analgesia was administered by patient-controlled pump
Ekblom A et al: Increased postoperative pain and consumption of analgesics following acupuncture, *Pain* 44(3):241, 1991.	Removal of third molars	110	No acupuncture control group (received lidocaine)	(1) Acupuncture presurgical (2) Acupuncture after surgery	Preacupuncture group 1 was significantly more tense and reported procedure more unpleasant than the other two groups Group 1 also had more intense pain than controls and had more pain immediately after surgery than group 2 and control group 15 of 24 groups, 1 subject needs lidocaine; none from other groups did Both acupuncture groups had higher total pain scores than controls and had more dry socket
Lao L et al: The effect of acupuncture on post-operative oral surgery pain: a pilot study, *Acupunct Med* 2(1):13, 1994.	Postoperative dental surgical pain (e.g., third molar extraction)	10	Placebo acupuncture	"Real" acupuncture, 2 sessions	3 of 7 "real" acupuncture patients never experienced even moderate pain; 6 of 7 reported little swelling and did not need ice packs with sham acupuncture; all 3 had swelling and required ice packs, suggesting an anti-inflammatory effect for acupuncture
Lao L et al: Efficacy of Chinese acupuncture on postoperative oral surgery pain, *Oral Surg Oral Med Oral Pathol Oral Radiol Endodontics* 79(4):423, 1995.	Third molar extraction postoperative pain	19	Placebo acupuncture	"Real" acupuncture	Acupuncture subjects reported longer pain-free duration (mean 181 vs 71 mins p,0.05) and experienced less pain that placebo acupuncture
Sung YF et al: Comparison of the effects of acupuncture and codeine on postoperative dental pain, *Anesth Analg Curr Res* 56(4):473, 1977.	Postoperative analgesia after dental surgery	40	Placebo acupuncture plus placebo medication; placebo acupuncture plus codeine	"Real" acupuncture plus placebo medication	Acupuncture significantly more effective than placebo acupuncture ($p < 0.05$); codeine was significantly more effective than placebo medication ($p < 0.01$) Further, acupuncture plus placebo was significantly more effective than acupuncture plus codeine in first $1/2$ hr after surgery; this reversed for the 1-3 hrs post-surgical period

portion of the large intestine is called *colonoscopy*; when the stomach is examined with a flexible tube, the procedure is called *gastroscopy*. Although necessary, these procedures can be extremely uncomfortable and sometimes painful. Wang, Chang, and Liu assessed acupuncture for the control of procedural pain. They concluded that acupuncture and analgesics were equally effective for relieving the discomfort of colonoscopy; acupuncture produced less side effects.[172] Cahn and colleagues determined that treatment of

patients with acupuncture before gastroscopy significantly reduced pain and consumption of sedatives and analgesics, as compared with sham acupuncture (i.e., placebo) or no acupuncture.[17]

Postoperative Pain
Christensen and associates concluded that acupuncture is more effective in managing postoperative pain than medication alone.[27] Studies of oral surgery by Sung and others (1994) and Lao and associates (1995) found that acupuncture sig-

nificantly reduced pain during the postsurgical period.[92,93,155] An interesting study by Lee and others assessed acupuncture as the only form of anesthetic for a dental procedure and found the method effective for 16 of 20 patients (80%).[95] Chen and colleagues found acupuncture and TENS equally effective for decreasing opioid requirements and side effects and both more effective than sham acupuncture.[21] A perplexing study by Ekblom and others found acupuncture administered to subjects before or after surgery resulted in more pain and dry socket problems than the number that occurred for a control group receiving lidocaine analgesia.[50]

It is unlikely that acupuncture as a surgical and postsurgical analgesia will be used in the West with frequency. Exceptions may be its use with dental procedures and to benefit patients who are highly allergic to anesthetic and analgesic compounds. Nonetheless, acupuncture's success in blunting the pain of these procedures in some patients is unquestionable.

Postoperative and Chemotherapy-Induced Nausea

Acupuncture has been evaluated for its effectiveness in reducing postsurgical nausea. Several studies have compared acupuncture with control groups receiving sham acupuncture (i.e., placebo), TENS, or preoperative medication.[44-46,60,73] These studies typically found acupuncture superior to the control groups for reducing postoperative nausea. Yentis and Bissonnette (1992) found acupuncture as effective as, but not superior to, postoperative medication for controlling nausea.[179] Ghaly and colleagues found acupuncture more effective in reducing nausea than medication, but not significantly so.[61] Two studies by Weightman (1987) and by Yentis and Bissonnette (1991) concluded that acupuncture was ineffectual for the treatment of postoperative nausea.[177,180]

Dundee and associates demonstrated acupuncture to be significantly more effective for reducing chemotherapy-induced nausea than sham acupuncture or no treatment.[43] Aglietti and colleagues found acupuncture combined with antiemetic (i.e., nausea-reducing) drug treatment more effective than antiemetic drugs alone.[2] A study by Dundee and Yang, in which acupressure was repeatedly applied after the initial acupuncture treatment, found that the antiemetic effect of acupuncture was prolonged.[47]

Acupressure, the application of pressure without needling, at the P6 acupoint has also been used to relieve nausea and vomiting, although it does not produce as strong an effect as the more invasive acupuncture. Acupressure has been found effective for visually induced motion sickness and pregnancy-induced morning sickness.[37,77,144]

A systematic review of the 29 antiemesis trials revealed that 27 found acupuncture statistically superior to placebo, comparison treatments, and no treatment. A second analysis of the 12 highest quality studies representing 2000 patients found a statistically significant effect for P6 stimulation. Interestingly, in four trials where acupuncture was administered under anaesthesia, all four trials failed to produce a nausea-reducing effect.[168] Except when administered under anesthesia, P6 acupuncture point stimulation seems to be an effective antiemetic technique for a variety of nausea complaints (Table 11-6).

Neurologic Impairment

Several studies found that neurologic impairment in stroke victims occurred more rapidly and that patients improved more with acupuncture than with sham acupuncture or traditional treatment alone.[75,81,124-126,182] A 1976 study by Frost found acupuncture more beneficial than no treatment in posttraumatic comatose patients.[55] Some of these studies are illustrated in Table 11-7.

Gynecologic and Obstetric Conditions

In a study by Helms, acupuncture was demonstrated significantly more effective in relieving the pain of primary *dysmenorrhea* (i.e., uterine cramps during the menstrual period) as compared with sham acupuncture or no treatment.[72] In a study by Gerhard and Postneck, auricular (ear) acupuncture was compared with hormone therapy. Approximately the same number of pregnancies were achieved with both treatments, but the hormone patients had fewer menstrual irregularities than acupuncture subjects.[59]

Kubista and colleagues found that contractions could be induced and frequency of labor contractions intensified by acupuncture.[89] By contrast, a controlled study by Lyrenas and associates comparing acupuncture with no treatment concluded that acupuncture was ineffective for controlling labor pain.[109]

Treatment of Breathlessness in Asthmatics

Acupuncture has been evaluated for its efficacy in the treatment of asthma. Studies by Berger and Fung and others reported acupuncture superior to sham acupuncture for the relief of acute symp-

TABLE 11-6	Acupuncture for Treatment of Chemotherapy-Induced and Surgically Induced Nausea		

STUDY	NUMBER	GROUPS	RESULTS
ACUPUNCTURE FOR CHEMOTHERAPY-INDUCED NAUSEA AND VOMITING			
Aglietti L et al: A pilot study of metoclopramide, dexamethasone, diphenhydramine and acupuncture in women treated with cisplatin, *Cancer Chemother Pharmacol* 26(3):239, 1990.	26	(1) Antiemetic drugs plus traditional acupuncture (2) Antiemetic drugs; no acupuncture	A combination of antiemetic treatment of metoclopramide, dexamethasone, and diphenhydramine plus acupuncture were provided; outcomes were compared with matched subjects receiving the same antiemetic drugs but no acupuncture Acupuncture increased complete protection from nausea and decreased intensity and duration of nausea and vomiting Difficulties of performing acupuncture routinely in daily practice proved a hindrance to its wider clinical use
Dundee JW et al: Effect of stimulation of the P6 antiemetic point on postoperative nausea and vomiting, *Br J Anaesth* 63:612, 1989. Dundee JW et al: Acupuncture prophylaxis of cancer chemotherapy-induced sickness, *J Royal Soc Med* 82:268, 1989.	130	(1) Electroacupuncture 10 hz for 5 minutes applied to P6 point (2) Electroacupuncture applied to a limited number of persons to a "dummy" position	Patients with a history of sickness at previous chemotherapy sessions, with a 96% change of nausea/vomiting, received acupuncture With 97%, sickness was either completely absent or considerably reduced with no side effects "Dummy" acupuncture provided little benefit Because of time involved and brevity of action (8 hrs) an alternative approach to electroacupuncture will be required before it is clinically adopted
Dundee JW, Yang J: Prolongation of the antiemetic action of P6 acupuncture by acupressure in patients having cancer chemotherapy, *J Royal Soc Med* 8(6):360, 1990.	35	After receiving acupuncture, subjects receive an elasticized wrist band with a stud placed over the acupoint	In Dundee's previous work (1989) it was clear that the antiemetic effect was too short term to be adopted clinically Dundee applied the wrist band AFTER acupuncture and instructed patients to press it regularly every 2 hrs 100% of 20 hospitalized patients and 75% of 20 outpatients extended the antinausea effects with the use of a seaband; it was hypothesized that hospitalized patients were more accurate in applying 2-hr pressure because of encouragement by staff
ACUPUNCTURE FOR TREATMENT OF SURGICALLY INDUCED NAUSEA AND VOMITING			
al-Sadi M et al: Acupuncture in the prevention of postoperative nausea and vomiting, *Anaesthesia* 52(7):658, 1977.	81	(1) Acupuncture (2) Placebo acupuncture	Patients received laparoscopic surgery; nausea and vomiting was monitored for 24 hrs after surgery Acupuncture reduced postoperative nausea/vomiting in hospital from 65% to 35% compared with placebo; after discharge, from 69% to 31% compared with placebo
Dundee JW et al: Reduction in emetic effects of opioid preanaesthetic medication by acupuncture, *Br J Clin Pharmacol* 22:583, 1986.	125	(1) No treatment (2) Electroacupuncture (3) TENS (4) 5 mg intravenous	Two studies were undertaken consecutively of patients undergoing gynecologic surgery The first 50 subjects received acupuncture after medication or drug alone 75 other patients received the drug nalbuphine with acupuncture, with dummy acupuncture, or alone Manual needling resulted in a significant reduction in nausea and vomiting in 50 patients who received acupuncture compared with 75 who did not (results from both groups combined)

TENS, Transcutaneous electrical stimulation.

| TABLE 11-6 | Acupuncture for Treatment of Chemotherapy and Surgically Induced Nausea—cont'd |

STUDY	NUMBER	GROUPS	RESULTS
Ho RT et al: Electroacupuncture and postoperative emesis, *Anaesth* 45:327, 1990.	100	(1) Acupuncture after premedication with meptazinol (2) Meptazinol alone (3) Nalbuphine plus acupuncture (4) Nalbuphine plus dummy acupuncture (30 nalbuphine alone)	Patients were females who underwent laparoscopy All received anesthesia in the recovery room, patients received one of three treatments (2, 3, 4) or prochlorperazine or no treatment Postoperative vomiting was 44% for no treatment; 12% (p<0.05) for electroacupuncture; 36% for TENS, and 12% for antiemetic prochlorperazine Electroacupuncture was as effective as prochlorperazine and more effective than TENS in preventing post-operative vomiting
Yentis SM, Bissonnette B: P6 acupuncture and postoperative vomiting after tonsillectomy in children, *Br J Anaesth* 67(6):779, 1991.	45	(1) Acupuncture (2) No acupuncture	Children undergoing tonsillectomy received acupuncture or no treatment after induction of anesthesia There was no difference in incidence of vomiting between acupuncture group (39%) and no-acupuncture group (36%) Authors concluded that when administered AFTER anesthesia, acupuncture is ineffective in reducing vomiting after tonsillectomy in children
Yentis SM, Bissonette B: Ineffectiveness of acupuncture and droperidol in preventing vomiting following strabismus repair in children, *Can J Anaesth* 39(2):151, 1992.	90	(1) Droperidol (2) Acupuncture plus droperidol (3) Acupuncture alone	Patients were children undergoing outpatient strabismus repair They received droperidol, medication with acupuncture, or acupuncture alone There was no significant difference in vomiting between the 3 groups; (e.g., for group 1, 17% before discharge and 41% up to 48 hrs after discharge; for group 2, 17% and 34%, respectively; and group 3, 27% and 45%, respectively The incidence in restlessness was significantly less in acupuncture-only group compared with both treatments or drug treatment (p=0.007) Droperidol and acupuncture were equally ineffective in preventing vomiting after pediatric strabismus repair; droperidol is associated with increased incidence of postoperative restlessness

ACUPRESSURE FOR MOTION SICKNESS AND PREGNANCY-INDUCED NAUSEA

STUDY	NUMBER	GROUPS	RESULTS
Senqu H et al: P6 acupressure reduces symptoms of vection-induced motion sickness, *Aviat Space Environ Med* 66:631, 1995.	64	(1) P6 acupressure (2) P6 sham acupressure (3) Dummy point (4) No treatment	Subjects sat in a rotational drum for 12 min to induce nausea "Real" P6 acupressure subjects reported acupressure significantly less nausea than other groups (p<0.0001) during drum rotation
De Aloysio D, Penacchioni: Morning sickness control in early pregnancy by Neiguan Point Acupressure, *Obstetr Gynecol* 80:852, 1992.	60	*Unilateral:* (1) A-band on right wrist placebo on left wrist (2) B-band on left wrist, placebo on right wrist *Bilateral:* (1) Acupressure bands on both wrists (2) Placebo bands on both wrists	This was a crossover trial; a 12-day period organized into 4 steps of 3 days each More than 60% received positive effect with both unilateral and bilateral acupressure compared with 30% improvement from placebo acupressure Changing from unilateral to bilateral provided no significant differences, nor did the wrist choice in the unilateral substudy effect outcomes; either wrist provided equal benefit
Hyde E: Acupressure therapy for morning sickness, *J Nurse Midwifery* 34(4):171, 1989.	16	(1) Acupressure for 5 days followed by no treatment (2) No therapy for 5 days followed by acupressure	Twelve of 16 subjects had relief of morning sickness with acupressure (p<0.025) There were also significant reductions in anxiety, depression, behavioral dysfunction, and nausea (p<0.05)

toms of *dyspnea* (i.e., breathlessness).[10,56,160,181] A large study by Aleksandrova and colleagues found that acupuncture reduced nonspecific bronchial hyperreactivity.[4]

The outcomes of acupuncture for chronic asthma are mixed. Luu and associates and Jobst and colleagues found that acupuncture is more effective than sham acupuncture.[80,108] Studies by Dias and others, Tashkin and others, Tandon and others, Tandon and Soh, and Biernacki and Peake found acupuncture was not more effective than sham acupuncture.[11,39,157-159] Christensen and colleagues found acupuncture more effective than sham acupuncture for some measurements, but not for others.[28]

Although Sliwinski and Matusiewicz found that acupuncture reduced corticosteroid use and that electroacupuncture improved lung function and reduced asthma attacks, their study was uncontrolled.[146] Further, in these and all other cited studies, no measurements of lung inflammation were conducted. Since inflammation is the underlying cause of asthma, it was not determined whether the clinical course of asthma was altered. Reductions in the use of medication by asthmatic patients can represent desensitization to the symptoms rather than the control or improvement of the condition.

A systematic review of 18 asthmatic trials found that even the eight best designed and con-

TABLE 11-7   Acupuncture for Treatment of Neurologic Disorders

STUDY	NUMBER	GROUPS	RESULTS
Kjendahl A et al: A one year follow-up study on the effects of acupuncture in the treatment of stroke patients in the subacute stage: a randomized, controlled study, *Clin Rehabil* 11(3):192, 1997.	41	(1) Classical acupuncture (2) Control no acupuncture	Patients were randomized with consideration for gender and hemispheral localization of lesion. Patients were stroke victims in the subacute stage. Acupuncture for 30 minutes, 3-4 times a wk for 6 wks. Acupuncture improved significantly more than controls, both during the 6-wk treatment period and even more so during the following year as assessed by the Motor Assessment Scale, the activity of Daily Living Scale, Nottingham Health Profile, and social situation
Hu HH et al: A randomized controlled trial on the treatment for acute atrial ischemic stroke with acupuncture, *Neuroepidemiol* 12:106, 1993.	30	(1) Classical acupuncture (2) Control no acupuncture	Stroke victims within 36 hrs of onset of symptoms received acupuncture 3-4 times a wk for 4 wks. Improvement was greatest in those patients with a poor neurologic score at baseline. Significantly greater benefit was observed for the acupuncture group on day 28 and at 90-day follow-up
Naeser MA et al: Acupuncture in the treatment of paralysis in chronic and acute stroke patients: improvement observed in all cases, *Clin Rehab* 8:127. 1994.	20	(1) Acupuncture—all patients	Stroke patients included 10 chronic and 10 acute patients. 19 of 20 patients (95%) could be correctly classified as receiving beneficial vs poor response based on CT scan. 8 of 20 had beneficial response as measured by improved motor function, including 3 of 10 chronic patients treated longer than 3 mos since stroke and 5 of 10 acute patients treated at less than 3 mos after stroke
Johansson K et al: Can sensory stimulation improve the functional outcome in stroke patients? *Neurology* 43:2189, 1993.	78	(1) Physiotherapy and occupational therapy (2) Above plus acupuncture	Of 8 patients that improved, significant improvements were observed for knee flexion and extension and abduction. Neither age nor months after stroke were correlated with improved tests post-acupuncture. Most improvements were sustained for at least 4 mos after the last treatment. Two chronic patients with benefits received acupuncture 3 and 6 yrs after stroke

trolled studies were, at best, mediocre, and the results from the better studies were contradictory. Kleijnen, ter Riet, and Knipschild concluded that the literature, as it existed at the time of the study, did not support acupuncture as an effective treatment for asthma[86] (Table 11-8).

Substance Abuse

In 1973, a neurosurgeon in Hong Kong was using acupuncture for surgical analgesia. His patients began reporting that cravings for opium, heroin, morphine, nicotine, or alcohol declined after they received their preoperative acupuncture treatments.[178] Since that time, acupuncture as treatment for substance abuse has received considerable attention from the research and medical communities.[85] Needles positioned in the auricle of the ear are typically used for detoxification of substance-abuse patients and to lower the craving for abusive substances.[135] In 1987 and 1989, randomized, placebo-controlled studies by Bullock

demonstrated the efficacy of acupuncture for treating severe alcoholism.[15,16]

Beginning in 1979, Smith, a drug abuse researcher, and others observed successful results in outpatient treatments of addicts at the Lincoln Hospital substance abuse program in the Bronx, New York City.[147-153] Soon, other programs, began springing up in clinics and in penal systems around the United States.[87]

Substance abuse is a complex problem involving known or suspected biochemical, behavioral, social, and genetic causal determinants. Those addicted to chemical substances must (1) experience withdrawal from the drug, an unpleasant process called detoxification; (2) receive treatment to help them develop the skills necessary for staying drug free; and, finally, (3) avoid relapse into drug use. It is commonly reported that acupuncture reduces withdrawal symptoms during the detoxification stage. Since the 1970s, more than 250 acupuncture programs modeled on the New

TABLE 11-8	Acupuncture for Treatment of Asthma		
STUDY	**NUMBER**	**GROUPS**	**RESULTS**
Aleksandrova RA et al: Bronchial nonspecific reactivity in patients with bronchial asthma and in the preasthmatic state and its alteration under the influence of acupuncture, *Ter Ark (Moskva)* 67(8):42, 1995.	152	(1) 94=Acupuncture (2) 58=Controls	Authors employed 241 parameters, diagnostic parameters, processed with the use of systematic modeling Acupuncture reduced nonspecific bronchial hyperreactivity Normalization of blood acetylcholine, resensitization of cell beta-adrenergic receptors, elevation of mean concentrations of T-lymphocytes and 11-OCS
Berger D, Nolte D: Acupuncture in bronchial asthma: body plethysmographic measurements of bronchospasmolytic effects, *Alternative Med East West* 5:265. 1975.	12	Effects of acupuncture on airway resistance was tested on all patients	45 tests of airway resistance were performed before and after acupuncture In 9 patients, there was significant decrease of airway resistance 10 min, 1 and 2 hrs after acupuncture, whereas placebo acupuncture did not change airway resistance significantly Acupuncture demonstrated a somewhat weaker bronchospasmolytic effect than Atrovent, an asthma medication for bronchodilation. 3 patients showed no change after repeated attempts with acupuncture
Biernacki W, Peake MD: Acupuncture in treatment of stable asthma, *Res Med* 92:9, 1998.	23	(1) "Real" acupuncture (2) Sham acupuncture	There was no improvement in any aspect of respiratory function after either form of acupuncture; subjects did report significant improvement in quality of life and reduction in bronchodilator use
Christensen PA et al: Acupuncture for bronchial asthma, *Allergy* 39:379, 1984.	17	(1) "Correct" acupuncture (2) Placebo-acupuncture	Objective assessments (morning and evening peak flows, and beta-agonist use) increased (both 10 sessions) in the treated group at wk 4 (p<0.01) and wk 11 (p<0.05) compared with baseline Compared to placebo, "real" acupuncture was significantly more effective at wk 2 After wk 2, no differences could be found Placebo acupuncture produced no improvements throughout the study

FEV$_1$, Forced expiratory volume per 1 second; *FVC,* forced vital capacity; *MMFR,* maximal midexpiratory flow rate; *PERF,* peak expiratory flow rate.

Continued

TABLE 11-8	Acupuncture for Treatment of Asthma—cont'd	
STUDY	**NUMBER GROUPS**	**RESULTS**
Dias PLR et al: Effects of acupuncture in bronchial asthma: preliminary communication, *J Royal Soc Med* 75:245, 1982.	20	(1) Acupuncture (2) Sham acupuncture	Sham group significantly improved peak expiratory flow; only 3 acupuncture patients showed improvement Subjective improvement and reduction in drug dosages were observed in both groups; authors concluded acupuncture has a placebo effect in bronchial asthma
Fung KP et al: Attenuation of exercise-induced asthma by acupuncture, *Lancet* 2:1419, 1986.	19	(1) "Real" acupuncture (2) Sham acupuncture	Subjects were exercise-induced asthmatic children During exercise sessions, patients had acupuncture (real or sham in random order) 20 minutes before exercise Lung function was assessed before, during, and after exercise Neither real nor sham acupuncture affected the basal bronchomotor tone but both, when applied 20 minutes before exercise, attenuated exercise-induced asthma Mean maximum % falls in FEV_1 FVC, and PERF were 44.4%, 33.3%, and 49.9% without acupuncture; and 23.8%, 15.8%, and 25.9% after "real" acupuncture; and 32.6%, 26.1%, and 34.3% after sham acupuncture "Real" acupuncture was significantly more effective in preventing exercise-induced asthma than has sham acupuncture ($p<0.05$)
Jobst K et al: Controlled trial of acupuncture for disabling breathlessness, *Lancet* 2:1416, 1986.	24	(1) Traditional acupucture (2) Placebo acupuncture	After 3 weeks, traditional acupuncture subjects demonstrated significantly greater benefits in subjective scores of breathlessness and 6-minute walking distance Objective measures of lung function were unchanged in either group
Luu M et al: Controle spirometrique dans la maladie asthmatique des effets de la puncture de points douloureux thoraciques, *Respiration* 48:340, 1985.	17	(1) Acupoints chosen by painful characteristics for treatment group (2) Acupoints chosen for controls were in lower limbs	Reference to classical acupuncture points were not made in this study; only pain characteristics vs lower limb placement Although vital capacity was not altered, expiratory flow rates were significantly higher ($p<0.05$) after puncture of thoracic pain points, with no shift observed after puncture of extrathoracic zone (lower limbs)
Sliwinski J, Matusiewicz R: The effects of acupuncture on the clinical state of patients suffering from chronic spastic bronchitis and undergoing long-term treatment with corticosteroids, *Acupunct Electrother Res* 9:203, 1984.	51	(1) Acupuncture (2) No acupuncture	Acupuncture was given for 2-3 mos followed by 2-3 mos of no treatment 36 of 51 patients completed 3 yrs of treatment 63.8% were able to eliminate corticosteroids from 3-26 mos In 19.5% of patients, all previously required drugs were eliminated during the last 3-15 mos

FEV₁, Forced expiratory volume per 1 second; *FVC*, forced vital capacity; *MMFR*, maximal midexpiratory flow rate; *PERF*, peak expiratory flow rate.

York City Lincoln Hospital program have evolved worldwide to address treatment and relapse issues.[14] The research supporting the efficacy of these programs is, however, quite thin.

Clinically controlled trials reported some positive benefits from acupuncture for the treatment of cocaine, heroin, opiate, and mixed drug user populations.[6,67,87,88,176] A large study by Lipton, Brewington, and Smith of 150 cocaine abusers found that patients receiving "real" acupuncture produced cleaner urinalysis tests than did those receiving placebo acupuncture (nonpoints).[102] Based on outcomes of urinalysis with heroin addicts, a study by Man and Chuang concluded that acupuncture was not a valid intervention for addicts; 82.9% of acupuncture-treated patients used illicit drugs during the research period.[113] A study by Otto, Quinn, and Sung with cocaine-dependent subjects found no difference between "real" and sham acupuncture-treated clients, whereas another study by Margolin and others found that cocaine users who completed acupuncture treatment provided cleaner urinalysis results than with other forms of pharmacotherapy.[114,133]

Although some studies have emerged that were experimentally and clinically supportive,

TABLE 11-8	Acupuncture for Treatment of Asthma—cont'd		

STUDY	NUMBER	GROUPS	RESULTS
Tandon MK, Soh PFT: Comparison of real and placebo acupuncture in histamine-induced asthma: a double-blind crossover study, *Chest* 96:102, 1989.	16	(1) "Real" acupuncture (2) Sham acupuncture	Both real and sham acupuncture failed to modulate bronchial hyperreactivity to histamine
Tandon M et al: Acupuncture for bronchial asthma? A double-blind crossover study, *Med J Aust* 154:409, 1991.	15	(1) "Real" acupuncture (2) Sham acupuncture	Patients received both treatments in randomorder, in a crossover design Both treatments were preceded by 3 wks of no, "real," or sham acupuncture When compared with no treatment and sham, "real" acupuncture failed to provide any improvements in daily peak flows, asthma symptom scores, beta 2–agonist use, and pulmonary function results
Tashkin DP et al: Comparison of real and stimulated acupuncture and isoproterenol in methacholine-induced asthma, *Ann Allergy* 396:379, 1977.	12	(1) "Real" acupuncture (2) Sham acupuncture (3) Nebulized isoproterenol (4) Nebulized saline (5) No treatment	All subjects received all treatments in a crossover design Saline and simulated acupuncture did not result in any significant improvement in airway conductance, thoracic gas volume, or forced expiratory flow rates compared with no treatment after methacholine-induced bronchospasm Isoproterenol and "real" acupuncture were both followed by increases in airway conductance, flow rates, and decreases in thoracic gas volume; changes were significant as compared with real acupuncture and isoproterenol Isoproterenol still produced greater improvement as compared with acupuncture Authors concluded acupuncture reduces methacholine-induced bronchospasm and hyperinflation to an extent greater than can be attributed to placebo phenomena
Tashkin DP et al: Comparison of real and stimulated acupuncture and isoproterenol in methacholine-induced asthma, *Ann Allergy* 396:379, 1977.	25	(1) Classical acupuncture (2) Placebo acupuncture (3) 3-4 wks with no acupuncture, real or sham	There was no significant acute effect of acupuncture on symptoms, medication use, lung function, self-ratings of efficacy, or physician's physical findings; neither "real" nor sham acupuncture produced change
Yu DYC, Lee SP: Effect of acupuncture on bronchial asthma, *Clin Sci Mol Sci* 51:503, 1976.	20	(1) Correct acupoint (2) Two other sites	In all patients the symptoms of bronchoconstriction improved during attack when the correct site was stimulated; in 5 patients, wheezing was abolished Correct-site stimulation increased FEV_1 by 58% and FVC by 29% After acupuncture, a still greater increase in FEV_1, FVC, and MMFR was produced by inhaling isoprenaline No change occurred in FEV_1, FVC, or MMFR when incorrect sites of acupuncture were stimulated Authors concluded acupuncture reduced reflex affect of bronchoconstriction, but not direct smooth muscle constriction caused by histamine

there is currently no compelling evidence for the efficacy of acupuncture in the treatment of either opiate or cocaine dependence.[117] In 1991, the National Institute on Drug Abuse (NIDA) sponsored a technical review to determine the efficacy of the acupuncture research to date. After presentations on the research (many by the researchers themselves), it was determined that at the time of the meeting, the work of Bullock in the field of alcohol dependence represented the only method-

ologically sound research suggestive of acupuncture efficacy for the treatment of any dependence disorder. This work, they determined, also needs to be replicated. A review of the data indicated no clear evidence that acupuncture is effective as treatment for opiate or cocaine dependence.[161]

It is important to note that there is very little evidence that acupuncture is **not** effective in the treatment of drug abuse or that acupuncture is in any way harmful; there is simply not the methodologic data needed to draw a conclusion in acupuncture's favor. As mentioned earlier, there are numerous methodologic problems in the acupuncture research. Does one use traditional (individualized) or formula acupuncture? Is electroacupuncture more effective than standard needling? Are the effects of electroacupuncture potentially the result of the generalized stimulation of the nervous system and not acupoint stimulation at all? What is placebo acupuncture, as opposed to a "treatment effect?"

Addiction is a multidimensional problem. To expect that acupuncture—or any one treatment, for that matter—will prevent substance abuse relapse is, perhaps, expecting too much. Nonetheless, until the methodologic issues are resolved and solid studies are replicated numerous times, it will be difficult to define the benefits of acupuncture as a treatment of drug abuse (Table 11-9).

An Expert Speaks: Dr. Skya Gardner-Abbata

Skya Gardner-Abbata, M.A., D.O.M., Dipl.Ac. Dipl. C.H., is a licensed Doctor of Oriental medicine in New Mexico, Executive Director of Southwest Acupuncture College, former President of the New Mexico Association of Acupuncture and Oriental Medicine, and has served as an educational expert and Commissioner for the Accreditation Commission for Acupuncture and Oriental Medicine. Dr. Garner-Abbata is the author of *Beijing: The New Forbidden City* (1991), *Holding the Tiger's Tail: A Techniques Manual in the Treatment of Disease* (1996), and *The Magic Hand Returns Spring, The Art of Palpatory Diagnosis* (1999). She is also a regular contributor to the *American Journal of Acupuncture*. Dr. Gardner-Abbata is also in private practice, specializing in the treatment of side effects of chemotherapy and radiation with cancer patients.

Question. Can you tell us how and why you become involved in acupuncture?

Answer. My interest in acupuncture and Oriental medicine began with a rather circuitous route beginning with my intrigue with culture and social organization. The simultaneous existence of various realities, values, and ways of doing things always fascinated me throughout much of my life. This lead to [my] undergraduate college education in sociology, anthropology, psychology, and political science. Entering the Peace Corps was a natural extension of this fascination.

Following my experience as a Peace Corps volunteer in Brazil, I was more acutely aware of how culture shapes every aspect of our lives and quite intimately our health. This awareness lead to my master's degree in sociology and shortly thereafter a new track in "pre-med."

My interest in medicine was never purely professional but always personal. I was searching for an approach and a philosophy of the human body that supported the empowerment of one's health care. I found this in the world of Oriental medicine.

It was both the exquisite logic and the profound simplicity of Oriental medicine, with its emphasis on naturalistic laws of the universe and man's relationship to them, that captured both my mind and soul. Acupuncture was just one of its many tools that could redress that balance in the human body, which we call disease.

The augmentation of acupuncture with breathing and bodily exercise, nutrition, and bodywork that are part of the repertoire of Oriental medicine were the lifestyle tools I was looking for, which correspond with my idea of medicine. To this day, choosing the study of Oriental medicine has changed my life and deepened my development, not just as an effective practitioner but, more importantly, as a whole person.

Question. Can you describe what acupuncture is and how it works?

Answer. Acupuncture, simply put, is a therapy [that] affects energy. It can strengthen it if it is weak (as in the case of fatigue or immune weakness), break it up if it is stagnant or blocked (such as in the case of various types of pain), or decrease it if it is excessive (such as high blood pressure or obesity). In oriental medicine, all disease fits into one or a combination of these energy patterns. This elegant simplicity—to be able to reduce all illness to an energy pattern—greatly empowers the acupuncture physician to correct these imbalances because the cause and hence its logical treatment plan can be identified. This is not to say that it is easy to treat all diseases, only that their etiology provides a broad yet accurate picture of the problem.

Acupuncture works on a multitude of illnesses. From acne and allergies, to fatigue and multiple sclerosis, from the infinite varieties of pain to periodontal gum disease, from Alzheimer's to depression—acupuncture can address all of these energy imbalances. In short, it works on a vast array of conditions—be they musculoskeletal, internal, or emotional.

In general, the more "energetic" the illness is, that is, the least physical in the sense of physical evidence such as that obtained from MRIs, CAT scans, [and] x-rays [films], the more efficacious

TABLE 11-9	Acupuncture for Treatment of Substance Abuse

STUDY	NUMBER	GROUPS	RESULTS
Avants SK et al: Acupuncture for the treatment of cocaine addiction. Investigation of a needle puncture control, *J Subst Abuse* 12(3):195, 1995.	40	(1) Daily acupuncture in 4 "correct" auricular sites (2) Daily acupuncture in 3 sites 2-3 mm from "correct" site	**Cocaine** use decreased significantly for both groups but the only statistically significant difference was noted for the category of "cravings" Subjects in this study were addicted to cocaine
Bullock ML et al: Acupuncture treatment of alcoholic recidivism: a pilot study, *Alcohol Clin Exp Res* 11(3):292, 1987.	54	(1) Acupuncture to points for substance abuse (2) Acupuncture to nonspecific points	Patients in treatment group reported less desire for **alcohol** (p<0.003); had fewer drinking episodes (p<0.0076); and fewer admission to detox (p<0.03) than non-specific point patients Treated patients reported acupuncture had a definite effect on their need for alcohol (p<0.015)
Bullock ML et al: Controlled trial of acupuncture for severe recidivist alcoholism, *Lancet* 1:1435, 1989.	80	(1) Acupuncture at site specific to treatment of alcoholism (2) Acupuncture at nonspecific points	21 of 40 patients in treatment group completed the program; only one of 40 in control group completed program (p<0.001) 12 treatment patients asked for and received, additional treatments during follow-up period; only 1 control asked for additional treatments (p<0.001) At 6 mos, control patients expressed a stronger need for alcohol (p<0.01); had more than twice the number of drinking episodes (241 vs 100, p<0.01); a fewer admissions to detox (62 vs 26, p<0.05)
Gurevich MI et al: Is auricular acupuncture beneficial in the inpatient treatment of substance-abusing patients? A pilot study, *J Subst Abuse* 13(2):165, 1996.	77	(1) Patients having acupuncture 5 or more times (treatment) (2) Patients refusing acupuncture or having 4 or less treatments (control)	Treatment group did significantly better controls in the following ways: compliance with treatment=75% vs 20%; noncompliance discharge rate=2% vs. 40%; acceptance of staff's discharge recommendations=77% vs 37%; remained in follow-up treatment for at least 4 months=58% vs 26% **Mixed drug population in a psychiatric unit**
Konefal J et al: The impact of the addition of an acupuncture treatment program to an existing Metro-Dade County outpatient substance abuse treatment facility, *J Addict Dis* 13(3):71, 1994.		(1) Usual care (2) Usual care plus frequent urine testing (3) Usual care, frequent urine testing and acupuncture	The Metropolitan Dade County outpatient substance abuse clinic reported that patients receiving acupuncture produced "clean" urinalysis results 57% faster than those who did not receive acupuncture Drop out rate was, nonetheless, high **Mixed drug use**
Kroenig RJ, Oleson TF: Rapid narcotic detoxification in chronic pain patients treated with auricular electroacupuncture and nalaoxone, *Int J Addict* 20(9):1347, 1985.	14	These were all chronic pain patients who had become **addicted to pain killing opiate medication**	Patients were first switched to methadone and then given bilateral electrical stimulation to needles inserted in acupoints on ear, followed by periodic intravenous injections of low doses of naloxone 12 of the patients (85.7%) were completely withdrawn from narcotic medications in 2-7 days; they experienced little or no side effects
Lipton DS et al: Acupuncture for crack-cocaine detoxification: experimental evaluation of efficacy, *J Subst Abuse* 11(3):205, 1994.	150	(1) "Real" acupuncture (2) Placebo acupuncture	**Cocaine/crack addicts** received accurate points treatment or treatment to points not related to drug treatment Urinalysis over a 1-mo period favored those who received "real" acupuncture Treatment retention in both groups was similar; significant decrease in use reported by both groups; urinalysis was definitive

AMA, Amatadine; *DMI*, desipramine.

Continued

TABLE 11-9		Acupuncture for Treatment of Substance Abuse—cont'd	

STUDY	NUMBER	GROUPS	RESULTS
Man Pl, Chuang MY: Acupuncture in methadone withdrawal, *Int J Addict* 15(6):921, 1980.	35	(1) Electroacupuncture (2) No treatment	Urinalysis identified that 82.9% of patients receiving acupuncture used illicit drugs during the research period Authors concluded that acupuncture was not a valid intervention for addicts going through methadone withdrawal Urinalysis was performed on all patients for 6-mo period Only 3 controls and 3 treatment patients remained drug free Subjects were male veterans with a long history of drug abuse, particularly **heroin**
Margolin et al: Effects of sham and real auricular needling: implications for trials of acupuncture for cocaine addiction, *Am J Addict* 2(3):194, 1993.	32	Auricular acupuncture	**Cocaine-dependent,** methadone-maintained clients received 8-wk course of auricular acupuncture 50% completed treatment; 88% of those completing course provided drug-free urinalysis for last 2 wks of study Post hoc comparison to pharmacotherapy with DMI, AMA, and placebo showed an abstinence rate for acupuncture of 44% compared with 15% for AMA, 135 for placebo, and 26% for DMI
Otto KC et al: Auricular acupuncture as an adjunctive treatment for cocaine addiction. A pilot study, *Am J Addict* 7(2):164, 1998.	36	(1) "Real" acupuncture (2) Sham acupuncture	Study failed to show any significant difference between treatment and control groups Both groups did remain longer in treatment than an analyzed group who received no, "real," or sham acupuncture Subjects were **cocaine-dependent**
Washburn AM et al: Acupuncture heroin detoxification: a single-blind clinical trial, *J Subst Abuse* 10(4):345, 1993.	100	(1) Standard auricular acupuncture for addiction (2) Sham acupuncture with points close to standard points	Subjects assigned to standard treatment attended the clinic more days and stayed in treatment longer than sham controls Attrition was high and those with lighter habits found the treatment most helpful Only 20 subjects completed the study Self-report of heroin use favored the true acupuncture treatment group
Wen HL, Cheung YC: Treatment of drug addiction by acupuncture and electrical stimulation, *Asian J Med* 9:138, 1973.	40	Acupuncture using a single ear point and patient-adjusted electrical stimulation	Patients were 30 **opium addicts** and 10 **heroin abusers** Relief of withdrawal symptoms was reported, with all patients reporting "good" response An earlier study and therefore lacks the rigor that allows definitive conclusions to be drawn

[acupuncture] is. Many of our maladies as human beings fall into this "energetic" category, and acupuncture is suitable for all of them.

Question. How should acupuncture be integrated into traditional medical practices?

Answer. Ever since I began the study of Oriental medicine, I believed the day would come when it would become part of an integrative health care system. It always stood on its own, in terms of its time-testedness and clinical validity; indeed, it has been practiced for centuries because of this; but, from my perspective

and that of most health care practitioners, we want what is best for each patient. Today, we have the experience and the consciousness to know that an integrative approach to medicine is the most comprehensive care we can offer.

This combination of world views and specialists who work together can only benefit the patient. In addition to this comprehensiveness, most duplication of effort and financial burdens can be significantly reduced. Apart from private practice, acupuncturists are well-equipped to work in private Western medical clinics, hospital settings, and other similar environments. Their roles may range from somewhat limited to full-scale patient care, for instance in an oncology clinic treating patients for the side effects of chemotherapy and radiation, to improvement in the quality of life, to the treatment of cancer. As a practitioner who heads up an acupuncture college and actively works on the national level, integration of health care systems is a personal goal.

Question. How difficult will it be to integrate acupuncture with conventional medicine?

Answer. There are challenges to this integration, but they are not insurmountable. They do require an openness on the part of Western health care physicians to learn about acupuncture and to consider it a viable, proven option as the National Institute of Health (NIH) Consensus Report, 1998, has indicated.[129] This challenge, likewise, necessitates that acupuncturists are comfortable with the terrain of the Western world view, its language and therapies. They must be comfortable in this world if they are to work within it. A certain degree of specialization on their part is required to treat in specialized Western health care settings. [Although] there are other minor challenges, to me these are essentially the ones upon which everything else depends. In the spirit of compassion for our patients and a desire to know more about the human body, I know we will all mutually create a new medicine for the 2000s.

■ Indications and Contraindications

Acupuncture is indicated for many common clinical conditions including headache, allergies, and most forms of pain (Table 11-10). In Chinese medicine, virtually all illnesses are treated with acupuncture. There are a few conditions, however, where acupuncture in not recommended.

Acupuncture is contraindicated in:
1. Children under 7 years of age
2. Patients who are intoxicated or under the influence of a narcotic drug (acupuncture enhances the effects of drugs)
3. Immediately after eating or when extremely hungry (movement of energy, via acupuncture, can lead to nausea or dizziness in either condition)
4. Patients who are pregnant
5. Patients who are senile (patients with senility or dementia cannot give accurate feedback concerning the effect of needling)
6. Hemophiliacs or patients with clotting disorders
7. Patients with needle phobias

■ Chapter Review

In this chapter, the clinically controlled trials of acupuncture as medical intervention for pain have been reviewed. Acupuncture has been researched and demonstrated effective, to varying degrees, in alleviating low back pain, headache pain, pain from osteoarthritis, neck pain, musculoskeletal and myofascial pain, organic pain, and presurgical and postsurgical pain. Acupuncture has also been found effective in the treatment of postoperative and chemotherapy-induced nausea, neurologic dysfunction, gynecologic and obstetric conditions, and as a potential treatment for substance abuse.

The methodology of many of the studies have been flawed, in no small part because Chinese medical theory is not designed or intended to treat conditions apart from the evaluation of the individualized pattern of symptoms in each patient. The benefits of acupuncture specifically and Chinese medicine as a whole extend far beyond the conditions reviewed in this chapter. Nonetheless, from the viewpoint of the Western research paradigm, acupuncture has still withstood the light of clinically controlled trials and demonstrated itself a worthy and beneficial intervention. More trials designed with a black-box structure and in harmony with the original theory of Chinese medicine are needed. Only then will the full benefits of acupuncture be delineated to the Western reader.

TABLE 11-10	Acupuncture for the Relief of Other Types of Pain				
AUTHOR	**TYPE PROCEDURE**	**NUMBER**	**CONTROL**	**TYPE**	**RESULTS**
Richter A et al: Effect of acupuncture in patients with angina pectoris, *Eur Heart J* 12(2):175, 1991.	Stable effort angina pectoris	21	Placebo tablet (crossover)	Classical acupuncture crossover	Anginal attacks per week reduced from 10.6 to 6.1 during the acupuncture Crossover period vs placebo crossover period (p<0.01)

Matching Terms and Definitions

Match each numbered definition with the correct term. Place the corresponding letter in the space provided.

a. Acupuncture
b. Five elements
c. *Jing*
d. Three treasures
e. Meridians
f. *Yellow Emperor's Inner Classic*
g. *Yin* and *yang*
h. Tao
i. Shen
j. James Reston
k. Eight principles
l. *Qi*

_____ 1. Name for the twelve major energy pathways; each is related to or named for an organ or function

_____ 2. Life force that drives every cell in the body

_____ 3. Stimulation of specific anatomic points in the body for therapeutic purposes

_____ 4. Subject of a *New York Times* article on acupuncture for the relief of postoperative pain

_____ 5. Path or the way of life; emphasizes moderation in all things and living in harmony with nature

_____ 6. *Shen, jing, qi*

_____ 7. Represents the spirit and brings light and joy to life

_____ 8. Essence of being, substance that makes growth, development, and reproduction possible

_____ 9. Opposing but complementary forces

_____ 10. *Yin, yang, cold, heat, internal, external, deficiency,* and *excess*

_____ 11. Wood, fire, earth, metal, and water; each is associated with a color, an emotion, a sound, a smell, a taste, a season, a climate, a body part, and an organ

_____ 12. One of the earliest source of information on acupuncture

CRITICAL THINKING AND CLINICAL APPLICATION EXERCISES

1. Outline and describe the research on mechanisms that underpin the practice of acupuncture including electrical resistance of acupoints and acupuncture channels and radioactive tracers. Are these findings correlational or causal? Defend your choice.

2. The philosophy of acupuncture is based on the principles of Tao (Dao); yin and yang; the eight principles; the three treasures; and the five elements. Discuss these principles and relate them to traditional Western medical thought. What do they have in common, and how do they differ?

References

1. *A barefoot doctor's manual: the American translation of the official Chinese paramedical manual,* Philadelphia, 1977, Running Press.
2. Aglietti L et al: A pilot study of metoclopramide, dexamethasone, diphenhydramine and acupuncture in women treated with cisplatin, *Cancer Chemother Pharmacol* 26(3):239, 1990.
3. Ahon E et al: Acupuncture and physiotherapy for the treatment of myogenic headache patients: pain relief and EMG activity, *Adv Pain Res Ther* 5:571, 1983.
4. Aleksandrova RA et al: Bronchial nonspecific reactivity in patients with bronchial asthma and in the preasthmatic state and its alteration under the influence of acupuncture *Ter Arkh* 67(8):42, 1995.
5. Alternative medicine: expanding medical horizons, Chintilly, VA, 1992, Workshop on Alternative Medicine.
6. Avants SK, Margolin A, Chang P, Kosten TR, Birch S: Acupuncture for the treatment of cocaine addiction. Investigation of a needle puncture control, *J Subst Abuse* 12(3):195, 1995.
7. Bache F: Cases illustrative of the remedial effects of acupuncture, *North Am Med Surg J* 1:311, 1826.
8. Ballegaard S, Christophersen SJ: Acupuncture and transcutaneous electric nerve stimulation in the treatment of pain associated with chronic pancreatitis, *Scand J Gastroenterol* 20:1249, 1985.
9. Bennett S: Chinese science: theory and practice, *Philos East West* 28(4):439, 1978.
10. Berger D, Nolte D: Acupuncture in bronchial asthma: body plethysmographic measurements of bronchospasmolytic effects, *Alternative Med East West* 5:265. 1975.
11. Biernacki W, Peake MD: Acupuncture in treatment of stable asthma, *Res Med* 92:9, 1998.

12. Borglum-Jensen et al: Effect of acupuncture on myogenic headache, *Scand J Dent Res* 87:373, 1979.

13. Bossy J, Sambuc P: *Acupuncture et systeme nerveux: les acquis. Acupuncture et medecine traditionnelle Chinoise,* Paris, 1989, Encyclopedie des Medecines Naturelles.

14. Brumbaugh AG: Acupuncture: new perspectives in chemical dependency treatment, *J Subst Abuse* 10:35, 1993.

15. Bullock M et al: Controlled trial of acupuncture for severe recidivist alcoholism, *Lancet* 1:1435, 1989.

16. Bullock ML, Umen AJ et al: Acupuncture treatment of alcoholic recidivism: a pilot study, *Alcohol Clin Exp Res* 11(3):292, 1987.

17. Cahn AM et al: Acupuncture in gastroscopy, *Lancet* 1(8057):182, 1978.

18. Carlsson J et al: Muscle tenderness in tension headache treated with acupuncture or physiotherapy, *Cephalalgia* 10:131, 1990.

19. Carlsson J, Rosenhall U: Oculomotor disturbances in patients with tension headache treated with acupuncture or physiotherapy, *Cephalalgia* 10:123, 1990.

20. Chan Wing-tsit, translator: *A source book in Chinese philosophy,* Princeton, NJ, 1963, Princeton University Press.

21. Chen et al: The effect of location of transcutaneous electrical nerve stimulation on postoperative opioid analgesic requirement: acupoint versus nonacupoint stimulation, *Anesth Analg* 87(5):1129, 1998.

22. Chen JYP: Acupuncture. In Quinn JR, editor: *Medicine and public health in the People's Republic of China,* US Dept of Health, Education and Welfare: John S Fogarty International Center, 1972, NIH.

23. Chen JYT: *Acupuncture anesthesia in the People's Republic of China,* Bethesda, MD, 1973, NIH.

24. Cheng ACK: The treatment of headaches employing acupuncture, *Am J Chin Med* 3:181, 1975.

25. Christensen BV et al: Acupuncture treatment of severe knee osteoarthritis: a long-term study, *Acta Anaesthesiol Scand* 36:519, 1992.

26. Christensen et al: Acupuncture treatment of knee arthrosis. A long-term study (abstract), *Ugeskrift for Laeger* (Copenhagen) 155(49):4007, 1993.

27. Christensen PA et al: Electroacupuncture and postoperative pain, *Br J Anaesth* 62:258, 1989.

28. Christensen PA et al: Acupuncture for bronchial asthma, *Allergy* 39:379, 1984.

29. Clement-Jones V et al: Increased beta-endorphin but not met—enkephalin levels in human cerebrospinal fluid after acupuncture for recurrent pain, *Lancet* 2:946, 1980.

30. Co LL et al: Acupuncture: an evaluation in the painful crises of sickle cell anemia, *Pain* 7:181, 1979.

31. Coan RM et al: The acupuncture treatment of low back pain: a randomized controlled treatment, *Am J Chin Med* 8:181, 1980.

32. Coan RM et al: The acupuncture treatment of neck pain: a randomized controlled study, *Am J Chin Med* 9(4):326, 1982.

33. Darras JC: Isotopic and cytologic assays in acupuncture. In *Energy fields in medicine,* Kalamazoo, 1989, John E. Fetzer Foundation.

34. Darras JC et al: Nuclear medicine investigation of transmission of acupuncture information, *Acupunct Med* 11(1):22, 1993.

35. Darras JC et al: Visualisation isotopique des meridiens d'acupuncture, *Cahiers de Biotherapie* 95:13, 1993.

36. Deluze C et al: Electroacupuncture in fibromyalgia: results of controlled trial, *BMJ* 305:1249, 1993.

37. De Aloysio D, Penacchioni: Morning sickness control in early pregnancy by Neiguan Point Acupressure, *Obstet Gynecol* 80:852, 1992.

38. De Vernejoul P et al: Study of acupuncture meridians using radioactive tracers, *Bull L'Acad Natl Med* 169(7):1071, 1985.

39. Dias PLR et al: Effects of acupuncture in bronchial asthma: preliminary communication, *J Royal Soc Med* 75:245, 1982.

40. Dickens W, Lewith GT: A single-blind, controlled and randomized clinical trial to evaluate the effect of acupuncture for the treatment of trapezio-metacarpal osteoarthritis, *Complementary Med Res* 3(2):5, 1989.

41. Dimond EG: Acupuncture anesthesia: western medicine and Chinese traditional medicine, *JAMA* 218:1558, 1971.

42. Dowson D et al: The effects of acupuncture versus placebo in the treatment of headache, *Pain* 21:35, 1985.

43. Dundee JW et al: Acupuncture prophylaxis of cancer chemotherapy-induced sickness, *J Royal Soc Med* 82:268, 1989.

44. Dundee JW et al: Effect of stimulation of the P6 antiemetic point on postoperative nausea and vomiting, *Br J Anaesth* 63:612, 1989.

45. Dundee JW et al: Reduction in emetic effects of opioid pre-anaesthetic medication by acupuncture, *Br J Clin Pharmacol* 22:583, 1986.

46. Dundee JW et al: Traditional Chinese acupuncture: a potentially useful antiemetic, *BMJ* 293, 1986.

47. Dundee JW, Yang J: Prolongation of the antiemetic action of P6 acupuncture by acupressure in patients having cancer chemotherapy, *J Royal Soc Med* 8(6):360, 1990.

48. Dung HC: Three principles of acupuncture points, *Am J Acupunct* 12(3):263, 1984.

49. Edelist G et al: Treatment of low back pain with acupuncture, *Can Anaesthesiol Soc J* 23:303, 1976.

50. Ekblom A et al: Increased postoperative pain and consumption of analgesics following acupuncture, *Pain* 44(3):241, 1991.

51. Emery P, Lythgoe S: The effect of acupuncture on ankylosing spondylitis, *Br J Rheumatol* 25:132, 1986.

52. Ernst E: Acupuncture as a symptomatic treatment of osteoarthritis: a systematic review, *Scand J Rheumatol* 26:444, 1997.

53. Fox E, Melzack R: Transcutaneous electrical stimulation and acupuncture: comparison of treatment for low-back pain, *Pain* 2:141, 1976.

54. Freling DL: *Anthropological perspectives on artificial intelligence and traditional Chinese medicine in the People's Republic of China,* Stanford, CA, 1988, Stanford University.

55. Frost EAM: Acupuncture for the comatose patient, *Am J Acupunct* 4:45, 1976.

56. Fung KP et al: Attenuation of exercise-induced asthma by acupuncture, *Lancet* 2:1419, 1986.

57. Garvey TA et al: A prospective, randomized, double-blind evaluation of trigger-point injection therapy for low-back pain, *Spine* 14:962, 1989.

58. Gaw AC et al: Efficacy of acupuncture on osteoarthritic pain, *N Engl J Med* 293(8):375, 1975.

59. Gerhard I, Postneck F: Auricular acupuncture in the treatment of female infertility, *Gynecolog Endocrinol* 6(3):171, 1992.

60. Ghaly RG et al: Antiemetic studies with traditional Chinese acupuncture: a comparison of manual needling with electrical stimulation and commonly used antiemetics, *Anesthesia* 42:1108, 1987.

61. Ghaly RG et al: Acupuncture also reduces the emetic effects of pethidine, *Br J Anaesth* 59:135, 1987.

62. Ghia JN et al: Acupuncture and chronic pain mechanisms, *Pain* 2:285, 1976.

63. Ghia JN, Mao W, Toomey TC, Gregg JM: Acupuncture and chronic pain mechanisms, *Pain* 2(3):285, 1976.

64. Godfrey CM, Morgan P: A controlled trial of the theory of acupuncture in musculoskeletal pain, *J Rheumatol* 2:121, 1978.

65. Grall Y: *Contribution a l'etude de la conductibilite electrique de la peau,* Algiers, 1962, These de Medecine.

66. Gunn CC et al: Dry needling of muscle motor points for chronic low back pain, *Spine* 5(3):279, 1980.

67. Gurevich MI, Duckworth D, Omhof JE, Katz JL: Is auricular acupuncture beneficial in the inpatient treatment of substance-abusing patients? A pilot study, *J Subst Abuse* 13(2):165, 1996.

68. Hansen PE, Hansen JH: Acupuncture treatment of chronic tension headache: a controlled cross-over trial, *Cephalalgia* 5:137, 1985.

69. Hansson P et al: Is acupuncture sufficient as the sole analgesic in oral surgery? *Oral Surg Oral Med Oral Pathol* 64:283, 1987.

70. Heine H: The morphological basis of the acupuncture points, *Acupunct* 1:1, 1990.

71. Helms JM: *Acupuncture energetics: a clinical approach for physicians,* Berkeley, CA, 1997, Medical Acupuncture Publishers.

72. Helms JM: Acupuncture for the management of primary dysmenorrhea, *Obstet Gynecol* 69:51, 1987.

73. Ho RT et al: Electroacupuncture and postoperative emesis, *Anaesthesia* 45:327, 1990.

74. Huard P, Wong M, Fielding B, translator: *Chinese medicine,* New York, 1968, McGraw Hill.

75. Hu HH et al: A randomized controlled trial on the treatment for acute atrial ischemic stroke with acupuncture, *Neuroepidemiology* 12:106. 1993.

76. Human Anatomy Department of Shanghai Medical University: *A relationship between points of meridian and peripheral nerves, acupuncture anaesthetic theory study,* Shanghai, 1973, Shanghai People's Publishing House.

77. Hyde E: Acupressure therapy for morning sickness, *J Nurse Midwifery* 34(4):171, 1989.

78. Hyvarinen J, Karlsson M: Low resistance skin points that may coincide with acupuncture loci, *Med Biol* 55:8, 1977.

79. Jensen LB et al: Effect of acupuncture of headache measured by reduction in number of attacks and use of drugs, *Scand J Dent Res* 87:373, 1979.

80. Jobst K et al: Controlled trial of acupuncture for disabling breathlessness, *Lancet* 2:1416, 1986.

81. Johansson K et al: Can sensory stimulation improve the functional outcome in stroke patients? *Neurology* 43:2189, 1993.

82. Johansson K et al: Effect of acupuncture in tension headache and brainstem reflexes, *Adv Pain Res Ther* (abstract):839, 1977.

83. Junnila SYT: Acupuncture superior to piroxicam for the treatment of osteoarthritis, *Am J Acupunct* 10(4):341, 1982.

84. Kaptchuk T: *The web that had no weaver,* New York, 1983, Congdon and Weed.

85. Kiresuk TJ, Colliton PD: *Overview of substance abuse acupuncture treatment research,* Workshop on acupuncture, Bethesda, 1994, Office of Alternative Medicine, NIH.

86. Kleijnen J, ter Riet G, Knipschild P: Acupuncture and asthma: a review of controlled trials, *Thorax* 46:799, 1991.

87. Konefal J, Dunca R, Clemence C: The impact of the addition of an acupuncture treatment program to an existing Metro-Dade County outpatient substance abuse treatment facility, *J Addict Dis* 13(3):71, 1994.

88. Kroenig RJ, Oleson TF: Rapid narcotic detoxification in chronic pain patients treated with auricular electroacupuncture and nalaoxone, *Int J Addict* 20(9):1347, 1985.

89. Kubista E et al: Initiating contractions of the gravid uterus through electroacupuncture, *Am J Chin Med* (4):343, 1975.

90. Laitinen J: Acupuncture for migraine prophylaxis: a prospective clinical study with six months' follow-up, *Am J Chin Med* 3:27, 1975.

91. Laitinen J: Acupuncture and TENS in the treatment of chronic sacrolumbalgia and ishialgia, *Am J Chin Med* 4:169, 1976.

92. Lao L et al: The effect of acupuncture on post-operative oral surgery pain: a pilot study, *Acupunct Med* 2(1):13, 1994.

93. Lao L et al: Efficacy of Chinese acupuncture on postoperative oral surgery pain, *Oral Surg Oral Med Oral Pathol Oral* 79(4):423, 1995.

94. Le Bars D et al: Diffuse noxious inhibitory controls. Part I: Effects on dorsal horn convergent neurones in the rat. Part II: Lack of effect on nonconvergent neurones, supraspinal involvement and theoretical implications, *Pain* 6:283, 1979.

95. Lee MHM et al: Acupuncture anesthesia in dentistry: a clinical investigation, *N Y State Dent J* 39(5):299, 1973.

96. Lee MHM, Liao SJ: Acupuncture in psychiatry. In Kottke F, Lehmann JF, editors: *Krusen's handbook of physical medicine and rehabilitation,* Philadelphia, 1990, WB Saunders.

97. Lee YH et al: Acupuncture in the treatment of renal colic, *J Urology* 147:16, 1992.

98. Lehmann TR et al: Efficacy of electroacupuncture and TENS in the rehabilitation of chronic low back pain patients, *Pain* 26:277, 1986.

99. Lehmann TR et al: The impact of patients with nonorganic physical findings on a controlled trial of transcutaneous electrical nerve stimulation and electroacupuncture, *Spine* 8(6):625, 1983.

100. Lewith GT, Machin D: On the evaluation of the clinical effects of acupuncture, *Pain* 16:111, 1983.

101. Lewith GT, Vincent C: Evaluation of the clinical effects of acupuncture. A problem reassessed and a framework for future research, *Pain Forum* 4(1):29, 1995.

102. Lipton DS, Brewington V, Smith M: Acupuncture for crack-cocaine detoxification: experimental evaluation of efficacy, *J Subst Abuse* 11(3):205, 1994.

103. Loh L et al: Acupuncture versus medical treatment for migraine and muscle tension headaches, *J Neurol Neurosurg Psychiatry* 47:333, 1984.

104. Longworth W, McCarthy PW: A review of research on acupuncture for the treatment of lumbar disk protrusions and associated neurological symptomology, *J Alternative Complement Med* 3(1):55, 1997.

105. Loy TT: Treatment of cervical spondylosis: electroacupuncture versus physiotherapy, *Med J Aust* 2:32, 1983.

106. Lundenberg T: A comparative study of the pain alleviating effect of vibratory stimulation, TENS, electroacupuncture, and placebo, *Am J Chin Med* 12:1, 1984.

107. Lu HC, translator: *The yellow emperor's classic of internal medicine and the difficult classic,* Vancouver, 1978, Academy of Oriental Heritage.

108. Luu M et al: Controle spirometrique dans la maladie asthmatique des effets de la puncture de points douloureux thoraciques, *Respir* 48:340, 1985.

109. Lyrenas S et al: Acupuncture before delivery: effect on pain perception and the need for analgesics, *Gynecol Obstet Invest* 29:188, 1990.

110. Lytle CD: *An overview of acupuncture,* Rockville, MD, 1993, Center for Devices and Radiological Health, US Dept of Health and Human Services, Public Health Service, FDA.

111. MacDonald AJR et al: Superficial acupuncture in the relief of chronic low back pain: a placebo-controlled randomized trial, *Ann Royal Coll Surg England* 65:44, 1983.

112. Maciocia G: The foundations of Chinese medicine, Edinburgh, 1989, Churchill Livingstone.

113. Man Pl, Chuang MY: Acupuncture in methadone withdrawal, *Int J Addict* 15(6):921, 1980.

114. Margolin A, Chang P, Avants SK, Kosten TR: Effects of sham and real auricular needling: implications for trials of acupuncture for cocaine addiction, *Am J Addict* 2(3):194, 1993.

115. Matsumoto T: *Acupuncture for physicians,* Springfield, IL, 1974, Charles C Thomas.

116. Mayer DJ et al: Antagonism of acupuncture analgesia in man by the narcotic antagonist naloxone, *Brain Res* 121:368, 1977.

117. McClellan AT et al: Acupuncture treatment for drug abuse: a technical review, *J Subst Abuse* 10:569, 1993.

118. Mendelson G et al: Acupuncture analgesia for chronic low back pain, *Clin Exp Neurol* 15:182, 1978.

119. Mendelson G et al: Acupuncture treatment of chronic back pain: a double-blind, placebo-controlled trial, *Am J Med* 74:49, 1983.

120. Mendelson G et al: Acupuncture treatment of chronic back pain, a double-blind, placebo-controlled trial, *Am J Med* 74(1):49, 1983.

121. Melzack R: Acupuncture and related forms of folk medicine. In Wall PD, Melzack R, editors: *Textbook of pain,* Edinburgh, 1984, Churchill Livingstone.

122. Morand S: Memoire sur l'acupuncture, suivi d'une serie d'observations recueillies sous les yeux de M.J. Cloquet, Paris. In Bache F, translator: *Memoir on acupuncturation: embracing a series of cases,* Philadelphia, 1825, Robert De Silver.

123. Mussat M: *Les reseaux d'acupuncture: stude critique et experimentale,* Paris, 1974, Librairie Le Francois.

124. Naeser MA et al: Acupuncture in the treatment of paralysis in chronic and acute stroke patients: improvement observed in all cases, *Clin Rehabil* 8:127, 1994.

125. Naeser MA et al: Acupuncture in the treatment of paralysis in chronic and acute stroke patients: improvement correlated with specific CT scan lesion sites, *Acupunct Electrother Res* 19:227, 1994.

126. Naeser MA et al: Real vs sham acupuncture in the treatment of paralysis in acute stroke patients: a CT scan lesion site study, *J Neurol Rehabil* 6:163, 1992.

127. National Academy of Sciences: *Institute of Medicine: report of the medical delegation to the People's Republic of China,* Washington, DC, 1973, The Academy.

128. National Institutes of Health: *National Institutes of Health Acupuncture research conference,* Bethesda, MD, 1994, DHEW Publication no 74-165, NIH.

129. National Institutes of Health: Acupuncture, *NIH Consens Statement* 15(5):1, 1997.

130. Niboyet JEH, Mery A: Compte-rendu de recherches experimentales sur les meridiens; chez levivant et chez le cadavre, Actes des Illeme, *Journees Internationales d Acupuncture* 47, 1957.

131. Omura Y: Pathophysiology of acupuncture treatment: effects of acupuncture of cardiovascular and nervous systems, *Acupunct Electrother Res* 1:51, 1976.

132. Osler W: *The principles and practices of medicine,* ed 1, New York, 1892, Appleton.

133. Otto KC, Quinn C, Sung YF: Auricular acupuncture as an adjunctive treatment for cocaine addiction. A pilot study, *Am J Addict* 7(2):164, 1998.

134. Patel M et al: A meta-analysis of acupuncture for chronic pain, *Int J Epidemiol* 18(4):900, 1989.

135. Patterson MA: *Getting off the hook: addictions can be cured. The treatment of drug addiction by neuro-electric stimulation,* Herts, Eng, 1975, Lion Publications.

136. Petrie J, Hazelman B: A controlled study of acupuncture in neck pain, *Br J Rheumatol* 25:271, 1986.

137. Petrie JP, Langley GB: Acupuncture in the treatment of chronic cervical pain: a pilot study, *Clin Exp Rheumatol* 1:333, 1983.

138. Pomeranz B, Clui D: Naloxone blocks acupuncture analgesia and causes hyperalgesia: endorphin is implicated, *Life Sci* 19:1757, 1976.

139. Pomeranz B, Warma N: Electroacupuncture suppression or nociceptive reflex is potentiated by two repeated electroacupuncture treatments: the first opioid effect potentiates a second non-opioid effect, *Brain Res* 452:232, 1988.

140. Reichmanis M et al: Skin conductance variation at acupuncture loci, *Am J Chin Med* 4:69, 1976.

141. Reston J: *Now about my operation in Peking,* New York, 1971, The New York Times.

142. Roppel RM, Mitchell F Jr: Skin points of anomalously low electrical resistance: current-voltage characteristics and relationships to peripheral stimulation therapies, *J Am Osteopath Assoc* 74:877, 1975.

143. Rotchford J: Medical outcome research and acupuncture, *Am Assoc Med Acupunct Rev* 3(1):3, 1991.

144. Senqu H et al: P6 acupressure reduces symptoms of vection-induced motion sickness, *Aviat Space Environ Med* 66:631, 1995.

145. Simon J et al: Acupuncture meridians demystified. Contribution of radiotracer methodology, *Presse Med* 17(26):1341, 1990.

146. Sliwinski J, Matusiewicz R: The effects of acupuncture on the clinical state of patients suffering from chronic spastic bronchitis and undergoing long term treatment with corticosteroids, *Acupunct Electrother Res* 9:203, 1984.

147. Smith MO: Acupuncture and natural healing in drug detoxification, *Am J Acupunct* 7(3):97, 1979.

148. Smith MO: Acupuncture treatment for crack: clinical survey of 1,500 patients treated, *Am J Acupunct* 241, 1988.

149. Smith MO: Creating a substance abuse treatment program incorporating acupuncture, *Am Acad Med Acupunct Rev* 2(1):25, 1990.

150. Smith MO: *Use of acupuncture in the criminal justice system,* New York, 1988, NADA.

151. Smith MO et al: Acupuncture treatment of drug addiction and alcohol abuse, *Am J Acupunct* 10(2):161, 1982.

152. Smith MO et al: *Evaluation of the maternal substance abuse program,* New York, 1989, New York Department of Health, Health Research Training.

153. Smith MO, Aponte J: Acupuncture detoxification in a drug and alcohol abuse treatment setting, *Am J Acupunct* 12(3):251, 1984.

154. Stux G, Pomeranz B: *Acupuncture: textbook and atlas,* Berlin, 1987, Springer-Verlag.

155. Sung YF et al: Comparison of the effects of acupuncture and codeine on postoperative dental pain, *Anesth Analg Curr Res* 56(4):473, 1977.

156. Takeda W, Wessel J: Acupuncture for the treatment of pain of osteoarthritic knees, *Arthritis Care Res* 7(3):118, 1994.

157. Tandon MK et al: Acupuncture for bronchial asthma? A double-blind crossover study, *Med J Aust* 154:409, 1991.

158. Tandon MK, Soh PFT: Comparison of real and placebo acupuncture in histamine-induced asthma: a double-blind crossover study, *Chest* 96:102, 1989.

159. Tashkin DP et al: A controlled trial of real and simulated acupuncture in the management of chronic asthma, *J Allergy Clin Immunol* 76(6):855, 1985.

160. Tashkin DP et al: Comparison of real and stimulated acupuncture and isoproterenol in methacholine-induced asthma, *Ann Allergy* 396:379, 1977.

161. ter Riet G, Kleijnen J, Knipschil P: A meta-analysis of studies into the effect of acupuncture on addition, *Br J Gen Pract* 40:379, 1990.

162. Thomas M et al: A comparative study of diazepam and acupuncture in patients with osteoarthritis pain: a placebo controlled study, *Am J Chin Med* 19(2):95, 1991.

163. Tkach W: I have seen acupuncture work, *Today's Health* 50:50, 1972.

164. Tavola T et al: Traditional Chinese acupuncture in tension-type headache: a controlled study, *Pain* 48:325, 1992.

165. Unschuld PU: *Medicine in China: history of ideas,* Berkeley, 1985, University of California Press.

166. Unschuld PU, translator: *Nan-Ching: The classic of difficult issues,* Ann Arbor, 1987, Center of Chinese Studies.

167. Unschuld PU: Prolegomena. In Unschuld PU, translator: *Forgotten traditions of ancient Chinese medicine: a Chinese view from the eighteenth century,* Brookline, MA, 1990, Paradigm Publications.

168. Vickers AJ: Can acupuncture have specific effects on health? A systematic review of acupuncture antiemesis trials, *J Royal Soc Med* 89:303, 1996.

169. Vincent CA: A controlled trial of the treatment of migraine by acupuncture, *Clin J Pain* 5:305, 1989.

170. Vincent CA: The treatment of tension headache by acupuncture: a controlled single case design with time series analysis, *J Psychosom Res* 34(5):553, 1990.

171. Vincent CA, Richardson PH: The evaluation of therapeutic acupuncture: concepts and methods, *Pain* 24:1, 1986.

172. Wang HH, Chang YH, Liu DM: A study in the effectiveness of acupuncture analgesia for colonoscopic examination compared with conventional premedication, *Am J Acupunct* 20(3):217, 1992.

173. Wang X: Research on the origin and development of Chinese acupuncture and moxibustion. In Zhang X-T, editor: *Research on acupuncture, moxibustion, and acupuncture anesthesia,* Berlin, 1986, Springer-Verlag.

174. Warren E: *An epitome of practical surgery,* Richmond, VA, 1863, West and Johnston.

175. Warren FZ: *Handbook of medical acupuncture,* New York, 1976, Van Nostrand Reinhold.

176. Washburn AM, Fullilove RE et al: Acupuncture heroin detoxification: a single-blind clinical trial, *J Subst Abuse* 10(4):345, 1993.

177. Weightman WM: Traditional Chinese acupuncture as an antiemetic, *BMJ* 295:1379, 1987.

178. Wen HL, Cheung YC: Treatment of drug addiction by acupuncture and electrical stimulation, *Asian J Med* 9:138, 1973.

179. Yentis SM, Bissonnette B: Ineffectiveness of acupuncture and droperidol in preventing vomiting following strabismus repair in children, *Can J Anaesth* 39(2):151, 1992.

180. Yentis SM, Bissonnette B: P6 acupuncture and postoperative vomiting after tonsillectomy in children, *Br J Anaesth* 67(6):779, 1991.

181. Yu DYC, Lee SP: Effect of acupuncture on bronchial asthma, *Clin Sci Mol Sci* 51:503, 1976.

182. Zhang WX et al: Acupuncture treatment of apoplectic hemiplegia, *J Tradit Chin Med* 7(3):157, 1987.

183. Zhang Z-J: *Shang Han Lun: treatise on febrile diseases caused by cold,* Bejing, 1986, New World Press.

184. *Zhen Jiu Da Cheng.* Darris J-C, editor. Paris, 1981, Editions Darras.

185. Zmiewski P: Introduction. In Soulie de Morant G: *L'acupuncture Chinoise,* Engl ed, Brookline, MA, 1994, Redwing Books.

12

Homeopathy: Like Cures Like

Lyn W. Freeman

WHY READ THIS CHAPTER?

Worldwide, more than 500 million people use homeopathic remedies. More than 2.5 million Americans took homeopathic medicines in 1990. The World Health Organization (WHO) has recommended that homeopathy be integrated with conventional medicine by the year 2000. Yet, in the scientific community, homeopathy is highly controversial and its mechanisms unexplainable by modern-day science. This chapter allows the reader to assess the available information and research on homeopathy. The mechanisms and outcomes of homeopathy are paradoxical and fascinating and will provide the discerning reader with much "food for thought."

CHAPTER AT A GLANCE

Homeopathy teaches that a disease is cured by introducing a miniscule amount of a substance into the body that, in larger doses, induces symptoms similar to the disease in a healthy person. This effect is referred to as "like cures like."

Samuel Hahnemann, a German physician, founded homeopathy. Hahnemann tested the concept of "like cures like" by ingesting a substance containing quinine and observing its effects on himself and then on others.

Hahnemann developed three essential principles of homeopathy: (1) the Principle of Similars, (2) the Principle of Infinitesimal Dose, and (3) the Principle of Specificity of the Individual. The Principle of Similars teaches that "like cures like." The Principle of Infinitesimal Dose teaches that, the more diluted the dose, the more potent its curative effects. The Principle of Specificity of the Individual teaches that, if the remedy is to cure, it must match the symptom profile of the patient.

Homeopathic remedies are often diluted until not a molecule of the original substance remains. Homeopaths believe that continued dilution and shaking can imprint the electromagnetic signal of a substance in the water. The selected remedy matches the signal of the sick person's electromagnetic field, resulting in a stimulation of the body's healing force.

Individual clinical controlled trials, some double-blinded and placebo-controlled, have found homeopathic remedies to be effective in the treatment of migraine pain, allergy, asthma, fibromyalgia, influenza, hepatitis B carriers, diarrhea, arthritis, and dental pain. More research that replicates these findings is needed.

> The introduction of homeopathy forced the old school doctor to stir around and learn something of a rational nature about his business. You may honestly feel grateful that homeopathy survived the attempts of allopathists (orthodox physicians) to destroy it.
>
> MARK TWAIN, FEB, 1890, A MAJESTIC LITERARY FOSSIL, HARPER'S MAGAZINE.

CHAPTER OBJECTIVES

1. Define homeopathy.
2. Explain how homeopathy evolved into a medical discipline.
3. Define and explain the Principle of Similars.
4. Define and explain the Principle of Infinitesimal Dose.
5. Define and explain the Principle of Specificity of the Individual.
6. Define and explain Hering's Law of Cures.
7. Explain, in detail, how homeopathic remedies are formulated.
8. Describe and discuss the studies that examine the mechanisms of homeopathy.
9. Explain the theories of how homeopathic remedies induce healing.
10. Describe the homeopathic studies related to the placebo effect.
11. Describe the homeopathic studies related to the control of viral illnesses.
12. Describe the homeopathic studies related to the treatment of pain.

■ Homeopathy Defined

The word *homeopathy* is derived from the Greek words *homios,* which means "similar" and *pathos,* which means "suffering." In simple terms, homeopathy teaches that stimulating the natural healing properties in the body cures a disease. This is accomplished by introducing into the body a substance that, in a healthy person, induces symptoms identical to the symptoms of the disease. Emulating the same disease symptoms in the body stimulates the person's healing energy and results in a cure. The phrase "like cures like" is often used to explain why this occurs.

The substances given to stimulate healing are homeopathic remedies. Homeopathic remedies are dilutions of natural substances from plants, minerals, and animals. Dilutions are prescribed that specifically match the patient's illness-symptom profile. The remedy that most closely fits all the symptoms of the individual is called the *similimum* for that person. Since homeopathic treatment is individualized, two persons with the same diagnosis may be given different medicines because their symptoms are different.

After the initial symptoms are alleviated, the practitioner progresses to the treatment of underlying symptoms (i.e., residues of fever, trauma, or chronic disease that may have been treated unsuccessfully in the past). During the treatment process, the patient may worsen temporarily, a condition called the "healing crisis." This is considered a good sign and one that will soon be followed by complete healing.

■ History of Homeopathy

Birth of Homeopathy

Homeopathy can trace its roots to Hippocrates who taught the Law of Similars, or "like cures like," over 2400 years ago. Samuel Hahnemann, a German physician, initially developed homeopathy in the 1790s. Hahnemann was known at the time for his papers on medicine and chemistry and his work in pharmacology, hygiene, public health, industrial toxicology, and psychiatry (Figure 12-1). Unfortunately, the accepted medical practices of the day included bloodletting, cathartics, leeches, and the administration of highly toxic chemicals. Often the treatment was more deadly than the disease.[35] Repulsed by these practices, Hahnemann gave up medicine (Figure 12-2).

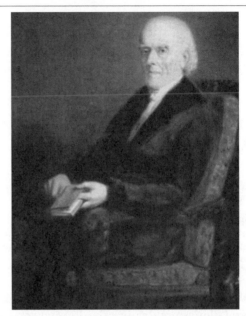

■ **Figure 12-1.** Dr. Samuel Hahnemann (1755-1843) founded homeopathy on the premise that drugs producing certain symptoms in healthy people will cause the same symptoms in those who are sick. *From Peterson, Weiss:* Chiropractic: an illustrated history, *St Louis, 1995, Mosby.*

It was agony for me to walk always in darkness, when I had to heal the sick, and to prescribe, according to such or such an hypothesis concerning diseases, substances which owed their place in the materia medica to an arbitrary decision. Soon after my marriage, I renounced the practice of medicine, that I might no longer incur the risk of doing injury, and I engaged exclusively in chemistry, and in literary occupations. But I became a father, serious diseases threatened my beloved children.... My scruples redoubled when I saw that I could afford them no certain relief.[2]

A gifted linguist, Hahnemann turned to the profession of translating medical works, while continuing to seek the fundamental principles of healing.

While translating *A Treatise of Materia Medica* by Dr. William Cullen, Hahnemann became troubled by Cullen's assertions that quinine cured malaria because of its astringent (bitter) properties. The idea seemed illogical to Hahnemann. He was determined to test this assertion by undertaking a medical experiment using himself as the subject.

Twice a day, Hahnemann ingested cinchona, a Peruvian bark that contains quinine and is well known as a cure for malaria (Figure 12-3). Each time he ingested the bark, he developed periodic fevers, symptoms common to patients with malaria. When he stopped taking the medication, his symptoms disappeared. Hahnemann theorized

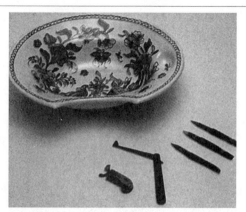

■ *Figure* 12-2. These bowls and lancets are examples of those used for the medical practice of bloodletting. *Courtesy of Pearson Museum, School of Medicine, Southern Illinois University, Springfield, Illinois.*

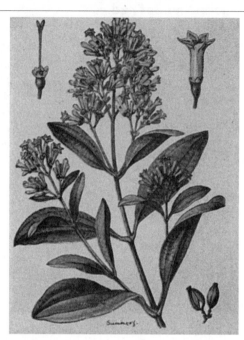

■ *Figure* 12-3. The cinchona plant is the source of the bark powder that for centuries was known as a miracle cure for malaria. *From Peterson, Weiss:* Chiropractic: an illustrated history, *St Louis, 1995, Mosby.*

that if taking a large dose of cinchona created malaria-like symptoms in a healthy person, perhaps smaller doses would stimulate bodily healing properties in a person sick with malaria. He then conducted experimental tests on other like-minded physicians and on healthy volunteers, noting their reaction to cinchona and meticulously and systematically recording the results. This systematic process of testing substances on healthy human beings to determine which symptoms the substance brings forth is called *proving*. He then conducted similar tests with arsenic and other poisonous substances.

Hahnemann's initial experimentation period lasted 6 years, during which time he also compiled an exhaustive list of "poisonings."

He noted, as Hippocrates had before him, that the severity of the symptoms and the healing responses elicited by these substances depended on the individual. Some symptoms, however, were common for most subjects, and these he called *keynote* or first-line symptoms. Observed and recorded symptoms were not only physical, but these symptoms were also of an emotional and mental nature. It was believed that the symptoms of disease and illness always manifest on all three levels, and treating the physical level only, as occurs in allopathic medicine, represented an incomplete treatment.

As Hahnemann continued to experiment with hundreds of substances and to treat illness with the substances that matched the symptom profile, he discovered that he could produce similar and beneficial results again and again.[14] Hahnemann's methods soon attracted the interest of physicians and medical students, many of whom would carry on his work (Figure 12-4).

Development of Homeopathy in the United States

Homeopathy as a medical treatment was soon introduced into the United States. Dr. Constantine Hering, a student of Hahnemann, established the first U.S. homeopathic medical school in 1835 in Allentown, Pennsylvania. By 1900, there were 22 homeopathic medical schools, nearly 100 homeopathic hospitals, and over 1000 homeopathic pharmacies in the United States. Approximately 15% of all U.S. physicians were homeopathic practitioners.[5] By the 1930s, the growth of conventional pharmaceutical medications and the political power of a conventional medical movement, represented by the American Medical Association (AMA), challenged homeopathy as a viable medical system.[5] Quickly, homeopathy virtually disappeared as a visible force in American medicine. Although homeopathy was severely curtailed in the United States, this was not the case in other parts of the world.

> **Points to Ponder**   By 1900, there were 22 homeopathic medical schools, nearly 100 homeopathic hospitals, and over 1000 homeopathic pharmacies in the United States. Approximately 15% of all U.S. physicians were homeopathic practitioners.

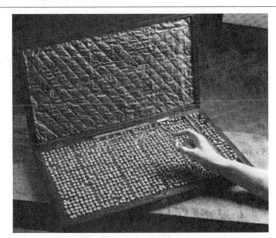

■ **Figure 12-4.** Samuel Hahnemann's remedy box. Many homeopathic practitioners kept their remedies in a similar box. *From Richardson S: Homeopathy: the illustrated guide. In Peterson, Weiss:* Chiropractic: an illustrated history, *St Louis, 1995, Mosby.*

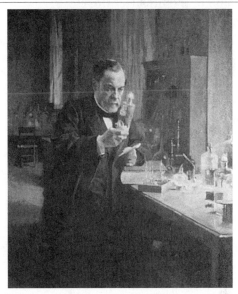

■ **Figure 12-5.** "Louis Pasteur in his Laboratory," an oil painting by Albert-Gustaf Edelfelt. Pasteur was responsible for laying the groundwork of modern immunity theory and immunization. *Courtesy Musee Pasteur, Institut Pasteur, Paris.*

Homeopathy Today

Today, homeopathy is practiced worldwide. It is estimated that more than 500 million people receive homeopathic treatments. The WHO recommended that homeopathy be integrated with conventional medicine to provide adequate global health care by the year 2000.[1]

In Europe, the birthplace of homeopathy, there are more than 6000 German and 5000 French practitioners. All French pharmacies are required to carry homeopathic remedies, as well as conventional drugs. In Great Britain, homeopathic hospitals and outpatient clinics are part of the national health care system. An act of Parliament ensures that homeopathy is recognized as a medical specialty, and homeopathy has enjoyed the support of the royal family for more than four generations. India uses homeopathy as part of its national health service and maintains more than 100 homeopathic colleges.[20]

It has been estimated that as many as 3000 homeopaths practice in North America, including 500 physicians. In Eisenberg's survey of complementary medical use, it was estimated that 2.5 million Americans used homeopathic medicines and 800,000 visited a homeopathic practitioner in 1990.[11]

■ Essential Principles of Homeopathy

Hahnemann developed three essential principles of homeopathy: (1) the Principle of Similars, (2) the Principle of Infinitesimal Dose, and (3) the Principle of Specificity of the Individual.

> **Points to Ponder**   The "Principal of Similars" is based on the principle of "like cures like." This law states that if a substance, given in large doses, induces specific disease symptoms in a healthy person, that same substance, given in small doses, will cure the disease in those who are ill.

Principle of Similars

The *Principal of Similars* is based on the principle of "like cures like." This law states that if a substance, given in large doses, induces specific disease symptoms in a healthy person, that same substance, given in small doses, will cure the disease in those who are ill.[16]

The Principle of Similars was also the theoretical basis for the development of vaccines by Jonas Salk and Louis Pasteur (Figure 12-5). For example, if a small amount of a disease component (e.g., a virus) is introduced into the body, but a component too weak to cause the disease, this exposure may strengthen the immune system's ability to fight off the related disease (e g., impart immunity). Today, allergies are often treated in a similar manner. Very small amounts of the allergen are introduced into the body, in tiny but increasing doses, resulting in increased resistance to the allergen.

Principle of Infinitesimal Dose

Through experimentation, Dr. Hahnemann discovered that the more times he diluted the substance, the more effective it became. This also avoided the toxic side effects of the stronger remedies of the time.

In homeopathy today, it is still accepted that the more a substance is diluted, the more potent it will be. Homeopaths assert that the more dilute the remedy, the longer the effect will last; the deeper the effect will be; and fewer doses will be required to provide a cure. The following text provides an explanation of how these dilute remedies are prepared.

Preparing Homeopathic Remedies

Tinctures of plants are dissolved in a mixture of alcohol and water and left to stand for 2 to 4 weeks. During that time, they are shaken occasionally and then strained. The strained solution is known as *mother of tincture*. The mother of tincture is then used to make different potencies. Homeopathic remedies are prepared by repeatedly diluting the substance with pure water or alcohol and then *succussing*, which means vigorously shaking, the solution until only an extremely dilute amount or none of the original substance remains. This process is called *potentization*. In potentization, a drop of the homeopathic solution is placed into a 1:10, 1:100, or 1:1000 ratio of distilled water, designated as 1x (decimal), 1c (centesimal) or 1m (millesimal). Successive dilutions of one drop of each proceeding solution are then placed into a fresh solution of 1:10 or 1:100 distilled water. Often, the progression of these dilutions results in an atomic concentration of the original preparation of less than 10^{24}. According to Avogadro's law, at this dilution level, it is unlikely that even a single atom of the original substance is left in the dilution.[14] It is this fact that has caused medical controversy concerning homeopathic treatments. If not a single atom of the medicinal substance remains in many homeopathic remedies, this fact defies current-day medical understanding of how such a remedy could affect health outcomes.

Today, homeopathic practitioners have more than 2000 of these dilute remedies from which to choose when treating their patients.

Points to Ponder   Often, the progression of these dilutions results in an atomic concentration of the original preparation of less than 10^{24}. According to Avegadro's law, at this dilution level, it is unlikely that even a single atom of the original substance is left in the dilution. ■

The official compendium containing the body of information on homeopathic remedies is called the *Homeopathic Pharmacopoeia of the United States*. This compendium is used by homeopaths to match symptom profiles of patients with the appropriate homeopathic remedy.

Homeopathic Remedies: Monitoring Quality, Preparation, and Distribution

In spite of the fact that the effectiveness of homeopathic remedies are questioned by the medical establishment, the Food and Drug Administration (FDA) still recognizes homeopathic dilutions as official drugs and regulates the manufacturing, labeling, and dispensing of homeopathic medications. Some simple homeopathic remedies, such as those for colds and influenza, are available as over-the-counter medications. Other dilutions for more complicated conditions are available only from a homeopathic practitioner. Sales of homeopathic medicines in the United States has been estimated at more than 250 million dollars per year.[33]

Explaining Effects of Homeopathy

If many homeopathic remedies contain no molecules of the treating substance, how, then, do these homeopathic remedies have any effect on the body? Trevor Cook, President of the United Kingdom Homeopathic Medical Association, stated that we must look to the domains of quantum physics and the field of energy medicine for the answer. A study using nuclear magnetic resonance imaging (NMRI) found distinctive readings of subatomic activity in 23 different homeopathic remedies, an activity not found in placebo substances.[30] It was hypothesized that the specific electromagnetic frequency of the original substance was imprinted in the remedy during the continued diluting-shaking process.

An Italian physicist, Emilio del Giudici, theorized that water molecules form structures that store electromagnetic signals. This theory obtains some support by the fact that a German biophysicist, Dr. Wolfgang Ludwig, found that homeopathic remedies give off measurable electromagnetic signals. Further, these signals demonstrate specific dominant frequencies for each homeopathic substance tested.[10,26]

Dr. Shin-Yin Lo, a senior researcher at American Technologies Group, identified and characterized a unique type of stable (nonmelting) ice crystal that maintains an electrical field (IE). These rod-shaped water clusters are created when a substance is placed in distilled water, then vigorously shaken or stirred, and repeatedly diluted and then shaken or stirred again. These water clusters or ice crystals remain stable at high temperatures and, with varying fluctuation, after repeated dilutions. Dr. Lo noted, "There seems to be something unique in water that undergoes extreme dilution, and we now have the laboratory evidence and even the photographic evidence to verify it. Thus far, we have only systematically tested substances which have been diluted one to ten[13] times. Homeopathic doctors sometimes use medicines which are diluted one to ten[30], 200 or 1000 or more times, and we have not tested these extreme dilutions yet. However, I would not be surprised if IE crystals are also observed in these doses. Based on our research to date, every dilution beyond the sixth has found IE crystals in them."[28,29,35]

It has been suggested that homeopathic remedies convey an electromagnetic message to the body, one that matches the frequency of the illness, thereby stimulating the body to heal itself.[14] Essentially, one subtle energy (that of the remedy) affects another subtle energy (that of the human energy field). Hahnemann called the subtle energy field in the body the vital force. The *vital force* is the healing energy that exists in all of us.

These hypotheses and theories raise another question that needs to be answered. Even if this subtle energy can be transferred into a homeopathic remedy, what evidence do we have that this energy actually affects bodily functions? The following is an overview of several studies that sought to provide evidence of the ability of homeopathic remedies to affect bodily functions, specifically, immune function.

A closer look: Magnetic resonance imaging

Magnetic resonance imaging (MRI) is a type of scanning that uses a magnetic field to induce tissues and substances to emit radio frequency (RF) waves. An RF detector coil senses the waves and sends the information to a computer that constructs images. Different tissues and substances can be distinguished because each emits different RF signals.

MRI, also called NMRI, is most typically used for diagnosis of brain disorders. The use of MRI in human patients avoids potentially harmful x-radiation and often produces sharper images of soft tissues than other imaging methods[31] (Figure 12-6).

Effects of Homeopathic Remedies on Immune Cell Activity

Homeopathic Remedy and Release of Histamine. In a study by Davenas and others, basophils were isolated from human blood and exposed to a homeopathic dilution of immunoglobulin E (IgE) antiserum. This exposure resulted in a release of histamine.[7] Although larger doses of IgE are known to stimulate histamine release, the fact that the homeopathic version achieved this effect stunned mainstream science, because the dilutions tested (as low as $1 \times 10_{120}$) no longer contained a single molecule of the original serum. The authors proposed that as each dilution was vigorously agitated, molecular information might have been transmitted during the dilution-shaking process, with water acting as a template by an infinite hydrogen-bonded network or an electromagnetic field.

This study was conducted under stringent experimental conditions, using blind double-coded procedures involving six laboratories in four countries.

Homeopathic Remedy Stimulates Macrophage Activity. Silica is a substance known to lead to cell death if ingested by macrophages. In this randomized, double-blind, placebo-controlled study,

Points to Ponder Although larger doses of IgE are known to stimulate histamine release, the fact that the homeopathic version achieved this effect stunned mainstream science, because the dilutions tested (as low as $1 \times 10_{120}$) no longer contained a single molecule of the original serum.

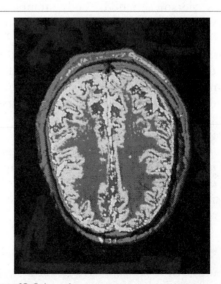

■ *Figure 12-6.* In nuclear magnetic resonance imaging, a magnetic field surrounding the head induces brain tissues to emit radio waves that can be used by a computer to construct a sectional image. *From Peterson, Weiss:* Chiropractic: an illustrated history, *St Louis, 1995, Mosby.*

female mice received silica dilution of either 1.66 $\times 10^{11}$ or 1.66×10^{19} for 25 days; control mice received tap water.[8]

Normally toxic to macrophages, silica in these extreme dilutions (1000 molecules or less per day) stimulated the production of the macrophage mediator, platelet-activating factor (PAF) acether. (Note: PAF is synthesized and released from a variety of cells when they are immunologically activated including, in this case, macrophages.) The effect was paradoxical, increasing in parallel with the continued dilution of the compound.

These studies suggest that some homeopathic remedies may, in fact, have biological effects on the body's immune system, even though these outcomes defy medical logic.

Principle of Specificity of the Individual

Homeopathic practitioners believe that the treatment for a physical condition must be matched to the unique symptoms of the individual. The influenza or headache is not treated; rather, the person with flulike or headachelike symptoms is treated.

For example, there are more than 200 symptom patterns associated with headache, and each has its own corresponding remedy. The headache may be in the front or the back of the head; it may get worse with cold and improve with heat; it may be better when sitting up or lying down; the patient may be thin and excitable or docile and sedentary. Additional considerations include the time of day when the symptoms worsen, as well as person's mood, body temperature, appetite, and thirst. These and other factors are carefully considered when "profiling" the patient.[33] In other words, all physical, emotional, and mental qualities must be considered when choosing the remedy. Then, multiple remedies (but not all at the same time) may be used to treat the person.[18]

Practitioners consult compendiums called *repertories* and *materia medicas* to determine which remedy "matches" the patient's symptoms. These compendiums represent thousands of tests or *provings* on healthy individuals, gathered over a 200-year period.

> **Points to Ponder**   Homeopathic practitioners believe that the treatment for a physical condition must be matched to the unique symptoms of the individual. The influenza or headache is not treated; rather, the person with flulike or headachelike symptoms is treated. ■

Laws of Cure

In addition to the three principles, there are *Hering's Laws of Cure.* Dr. Constantine Hering, the father of American homeopathy, taught that the healing process progresses as follows:
- From the deepest part of the body to the extremities
- From the emotional and mental to the physical
- From the upper body parts (e.g., head, neck, ears, throat) to the lower body parts (e.g., fingers, abdomen, legs, feet)

Hering's Laws of Cure also states that healing progresses in reverse order and from the most recent condition to the oldest.

■ Clinical Trials of Homeopathy

There are essentially three questions at issue concerning homeopathy.
1. What is the underlying mechanism of homeopathy?
2. Is homeopathy more effective than placebo?
3. If homeopathy is not a placebo effect, is it clinically effective for the treatment of disease?

The data available to address the first question have been discussed in previous sections. The following sections address the last two questions.

Challenges of Homeopathic Research

Homeopathic practitioners often prescribe different medications or combination of medication for patients suffering from the same problem. They select different medications based on history, patient characteristics, and reactivity. Essentially, homeopathy holds that the individuality of the patient is the ultimate factor for determining prescription. Historically, this has led many researchers to believe that controlled trials were not possible with homeopathy because the treatment, (e.g., medication) would differ patient to patient.

This problem is normal for the researchers of alternative therapies. For example, acupuncturists choose different acupuncture points and/or different herbal compounds or treatments or a combination of these, based on patient characteristics (e.g., pulses, tongue color) and complaint. Traditional native healers also vary their treatments for the same illness, based on patient characteristics. In such cases, research can be performed that is referred to as *black box* research. The patient outcome is the determination of efficacy, not the specific treatment prescribed. It is the medical system or approach (e.g., homeopathy, traditional Chinese acupuncture) that is being assessed, not a single remedy. In this chapter, we review the trials that address homeopathic treatment outcomes, using both individualized research designs (e.g., black box), and one-treatment designs.

Conventional medicine continues to reject the validity of homeopathy, based on the argument that no double-blind, placebo-controlled studies that demonstrate clinically significant health improvements have been successfully replicated.[4]

Three of the best-controlled homeopathic trials have, nonetheless, provided evidence for the clinical effectiveness of homeopathy in the treatment of hay fever, migraine pain, and fibromyalgia.[3,13,25] The text that follows reviews these trials.

Homeopathy for the Treatment of Migraine Pain

Claims are often made that the efficacy of homeopathy cannot be proven with strict scientific methods, because of the true nature of homeopathic medicine (i.e., drug prescription must be individualized to be truly homeopathic in nature, and more than one homeopathic remedy per patient may be prescribed). The following is an excellent example of how homeopathic research, true to the philosophy and nature of homeopathy, can still be conducted using the "black box" research design.

Brigo and Serpelloni conducted a randomized, double-blind, placebo-controlled study. They sought to demonstrate (1) whether homeopathic treatment of migraine attacks was superior to a placebo effect, and (2) whether an effective homeopathic study could be designed using the "black box" approach, while still meeting classical exper-

imental model requirements.[3] The study divided 60 individuals (aged 12 to 70 years old; 10 male and 50 female subjects) into either a treatment or control group. Group characteristics were virtually identical.

The treatment group was given a single dose of 30C potency, four separate times, 2 weeks apart. (The *centisimal* is commonly used in homeopathy and is based on serial dilutions of 1/100.) The control group received a placebo during the same time (Figure 12-7). The authors administered one of eight drugs with the option of associating any two, based on patient history, characteristics, and reactivity.

As expected, based on placebo response, the control group experienced a slight decrease in the number of migraine attacks per month. They experienced 9.9 attacks per month during the evaluation period and 7.9 attacks per month at the 2-month mark (i.e., 8 weeks after beginning treatment and the week of the last dose) and at the 4-month period (p=0.04). The treatment group reduced migraine attacks from 10 per month to 3 and 1.8 per month at the 2- and 4-month periods (p=0.000001). Analysis of the intensity of the migraine pain demonstrated an insignificant reduction for the placebo group; the treatment group experienced a significant reduction of pain intensity at the end of treatment (p=0.00001).

At 4 months, 78.8% of placebo patients needed medication to eliminate migraine pain, whereas 21.2% of treatment group required medication (p=0.001). The treatment group reported a greater sense of bodily well being than the placebo group (p=0.0001) and judged treatment as more efficacious (p=0.000003).

Analysis of the homeopathically treated patients found a significant reduction in the periodicity, frequency, and duration of migraine attacks,

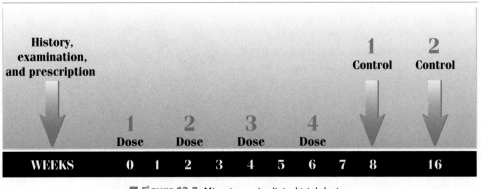

■ *Figure 12-7.* Migraine pain clinical trial design.

demonstrating efficacy of homeopathy in comparison with classical experimental study models adapted to the specific character of homeopathy.

■ Placebo Response? Putting Homeopathy to the Test

Reilly and others performed three studies to test the hypothesis that the responses to homeopathic therapy are the result of the placebo effect. The first trial was a pilot study, followed by two randomized, double-blind, placebo-controlled trials. The last two trials are presented in the text that follows.

Homeopathic Treatment of Allergies

In a 5-week study by Reilly and others, the hypothesis that homeopathic potencies function only as a placebo response was tested in a randomized, double-blind, placebo-controlled trial.[24] After randomization, a 1-week, placebo run-in period was conducted to obtain a baseline for both groups (i.e., all subjects received placebo pills). For weeks 2 and 3, a 30C homeopathic mixture of grass pollens **or** placebo was given to the 144 hay fever sufferers, twice daily. (Skin testing and/or IgE antibody measurements confirmed supplementary objective evidence of diagnosis). Symptoms were then observed during weeks 4 and 5.

Patients receiving the homeopathic remedy significantly reduced patient- and physician-assessed symptom scores (e.g., sneezing; blocked and runny nose; watery, red, and irritated eyes). Significance of response was increased when results were corrected for pollen count. The response was associated with a 50% reduction of antihistamines for the homeopathic group. Symptoms and antihistamine use in those receiving the placebo mixture did not significantly alter.

As occurs with homeopathic treatments, an initial aggravation of symptoms was noted on day 7 of treatment in homeopathically treated subjects, followed by consistent improvement in weeks 3 through 5. In week 5, the homeopathic group demonstrated significantly greater symptom reduction than the placebo group, as determined by both patient and physician assessment (p=0.02).

> **Points to Ponder** Patients receiving the homeopathic remedy significantly reduced patient- and physician-assessed symptom scores (e.g., sneezing; blocked and runny nose; watery, red, and irritated eyes). ■

Homeopathic Treatment of Asthmatics Sensitive to House Dust Mites

To again test the hypothesis that the effects of homeopathy are caused by the placebo effect, authors used a homeopathic immunotherapeutic approach to treat dust-mite sensitivity in asthmatics[24] (Figure 12-8). The trial was a randomized, double-blind assessment of 24 patients with asthma. The patients were randomized and stratified for indicated allergen and daily dose of inhaled steroid. The trial began in February to avoid the confounding variable of pollen. Skin tests, pulmonary function, and bronchial reactivity to histamine were conducted. The patients were assessed by homeopathic and asthma-clinic physicians.

The patients were then given one dose of either placebo or homeopathic remedy. The remedy was determined on the basis of the largest skin-test weal concordant with allergy history. Approximately 4 weeks later, patients returned for assessment. Reported asthma symptoms favored the homeopathic group, with the difference between groups averaging 33% over 4 weeks of treatment (p=0.03 for force vital capacity [FVC], p=0.08 for forced expiratory volume per second [FEV_1]). There was also a greater reduction in bronchial reactivity for the homeopathic group, with a 53% increase in histamine resistance compared with a median decrease of 7% in the placebo group. Of the 9 homeopathic patients, 7 (77%) showed improvement on the PC_{20} results, compared with 4 of 11 (36%) placebo patients (p=0.08). PC_{20} refers to the amount of histamine required to cause a 20% drop in FEV_1. Patients

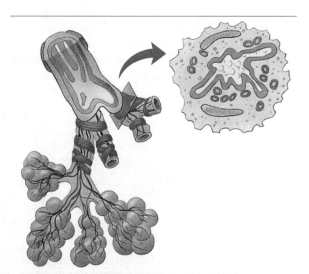

■ **Figure 12-8.** In asthma, edema of respiratory mucosa and excessive mucous production obstruct airways. *From Thibodeau:* Anatomy & physiology, ed 4, *St Louis, 1999, Mosby.*

and homeopathic physicians rated homeopathic treatment more effective (p=0.05 and p=0.09).

Summary of Placebo Tests

The authors performed a metaanalysis of the visual analog scales of symptoms for the pilot study and the two studies previously reviewed in this text.[23] All three studies, representing 202 patients, used a model of homeopathic immunotherapy in inhalant allergy and used identical visual analog scale scores. The authors found homeopathy significantly improved symptoms compared with those in the placebo group (p=0.0004).

Homeopathic Treatment of Fibromyalgia

In a double-blind, placebo-controlled, crossover study, 30 patients with fibromyalgia received 1 month of remedy followed by 1 month of placebo, each in random sequence.[13] The number of tender spots and pain, sleep, and overall assessment scores were calculated. While taking the homeopathic remedy, patients reduced tender spots by 25% (p<0.005) and improved pain or sleep (p<0.0052). Although crossover studies are not typically recommended for homeopathic remedies, this study produced positive results for homeopathy.

Supporters of homeopathy point to the studies reviewed as the best examples of the efficacy of homeopathy. The following studies are also worthy of consideration.

■ Homeopathic Treatment of Viral Conditions

Influenza

Ferley and others performed a controlled clinical trial of 481 patients with influenza.[12] The patients recorded rectal temperatures twice daily and the presence or absence of the five cardinal symptoms—headache, stiffness, lumbar and articular pain, and shivers. Recovery was defined as rectal temperature of less than 37.5° C and complete resolution of the five cardinal symptoms. Proportion of patients resolving within 48 hours was greatest for the active homeopathic drug group as compared with those in the placebo groups (17.1% versus 10.3%, p=0.03). Treatment was five doses of a single remedy, a form of nonclassical homeopathic treatment.

Chronic Carriers of Hepatitis B Virus

In an intriguing study, 60 chronic carriers of hepatitis B virus were randomized to receive a placebo or a homeopathic remedy known to inhibit surface antigen of hepatitis B virus. Of the treated patients, 59% lost hepatitis B surface antigen 15 to 20 days later, whereas only 1 of 23 placebo patients (4%) lost surface antigen. Some subjects were followed for 9 months. In no case did the surface antigen return.[32]

■ Homeopathic Treatment of Rheumatoid Arthritis

In a study by Gibson and others, 23 patients with rheumatoid arthritis taking first-line antiinflammatory treatment plus homeopathic remedies were matched with a similar group of 23 patients taking first-line treatment plus an inert placebo.[15] Matching was based on good versus poor prescribing symptoms, as well as age, gender, and clinical and laboratory features, which were balanced between the groups. Patients and homeopathic physicians were blind to group placement. At 3 months, there was significant improvement in subjective pain, articular index, stiffness, and grip strength for the homeopathic group; there was no significant change in patients who received the placebo (p=0.001).

■ Homeopathic Treatment of Childhood Diarrhea

A randomized, double-blind, placebo-controlled study was performed with 81 Nicaraguan children (6 months to 5 years old) who were experiencing mild-to-moderate diarrhea.[17] Treatment was individualized, with children receiving different medicines as prescribed by homeopathic procedures and daily follow-up for 5 days. Compared with the placebo group, homeopathic patients experienced significantly fewer days of diarrhea and number of unformed stools per day after 72 hours of treatment (p<0.05).

■ Unsuccessful Homeopathic Treatments

Not all studies support the efficacy of homeopathic treatments.

In a nonclassical, randomized, double-blind, placebo-controlled 26-week study, 170 Dutch children (1.5 to 10 years old) with recurring upper respiratory tract infections received either a homeopathic remedy or a placebo.[9] Individually prescribed homeopathic medicines did not significantly or clinically alter the effects of symptoms, the use of antibiotics, or the need for adenoidectomy and tonsillectomy as compared with the placebo group. However, the difference in mean daily scores over the year demonstrated a trend of greater improvement for the homeopathic group (p=0.06).

In a double-blind, placebo-controlled crossover trial, a homeopathic remedy was compared with fenoprofen, a standard antiinflammatory analgesic for the treatment of osteoarthritis of the hip and knee (N=33).[27] The effects of a homeopathic treatment and placebo did not differ significantly. Patient preference was for fenoprofen. The homeopathic treatment used in this study was nonindividualized (i.e., the remedy was not individually selected for the homeopathic subjects).

Finally, in a randomized, double-blind, placebo-controlled crossover trial (N=24), two identical surgical procedures (removal of bilaterally impacted wisdom teeth) were performed per patient. The patients were treated once with placebo and once with homeopathic medications. No differences were found between groups when comparing postoperative bleeding, painful side effects, or complaints.[22] However, homeopathic treatment provided an improved ability to open the mouth (p=0.05).

■ Efficacy of Homeopathic Treatments

A review of clinical trials in homeopathy included 107 controlled trials, published between 1966 and 1990. In 14 trials, classical homeopathy was tested, whereas a single homeopathic treatment was given to patients with comparable conventional diagnoses in 58 trials. Combinations of homeopathic treatments were tested in 26 trials. Most trials were of very low quality. There was a positive trend, regardless of trial quality. Of the 107 trials, 81 of these demonstrated improvements in the treatment of headaches, respiratory infections, diseases of the digestive tract, postoperative infections and symptoms, and other disorders; 24 trials found no positive effects of homeopathy. The authors reached the conclusion that, because of low trial quality and because of possible publication bias, the evidence from the clinical trials is positive at the moment but not sufficient to draw definitive conclusions.[19]

In a more recent review, Linde and others evaluated 186 homeopathic studies—all languages, double-blind, and/or randomized placebo-controlled trials—and found that 89 met inclusion criteria for metaanalysis. They found that the clinical effects of homeopathy were not explained by the placebo effect and that homeopathic treatment was 2.24 times more likely to result in ther-

apeutic effects than was placebo. However, the authors still believed that the evidence was insufficient to determine homeopathy's efficacy for individual clinical conditions.[21]

An Expert Speaks: Dr. David Reilly*

David Reilly is a Scottish physician and is well known for his published articles on homeopathy in the *Lancet*. Dr. Reilly's medical background is a traditional one. He graduated from Glasgow Medical University in 1973 and is a member of the Royal College of Physicians and the Royal College of General Practitioners. He is currently Honorary Senior Lecturer at the Royal Infirmary in Glasgow and consulting physician at Glasgow Homeopathic Hospital. In 1992, he was elected as a Fellow to the Royal College of Physicians and Surgeons, one of Britain's highest medical honors.

The following interview is particularly meaningful for several reasons. It is a model of the breadth and depth of thinking that should be used by any individual who performs research in alternative medicine—especially in areas that provoke great controversy, such as homeopathy. It also paints a clear and riveting picture of the kinds of "sacrifices" that must be paid if a researcher is to change, even in a small way, a cultural way of thinking about healing.

Dr. Reilly's interview reveals the type of thinking and the type of research that should be emulated by those performing research on complementary medicine and alternative therapies.

Question. Can you describe how you came to be involved in homeopathy and homeopathic research?

Answer. I see myself first as a doctor, maybe with a small "d," as in the traditional sense of that word. Before I went to medical school, I read a lot about human beings, and experience, and illness and health. I was intrigued by hypnosis and inner mind work. I had to put it on the back burner, but eventually I reached a crisis point.

My first water in the desert was the British Society of Medical and Dental Hypnosis. I did some of their postgraduate courses. It was the first chance I had to bring together more systematically some of the strands I'd been studying and thinking of and spontaneously developing with my patients. Right after that, there was an adver-

*Original article, "FRCP, MRCGP, FFHom: Research, Homeopathy, and Therapeutic Consultation," modified and updated by Dr. Reilly with permission from *Alternative Therapies in Health and Medicine*, 1(4):64, 1995.

tisement in the *British Medical Journal* for a registrar at the homeopathic hospital in Glasgow. I had never been there and knew nothing about homeopathy.

Question. But you applied for the job?

Answer. Yes, I crossed the door and thought, "I like it." The people I met had a more flexible, open attitude and feeling. I joined the unit and watched and listened. I had no confidence whatsoever in homeopathy in terms of the dilutions, but I was very intrigued by the system of care.

The funny thing is [that] the dilutions are often the least part of homeopathy. The biggest part is human engagement and a system for approaching illness and disease that is not based on judgment and theory. Homeopaths try to match up the physiological and emotional disturbances of the person, at a particular time, with a pattern of disturbance recognized with different drugs. If a headache comes in the evening or morning; suddenly or gradually; if it's helped by heat or by cold; or if it changes with barometric pressure; it's recorded. What's the mental content during the headache? Is the person withdrawn or sad? So the patient suddenly realizes this practitioner is interested in what they are saying. That's powerful medicine.

The other thing is that homeopathic medicine never perceived the mind and body as separate, so it never went down the tracks of conventional medicine and many of the dead ends of conventional medicine in that regard.

Question. How difficult was it for you to get published in the *Lancet*?

Answer. Extremely difficult on one level. But they have a saying in Britain: "If you can't stand the heat, get out of the kitchen."

I thought a lot about what research is, and the best thing I can say is that it is an act of communication. As an act of communication, therefore, it behooves you to resonate with the people with whom you would like to communicate. I understood that.

In 1983, when I first went to the homeopathic hospital, I stood in the library. It was a remarkable experience, because of these books, published in continuity for 200 years. I thought, "Is this crazy? Imagine if 10% of it is accurate. Think of the implications for health care.

So, I began to construct my intent. I began to think, what moves a culture? What shifts attitudes? I reckoned that human beings are the same everywhere, and they're locked into the same constraints, which includes culture, peer pressure, belief, and exposure. Medicine's belief

system has its own religious roots, the ritualistic or symbolic, and the catalysts that would move it, such as articles in the *Lancet*. So I took on the board and set it as a goal for the inquiry. I picked models of research that were easily communicable and understood. That is why I chose pollen and hay fever.

Most people have been exposed to the idea that you can give pollen shots for hay fever. Therefore the only new concept was the homeopathic dilution. I used standard methodology and off-the-shelf, validated outcome measures. I visited multiple university departments. I presented the idea for the research to skeptical colleagues, because I think it's important to go to people who are your worst enemies rather than your best friends and try to understand where they're coming from. So, every step along the way was very carefully constructed. When the pilot study worked, I must confess, I was very shocked.

Question. You were shocked?

Answer. Very shocked. My preconception was that homeopathic dilutions, not the system of homeopathy but homeopathic dilutions, were definitely a placebo. I wanted, however, to put flesh on the bones of my prejudice. I wanted to test my hypothesis, which is what science is. So, the title of the project was, "Is Homeopathy a Placebo Response?" and the pollen and hay fever were just models to address the specific question. When it came out positive, my gut level said, "This is a mistake."

I wrote to all the departments that had given me the advice to start and said, "What do you think? What could be the flaw here? What's the mistake? What does it mean?" I sent the pilot study to the *Lancet*. [It] refused it. So we took on board all the criticisms from every forum that we could gather, we incorporated them and re-ran the study a second time the next year, five times bigger.

We built into it solid protection against the possibility of fraud. We had one of the senior lecturers from the university department of medicine personally look at every diary and check results off the visual analog scales in the diary against the computer printout. This was a duplicate of the printout that the statistician had already received, which was independently correlated; and the statistician was not a homeopath and not interested, so he was neutral.

It all came out positive, clinically and statistically significant. So I was able to write back to the editor of the *Lancet* and say "You recall the pilot paper? Your referee's comments? Well, here's the second piece of work, taking on board the ideas." And they [printed] it.

Then the feedback, the criticisms rolled in. Things like, "Who cares about hay fever?" which missed the point. It had nothing to do with hay fever. Also, I was now tainted and called a "homeopathic researcher."

I was then awarded, with my co-worker, Morag Taylor, the RCCM/MRC Research Fellowship at Glasgow University. So I went to Robin Stephenson, head of the department of respiratory medicine, and said, "How would you like to be the man that proves homeopathy doesn't work? I have the grant."

So what we set up was still allergy, treated with the allergen, but it was asthmatic patients, principally with house dust-mite allergy. And this time we didn't do it with homeopathic researchers, we did it with conventional researchers. We didn't do it with homeopathic patients but with conventional patients already attending the department. We had them rediagnosed by the respiratory people, including laboratory tests and histamine provocation. We had the drugs made independently in France, sent straight to the pharmacists, double-blinded, who recoded them and administered them to the patients. The respiratory doctor monitored them throughout, and the homeopathic doctor, Neal Beattie, chose the allergen.

Within 7 days of receiving the randomized active medicine, those patients showed a clinically and statistically, significantly greater drop in symptoms. We sent it back to the *Lancet* after we took over 2 years in the analysis of it, and they [published] it.

By now, there was a cultural debate growing as to whether the clinical trial evidence was proving sufficient to validate an unconventional therapy. A review was published after 100 trials of homeopathy, with 77% showing results in favor of the therapy. I began to wonder, would 200 trials be evidence? Would 300 trials be evidence? What is evidence? So, I sat down in the last month before sending the paper to the *Lancet* and thought, "What do three positives in a row mean?" And a very simple answer came back. It's one of two things: either we have shown homeopathy works and that it works more than placebo, or we've shown the clinical trial doesn't work. We've shown the clinical trial, with predictability, reproducibility, clinical and statistical significance, can produce three false-positives in a row. I put that in the paper and the editor,

much to my surprise, ran an editorial called, "Reilly's Challenge."

Question. Do you think you took a step toward change in your culture?

Answer. I would say the first paper in particular did change the culture. What I learned is that conventional medicine and religion have the same roots. The high alter is the Lancet and a sacrifice has to be laid upon the alter with certain validating rituals occurring before the moment that it's placed there; and there must be magical symbols with the paper. There's a small one, and it's the letter "p," for example. [Here, Dr. Reilly refers to the statistical symbol p].

I've seen people take homeopathy with much more seriousness than before. That's why I searched my heart very deeply and why Morag, my partner, and I had to have the highest possible standard of science; because think of the responsibility if this was sloppy science, if that were bad results, if this was distorted datum? The cultural implication for me would be unthinkable.

I know now that homeopathy works, clinically. I accept that. But I know, actually, good consulting often works even better, which is my big interest in medicine; and I know the results of these trials are accurate. What it all adds up to? I wait to see.

■ Indications and Contraindications

Homeopathy is contraindicated as treatment for the following:
- Advanced stages of disease as the only line of treatment
- Cancers, syphilis, or gonorrhea (these are legally prohibited)
- Irreparable bodily damage, such as defective heart valves or brain damage because of stroke

Homeopathy has been reported as an effective treatment for the following:
- Short-term, acute illnesses, such as influenza
- Chronic pain syndromes, such as migraine pain
- Allergies
- Chronic fatigue
- Acute or chronic otitis media
- Immune dysfunction
- Digestive disorders
- Colic in infants

■ Summary

Although rejected by conventional medicine in the United States, homeopathy is used extensively in other countries. However, more studies and several replications of these studies (e.g., double-blind, placebo-controlled) are needed. Studies need to be high in quality—similar in design to those performed by Reilly and others. Studies need to be replicated for specific disease condi-tions, so it can be determined where homeopa-thy's greatest clinical strengths lie. These trials will have to be performed before homeopathy will be accepted as standard treatment in most U.S. medical settings.

Chapter Review

Matching Terms and Definitions

Match each numbered definition with the correct term. Place the corresponding letter in the space provided.

a. Principle of Similars
b. Hering's Law of Cures
c. Samuel Hahnemann
d. Cinchona
e. Proving
f. Keynote
g. Constantine Hering
h. Principle of Infinitesimal Dose
i. Mother of Tincture
j. Hippocrates
k. Potentization
l. Black box
m. Principle of Specificity
n. Successing

_____ 1. Originator of homeopathy
_____ 2. Substance from which homeopathic dilutions are made
_____ 3. Systematic process of testing substances on human beings to determine which symptoms the substance brings forth
_____ 4. Established the first U.S. school of homeopathy
_____ 5. Symptoms experienced by most healthy persons in response to a homeopathic remedy
_____ 6. What, in large doses, induces symptoms in a healthy person that will cure, in small doses, those symptoms in a sick person
_____ 7. Selected remedy must be matched to the individual's symptom-profile
_____ 8. Healing progresses in reverse order
_____ 9. The more dilute the remedy, the more potent its effects
_____ 10. Research design that tests the healing system rather than a specific remedy
_____ 11. Substance containing quinine that is used to treat malaria
_____ 12. Repeatedly shaking and diluting a homeopathic remedy
_____ 13. Vigorous shaking
_____ 14. First taught the Law of Similars 2400 years ago

CRITICAL THINKING AND CLINICAL APPLICATION EXERCISES

1. Compare and contrast the "energy" mechanisms used to explain homeopathy with the "energy" mechanisms used to explain acupuncture.
2. Design a "black box," placebo-controlled study to test the efficacy of homeopathy to treat the common cold.
3. Describe what you find most believable about homeopathic principles and what you find least believable. Defend your assertions.

References

1. Bannerman RH, Burton J, Wen Chieh C, editors: *Traditional medicine and health care coverage,* Geneva, Switzerland, 1983, World Health Organization.
2. Bradford TL: *Life and letters of Dr. Samuel Hahnemann,* Philadelphia, 1895, Boericke and Tafel.
3. Brigo B, Serpelloni G: Homeopathic treatment of migraines: a randomized double-blind controlled study of sixty cases, *Berl J Res Homeopathy* 1:98, 1991.
4. Buckman R, Lewith G: What does homeopathy do—and how? *BMJ* 309:103, 1994.
5. Coulter H: *Divided legacy: a history of the schism in medical thought,* Washington, DC, 1977, Wehawken.
6. Coulter HL: *Divided legacy: the conflict between homeopathy and the American Medical Association,* Berkeley, 1973, North Atlantic.
7. Davenas E et al: Human basophil degranulation triggered by very dilute antiserum against IgE, *Nature* 333:816, 1988.
8. Davenas E, Poitevin B, Beneveiste J: Effect of mouse peritoneal macrophages of orally administered very high dilutions of silica, *Eur J Pharmacol* 135:313, 1987.
9. de Lange de Klerk ESM, Blommers J, Kui DJ, Bezemer PD, Feenstra L: Effect of homeopathic medicines on daily burden of symptoms in children with recurrent upper respiratory tract infections, *BMJ* 309:1329, 1994.
10. del Giudici E, Preparata G: *Superradiance: a new approach to coherent dynamical behaviors of condenses matter, Frontier Perspectives,* Philadelphia, 1990, Temple University, Center for Frontier Sciences.
11. Eisenberg D et al: Unconventional medicine in the United States, *N Engl J Med* 324(4):246, 1993.
12. Ferley JP, Zmirou D, Adhemar D, Balducci F: A controlled evaluation of a homeopathic preparation in the treatment of influenza-like syndromes, *Br J Clin Pharmacol* 27:329, 1989.
13. Fisher P, Greenwood A, Huskisson EC, Turner P, Belon P: Effect of homeopathic treatment of fibrositis (primary fibromyalgia), *BMJ* 299:365, 1989.
14. Gerber R: *Vibrational medicine,* Santa Fe, NM, 1988, Bear & Co.
15. Gibson RG, Gibson LM, MacNeill AD, Buchanan WW: Homeopathic therapy in rheumatoid arthritis: evaluation by double-blind clinical therapeutic trial, *Br J Clin Pharmacol* 9:453, 1980.
16. Hahnemann S: Organon of medicine, Boercke W, translator, *Organon of medicine,* New Delhi, 1992, B. Jain Publishing.
17. Jacobs J, Jiminez M, Gloyd SS, Gale JL, Crothers D: Treatment of acute childhood diarrhea with homeopathic medicine: a randomized clinical trial in Nicaragua, *Pediatrics* 93:719, 1994.
18. Jouanny J: The essentials of homeopathic therapeutics, Ste-Foy-les-Lyon, France, 1980, Laboratories Boiron.
19. Kleijnen J, Knipschild P, ter Reit G: Clinical trials of homeopathy, *BMJ* 302(6772):316, 1991.
210. Lange A: Homeopathy. In Pizzorno JE, Murray MT, editors: *A textbook of natural medicine,* Seattle, WA, 1989, Bastyr College Publications.
21. Linde K, Clausius N, Ramirez G, Melchart D, Eitel F, Hedges LV, Jonas WB: Are the clinical effects of homeopathy placebo effects? A meta-analysis of placebo-controlled trials, *Lancet* 350:834, 1997.
22. Lokken P, Straumsheim PA, Tveiten D, Skjelbred P, Borchgrevink CF: Effect of homeopathy on pain and other events after acute trauma: placebo controlled trial with bilateral oral surgery, *BMJ* 310:1439, 1995.
23. Reilly D, Taylor MA, Beattie NGM, Campbell JH, McSharry C, Aitchison TC, Carter R, Stevenson RD: Is evidence for homeopathy reproducible? *Lancet* 344:1601, 1994.
24. Reilly DT, McSharry C, Taylor MA, Atchison T: Is homeopathy a placebo response? Controlled trial of homeopathic potencies, *Lancet* 2:881, 1986.
25. Reilly DT, Taylor MA, McSharry C, Atchison T: Is homeopathy a placebo response? Controlled trial of homeopathic potency with pollen and hay fever as a model, *Lancet* ii:881, 1986.
26. Rubic B: *Frontiers of homeopathic research, Frontier Perspectives,* Philadelphia, 1991, Temple University, Center for Frontier Science.
27. Shipley M et al: Controlled trial of homeopathic treatment of osteoarthritis, *Lancet* 1:97, 1983.
28. Shui-Yin Lo, Angela Lo, Li-Wen Chong et al: Physical properties of water with Ie structures, *Mod Phys Lett* 19:921, 1996.
29. Shui-Yin Lo: Anomalous state of ice, *Mod Phys Lett* 19:909, 1996.
30. Smith RB, Boericke GW: Changes caused by succussion on N.M.R. patterns and bioassay of Bradykinin Triacetate (BKTA) succussions and dilution, *J Am Inst Homeopathy* 61:197, 1968.
31. Thibodeau GA, Patton KT: (1999). *Anatomy and physiology,* St Louis, 1999, Mosby.
32. Thyagarajan SP, Subramanian S, Thirunalasundari T, Venkateswaran PS, Blumberg BS: Effect of phyllanthus amarus on chronic carriers of hepatitis B virus, *Lancet* 764, 1988.
33. Ullman D: *Consumer's guide to homeopathy,* New York, 1995, Jeramy Tarcher/Putnam.
34. Ullman D: *Extremely dilute solutions create non-melting ice crystals in room temperature water: the implications on homeopathic medicine,* 1997, http://www.homeopathic. com.
35. Vithoulkas G: *The science of homeopathy,* New York, 1980, Grove Press.

13

Massage Therapy

Lyn W. Freeman

WHY READ THIS CHAPTER?

Human touch is one of our most primal needs. Without touch, infants fail to thrive, depressed persons are denied comfort, and maximal pain relief is often not provided. Can touch really heal? There is excellent research to suggest that it can. Massage seems to stimulate and strengthen one's natural healing capacities. In these times of medical technology, when touch is avoided, massage is a complementary treatment that offers benefits not provided by approaches that are more orthodox. It behooves the medical provider and the patient to be aware of the benefits of massage.

CHAPTER AT A GLANCE

Massage is defined as the intentional and systematic manipulation of the soft tissues of the body, that is, the normalization of soft tissues, to enhance health and healing. It is one of the oldest forms of health practice and has been used since ancient times in the cultures of India, Persia, Arabia, Egypt, and Greece.

The mechanics used to explain the benefits of massage are the following:
1. Mechanical—compressing, stretching, shearing, and broadening tissues
2. Physiologic—cellular, tissue, and organ system effects
3. Reflex—pressure and movement in one body part affecting another
4. Body-mind interactions—between the mind and the emotion and disease processes
5. Energetic—flow of our life energy or chi

Massage has been found beneficial as an intervention in or for the treatment of anxiety, depression, acute and chronic pain, childbirth, neonatal development, and infants exposed to cocaine and human immunodeficiency virus (HIV).

The preservation of health is a DUTY. Few seem conscious that there is such a thing as physical morality.

HERBERT SPENCER, ENGLISH PHILOSOPHER, 1861.

CHAPTER OBJECTIVES

After completing this chapter, you should be able to:

1. Define massage and massage techniques.
2. Discuss the history of massage.
3. Describe the mechanisms that account for the benefits of massage.
4. Describe the research outcomes of massage for the treatment of depression and anxiety.
5. Explain the benefits of massage for the treatment of acute and chronic pain.
6. Compare and contrast the research outcomes of massage for premature infants and full-term infants exposed to HIV and cocaine.
7. Discuss the indications and contraindications for the use of massage.

■ Massage Defined

Massage is defined as the intentional and systematic manipulation of the soft tissues of the body, that is, the normalization of soft tissues, to enhance health and healing. The primary characteristics of massage are the applications of touch and movement.[67] Massage consists of a group of manual techniques that include applying fixed or movable pressure and/or causing movement of or to the body. Massage is primarily delivered by the use of hands, but it may also be delivered using other body parts such as the forearms, elbows, or feet (Figure 13-1).

Today, massage is used in a variety of health professions that include therapeutic massage, body work, physical therapy, sports training, nursing, chiropractic, osteopathy, and naturopathy.

In this chapter, clinical outcomes demonstrating what is termed as classical Western massage techniques are emphasized. "Classical" refers to massage techniques that have endured the test of time and that have been traditionally used since the late nineteenth century in Europe and the United States. In addition, numerous massage techniques have emerged in the last few decades. Of the 80 different methods classified as massage

therapy, more than 60 are techniques that were developed in the last 20 years. Research on emerging techniques is extremely limited compared with the research on the classical methods. Emerging techniques include but are not limited to the structural, functional, and movement integration methods known as Rolfing, Hellerwork, Aston patterning, Trager, Feldenkrais, and Alexander. These methods seek to organize and integrate the body in relation to gravity by manipulating the soft tissues or by correcting inappropriate patterns of movement. The expected outcome is a more balanced use of the nervous system, brought about by creating new, integrated possibilities of movement.[9]

The bulk of the research has evaluated the classical methods of massage, rather than the emerging techniques, and the effects these methods have on illness and disease states. Therefore the research on the classical methods is reviewed in this chapter.

■ History of Massage

Massage therapy is one of the oldest forms of health practice and has been used to enhance

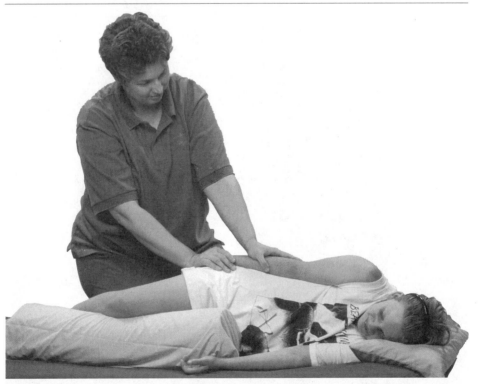

■ **Figure 13-1.** Massage is most typically delivered with the hands, although forearms, elbows, or feet may be used as well. *Modified from Fritz S:* Mosby's visual guide to massage essentials, *St Louis, 1996, Mosby.*

health, general well being, and healing since ancient times. Massage has been a part of the health practices of many ancient cultures, including India, Persia, Arabia, and Greece.[9] Some of the earliest references to massage are found in ancient Chinese medical texts. The *Yellow Emperor's Classic of Internal Medicine,* believed to be the first book on Chinese medicine, was written more than 2500 years ago. This text includes information on *Tuina,* an ancient form of massage, and *acupressure,* the application of finger pressure to points that are sensitized by organ impairment.[51] Anma, or amma, is a form of Japanese massage brought from China by way of the Korean peninsula in the sixth century BC. The Japanese then incorporated Chinese medical philosophies into their own medical practices, and amma became an accepted Japanese healing modality.

In India, traditional medicine is based on the Ayurvedic system that dates back at least to the fifth century BC. The Ayurvedic health practices include forms of cleansing, movements, and postures (Hatha yoga), meditation, and massage. Many of these health practices have been popularized in the United States by Deepok Chopra.[12] The recent revival of infant massage in the United

States has been patterned in part on the ancient practice of baby massage in India[44] (Figure 13-2).

In ancient Greece, the use of massage was advanced. Hippocrates (425-377 BC), the father of modern medicine, wrote of the use of friction for the treatment of sprains and dislocations and recommended chest clapping. Aristotle, philosopher and tutor to Alexander the Great, recommended rubbing the body with oil and water as a remedy for weariness. The gymnasia in Athens and Sparta, free facilities for men and youth, offered massage with oil to prepare the men for their exercises and to refresh them after their baths.[41] In Rome, Aulus Cornelius Celsius (25-50 AD), a Roman physician, compiled a textbook known as *De Medicina,* eight books covering all the medical knowledge of his time. In this textbook, massage techniques including frictions, oil and ointment application, rubbing, brushing, and dry cupping are recommended for the treatment of illness.[32] Avicenna, an Arabic physician (980-1037) also wrote about massage in his medical texts. He believed that massage dispersed the toxic matter formed in the muscles and not expelled by exercise, resulting in improved health and a reduction of fatigue.[74]

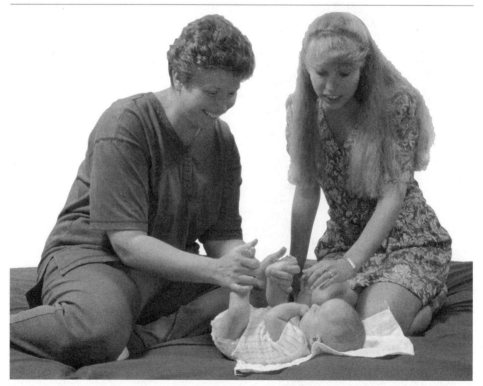

■ **Figure 13-2.** A parent is taught infant massage by her massage practitioner. *Modified from Fritz S: Mosby's visual guide to massage essentials, St Louis, 1996, Mosby.*

Evolution of Classical Massage

The evolution of classical Western massage is attributed to two men, Pehr Henrik Ling and Johann Mezger. Pehr Henrik Ling (1776-1839) developed four systems of movement described in his treatise, *The General Principles of Gymnastics.* Ling's medical gymnastics emphasized both active and passive movements. His passive movements were described as shaking, hacking, pressing, stroking, pinching, kneading, clapping, vibrating, and rolling. He instructed that oil should be used to decrease skin friction. In the nineteenth century, disease and illness reportedly treated by Ling's methods included head congestion, asthma, emphysema, constipation, incontinence, hernia, epilepsy, neuralgic pain, and paralysis.[60] Ling taught that a combination of active and passive movements could restore health and balance to the body. His work was a precursor to many of the Swedish movements used later in physical therapy.

Johann Mezger (1838-1909), a physician from Amsterdam, also believed that passive movements had the power to improve health. Mezger categorized soft-tissue manipulation into effleurage (stroking), petrissage (kneading), friction (rubbing), and tapotement (tapping). Mezger's work was instrumental in reviving interest in the use of massage in medical settings, and his general categories of movements form the basis of today's classical Western massage.[53]

Swedish Massage

In 1854, two New York physicians, Dr. George Taylor and his brother, Dr. Charles Taylor, brought the "Swedish movement cure" to the United States. Both had previously studied massage techniques in Sweden. Swedish massage can be defined as the manipulation of soft tissues for therapeutic purposes, both psychologic and physical. The various movements are said to affect skin, muscle, blood and lymph vessels, nerves, and some internal organs.[49,68]

Two Swedes opened the first massage therapy clinics in the United States after the Civil War. Baron Nils Posse ran the Posse Institute in Boston, and Hartwig Nissen opened the Swedish Health Institute near Washington, D.C. Members of Congress and American presidents, including Benjamin Harrison and Ulysses S. Grant, were among the massage therapy clientele of the day.[9]

After that time and into the early twentieth century, practitioners of the "Swedish movement cure" adopted Mezger's massage forms, and the merged forms became known as Swedish massage. Swedish massage was most popular between 1920 and 1950 and included massage, Swedish movements, hydrotherapy, heat lamps, diathermy, and colonic irrigation. Practitioners were trained in "colleges," and graduates often found jobs in the Young Men's Christian Association (YMCA), private health clubs, resorts, and hospitals or with professional sports teams.[67]

Decline of Massage

In the 1940s and 1950s, massage entered a period of decline. A contributing factor to this decline was the fact that massage parlors were often used as a cover for prostitution. The biggest contributor to the decline, however, was that other interventions were taking the place of massage. The value of physical therapy and massage was being challenged.

Beginning in the early 1900s, physicians influenced by biomedicine and technology began assigning their massage duties to assistants, nurses, and physical therapists. In the 1930s and 1940s, nurses and physical therapists lost interest in massage therapy, virtually abandoning it.

In the sports world, trainers began to specialize in the treatment of sports injuries and massage as a training aid was neglected. The social conservatism of the day left people reticent to undress for massage or to allow the touching necessary for the application of massage. During this period, only a small number of massage therapists carried on the profession. This disinterest in massage, however, was to last for only a short time.

Massage Bounces Back

During the human potential movement of the 1960s, young people rejected the more conservative views of their elders. Esalen Institute in Big Sur, California, became the meeting place for the leaders of the human potential movement. At Esalen, a form of massage was developed to help the recipient reconnect with the inner self and with others. This form of massage was loosely based on classical Western massage.

This renewed interest in massage had a positive effect on the emerging profession of massage therapy. The number of practitioners and recipients of massage exploded. Massage and body work training programs increased dramatically, and the concepts of holistic health and healing were revived.[8]

On the heels of the human potential movement came the wellness movement of the 1970s. Health professionals began to reevaluate the therapeutic value of methods of touch. The American Nurses Association recognized massage therapy as an official nursing subspecialty, and "therapeutic touch" was embraced by a large number of nurses as an energy work form.

■ Massage Therapy Today

Today, massage is enjoying unprecedented attention from professional researchers. The unchallenged leader in this arena is Dr. Tiffany Field of the Touch Research Institute at the University of Miami. This Institute was created in 1991 and is the first center devoted to basic and applied research in the use of touch for human health and development.[14] The research produced by Dr. Field and others is reviewed in detail in this chapter.

The creation of the Office of Alternative Medicine (OAM) in 1991 also contributed to the medical credibility of massage therapy. OAM became a source of grant funding for exploration of the medical benefits of massage. By January, 1993, Eisenberg's landmark survey of the use of alternative therapies revealed that massage was the third most used alternative modality in the United States, outranked only by relaxation techniques and chiropractic care.[19] Massage therapy had again come into its own.

■ Philosophy and Mechanisms of Massage

The basic philosophy of massage therapy is based on the concept of *vis medicatrix naturae*—or aiding the ability of the body to heal itself. Massage is aimed at achieving or increasing health and well being. The benefits of massage are attributed to its effects on the musculoskeletal, circulatory and lymphatic, nervous, and other bodily systems.[9] It also benefits the mental and emotional states of the individual.

Mechanisms Explaining the Effects of Massage

The mechanisms of massage are categorized as mechanical, physiologic, reflex, body mind, and energetic.

- *Mechanical mechanisms* result essentially from physical forces of compression, stretching, shearing, and broadening of tissues. Mechanical mechanisms occur at the gross level of the physical structure.
- *Physiologic mechanisms* refer to the organic processes of the body (e.g., changes at the cellular, tissue, or organ system level).
- *Reflex mechanisms* refer to the result of pressure or movement in one body part affecting another body part.

- *Mind-body mechanisms* refer to the interplay of mind, emotion, immunity, physiology, and health or disease processes.
- *Energetic mechanisms* refer to changes in the body's flow of energy, a mechanism related to acupuncture points, the meridian system, and the flow of chi (life energy).

Physical, Mental, and Emotional Effects of Massage

It is asserted that the mechanisms described in this text are responsible for specific, health-enhancing changes in the body, including improvements in immune function, pain relief, infant thriving, relaxation, and increasing sense of worth.[13,67] Yet, the research supporting these beliefs is conflicting and often confusing.[15] The following text is a summary of the stated effects of massage on the integumentary, circulatory, muscular, skeletal, nervous, endocrine, immune, and digestive systems, as well as on the connective tissues and the mental and emotional state. Available research supporting or refuting these findings is described.

It should be noted that researchers and health professionals do not claim that these effects occur with every massage session or for every individual. Rather, the massage techniques used, the quality of movement, the receptivity of the client, and the gender, age, and health condition of the client all determine which effects are most likely to occur (Figure 13-3).

Effects on Integumentary System and Connective Tissues

The skin, or integumentary system, is crucial to our survival (Figure 13-4). The skin protects us from harmful microorganisms and chemicals, regulates body temperature, synthesizes important chemicals and hormones, and functions as a sophisticated sense organ. The integumentary system includes skin and its appendages (e.g., hair, nails, specialized sweat glands, oil-producing glands). Massage affects the integumentary system by stimulating sensory receptors in the skin, increasing superficial circulation, removing dead skin, increasing sebaceous gland excretions, and adding moisture through the use of oil or lotion. The skin also performs a certain amount of respiration (i.e., exchange of carbon dioxide and oxygen), which can be assisted by the action of massage. Massage affects the connective tissues (the fascia) by separating these tissues and improving their pliability.

Effects on Circulatory and Muscular Systems

The circulatory system is benefited by increased local circulation and enhanced venous return (Figure 13-5). Research has demonstrated that capillary vessel dilation and increased blood flow occur as a result of massage, even with light pressure.[74] In one study, deep stroking and kneading doubled the blood flow to the calf, an effect that lasted for 40 minutes.[6]

Through relaxing the muscle and reducing the sensitivity of myofascial trigger points, the "milking" of metabolic wastes into venous and lymph flow channels benefits the muscular system (Figure 13-6 on pages 370 and 371). In one study, the following three methods of postmastectomy lymphedema (lymph swelling) treatments were compared:

1. Pneumatic pressure therapy with uniform pressure, 6 hours a day
2. Pneumatic pressure therapy with differentiated pressure, inflated in rhythmic cycles
3. Manual lymphatic massage for 1 hour, three times a week, for 4 weeks

Changes in arm circumference, mood, and visual analog scale ratings before treatment, at the end of treatment, and 3 months later were evaluated (N=60). A statistically significant and permanent reduction in swelling was observed in pneumatic pressure therapy with uniform pressure and in manual lymphatic massage; reduction in swelling was not observed in pneumatic pressure therapy with differentiated pressure.[75] Manual massage produced better results than pneumatic pressure with uniform pressure, although the differences were not statistically significant.

Effects on Muscle Soreness

Unaccustomed exercise often results in delayed onset muscle soreness and disruption of contractile and/or connective tissue. Acute inflammation occurs whenever muscle and associated connective tissues are injured. Massage is recommended as an aid to speed recovery. Within a few hours after injury, neutrophils (the first wave of white blood cells) accumulate at the injured site. This is preceded by an increase in blood neutrophils and followed by a decline in blood neutrophils. In a study of the effects of massage on muscle soreness, 14 subjects exercised the biceps and triceps of their nondominant arm for five exercise sets to exhaustion. Half of the subjects received massage and half served as controls. Muscle soreness ratings demonstrated that there were sufficient exercise sets to induce a delayed onset muscle sore-

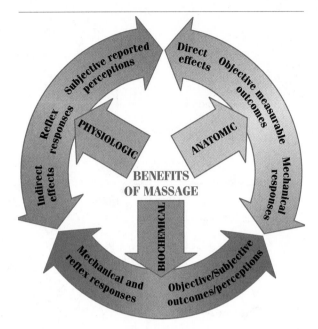

■ **Figure 13-3.** The benefits, effects, responses, and outcomes can occur separately, combined, or as a result of each other. *Modified from Fritz S:* Mosby's visual guide to massage essentials, *St Louis, 1996, Mosby.*

ness. The control subjects reported peak soreness 48 hours after exercise, whereas the massage subjects reported peak soreness 24 hours after exercise. Soreness levels were greater for those in the control group. Creatine kinase, a marker of muscle trauma, increased for both groups, but the control group demonstrated an earlier and a sharper curve for creatine kinase than did the massage group. Neutrophils were significantly more elevated from baseline for massage subjects, suggesting that massage may interfere with the emigration of circulating cells into the tissue spaces. This study suggests that delayed onset muscle soreness and creatine kinase levels may be significantly reduced if massage is rendered 2 hours after the termination of unaccustomed exercise.[65]

Effects on Skeletal System

Massage benefits the skeletal system by increasing joint mobility and flexibility (Figure 13-7 on page 372). For example, frozen shoulder is a common problem encountered in orthopedic clinics. Because of the pain and inability to use the shoulder, patients may not be able to live or work independently. In a series of case studies of patients with frozen shoulder, manipulation and massage (N=205) or sudden tearing by force of adhesion of

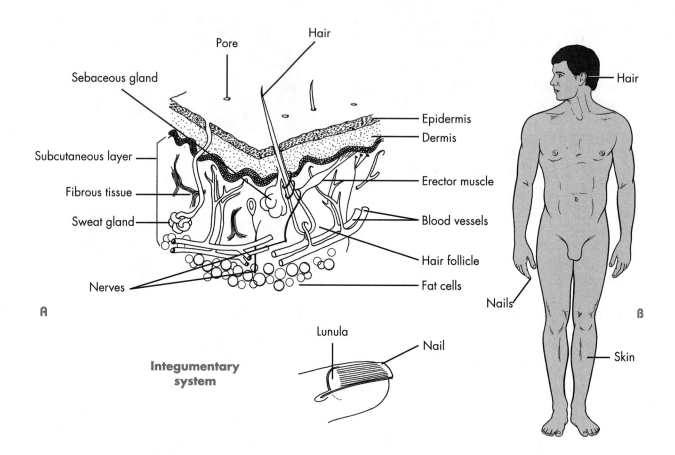

■ *Figure* 13-4. **A,** Integument means covering. The integumentary system covers the body and consists of skin and its appendages: hair, sebaceous (oil-producing) glands, sweat glands, nails, and breasts. It protects the internal organs and structures from trauma, sun exposure, chemicals and water loss. It prevents the entry of bacteria and viruses, synthesizes vitamin D when exposed to ultraviolet rays from the sun, helps regulate body temperature, and excretes sweat and salts. *Modified from Williams RW:* Basic health care terminology, *St Louis, 1995, Mosby.* **B,** The integumentary system covers and protects the body. *Modified from Thibodeau GA, Patton KT:* Anatomy & physiology, *St Louis, 1999, Mosby.*

tissues (N=30) was administered as treatment. Massage consisted of pressing, kneading, pinching, grasp-point massaging, and separating tissues for 20 minutes, once every 3 days for at least four sessions. Tearing by force of adhesion was administered under anesthesia and was intended to tear off the abnormal adhesion of the shoulder joint. The rate of complete recovery in the massage-manipulation group was 71.2%; in the tearing group, the rate of recovery was 10%.[77]

Effects on Nervous System
It is asserted that massage stimulates the parasympathetic nervous system, resulting in relaxation and a reduction in pain via a neural-gating mechanism and an increase in body awareness

(Figure 13-8 on page 373). Two theories explain how massage reduces pain. The first is referred to as "The Gate Theory of Pain Control." This theory states that a gate or series of gates exist throughout the length of the spinal cord. Pain messages that originate from the periphery travel to the gate in the spinal cord. If the gate is open, pain messages get through to the brain; if the gate is closed, the brain does not register the pain messages. Two types of nerves are relevant to the gate theory. They are A-delta, small diameter fibers that originate from pain receptors, and A-beta, large diameter fibers that are sensitive to touch, pressure, and warmth. Both the small and large fibers activate T-cells in the spinal cord, which then pass messages to the brain. Activity of T-cells

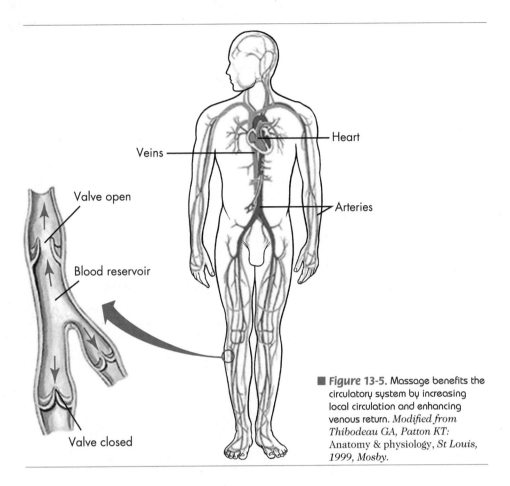

Veins

Valve open

Blood reservoir

Heart

Arteries

Valve closed

■ *Figure* 13-5. Massage benefits the circulatory system by increasing local circulation and enhancing venous return. *Modified from Thibodeau GA, Patton KT:* Anatomy & physiology, *St Louis, 1999, Mosby.*

is also affected by other types of cells in the *substantia gelatinosa,* an adjacent part of the spinal cord. Large diameter fibers, those that are sensitive to touch, pressure, and warmth (e.g., sensitive to massage), stimulate activity in the substantia gelatinosa. This affects the activity of the T-cells in such a way that no pain impulses can pass to the brain—the gate is closed. On the other hand, small diameter fibers sensitive to pain interfere with this activity in the substantia gelatinosa. The activity of certain T-cells is increased and the gate opens, allowing pain impulses to be relayed to the brain. It is believed that massage stimulates the large diameter A-beta fibers and succeeds in closing the gate so that pain impulses are reduced, decreasing the patient's perception of pain.[49,50] The second theory states that massage therapy increases restorative (deep or quiet) sleep, resulting in the decreased release of substance P, a pain transmitter.[66]

Relaxation Response
It is believed that soothing massage techniques are also effective relaxation interventions, triggering the relaxation response in many subjects. The

relaxation response has been demonstrated to result in the following:

1. Decreased oxygen consumption and metabolic rate, lessening the strain on energy resources
2. Increased alpha brain waves associated with deep relaxation
3. Reduced blood lactates, which are associated with anxiety
4. Decreased blood pressure in some individuals
5. Decreased muscle tension
6. Increased blood flow to the limbs
7. Improved mood state
8. Improved quality of sleep[59]

Yet, massage research outcomes related to autonomic responsivity are mixed. Four massage studies produced no significant changes in measurements of autonomic response, including blood pressure, heart rate, and galvanic skin response.[15,39,46,58] However, Corley found that massage improved mood state in residents living in a long-term care facility.

Madison reported a decrease in heart rate in older women, whereas Tyler and others found increased heart rates and decreased oxygen saturation in response to massage.[48,69] Fakouri and

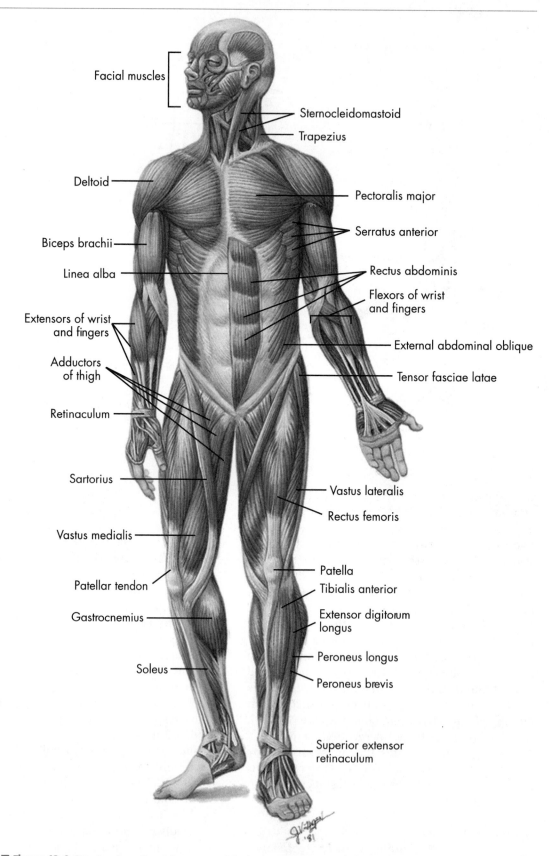

Facial muscles

Sternocleidomastoid

Trapezius

Deltoid

Pectoralis major

Serratus anterior

Biceps brachii

Rectus abdominis

Linea alba

Flexors of wrist
and fingers

Extensors of wrist
and fingers

External abdominal oblique

Adductors
of thigh

Tensor fasciae latae

Retinaculum

Sartorius

Vastus lateralis

Rectus femoris

Vastus medialis

Patella

Tibialis anterior

Patellar tendon

Extensor digitorum
longus

Gastrocnemius

Peroneus longus

Peroneus brevis

Soleus

Superior extensor
retinaculum

■ **Figure 13-6. Anterior view.** General overview of the body musculature. *Modified from Thibodeau GA, Patton KT:* Anatomy & physiology, *St Louis, 1999, Mosby.*

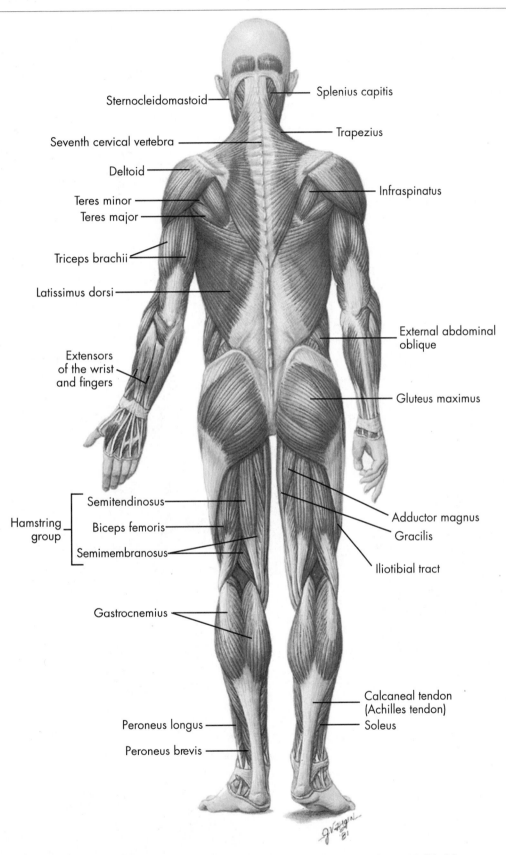

Sternocleidomastoid

Seventh cervical vertebra

Deltoid

Teres minor
Teres major

Triceps brachii

Latissimus dorsi

Extensors
of the wrist
and fingers

Hamstring
group

Semitendinosus

Biceps femoris

Semimembranosus

Gastrocnemius

Peroneus longus

Peroneus brevis

Splenius capitis

Trapezius

Infraspinatus

External abdominal
oblique

Gluteus maximus

Adductor magnus

Gracilis

Iliotibial tract

Calcaneal tendon
(Achilles tendon)

Soleus

■ **Figure 13-6—cont'd. Posterior view.** *General overview of the body musculature. Modified from* Thibodeau GA, Patton KT: *Anatomy & physiology, St Louis, 1999, Mosby.*

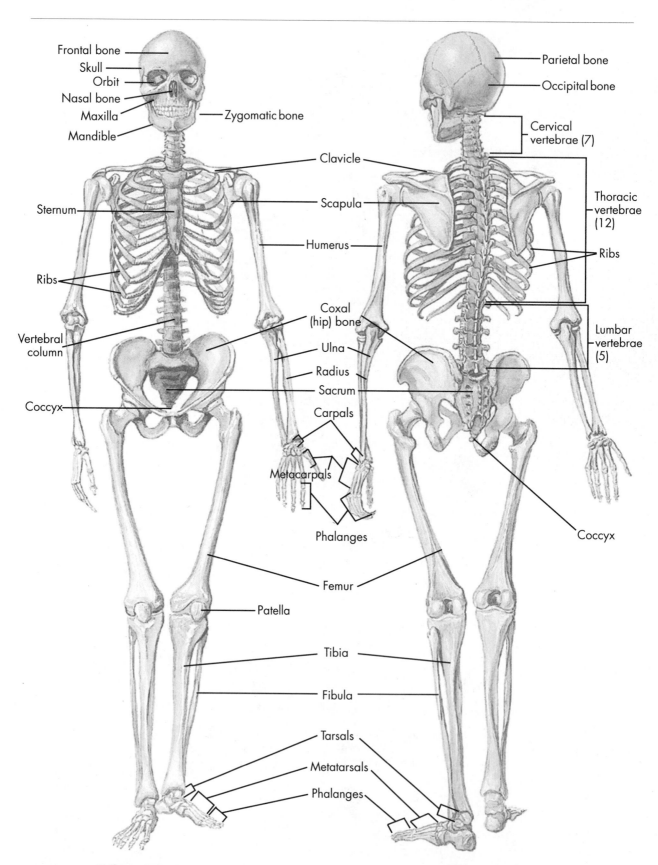

■ **Figure 13-7. Skeleton.** Anterior and posterior views. *Modified from Thibodeau GA, Patton KT: Anatomy & physiology, St Louis, 1999, Mosby.*

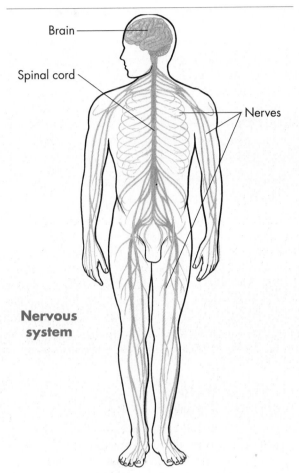

Brain

Spinal cord

Nerves

Nervous system

■ **Figure 13-8.** The nervous system. *Modified from Thibodeau GA, Patton KT:* Anatomy & physiology, *St Louis, 1999, Mosby.*

Jones supported massage's efficacy by demonstrating decreases in blood pressure and heart rate and an increase in skin temperature.[21]

Research Outcomes: Gender, Age, and Patient Receptivity

In an attempt to explain these contradictions, Labyak and Metzger performed a metaanalysis of nine studies examining autonomic nervous system response to massage. Differences in gender, age, and presence of cardiovascular disease were evaluated. Findings demonstrated that massage was significantly associated with a reduction in heart and respiratory rates for all subjects. However, effects of massage on systolic and diastolic blood pressure were gender-specific, with blood pressure initially increasing for women but decreasing consistently over time for men. When blood pressure was the variable being evaluated, men clearly benefited from massage more significantly than women. Additionally, whereas massage had positive effects on cardiovascular parameters for patients who has previously suffered heart attacks (postmyocardial infarction), blood pressure and heart rate in patients with coronary artery bypass grafting (CABG) rose in response to massage within the first 48 hours after surgery, contraindicating massage during this critical time period. The authors concluded that massage effects are situation-specific, depending on the length of the massage, gender, age, health status, and receptivity of the client. They further concluded that biological relaxation was significantly associated with reduction in heart and respiratory rates for both genders, in spite of the presence of cardiovascular disease or cardiovascular drugs.[43a]

Effects on Endocrine System

The endocrine system is composed of specialized glands that secrete a variety of hormones into the blood (Figure 13-9). Massage has been reported to result in the release of endorphins. Endorphins affect the nervous system, pain severity, and mood state.[38] However, when healthy massaged patients were compared with healthy patients who rested, no differences were found in endorphin or lipotropin levels.[17] Benefits to the endocrine system may occur only for those with compromised endocrine function, with little or no endocrine effects in healthy subjects.

Effects on Immune Function

It is asserted that the immune system is aided by massage because of an increase in lymphatic flow and potential improvements of immune function induced by the reduction of stress. Chronic stress has been demonstrated to have negative effects on immunity, which include increased susceptibility to infections, slow wound healing, and exacerbation of autoimmune diseases.[16,34] In studies by Groer and colleagues, Green and Green, and Field and others, massage produced increases in salivary immunoglobulin A concentrations, an indicator of stress reduction and immune enhancement.[24,33,35]

A study by Ironson, Field, and others demonstrated more direct effects of massage on chronic disease outcomes. Massage therapy was provided to HIV-positive men. Compared with HIV-positive controls, massaged HIV-positive men demonstrated a significant increase in the number of natural killer (NK) cells, NK cytoxicity, soluble CD8, and cytotoxic subset of CD8 cells.[37] Significant decreases in cortisol levels were observed before and after massage; no changes in HIV disease pro-

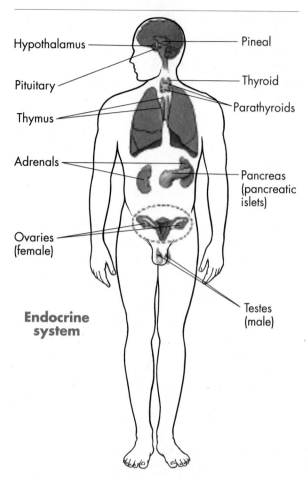

Hypothalamus

Pituitary

Thymus

Adrenals

Ovaries
(female)

Pineal

Thyroid

Parathyroids

Pancreas
(pancreatic
islets)

Testes
(male)

**Endocrine
system**

■ *Figure* **13-9.** The endocrine system is made up of specialized glands that secrete a variety of hormones into the blood. *Modified from Thibodeau GA, Patton KT:* Anatomy & physiology, *St Louis, 1999, Mosby.*

gression markers were demonstrated. Anxiety was significantly decreased and relaxation increased. These changes were significantly correlated with the increased number of NK cells. The authors concluded that increased cytotoxic capacity was associated with massage.

Another study sought to assess the effects of massage on stressed medical students. Students received a 1-hour body massage 1 day before an academic examination. Blood samples and self-report anxiety data were obtained before and after the massage treatment. Before and after massage, the total number of white blood cells significantly increased, whereas the number of T-cells significantly decreased. NK cell function significantly increased; and anxiety, which decreased, was significantly correlated with an increase in NK cell function. The authors concluded that immune function might be enhanced

by massage and that anxiety reduction may be an important mediating factor.[76]

Massage and Mood State

Massage is reported to increase mental clarity, reduce anxiety, increase general feelings of well being, and release unexpressed emotions. Sims found that patients with cancer experienced improvements in mood state because of massage.[64]

■ Research Outcomes: Classical Western Massage

Classical Western massage has been researched as an intervention for anxiety and depression and for pain from juvenile arthritis, burns, surgery, cancer, and labor. It has been researched as a preparation for childbirth, as well as an intervention for premature infant development, infants exposed to HIV and cocaine, and patients with attention deficit hyperactivity disorder (ADHD), asthma, and other conditions. This research is reviewed in the following text.

Massage as Treatment for Anxiety and Depression

In a study of postpartum depression, 32 adolescent mothers received either massage or relaxation therapy. Massage subjects received two massages a week for 5 weeks, whereas relaxation subjects received two relaxation sessions a week for 5 weeks. Preintervention to postintervention, the massage group demonstrated a decrease in anxious behaviors and pulse rate. A significant reduction in depression and urinary cortisol levels across the course of the study were also noted for the massage group but not for the relaxation group.[24]

In an earlier study, 52 hospitalized depressed and adjustment-disordered children and adolescents either received a 30-minute back rub daily for 5 days or viewed a relaxing videotape for the same period. At the end of treatment, massaged subjects were less depressed and anxious and had lower saliva cortisol levels; they were observed to be less anxious and more cooperative and had increased nighttime sleep. Urinary cortisol and norepinephrine levels also decreased significantly, but only for the depressed patients.[29]

An interesting study assessed outcomes in 50 working adults receiving chair massage for 15 minutes two times a week for 5 weeks or resting in the massage chair for the same periods (Figure 13-10). Electroencephalographic (EEG) patterns, depression and anxiety scores, cortisol in saliva, and math

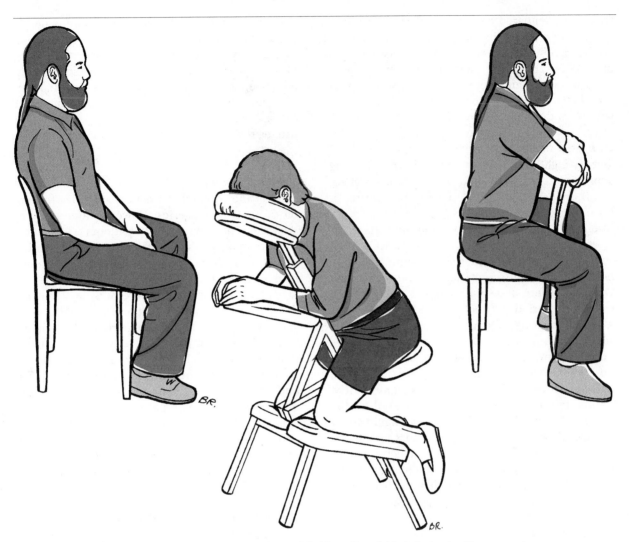

■ **Figure 13-10.** Forms of seated massage. *Modified from Fritz S:* Mosby's visual guide to massage essentials, *St Louis, 1996, Mosby.*

computation skills were evaluated before and after the sessions on the first and last days of massage. Frontal delta increased for both groups, suggesting relaxation. The massaged group demonstrated decreased frontal alpha and beta power, suggesting enhanced alertness, whereas control subjects increased these patterns, suggesting drowsiness. Further, the massage group demonstrated increased speed and accuracy on math computations, whereas the control scores did not change. Anxiety was reduced by massage but not by relaxation, although mood state was less depressed for both groups. Salivary cortisol levels decreased for massaged subjects, but only on the first day; controls demonstrated no cortisol changes. At the 5-week completion of the study, depression scores were lower for both groups, but job stress was lower for the massaged subjects only.[28]

Effects of Massage on Clinical Pain

Pain from Juvenile Rheumatoid Arthritis

Juvenile rheumatoid arthritis is the most common rheumatic disease of childhood and one of the most common chronic diseases of childhood.[10,47] Symptoms include night pain, joint stiffness during the morning, and pain after periods of inactivity. In a study by Field and others, 20 children with rheumatoid arthritis (1) were massaged by their parents for 15 minutes a day for 30 days, or (2) practiced relaxation 15 minutes a night with their parents. Relaxation involved conscious relaxation of large muscle groups. Parents were trained to administer both treatments. At the end of treatment, both the parents who massaged their children and the massaged children experienced lower anxiety, as determined by behavioral observation and lower stress hormone levels (e.g., salivary cortisol). As compared with those in the relaxation group, the children in the massage group experienced significantly less pain after massage, less pain over the week, and fewer severe pain episodes. Outcomes were based on observation of the child's anxiety level and by reports from the parents and the child's physician.[26]

Pain from Burns and Débridement Process

Twenty-eight adult patients with burns covering approximately 10% of their bodies were assigned, before débridement (the painful procedure of scrubbing off dead skin cells from a burn wound), to either a massage therapy group or a standard treatment control group. In the massage group, subjects were massaged for 20 minutes a day before their morning débridement session. Outcomes were assessed for day 1 and 5 of the treatment period. On both days, anxiety scores were significantly lower after the massage therapy session, and behavior observation ratings improved for pain effect, activity level, vocalization, and anxiety, but not for cooperation. Saliva cortisol levels also decreased significantly. Depression and anger scores, as assessed by the Profile of Mood States (POMS) also significantly decreased on both days. The authors concluded that massage reduced the pain of the débridement procedure because of the reduction in anxiety and that the clinical course was enhanced because of reductions in pain, anger, and depression.[30]

Pain from Surgery

In a study of the effects of massage on abdominal surgical pain, 39 patients admitted for abdominal surgery over a 5-month period were assigned to receive massage or to serve as control subjects.[54] The groups were equivalent in terms of age, gender, ethnicity, pain tolerance, medical and surgical history, dose and route of sedation and analgesia, surgical procedure, and previous experience with massage. A masseur, competent in Swedish massage techniques, trained 20 nurses who delivered the massage treatments. The quality of massage was monitored throughout the study. The experimental group was massaged for a minimum of 2 minutes a day, twice daily for 7 days or until discharge. No maximum time limit was set for delivery of massage. When controlled for age, perceptions of pain over the 24-hour postsurgical period were significantly lower for massaged patients (p=0.0037). Age was a significant covariate, with patients 41 to 60 years benefiting more from massage than other age groups. It was also noted that this older age group received massage an average of 13 minutes a day, whereas those younger than 41 received an average massage of only 5.77 minutes per day. Since the duration of massage may be a critical factor in its effectiveness, it cannot be assumed that the younger age groups would not have benefited equally had they received more massage time. Nurses reported they were more comfortable massaging older patients.

Pain from Cancer

Most of the research on cancer pain has focused on the use of analgesics. However, in a study by Weinrich and Weinrich, 28 patients with cancer were randomly assigned to a massage or control group. Massage patients were given a 10-minute back massage and control patients were visited for 10 minutes. For men, there was a significant decrease in the pain level immediately after massage, whereas the women experienced no significant reduction in pain. There was no significant difference in pain 1 and 2 hours after massage in comparison with the initial pain experience. The authors concluded that massage provided short-term relief of cancer pain for men but not for women.[71] Smaller studies reported similar outcomes. Ferrell-Torry and others, administering back massage to nine male patients with cancer, found that pain and anxiety were significantly decreased after massage.[22]

Labor, Delivery, and Massage

Touch and massage have been used during labor in nearly every culture for hundreds of years.[36] Massage during labor was used to improve or correct the position of the fetus, to stimulate uterine contractions, to prevent the fetus from rising back up in the abdomen, and to exert mechanical pressure to aid in the expulsion of the child.[20] Today, massage is typically centered on relaxation to reduce anxiety and alleviate pain during labor.

An association has been found between anxiety and labor discomfort. Fear of the unknown leads to sympathetic arousal, producing tension in the circular fibers of the uterus and rigidity at the opening of the cervix. This acts against the expulsive muscle fibers in labor.[57]

Prolonged uterine muscle tension can produce ischemia (local and temporary anemia caused by reduced blood flow), resulting in additional pain. Maternal anxiety can also result in increased catecholamines (sympathetic nervous system stimulators), producing a decrease in uterine contractility and blood flow and an increase in pain and maternal complications during delivery.[40]

During their last trimester of pregnancy, 28 women were recruited from Lamaze classes and randomly assigned to massage therapy or to a control group.[27] The groups did not differ on baseline variables. In the experimental group, a massage therapist taught partners how to massage their pregnant spouses. When the laboring women were cervically dilated approximately 3 cm to 5 cm, they received 20 minutes of head, shoulder, and back, and then hand and foot massage, respectively. The partner repeated the same 20 minutes of massage every hour for 5 hours. Women in the control group did not receive massage, but they were asked to engage in whatever activity they had been taught in class. Data from three sources—mother, partner, and trained observer—suggested that massage therapy reduced stress and pain during labor. The pregnant women reported that they experienced fewer depressed moods and less stress and labor pain, as well as feeling better after massage. By contrast, control mothers reported more labor pain during the same periods. Behavioral observers blinded to group assignment rated the massaged women as having lower activity and anxiety levels during labor.

Perineal Massage and Labor Outcomes

The perineum is the external surface area between the vulva and the anus in the woman. During a difficult labor, this area may tear or the physician may decide to perform an episiotomy—the surgical cutting of the vulva—to prevent it from tearing at the time of delivery. According to the 1990 National Hospital Discharge Survey, episiotomy is the most common surgical procedure in the United States, with 55.8 performed per 100 vaginal deliveries.[52]

Much has been written about perineal massage during pregnancy and during delivery as a method for reducing perineal tears. Information advocating the use of prebirth perineal massage has been widely disseminated by childbirth groups. The National Childbirth Trust advocates its use in its pregnancy book, as does the Active Birth Centre.[5] Some midwives and physicians also recommend this practice.

In one study, 10 women practiced perineal massage four times a week for several weeks, and 10 other women did not. The authors concluded that this practice lowered the incidence of episiotomies and lacerations.[3] However, the study sample was small and not limited to women experiencing their first childbirth. In a nonrandomized study of 55 nulliparous (first birth) women, those practicing perineal massage produced statistically better outcomes from those in the control group, leading the authors to suggest that perineal massage might be one technique to reduce the need for episiotomies.[4]

In a single-blind, randomized, controlled pilot study by Labrecque and others, 46 nulliparous women were randomized to practice perineal massage or to serve as controls.[43] Of the 22 assigned to the perineal massage group, 20 (91%) practiced their massage regularly. Although this study did not find that massage reduced perineal trauma, the number of subjects was too small to provide an adequate assessment of this fact. However, the women reported that perineal massage helped prepare them physically and psychologically for birth, and the study demonstrated that pregnant women appear to be motivated to practice their massage technique at least 60% of the time as a preparatory strategy for birth.

In a larger, randomized, single-blind prospective study, 861 nulliparous women were assigned to a massage or no-massage group.[63] Those practicing perineal massage demonstrated a reduction of 6.1% in second- and third-degree tears or episiotomies. There was a corresponding reduction in instrument deliveries of 6.3% (40.9% of the control group to 34.6% of the massage group). Both of these outcomes were statistically significant when adjusted for mother's age and infant's birth weight ($p=0.02$ and $p=0.03$, respectively). Analysis by mother's age demonstrated a much greater benefit of massage for those 30 years and older, as compared with mothers younger than 30 years of age. Women over 30, who practiced perineal massage, reduced perineal trauma by 12.1% and instrument delivery by 12.3%, as compared with unmassaged mothers over 30 years of age.

Massage Therapy for Infants

Beneficial effects have been recorded in infants as a function of neonatal stimulation, implying a potential plasticity in physical and behavioral development. The infant neonatal stimulation model, derived from the works of Denenberg and Levine, is now being applied in hospital nurseries to speed growth and development in premature infants.[18,45] Preliminary reports dealing with the effects of human neonatal stimulation began appearing in the literature in 1960 and have continued since that time. Most of the early data were merely suggestive, because research in this area is difficult to control. The following text reviews some of the studies related to massage and infant development.

Neonatal Development in Premature Infants

Problems with premature infants include unstable temperature regulation, inadequate respiration, feeding difficulties, poor sucking reflex, and poor weight gain. In 1960, Kulka began research to determine the effects of stimulation on infant weight gain. Her theory stated that a kinesthetic drive (i.e., the drive to alter position and produce sensation) developmentally predates the oral drive and is satisfied by means of stroking, fondling, cuddling, swaying motions, and rocking.[42] Since that time, studies have been forthcoming to assess the effects of tactile and kinesthetic stimulation on caloric intake, stooling, and weight gain in premature infants.

A study by White and Labarba sought to investigate the effects of tactile and kinesthetic stimulation on low–birth-weight babies in a hospital nursery.[73] The specific goal was to determine whether baby massage would result in weight gain. Twelve premature infants free from gross organic defects were assigned to an experimental or a control group by order of birth. All infants were bottle-fed from birth by choice of the mother. Within 48 hours of birth, each infant in the experimental group started the stimulation program. Massage was administered in 15-minute periods every hour for 4 consecutive hours beginning on day 2 after birth and ending on day 11. The infant's neck, shoulder, arms, legs, chest, and back were massaged and arms and legs passively flexed. Massagers remained silent during the massage period. Control infants received regular nursery care. At 10 days of treatment, the experimental infants gained significantly more weight, a gain of 257 grams for experimental infants as compared with 67 grams for control infants, representing 13.9% and 3.6% gains, respectively. Massaged babies also ingested more formula (mean increase 83 cc for massaged babies and 56 cc for control infants, an increase of 66% and 53%, respectively). The mean number of feedings over time was 7.9 for the experimental group and 8.6 for the control group. In spite of the fact that experimental babies were given fewer feedings, they were able to ingest more at each feeding than those in the control group. Although the number of infant subjects for this group was small, these findings suggested that touch may aid in the growth and development of premature infants.

Rausch reported similar findings in a study in which 40 premature infants were matched and divided into treatment and control groups.[56] Experimental infants received 15 minutes of massage once daily for the first 10 days after birth. Massage was administered in the morning when the infant was awake and receiving no therapy or feeding. Massage consisted of gentle rubbing of the infant's neck, back, chest, legs, thigh to foot, arms, shoulder to hand, head, and forehead to ear. At 10 days after birth, the control infants **lost** an average of 48 g and the massaged babies **gained** an average of 25 g. The difference, however, was not statistically significant. A statistically greater amount of food intake occurred for the massaged infants on days 6 through 10 (p<0.0001). By day 10, stooling frequency was significantly different between groups, with massaged infants producing 6.20 stools and controls 2.95 (p<0.004). The authors concluded that tactile and kinesthetic stimulation treatment improved the clinical course of premature infants.

A metaanalysis of 19 studies of infants receiving tactile stimulation found that 72% of infants receiving massage did better than control infants.[55] A delineation of which premature infants most benefited from massage had not yet been made. A study by Scafidi, Field, and Schanberg sought to remedy this issue.[62] Once considered medically stable, 93 preterm infants were randomly assigned to massage therapy or to a control group. Randomized stratification was undertaken to achieve equivalency between groups for gestational age, birth weight, duration of care in the intensive care unit, and entry weight. Gestational age of infants was between 26 and 36 weeks. Three 15-minute massage periods occurred once per hour for 3 consecutive hours. The first and third phases consisted of stroking different body parts, and the second phase involved moving the upper and lower limbs into flexion and extension. Massage was firmly administered with the flats of the fingers of both hands. The massaged infants gained significantly more weight per day than those in the control group (32 g versus 29 g). Both groups were then divided into high- and low-weight gainers. Of massaged infants, 70% were rated high-weight gainers and 40% of the control infants were rated high-weight gainers. Discriminate function analyses determined the characteristics that distinguished high- from low-weight gainers. For the massaged infants, the pattern of less caloric intake, more days in intermediate care, and more obstetric complications differentiated high- from low-weight gainers, suggesting that infants with more complications before the study benefited the most from massage. Control infants experienced the opposite effect (i.e., high-weight gainers consumed more calories, spent less time in intermediate care, and gained more weight prestudy enrollment). These variables accurately predicted 78% of the infants who benefited significantly from massage and are suggested as variables for selecting infants for enrollment in future massage therapy programs.

Special-Risk Infants

Perinatal transmission is responsible for approximately 80% of all pediatric patients with acquired immunodeficiency syndrome (AIDS), with pediatric AIDS and perinatal HIV infection becoming the leading infectious cause of developmental delays.[2,7,11,70] Only 22% to 39% of exposed infants are expected to be diagnosed as HIV positive. Very little research has been conducted on HIV-exposed but not HIV-positive infants. In an earlier study concerning Brazelton performance of HIV-exposed newborns, Field and others noted deficits in HIV-exposed versus nonexposed infants. Because exposed newborns showed inferior neonatal performance in the Scafidi and Field study and because at least 30% of a sample of exposed infants may be at risk for poor development because of infection, Scafidi and Field decided to investigate the effects of massage therapy on HIV-exposed infants.[61]

In this study, 24 neonates identified as exposed to HIV were randomly assigned to a massage or control group. Average gestational age was 29 weeks. All infants were bottle-fed. The same massage format was conducted as previously described—three 15-minute periods per hour for 3 consecutive hours for 10 days. Both groups were determined to be initially equivalent. At the end of the study, massaged infants had more optimal score changes for the Brazelton clusters of habituation, motor, range of state, and autonomic stability scores. Massaged infants also received better scores for excitability and stress behaviors. Finally, massaged infants averaged a significantly greater increase in weight. The results from this study are potentially surprising because these infants were essentially full term, unlike the previous studies for premature infants. The fact that the massaged infants improved while the control group infants remained the same or declined accounted for many of the score differences. In the absence of the compensatory treatment provided by stimulation, exposure to HIV may contribute to developmental delays and a failure to thrive as early as the newborn period. Deterioration in HIV-exposed infants apparently can be attenuated by massage therapy.

In another study, 30 preterm, cocaine-exposed infants (mean gestational age 30 weeks, intensive care duration 18 days) were randomly assigned to massage therapy or to a control group.[72] Random stratification occurred by gesta-

tional age, birth weight, intensive care duration, and entry weight. The same 15-minute massage per hour over 3 consecutive hours for 10 consecutive days was administered. Although the groups did not differ on calories or volume of food intake, the massage group averaged 28% greater weight gain per day (33 g versus 26 g). Massaged infants also demonstrated significantly fewer postnatal complications and stress behaviors than control infants and more mature motor behaviors, as determined by the Brazelton test.

Massage Therapy for Other Childhood Conditions

ADHD is a condition affecting 3% to 6% of the youthful population. ADHD is characterized by developmentally inappropriate degrees of inattention, impulsiveness, and hyperactivity, with overactivity its most prominent feature.[1] In a study by Field and others, 28 adolescents with ADHD were provided either massage therapy or relaxation therapy for 10 consecutive school days. Massaged adolescents rated themselves as happier, and observers rated them as fidgeting less. At 2 weeks, teachers reported the adolescents as spending more time on tasks and assigned them lower hyperactivity scores.[31]

In a study by Field and others, 16 children aged 4 to 8 and 16 children aged 9 to 14 were randomly assigned to receive massage or relaxation therapy.[25] The children's parents were trained to provide the treatments for 20 minutes before bedtime for 30 consecutive nights. The younger age group demonstrated an immediate decrease in anxiety and cortisol levels after massage, and their peak air flows and pulmonary functions improved over the course of the study. The older children also reduced anxiety, but only one pulmonary function improved (forced expiratory flow from 25% to 75%). Reductions in anxiety are key to the improvements demonstrated in this study, since anxiety is known to exacerbate asthma symptoms, especially in children. Although improvements were meaningful, no measurements of the actual underlying cause of asthma were performed. Caution must be taken in interpreting these outcomes as a "treatment" for asthma. Inflammation, the underlying cause of asthma and the cause of asthmatic deaths, was not evaluated in these studies.

Summary of Benefits of Massage for Infants and Children

Tactile or kinesthetic stimulation in the form of massage has been demonstrated to facilitate growth and development in healthy, preterm infants. These infants demonstrate greater weight gain, more mature awake and active behaviors, and more mature motor function.[72] HIV- and cocaine-exposed infants clearly benefit as well. In a review by Field, childhood conditions that have reportedly improved with massage included sexual and physical abuse, asthma, autism, burns, cancer, developmental delays, psoriasis, diabetes, bulimia, juvenile rheumatoid arthritis, posttraumatic stress disorder, and psychiatric problems.[23] Massage has generally demonstrated the capacity to lower anxiety and stress hormones and improve the clinical course for these conditions. Further, when grandparents, volunteers, and parents provided the massage therapy, their own sense of well being was benefited, as well as the well being of the patient.

An Expert Speaks: Dr. Tiffany Field

Tiffany Field, PhD, is currently the director of the Touch Research Institute (TRI), an institute she founded in 1992. Located at the University of Miami School of Medicine, TRI was the first center in the world devoted solely to the study of touch and its application in science and medicine.

Dr. Field has authored or co-authored numerous articles on the use of massage as therapeutic intervention. In the following interview, she describes her experiences with massage and the outcomes related to her research.

Question. Dr. Field, how did you become interested in research on touch therapy?

Answer. Some say that research is me-search. I became involved in massage therapy research when my daughter was born prematurely. We gave her massage therapy on a daily basis in an attempt to help her gain weight. Today she is 23 years old (going on 35) and is taller and smarter than I am, perhaps my best testimony to massage therapy being effective.

As a research psychologist, I have always needed to explore underlying mechanisms for why various therapies work. Many years have been spent exploring the question of why premature babies gain weight when they are massaged. These studies led to several other studies on other medical and psychiatric conditions, including growth and development, learning, depression, addictions, pain syndromes, autoimmune disorders, and job stress.

Question. Let's take them one at a time. Can you tell me about the growth and development studies?

Answer. In several studies in our lab and in at least three other labs, preterm babies gained in the range of 31% to 47% more weight following massage therapy. This resulted in their behavior also being improved and their being discharged earlier from the hospital (on an average of 5 to 10 days) with hospital cost savings approximating $10 to $15 thousand per day. If one considers that 470,000 preterm babies are born annually in the United States, the hospital cost savings associated with massage therapy would approximate $4 to $7 billion annually. Other types of preterm babies who have benefited from the massage therapy included cocaine-exposed preterm babies and HIV-exposed preterm babies.

We have discovered a cost-effective way to deliver the massage therapy, including having elderly volunteers massage the babies and teaching the parents massage. In one study on "grandparent" volunteers, we noted that the volunteers also benefited from massaging the infants. They were less depressed, their stress hormones were lower, and they engaged in better lifestyle habits, such as drinking less coffee, making more social phone calls, and taking fewer trips to the doctor's office. In a study where we massaged depressed mothers, we found that their depression levels and their stress hormones decreased; and [after] massaging their infants for a 1-month period, the infants became more interactive and they fell asleep sooner. The massage, in fact, was more effective than rocking to put the babies to sleep. When the massaged infants were followed out to 1 year of age, they continued to show a growth advantage—they were heavier babies—and at this time they showed a developmental advantage, performing better on infant mental and motor scales. Following several different possible underlying mechanisms, we have been able to show that massage therapy leads to a more physiologically organized state. Respiration, heart rate, and blood pressure are slower and stress hormones are decreased. This is probably explained by the increase in vagal activity—a slower, more relaxed state stimulated by the vagus nerve in the brain. In one study we measured vagal activity and noted that it was increased. The vegetative branch of the vagus nerve stimulated the release of food absorption hormones in the gastrointestinal tract, such as gastrin, glucose, and insulin. In the same study, we measured the levels of insulin, which significantly increased after massage therapy. The babies were gaining weight because of a relaxed state during which food absorption hormones were released. Food was then absorbed without any increases in formal intake.

Question. How does massage affect learning?

Answer. We know from studies with infants and young children that learning can be enhanced by massage therapy. In one study, the infant's limbs were massaged just before a learning task was given. The learning task was performed more quickly following the massage than when the infant was just allowed to play with a toy—a control condition. In a similar study with preschool children, briefly massaging the children [before] an I.Q. examination led to higher scores on the I.Q. tests.

Question. I understand that massage has also been researched for its effects on attention disorders. Can you describe some of that research for me?

Answer. One of the most difficult attention disorders is autism. Children with autism engage in stereotypical behaviors and are not very socially involved—they show more gaze aversion and touch aversion. In a study on children with autism, we were able to show that the children not only liked the massage, but they were also able to spend more time on task in the classroom; they related to their teachers better, and they showed fewer stereotypical behaviors.

In a similar study on children with attention deficit hyperactivity disorder, we were also able to show that following two 20-minute massages a week for 1 month, the children were able to stay on task in their classrooms more often and they also showed fewer disorderly behaviors.

One of the underlying mechanisms for these findings may also relate to enhanced vagal activity. The "smart" branch of the vagus slows down the heart and enables increased attentiveness. Typically, attention tasks are accompanied by increased vagal activity. This may explain the enhanced attentiveness observed in the children with autism and the children with attention deficit hyperactivity disorder.

Question. I understand that you have also researched the effects of massage on psychiatric disorders. Can you describe the findings from those studies?

Answer. In a study on children and adolescents who were hospitalized for depression, we provided 30-minute massages for 5 days. Following this period we noted that the children's sleep patterns were more organized, they spent more time in deep sleep and had fewer awakenings. They also showed a decrease in stress hormones including cortisol and norepinephrine levels.

In a study on children with posttraumatic stress disorder following hurricane Andrew, massage therapists visited their school and massaged them for 20 minutes twice a week for 1 month. Following this period, the children who received the massage versus children who sat on an adult's lap and watched a child video showed less depression, less anxiety, and fewer behavior problems; and their drawings were less disturbed. Their drawings were larger on the page, featured more colors and more animation, and their drawings of their faces were happier. One possible explanation for these data is the increase in serotonin levels noted following massage therapy. Serotonergic drugs, such as Prozac, are noted to have similar effects. Increasing the body's natural production of serotonin by massage therapy reduces the need for these antidepressant medications.

Question. How has massage been applied in the treatment of addictive behaviors?

Answer. To help people with smoking cravings, we taught them to massage their earlobes (or to massage their hands). We asked the subjects to massage themselves whenever they experienced a smoking craving. At the end of 1 month, the anxiety levels of the subjects decreased, the intensity of their smoking cravings decreased, and they were smoking one cigarette versus five cigarettes per hour; 27% of the subjects stop smoking.

In another study on eating disorders (anorexia and bulimia), adolescent girls were provided a 20-minute massage twice a week for 4 weeks. Their weight not only normalized, but they showed decreased depression and improved body image. The reduction of stress and stress hormones may lead to the lesser need for addictive behavior. Similarly, the increase in antidepressant natural hormones in the body, such as serotonin, may alleviate the craving intensity. Finally, a very simple behavioral explanation is that you are replacing one activity with another activity when you replace smoking with earlobe rubbing.

Question. Pain has become an increasing problem in our society. How is massage helpful for pain management?

Answer. Several theories exist as to why massage therapy may alleviate pain. In the "gate theory," the notion is that the pressure receptors stimulated by massage therapy are longer and more myelinated—better insulated—than pain receptors. So, when pain is experienced and the painful part is rubbed, the pressure message gets to the brain more quickly than the pain message and the gate is shut, thus disallowing the entry of the pain message. Much of this undoubtedly occurs via chemical messages. Another possibility is that the pain syndrome is being mediated by sleep disturbance. In the absence of adequate amounts of deep sleep, substance P, which transmits pain, is emitted. If massage therapy can enhance deep sleep, which we know it can, then substance P levels and the pain that it causes should be lower.

In one of the most excruciatingly painful procedures, skin brushing following burns, we have shown that if you massage the patients for 30 minutes before the skin brushing, their anxiety levels are lower and their pain thresholds are higher. They experience less pain in the procedure.

In a study on juvenile rheumatoid arthritis, we have been able to show that massage therapy by the parents of the children for 15 minutes every night before bedtime manages to decrease pain as reported by the child, the parents, and the physician. The pain-limiting activities are also increased.

In another study on lower back pain in which the massage focused on the lower back region, we noted fewer lower back pain days and increases in range of motion, such as being better able to touch one's toes and better able to perform activities of daily living.

There was a study on migraine headaches in which the massage focused on the area at the base of the skull. Migraine-free days increased. Similar data were noted for premenstrual syndrome. In addition, in that study the women had lower levels of water retention and reduced pain.

Chronic debilitating conditions that lead to significant absenteeism and worker's compensation are chronic fatigue syndrome and fibromyalgia. Both of these conditions appear to have an underlying component of depression that may be contributing to the syndrome, as well as resulting from the syndrome.

Following a month of two 20-minute massages per week—as compared with the control group who received transcutaneous electrical stimulation—the [patients with] chronic fatigue syndrome and fibromyalgia syndrome experienced less depression, lower anxiety levels, and lower stress hormones. In addition to their reporting less pain, they also reported significant improvement of sleep. As was already mentioned, massage therapy may facilitate pain reduction by enhancing sleep and thereby decreasing substances like substance P that cause pain that are emitted in the absence of sleep.

Question. Some of the toughest medical conditions facing us today involve autoimmune and immune disorders. Has massage been found to benefit these types of conditions?

Answer. We have studied a number of autoimmune conditions including asthma, dermatitis, and diabetes. In all of these studies, parents massaged their children for 15 minutes before bedtime so that it would become part of the bedtime ritual and so that parents would have a positive involvement in treatment. In diabetes, for example, parents often have the undesirable task of having to monitor blood glucose levels, provide insulin injections, and make sure their children comply with their diet. Teaching the parents to apply massage therapy gives them a positive form of treatment and makes them feel empowered by being part of the treatment process.

In children with asthma, the massage therapy over a 1-month period resulted in increased peak air flow and all the other functions measured by the pulmonologist, including forced vital capacity, forced expiratory volume, and peak expiratory flow. In children with eczema, parents were asked to massage their child in addition to applying the therapeutic ointments. The control group simply received the therapeutic ointments. After 1 month of massages, the children with dermatitis showed improvement on all the measures considered gold standard by the dermatologist, including redness, lichenification scaling, excoriation, and pruritus. In the cases of children with diabetes, the most salient measures that improved were a decrease in blood glucose levels from a high value of 158 to a value within the normal range of 118, and the parents' report that the children were more compliant with their diet.

In our studies on immune disorders we invariably note an increase in natural kill cell activity. Natural killer cells, being the front line of the defense system, are critical for killing off viral cells and cancer cells. When cortisol levels are decreased, immune cells are invariably increased, inasmuch as cortisol typically destroys immune cells.

In HIV studies on men and adolescents, we have noted not only a reduction in the stress hormones cortisol and norepinephrine after a month of massage, but also an increase in the number of natural killer cells, an increase in natural killer cell activity level, and, in the case of adolescents, we also noted an increase in the cells that are typically killed off by the HIV virus (CD4 cells). In studies on cancer—leukemia in children and breast cancer—we have noted a similar increase in natural killer cells, which presumably would slow down the disease as natural killer cells ward off cancer cells.

Question. We have discussed the chronic and life threatening diseases. What about the daily stresses we all face?

Answer. In one of the most exciting prevention studies, we provided hospital employees with 10-minute massages during their lunch hour. The massage not only led to decreased stress, but the subjects reported a sense of heightened alertness, much like a "runners' high." We monitored the EEG waves and noted that the EEG patterns also conformed to a state of heightened alertness. Namely, alpha waves, which normally increase during sleep, were decreased after massage. In addition, performance on a math computation—adding a series of numbers—improved after a massage. The subjects were able to perform the math test in half the time with half the errors.

Question. Is there anything else you would like the reader to know?

Answer. We have discussed some of the research highlights from the Touch Research Institutes. They strongly suggest the need for replications from other laboratories and for additional research on the underlying mechanisms. Nonetheless, the data are significantly rigorous to suggest that it is a good thing that massage therapy is one of the fastest growing professions in the United States. Following up on reports that some 48% of American people are buying alternative medicine out of their own pockets—one of the most popular being massage therapy—insurance companies and HMOs will presumably take this consumer preference seriously and cover these forms of therapy. They may not only be effective as treatments, but as potentiators of drug effects so that people have less need to take as much medication and as prevention measures to help people find wellness. In my view, massage therapy should be right up there with a good diet and daily exercise.

■ Indications and Contraindications

In summary, massage is indicated for:
1. Relaxation and anxiety reduction
2. Enhanced circulation, for example, in pregnant women with back and leg strain
3. Enhanced digestion and elimination
4. Enhanced development and growth of premature infants or children who are not thriving because of touch deprivation
5. Exercise recovery and preparation

6. The bedridden and those suffering from chronic diseases that prevent adequate exercise

Massage is contraindicated for the person who has:
1. Nausea, severe pain, fever, or has been seriously injured recently (a local contraindication).
2. Rashes, boils, open wounds, athlete's foot, herpes simplex—cold sores, or impetigo—skin infection caused by *Staphylococcus* or *Streptococcus*.
3. Pathologic condition that may spread through the lymph or circulatory systems, such as lymphangitis—an inflammation of the lymphatic vessels or blood poisoning; malignant melanoma—a cancerous mole or tumor that metastasizes or spreads easily through the bloodstream or lymph system; or swollen glands. (Swollen glands attempt to filter out bacteria and pathogens, and draining may cause an infection to spread.)
4. Bleeding, such as occurs in a bruised area, where whiplash or any other acute trauma has occurred (a local contraindication).
5. Acute inflammation, as demonstrated by fever; inflamed joints, because of rheumatoid arthritis; or locally inflamed tissues that demonstrate redness, heat, or swelling.
6. Cardiac arrhythmias or carotid bruit, phlebitis, severe arteriosclerosis, or severe varicose veins.
7. Decreased sensation because of stroke, diabetes, or medication (e.g., muscle relaxants). (Patient may be unable to provide adequate feedback on pressure. Caution must also be taken in persons with hyperesthesia or increased sensitivity to touch.)
8. Recently undergone surgery with artificial joint replacements, chronic sacroiliac joint subluxation, or severe rheumatoid arthritis. (Massage only on physician recommendation.)
9. Acute edema from trauma; inflammation from bacterial or viral infection; pitted edema indicating tissue fragility; lymphatic obstruction from parasites; and edema from deep vein thrombosis. (Edema or swelling in the interstitial spaces may be either an indication or contraindication for massage, depending on the circumstances.)
10. Under the influence of alcohol and recreational drugs. (Caution must be exercised if the patient is taking certain prescribed medications that result in numbing, prevent blood clotting, or significantly alter mood state. Massage only on physician recommendation.)

■ Ongoing Research

Research studies on the effects of massage continue to multiply. At the Touch Institute in Florida, studies underway include the following:

- Infant studies: cerebral palsy, sudden infant death syndrome, preterm birth
- Child studies: abuse, autism, burns, coma, Down syndrome, HIV, pediatric oncology, sickle cell anemia
- Adolescent studies: HIV, violence
- Adult studies: breast cancer, carpal tunnel syndrome, fibromyalgia sleep disorder, pregnancy depression, spinal cord injuries, fathers massaging infants

■ Chapter Review

Historically, massage was believed to be a curative treatment for a variety of medical and psychologic conditions. Today, research in this field seems to support many of those original beliefs. Touch can, in the right circumstances, result in increased healing capacities. It behooves the health practitioner and patients to familiarize themselves with massage research and its potential benefits.

Matching Terms and Definitions

Match each numbered definition with the correct term. Place the corresponding letter in the space provided.

a. Massage

b. Tiffany Field

c. Classical Western techniques

d. George Taylor

e. Massage parlors

f. Emerging techniques

g. Tuina

h. Vis medicatrix naturae

i. Anma

j. Hippocrates

k. Pehr Henrik Ling

_____ 1. Father of modern medicine

_____ 2. Group of manual techniques that include applying fixed or movable pressure, and/or causing movement of or to the body

_____ 3. Japanese form of massage

_____ 4. Ancient Chinese form of massage

_____ 5. Techniques traditionally used in Europe and the United States since the nineteenth century

_____ 6. Author of the General Principles of Gymnastics

_____ 7. One of the physician brothers who brought "Swedish movement cure" to the United States

_____ 8. One of the reasons massage declined

_____ 9. The current leader in massage therapy

_____ 10. Aiding the body in its ability to heal itself

_____ 11. Hellerwork, Trager, Feldenkrais

CRITICAL THINKING AND CLINICAL APPLICATION EXERCISES

1. Discuss the societal changes resulting in the reemergence of massage in the 1960s and later.
2. Describe and elaborate on the mechanisms explaining the effects of massage.
3. Explain the effects of massage on immune function.
4. Compare and contrast the effects of massage on premature infants and on special-risk infants.

References

1. Anderson, Williams, McGee, Silva: *DSM-III-R,* Washington, DC, 1987, American Psychiatric Association.
2. Armstrong FD, Seidel JF, Swales TP: Pediatric HIV infection: a neuropsychological and educational challenge, *J Learn Disabil* 26:92, 1993.
3. Avery M, Burke B: Effect of perineal massage on the incidence of episiotomy and perineal laceration in a nurse midwifery service, *J Nurse Midwifery* 31:128, 1986.
4. Avery M, Van Arsdale L: Perineal massage, effect on the incidence of episiotomy and laceration in a nulliparous population, *J Nurse Midwifery* 32:181, 1987.
5. Balaskas J: *New active birth: a concise guide to natural childbirth,* London, 1991, Thorsons.
6. Bell AJ: Massage and the physiotherapist, *Physiotherapy* 50:406, 1964.
7. Belman AL: AIDS and pediatric neurology, *Neurol Clin* 8:571, 1990.
8. Benjamin PJ: *The California revival: massage therapy in the 1970-80's,* Los Angeles, 1996, AMTA National Education Conference.
9. Brennen B, Demmerle A, Patterson M et al: Manual healing methods. In *Alternative medicine: expanding medical horizons: a report to the National Institutes of Health on alternative medicine systems and practices in the United States,* Bethesda, MD, 1994, National Institutes of Health.
10. Cassidy JT, Petty RE: *Textbook of pediatric rheumatology,* ed 3, Philadelphia, 1995, WB Saunders.
11. Centers for Disease Control: Update: acquired immunodeficiency syndrome—United States, *Morbidity Mortality Weekly* 39:81, 1989.
12. Chopra D: *Perfect health: the complete mind/body guide,* New York, 1991, Harmony Books.
13. Claire T: *Body work: what type of massage to get, and how to make the most of it,* New York, 1995, William Morrow.
14. Collinge W: *The American Holistic Health Association complete guide to alternative medicine,* New York, 1996, Warner Books.
15. Corley MC, Ferriter J, Zeh J, Gifford C: Physiological and psychological effects of back rubs, *Appl Nurs Res* 8(1):39, 1995.
16. Corwin EJ: *Handbook of pathophysiology,* Philadelphia, 1996, Lippincott.
17. Day JA, Mason RR, Chesrown SE: Effect of massage on serum level of B-endorphin in healthy adults, *Phys Ther* 67(6):926, 1987.
18. Denenberg VS: Critical periods, stimulus input, and emotional reactivity: a theory of infantile stimulation, *Psychol Rev* 71:335, 1964.
19. Eisenberg DM, Kessler RC, Foster C, Norlock FE, Calkins DR, Delblanco TL: Unconventional medicine in the United States, *N Engl J Med* 328(4):246, 1993.
20. Engelman G: *Labour among primitive peoples,* St Louis, 1982, JH Chambers.
21. Fakouri C, Jones P: Relaxation Rx: slow stroke back rub, *J Gerontol Nurs* 13(2):32, 1987.
22. Ferrell-Torry AT et al: The use of therapeutic massage as a nursing intervention to modify anxiety and the perception of cancer pain, *Cancer Nurs* 16(2):93, 1993.
23. Field T: Massage therapy for infants and children, *J Dev Behav Pediatr* 16(2):105, 1995.
24. Field T, Grizzle N, Scafidi F, Schanberg S: Massage and relaxation therapies' effects on depressed adolescent mothers, *Adolescence* 31(124):903, 1996.
25. Field T, Henteleff T, Hernandez-Reif M, Martinez E, Mavunda K, Kubn C, Schanberg S: Children with asthma have improved pulmonary functions after massage therapy, *J Pediatr* 132:854, 1998.
26. Field T, Hernandez-Reif M, Seligman S, Krasnegor J, Sunshine W, Rivas-Chacon R, Schanberg S, Kuhn C: Juvenile rheumatoid arthritis: benefits from massage therapy, *J Pediatr Psychol* 22:607, 1997.
27. Field T, Hernandez-Reif M, Taylor S, Quintino O, Burman I: Labor pain is reduced by massage therapy, *J Psychosom Obstetr Gynaecol* 18:286, 1997.
28. Field T, Ironson G, Scafidi F, Nawrocki T, Goncalves A, Burman I, Pickens J, Fox N, Schanberg S, Kuhn C: Massage therapy reduces anxiety and enhances EEG pattern of alertness and math computations, *Int J Neurosci* 86:197, 1996.
29. Field T, Morrow C, Valdeon C, Larson S, Kuhn C, Schanberg S: Massage reduces anxiety in child and adolescent psychiatric patients, *J Am Acad Child Adolesc Psychiatry* 31(1):125, 1992.
30. Field T, Peck M, Krugman S, Tuchel T, Schanberg S, Kuhn C, Burman I: Burn injuries benefit from massage therapy, *J Burn Care Rehabil* 19:241, 1998.
31. Field T, Quintino O, Hernandez-Reif M, Koslovsky G: Adolescents with attention deficit hypersensitivity disorder benefit from massage therapy, *Adolescence* 33(129):103, 1998.
32. Georgii A: *Kinetic jottings,* London, 1880, Henry Renshaw.
33. Green R, Green M: Relaxation increases salivary immunoglobulin A1, *Psycholog Rep* 61:623, 1987.
34. Greene E: Study links stress reduction with faster healing, *Massage Ther J* 35(1):16, 1996.
35. Groer M, Mozingo J, Droppleman P, Davis M, Jolly M, Boynton M, Davis K, Kay S: Measures of salivary secretory immunoglobulin A and state anxiety after a nursing back rub, *Appl Nurs Res* 7:2, 1994.
36. Hedstrom LW, Newton N: Touch in labor: a comparison of cultures and eras, *Birth* 13:181, 1986.
37. Ironson G, Field T, Scafidi F, Hashimoto M, Kurar M, Kumar A, Price A, Goncalves A, Burman I, Tetenman C, Patarca R, Fletcher MA: Massage therapy is associated with enhancement of the immune system's cytotoxic capacity, *Int J Neurosci* 84:205, 1996.
38. Kaard B, Tostinbo O: Increase of plasma beta endorphins in a connective tissue massage, *Gen Pharmacol* 20(4):487, 1989.
39. Kaufman MA: Autonomic responses as related to nursing comfort measures, *Nurs Res* 13:45, 1964.
40. Kennell J, Klaus M, McGrath S, Robertson S, Hickey C: Continuous emotional support during labor in a U.S. hospital, *JAMA* 265(2):197, 1991.
41. Kleen EA: *Massage and medical gymnastics,* New York, 1921, William Wood & Company.
42. Kulka AC, Fry ST, Goldstein FJ: Kinesthetic needs in infancy, *Am J Orthopsychiatry* 30:562, 1960.
43. Labrecque M, Arcoux S, Pinault J, Laroche C, Martin S: Prevention of perineal trauma by perineal massage during pregnancy: a pilot study, *Birth* 21(1):20, 1994.
43a. Labyak SE, Metzger BL: The effects of effleurage backrub on the physiological components of relaxation: a meta-analysis, *Nurs Res* 46(1):59, 1997.
44. Leboyer F: *Loving hands: the traditional art of baby massage,* New York, 1982, Alfred A. Knopf.
45. Levine S: The psychophysiological effects of infantile stimulation. In Bliss E, editor: *Roots of behavior: genetics, instinct and socialization in animal behavior,* New York, 1962, Hoeber.
46. Longworth J: Psychophysiological effects of slow stroke back massage in normotensive females, *Adv Nurs Sci* 4(4):44, 1982.
47. Lovell T, Walco G: Pain associated with juvenile rheumatoid arthritis, *Pediatr Clin North Am* 36:4, 1989.
48. Madison AS: Psychophysiological responses of female nursing home residents to back massage: an investigation of the effect of one type of touch. Doctoral Dissertation, University of Maryland, *Dissertation Abstr Int* 35:914B, 1973.
49. Malkin K: Use of massage in clinical practice, *Br J Nurs* 3(6):292, 1994.
50. Melzack R, Wall PD: Pain mechanisms: a new theory, *Science* 150:971, 1965.

51. Monte T: *World medicine: the East and West guide to healing your body,* New York, 1993, Putnam.
52. National Center for Health Statistics: *National hospital discharge survey: annual summary 1990,* Rockville, MD, 1992, The Center.
53. Nissen H: *Practical massage and corrective exercise with applied anatomy,* Philadelphia, 1920, FA Davis.
54. Nixon M, Teschendorff J, Finney J, Karnilowicz W: Expanding the nursing repertoire: the effect of massage on post-operative pain, *Aust J Adv Nurs* 14(3):21, 1997.
55. Ottenbacher KJ, Muller L, Brandt D et al: The effectiveness of tactile stimulation as a form of early intervention: a quantitative evaluation, *J Dev Behav Pediatr* 8:68, 1987.
56. Rausch PB: Effects of tactile and kinesthetic stimulation on premature infants, *J Obstetr Gynecol Neonatal Nurs* 34, 1981.
57. Read D: *Childbirth without fear: the principles and practices of natural childbirth,* New York, 1972, New York Press.
58. Reed BV, Held JM: Effects of sequential connective tissue massage on autonomic nervous system of middle-aged and elderly adults, *Phys Ther* 68(8):1231, 1988.
59. Robbins G, Powers D, Burgess S: *A wellness way of life,* ed 2, Madison, Wis. 1994, Brown 7 Benchmark.
60. Roth M: *The prevention and cure of many chronic diseases by movements,* London, 1851, John Churchill.
61. Scafidi FA, Field T: Massage therapy improves behavior in neonates born to HIV-positive mothers, *J Pediatr Psychol* 21(6):889, 1996.
62. Scafidi FA, Field T, Schanberg SM: Factors that predict which preterm infants benefit most from massage therapy, *Dev Behav Pediatr* 14(3):176, 1993.
63. Shipman MK, Boniface DR, Teff ME, McCloughry F: Antenatal perineal massage and subsequent perineal outcomes: a randomised controlled trial, *Br J Obstetr Gynaecol* 104:787, 1997.
64. Sims S: Slow stroke back massage for cancer patients, *Nurs Times* 82(13):47, 1986.
65. Smith L, Keating MN, Holbert D, Spratt DJ, McCammon MR, Smith SS, Israe RG: The effects of athletic massage on delayed onset muscle soreness, creatine kinase, and neutrophil count: a preliminary report, *J Sports Phys Ther* 19(2):93, 1994.
66. Sunshine W, Field T, Schanberg S, Quintino O, Kilmer T, Fierro K, Burman I, Hashimoto M, McBride C, Henteleff T: Massage therapy and transcutaneous electrical stimulation effects on fibromyalgia, *J Clin Rheumatol* 2:18, 1996.
67. Tappan FM, Benjamin PJ: *Tappan's handbook of healing massage techniques: classic, holistic, and emerging methods,* ed 3, Stamford, Conn, 1998, Appleton & Lange.
68. Taylor A: *The principles and practice of physical therapy,* ed 3, Stanley Thornes, 1991, Cheltenham.
69. Tyler D, Winslow E, Clark A, White K: Effects of a 1-minute back rub on mixed venous oxygen saturation and heart rate in critically ill patients, *Heart Lung* 19:562, 1990.
70. Ultmann MH, Belman AL, Ruff HA, Novick BE, Cone-Wesson B, Cohen HJ, Rubenstein A: Developmental abnormalities in children with acquired immunodeficiency syndrome (AIDS) and AIDS-related complex, *Dev Med Child Neurol* 27:563, 1985.
71. Weinrich SP, Weinrich MC: The effect of massage on pain in cancer patients, *Appl Nurs Res* 3(4):140, 1990.
72. Wheeden A, Scafidi FA, Field T, Ironson G, Valdeon C, Bandstra E: Massage effects on cocaine-exposed preterm neonates, *Dev Behav Pediatr* 14(5):318, 1993.
73. White JL, Labarba RC: The effects of tactile and kinesthetic stimulation on neonatal development in the premature infant, *Dev Psychobiol* 9(6):569, 1976.
74. Wood EC, Becker PD: *Beard's massage,* ed 3, Philadelphia, 1981, WB Saunders.
75. Zanolla R, Monzeglio C, Balzarini A, Martino G: Evaluations of the results of three different methods of postmastectomy lymphedema treatment, *J Surg Oncol* 26:210, 1984.
76. Zeitlin D, Keller SE, Shiflett SC, Schleifer SJ, Bartlett JA, Eckholdt HM, Niu H-L: Unpublished data, Kessler Medical Rehabilitation Research and Education Corporation, Center for Research in Complementary and Alternative Medicine West Orange, New Jersey.
77. Zumo Li: 235 cases of frozen shoulder treated by manipulation and massage, *J Tradit Chin Med* 4(3):213, 1984.

Complementary Self-Help Strategies

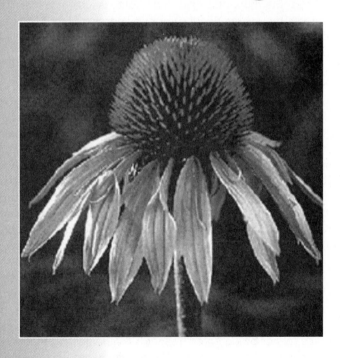

14

Herbs as Medical Intervention

Lyn W. Freeman

WHY READ THIS CHAPTER?

Herbal medicines are the fastest growing category of alternative therapies in the United States. Yet, there are challenging issues to be considered when using herbal phytomedicines. What are the benefits of a particular herb? Has an herbal product been controlled for quality? Are there side effects? Will a particular herb cross-react with a patient's prescription medication? What do the clinically controlled trials reveal about an herb's efficacy and its side effects? This chapter will answer these questions for 10 popular herbs sold in the United States today. Most importantly, this chapter assists the reader in the development of an herbal "thinking style" so that critical information can be sought concerning any herbal product the reader must evaluate. Can herbal medications be beneficial? Yes. Are there also risks and quality issues that must be addressed? Absolutely. This chapter delineates the informational categories necessary for evaluating the benefits and risks of herbal products.

CHAPTER AT A GLANCE

Plants used for medicinal purposes, rather than for food, are referred to as "herbs" or "medicinal herbs." Physical evidence of the use of herbal remedies dates back approximately 60,000 years, and more than one fourth of prescription medicines have been developed from herbs.

For centuries, it was believed that each herbal plant was a gift from God and contained a "sign," intended to give humankind clues as to the herb's healing effects. This belief was referred to as the "doctrine of signatures." Today, herbals are still used for their healing abilities, and herbal phytomedicine is the fastest growing alternative therapy in the United States.

Germany has been the premier world leader in developing a mechanism designed to ensure herbal safety and efficacy. Herbs, in Germany, are reviewed and approved in the same manner as drugs. The creation of the German Commission E expert panel resulted in the development of monographs, which provide the most accurate data in the world today on the safety and efficacy of herbals.

In the United States, the Food and Drug Administration (FDA) evaluates the safety and efficacy of new drugs based on data supplied by the drug manufacturer. The process of demonstrating new drug safety and efficacy takes approximately 15 years and costs an estimated $500 million. Since herbal remedies cannot be patented, research companies in the United States are unlikely to invest the time and money necessary to meet FDA requirements. This means that the quality of herbal products in the United States is not as controlled as it is in Europe.

In this chapter, 10 popular herbs are discussed in detail: bilberry, cranberry, echinacea, feverfew, Ginkgo biloba, goldenseal, kava kava, milk thistle, saw palmetto, and St. John's wort. The categories of information provided on these herbs include description and history; pharmacology and action; recommended key uses; and dosage, toxicity, and side effects. These informational categories should be evaluated when considering the use of any herbal as medical intervention.

> First the word, then the plant, lastly the knife.
>
> AESCULAPIUS OF THASSALY, GREEK GOD OF HEALING, CIRCA 1200 BC.

CHAPTER OBJECTIVES

After completing this chapter, you should be able to:

1. Describe 10 herbs and discuss the history of each.
2. Explain the pharmacology and actions of the herbs discussed in this chapter.
3. List the key recommended uses for these herbs.
4. Delineate their dosage, toxicity, and side effects.
5. Summarize the findings from clinically controlled trials for the 10 herbs discussed in this chapter.
6. Outline the key categories of information that should be gathered on herbal products before considering their use.

■ Description and History of Medicinal Herbs

Plants used for medicinal purposes, rather than for food, are referred to as "herbs" or "medicinal herbs." Physical evidence of the use of herbal remedies dates back approximately 60,000 years. In 1960, a burial site of a Neanderthal man was uncovered, along with the herbs used to treat him. This burial site revealed eight different species of plants that had been gathered by community members to treat the man. Seven of those species are still used for medicinal purposes today.[156]

Herbs have been used as medicine by all cultures; even animals in the wild "partake" of herbal medicines. Chimpanzees swallow, without chewing, a medicinal herb called *Aspilia*. The chimpanzees do not chew *Aspilia* because it tastes bad, and they are observed to grimace when they swallow it. Chimps chew the herb at dawn, before the sun activates certain dangerous chemical compounds. *Aspilia* has been demonstrated to kill parasites, fungi, and bacteria. Local villagers also use *Aspilia* for medicinal purposes, and both chimps and humans carefully select the same three species of *Aspilia* while neglecting a fourth, presumably because of the medicinal differences of the four species.[23] The African villagers swallow the leaves as treatment for stomachaches and rub crushed leaves on wounds or cuts.

Medications Developed from Herbs

We owe a great deal to herbs and their medicinal properties. For example, the chemical basis for aspirin was originally discovered in white willow bark *(Salix alba),* and aspirin was later synthesized from the same chemical in meadowsweet *(Spiraea ulmaria).* The opium poppy gave us our first narcotic, and the birth control pill was derived from a Mexican yam called *Dioscorea villosa.* Taxol, used to treat breast and ovarian cancers, was originally found in the Pacific yew called *Taxus* and later discovered in the more common ornamental yew used as a hedging bush. Vincristine and vinblastine, used in cancer treatments, come from the Madagascar periwinkle *Catharanthus roseus.*

Herbs Used as Treatments

Herbal medicine involves whole plants or parts of plants, such as the bark, fruit, stem, root, or seed. Herbs can be purchased fresh or dried, in pills or capsules, and in *tinctures* that are preserved in alcohol, glycerin, or some other liquid. The term *standardized extract* means that a herbal medicine is guaranteed to contain a specific amount of a particular active ingredient. This is an important consideration because the active ingredient can vary even in the same part of a particular plant grown in different seasons, soils, or climates. Obviously, extracts can only be standardized when the active ingredient is known.

■ Philosophy Underlying the Development of Herbal Medicine

Herbs have long been viewed in certain cultures as a healing "gift" from God. For centuries, it was believed that each herbal plant contained a "sign" left by God, intended to give humanity clues as to the herb's healing effects. This concept was called the *Doctrine of Signatures.* Examples of this include goldenseal, whose yellow-green root indicates its use for jaundice; lobelia, with flowers shaped like a stomach, reflecting its emetic (nausea-inducing) qualities; and cohosh, whose branches are arranged like limbs in spasm, representing its ability to treat muscular spasm.[62]

As reading and writing became more common, *Materia Medica,* or books that taught about herbs and their healing properties, became the best method for passing on the "art" of herbology. *Materia Medica* in China, Babylon, Egypt, India, Greece, and other parts of the world demonstrated the acceptance of the healing powers of plants.

In the 1500s, Paracelsus, an alchemist who believed in the Doctrine of Signatures, became the founder of modern pharmaceutical medicine. He is best remembered for prescribing laudanum (tincture of opium).

In the early 1600s, Nicholas Culpepper, an English pharmacist, published *The English Physician,* an herbal book that recommended that patients grow their own herbs rather than buy expensive exotic or imported drugs. Culpepper published his book during the time when professional physicians were beginning to become contemptuous of herbal medicine. Culpepper's book was the beginning of an established and strong English tradition of domestic herbal medicine. Even so, mercury for the treatment of syphilis, as well as bleeding and purging, were still "standard" medical practices of the day. During this same time, George Washington was reportedly bled to death by his physicians in an effort to treat his sore throat.

Flexner Report and the Downfall of Herbal Medicine

In the early 1800s, the *Eclectic Movement* became popular in the United States. This movement included an attempt to bridge the gap between standard medical thought and traditional herbal medicines. The herbal eclectics sought to educate physicians about herbal medicines and established several medical colleges.

In the mid 1800s, the medical system we now refer to as "biomedicine" began to dominate orthodox medicine in the United States. Its basic concepts were that bacteria and viruses cause disease; and certain substances, like vaccines and antitoxins, can improve health. With this movement, births and deaths, which typically occurred in the home, were moved to hospitals. Scientific research methods and adequate medical training for medical schools were sorely lacking during this time. In the late 1800s, the American Medical Association (AMA), which was first organized in 1847, sponsored and lobbied for enactment of state licensing laws. By 1900, every state had such an enactment.

The future of competing forms of medicine was sealed with the release of a report by Abraham Flexner, a U.S. educator and founder of the Institute for Advanced Study at Princeton, New Jersey. The report, "Medical Education in the United States and Canada," was funded by the Carnegie Foundation and was instrumental in upgrading medical education. It also enabled medical schools, with their greater orientation toward biomedicine research, to receive preferential treatment from large philanthropic foundations that were awarding money for medical education. Indirectly, this development led to the demise of more financially strapped schools of alternative medicine.

Although this report is properly credited with closing many substandard medical teaching establishments, an unfortunate side effect was a complete stifling of all competing schools of thought regarding the origins of illness and the appropriateness of therapies. This occurred even though Flexner had no knowledge of medical science, the scientific methods, or their potential shortcomings. In fact, years after his report was published, Flexner became increasingly disenchanted with the rigidity of educational standards that had become identified with his name. By 1938, all eclectic medical schools had closed.[126]

Meanwhile, traditional medical schools, supported by the Rockefeller Foundation, flourished. The growth of the modern pharmaceutical industry was assured by the downfall of natural forms of healing and the emphasis on biomedicine.

Herbal Use in Germany and the United States: A Twentieth Century Comparison

Germany has been the premier world leader in developing a mechanism to ensure herbal safety and efficacy. In 1976, the Federal Republic of Germany defined herbal remedies in the same manner as other drugs. In 1978, the Federal Health Agency established an expert committee on herbal remedies to evaluate the safety and efficacy of phytomedicines. This expert panel was called the *German Commission E,* and it included physicians, pharmacists, pharmacologists, toxicologists, representatives of the pharmaceutical industry, and lay persons.

Therapeutic use of herbs and phytomedicines is very popular in Germany, where 600 to 700 different plant drugs are currently sold in pharmacies, health food stores, and markets. Approximately 70% of physicians in general practice prescribe registered herbal remedies, and a significant portion of the $1.7 billion annual sales is paid for by government health insurance. In 1988, in excess of 5.4 million prescriptions were written for Ginkgo biloba extract alone.[18]

The German Commission E checks herbal data independently. Data are evaluated from clinical trials, field studies, case studies, and the expertise of medical associations. This process allows the German Commission E to determine, with "reasonable certainty," the safety and efficacy of the herb being evaluated.

The German Commission E's recommendations became available in English in 1998. The American Botanical Council's *The Complete German Commission E Monographs: Therapeutic Guide to Herbal Medicines* was published by Integrative Medicine and is considered the most accurate information available in the world on the safety and efficacy of herbs and phytomedicines.[18]

In the United States, the FDA evaluates the safety and efficacy of new drugs based on data supplied by the drug manufacturer. The process of demonstrating new drug safety and efficacy takes approximately 15 years and costs an estimated $500 million.[131] Since herbal remedies cannot be patented, research companies in the United States are unlikely to invest the time and money necessary to satisfy FDA requirements.[163]

European and American phytomedicine manufacturers petitioned the FDA to allow well-researched European herbs the status of "old drugs," so they would not have to withstand the prohibitively expensive new drug application process. To date, the FDA has not responded to this petition.[18]

In 1994, the United States' Dietary Supplement Health and Education Act (DSHEA) allowed herbal products to be labeled with potential safety problems, side effects, contraindications, and special warnings. Statements of nutritional support and how the product affects structure and function of the body can also be included. However, an herbal product cannot make a statement that implies that it is "therapeutic" or useful to diagnose, treat, cure, or prevent any disease. Herbal products are not permitted to have labeling that contains a drug claim, except for the few herbs that are approved for over-the-counter drug use.[129]

Pharmaceutical Medicine versus Herbal Medicine

Because plants cannot be patented, very little research has been performed in the United States on plants as medicinal agents. Rather, plants are typically screened for a biologically active ingredient; the ingredient is then isolated and patented as a drug. In many cases, the removed constituents are less biologically active than the crude herb, and side effects occur more often when elements are administered in isolation. In Europe, policies on herbal medicines make it economically feasible for companies to research and develop phytopharmaceuticals. For that reason, quality of herbal products is highly controlled, and herbal medicine is integrated with more conventional medical approaches.[50]

Prevalence of Herbal Medicine

Almost one fourth of pharmaceutical drugs currently available in the world are derived from herbs. The World Health Organization (WHO) estimates that 4 billion people—80% of the world population—use herbal medicine for some aspect of primary health care.[50] A recent survey by Eisenberg and others identified herbal use as the fastest growing category of complementary medicine in the United States and the second most used alternative therapy.[45] In 1997 it was estimated that the dollar total of herbs sold in mass-market outlets (e.g., grocery stores, pharmacies, mass merchandising retail stores) in the United States was $441.5 million. This was a dramatic 79.5% increase over the total 1996 sales of $246 million.[80] The dollar sales for herbal medicine is predicted to increase with each passing year.

U.S. citizens' interest in herbs and other natural products is reflected by the estimated 2 million letters, faxes, and telephone calls by Americans to members of Congress during 1993 and 1994 in support of legislation that would protect and increase access to the products and information on their use.[129]

■ Safety and Efficacy of Herbal Medicine

Some herbs are more dangerous than the drug derived from them. Digitalis, used to strengthen heart contractions, was originally isolated from foxglove (*Digitalis purpurea*). Since the active ingredient varies substantially in this plant and since an individual could accidentally take a fatal rather than a therapeutic dose, the consistent dose provided in pharmaceutical digitalis is far safer than foxglove alone. Although some herbs are harmless even in large quantities, there is still the potential for overdose or cross-reaction possibilities of herbal effects with other medications.

Compounds originally thought to be rare are often found in different and unrelated plants. The flavor of licorice (*Glycyrrhiza glabra*) is also found in fennel (*Foeniculum vulgare*) and in anise (*Pimpinella anisum*). Although these plants were originally used for culinary purposes, they also have medicinal value. Other culinary herbs now known to promote health include garlic, onions, ginger, parsley, sage, rosemary, and thyme. On the other hand, nutmeg, a delightful flavoring in many dishes, is toxic in amounts of more than one whole nutmeg. Unfortunately, adolescents have used it in toxic quantities because of its mind-altering properties.

The term *simples* refers to preparations made from a single herb. In Chinese medicine, Ayurvedic medicine, and other systems of herbal medicine, several herbs may be blended to treat a patient's condition. This blending must be performed carefully, however, since various ingredients modulate biochemical activity.

Quality control is one critical problem for those interested in using herbs in the United States. For example, an analysis of over five different commercial preparation of feverfew found wide variations in the amounts of parthenolide in commercial preparations. Most products contained no parthenolide or only trace amounts.[71]

Poor quality control of herbs often leads to misinterpretation of outcomes in U.S. herbal research, even when otherwise well-controlled research designs are employed. For example, a 1979 article in the *Journal of the American Medical Association* entitled "Ginseng Abuse Syndrome" reported side effects from Ginseng that included hypertension, euphoria, nervousness, insomnia, skin eruptions, and diarrhea. None of the preparations used in the trial had been subjected to controlled analysis. The species of ginseng used included *Panex ginseng* and *Panex quinquefolius*. Ginseng was delivered in a variety of forms (e.g., roots, capsules, teas, cigarettes, candies). More controlled studies performed with standardized extracts of *Panex ginseng* demonstrated an absence of side effects, suggesting the critical importance of both researching and using standardized herbal preparations.[153]

One of the most inaccurate assumptions concerning herbs is that scientists fully understand the pharmacologic pathways of herbs that are well researched. Because there are so many different compounds or elements in each and every herb and because they interact differently, based on the soil content, the time of year harvested, and the portion of the plant used, we can, in reality, only discuss a few of the components implicated in each herb's effects. The standardized "marker" compounds used to determine herbal quality only explains a small portion of the pharmacologic story.

■ Purpose of this Chapter

This chapter is not intended to provide an overview of all the major herbs in use today. Indeed, more than 600 herbal medications are currently sold in Germany alone, and unlimited herbal combinations are used as Chinese and Ayurvedic medicine. Rather, this chapter introduces 10 popular herbs and delineates the types of information with which you should become familiar when considering the use of any herbal product as medicine. The information you should seek includes the following:

1. Description and history
2. Pharmacology and actions
3. Recommended uses
4. Recommended doses
5. Potential toxicity
6. Side effects

For some herbs, information is available on indications, contraindications, and potential drug interactions. These categories of information are provided for the herbs discussed in this chapter. You are encouraged to develop an herbal "thinking style" that includes these essential categories.

For information on additional herbal products, *The Complete German Commission E Monographs* is an excellent reference manual. Other suggested readings are listed in the appendixes.

The remainder of this chapter is devoted to providing essential data on 10 popular herbs used in the United States. Although the ranking of herbs varies, depending on public response to the media or the type of survey used, these herbs have consistently ranked in the top 20 for several years.[18] The herbs reviewed include bilberry, cranberry, echinacea, feverfew, Ginkgo biloba, goldenseal, kava kava, milk thistle, saw palmetto, and St. John's wort.

■ Bilberry

Description and History

Bilberry is a member of the genus *Vaccinium,* as are the cranberry, American blueberry, and 200 other species (Figure 14-1). Historically, bilberry has served as a highly nutritious food. Medicinally, it has been used to treat scurvy and urinary complaints, including infection and stones. Because the dried berries have strong astringent properties, bilberry has often been recommended for the treatment of diarrhea and dysentery.[61]

Renewed interest in bilberry occurred during World War II. British Royal Air Force pilots forced to fly at night complained of poor visibility and therefore poor outcomes related to successful bombing raids. Pilots discovered by accident that if they ate significant quantities of bilberry jam before a raid, their night vision improved dramatically, resulting in better "hits."[82] Today, bilberry extracts are an accepted component of European medical treatment for eye disorders, including cataracts, macular degeneration, retinitis pigmentosis, diabetic retinopathy, and night blindness.

Pharmacology and Actions

The active components in bilberry include flavonoid compounds, known as *anthocyanosides.* Fif-

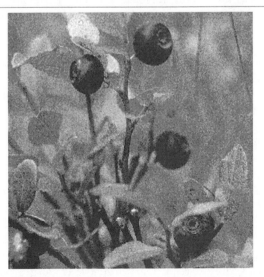

■ *Figure 14-1.* **Bilberry.** Treatment for eye disorders.

teen different anthocyanosides originate from five different *anthocyanidins* found in bilberry. The concentration of anthocyanosides in bilberry ranges from one tenth to one fourth of 1%. Concentrated extracts of bilberry yield an anthocyanidin content of almost 25%. For analytical purposes, anthocyanoside content should be expressed by amount of anthocyanidin. Bilberry also contains tannins and flavonoid glycides.[18]

Collagen-Stabilizing Properties of Anthocyanosides

Pharmacologic research has focused primarily on anthocyanosides, which possess significant collagen-stabilizing action. Collagen is the most abundant protein in the body, and collagen is destroyed during inflammatory processes (e.g., inflammation of bones, joints, cartilage and connective tissue; rheumatoid arthritis; other inflammatory-driven diseases).

Research studies have found that (1) anthocyanosides actually cross-link collagen fibers, reinforcing the matrix of connective tissue; (2) anthocyanosides and other flavonoid components of bilberry prevent the release and synthesis of compounds that promote inflammation, such as histamine, serine proteases, prostaglandins, and leukotrienes; and (3) anthocyanosides prevent free-radical damage with their antioxidant and free-radical scavenging action.[2,56,84,96,115,117]

Anthocyanosides Normalize Capillary Permeability

Anthocyanosides have strong "vitamin P" effects, including the ability to increase intracellular vitamin C levels and decrease capillary permeability (including that of the blood-brain barrier) and capillary fragility.[56,68,96]

These findings have implications for health because increased blood-brain permeability has been linked to autoimmune diseases of the central nervous system, schizophrenia, cerebral allergies, and other psychiatric disorders.

Effects on Atherosclerosis

Arteriosclerosis is a term for several diseases in which the wall of an artery becomes thicker and less elastic. The most common of these is *atherosclerosis,* where fatty materials accumulate under the inner lining of the arterial wall. When this develops in the arteries that supply the brain, a stroke can occur; when it develops in arteries supplying the heart, a heart attack may be the outcome. Atherosclerosis begins when monocytes, or white blood cells (WBCs), migrate into the wall of the artery and transform into cells that accumulate fatty materials; plaque then develops in the inner lining of the artery.

The oxidative modification of low-density lipoproteins (LDLs) represents one of the major mechanisms implicated in arteriosclerosis. Oxidized LDLs promote a number of processes leading to the formation of plaque in the arterial wall, including enhancement of macrophage uptake. In an in vitro study of the antioxidative potential of bilberry extract on human LDLs, it was found that the extract exerted potent protective action on LDL particles during in vitro copper-mediated oxidation. On a molar-to-molar basis, the extract was more potent than ascorbic acid (vitamin C) or butylated hydroxytoluene (BHT) in the protection of LDL particles from oxidative stress. Further, the protection was dose-specific; the higher the dose, the more the protection.[97]

Anthocyanosides have also been demonstrated to exert antiaggregation effects on platelets. Excessive platelet aggregation is linked to atherosclerosis and blood clot formation.[22,174]

Anthocyanosides also enhance antiaggregatory processes by stimulating the formation of *prostacyclin* (PGI2)–like substances by vascular tissue.[118] In animal studies, PGI2-like activity was measured in rat abdominal arteries after oral administration of *Vaccinium myrtillus* anthocyanosides (VMA) or acetylsalicylate (aspirin). PGI2 activity was evaluated by measuring the inhibition of adenosine diphosphate (ADP)-induced aggregation of blood platelets. Whereas aspirin inhibited the release of arterial PGI2-like activity, the anthocyanosides increased the formation of PGI2-like activity.

ADP- and collagen-induced aggregation of platelets obtained from human volunteers was then examined. Volunteers were treated for 30 and 60 days with VMA orally, alone, or with ascorbic acid. There was significant inhibition of platelet aggregation by VMA alone or with ascorbic acid after 30 days and still more after 60 days of treatment. After discontinuation of treatment for 120 days, the platelet aggregation values returned to baseline levels. These ex vivo findings confirmed other in vitro data; the release of prostacyclins from blood vessel walls, the release of histamine and serotonin, the removal of free radicals from platelets, and the decrease in platelet adhesiveness all seem to play important roles in the antiplatelet actions of VMA.[135]

Recommended Key Uses

Key uses cited for bilberry include varicose veins, cataract, macular degeneration, and glaucoma.[123] The German Commission E recognizes bilberry fruit as effective for the treatment of nonspecific, acute diarrhea and as local therapy for mild inflammation of the mucous membranes of the mouth and throat.[18]

Clinically Controlled Trials

Effects on Diabetes

Diabetes is a disorder in which blood levels of glucose (a simple sugar) are abnormally high because the body does not adequately release or use insulin. Bilberry leaves have been used as folk medicine for the treatment of diabetes. The VMA is the active hyperglycemic component in bilberry. On injection, *V. myrtillus* is somewhat weaker than insulin, but it is less toxic at even 50 times the therapeutic dose of 1 g per day. One study found that a single dose could produce some benefits lasting several weeks.[16]

A dried extract of the leaf was administered orally to diabetic rats for 4 days. Plasma glucose levels were consistently found to drop by approximately 26% at two different stages of diabetes. Unexpectedly, plasma triglycerides were also reduced by 39% after treatment.

It is important to note that the German Commission E panel of experts has not approved the use of the bilberry leaf for the treatment of diabetes, gastrointestinal tract disorders, and other conditions. The bilberry leaf monograph (published April 23, 1987) noted that higher doses or prolonged use can lead to chronic intoxication with the following symptoms:

1. Weight loss caused by chronic disease or emotional stress (cachexia)
2. Jaundice (icterus)
3. Acute excitation
4. Disturbances of tonus, which after chronic administration can lead to death

The efficacy of the claimed uses were not found compelling, and the German Commission E ruled that use of bilberry leaf is not justifiable in view of the possible risks involved.[18]

Effects on Lipid Levels

Hyperlipidemia refers to abnormally high levels of fats (e.g., cholesterol, triglycerides, or both) in the blood. Abnormally high levels of these fats in the bloodstream have implications for heart disease, stroke, and other health problems. Bilberry was therefore compared with ciprofibrate, a well-established hyperlipidemic drug. Both bilberry and ciprofibrate reduced triglyceride levels in a dose-dependent fashion. Only ciprofibrate reduced thrombus (clot) formation in diabetic rats. The findings indicate that active constituents of *V. myrtillus* leaves may prove potentially useful for the treatment of dyslipidemia associated with impaired triglyceride-rich lipoprotein clearance.[31]

Effects on Ulcers

Oral administration of bilberry anthocyanosides to rats demonstrated that this treatment provided a significant preventative and curative antiulcer activity without affecting gastric secretion.[35] Another animal study (rats) found VMA, given orally, antagonized gastric ulcerations induced by stress, nonsteroidal antiinflammatory drugs (NSAIDs), reserpine, and histamine, and duodenal ulceration induced by cysteamine. Given intravenously, it was more potent than when given orally. It did not affect gastric secretion, but it increased gastric mucus in normal animals.[104]

Effects on Health and Function of the Eye

The most significant clinical applications for bilberry extracts are in the field of ophthalmology. The health of the eye is dependent on a rich supply of nutrients and oxygen. When mechanisms responsible for nutrient and oxygen delivery and for protection of the eye fail, eye disorders develop, including cataracts and macular degeneration. These disorders are usually related to aging. Bilberry seems to benefit the eye by increasing oxygen and nutrient supply and by acting as an antioxidant.

Two studies found that Royal Air Force pilots who ingested bilberry fruit during World War II demonstrated improved nighttime visual acuity, adjustment to darkness, and restoration of visual acuity after glare exposure. Specifically, retinal purple increased.[82,160] Later studies supported these findings.[28,58,172]

A landmark study found that bilberry improved eyesight and increased ocular blood supply in approximately 75% of patients, and 80% of patients taking bilberry improved visual acuity examination scores for nighttime vision. Long-term improvements took an average of 6 weeks.[141]

In one clinical trial (N=50), bilberry extract plus vitamin E stopped cataract progression formation in 97% of patients with senile cortical cataracts.[26]

The macula is the portion of the eye responsible for fine vision. Risk factors to macular health include aging, atherosclerosis, and high blood pressure (BP). Currently, there is no medical treatment for common forms of macular degeneration. Laser surgery is used for a less common type (exudative) of macular degeneration.

Retinopathy is a condition in which the small arteries carrying blood to the eye become partially blocked because their walls have thickened. In a clinical trial (N=31), patients with different types of retinopathy (diabetic retinopathy=20; retinitis pigmentosa=5; macular degeneration=4, hemorrhagic retinopathy=2) treated with bilberry extract demonstrated less permeability and tendency to hemorrhage, with results most pronounced in those with diabetic retinopathy.[143]

Ischemic Reperfusion Injury

The effects of VMA on induced ischemia reperfusion injury in hamsters found that VMA decreased the number of leukocytes sticking to the venular wall and preserved the capillary perfusion; the increase in permeability was reduced after reperfusion. VMA maintained arteriolar tone and induced the appearance of rhythmic changes in arteriolar diameter. These results demonstrated the ability of VMA to reduce microvascular impairments caused by ischemia reperfusion injury, with preservation of endothelium, attenuation of leukocyte adhesion, and improvement of capillary perfusion.[15]

Dosage, Toxicity, and Side Effects

Anthocyanoside, calculated as 25% anthocyanidin content, is often recommended in dosages of 20 mg to 40 mg three times daily; or as bilberry extract, calculated as 25% anthocyanidin content, in dosages of 80 mg to 160 mg three times daily.[123] The German Commission E recommends a daily dose of 20 g to 60 g of dried drug for infusions and for external use, 10% decoction or equivalent preparation.[18] (Note: *Infusion* refers to the act of pouring boiling water over chopped herbs and allowing the mixture to steep for several minutes. A tea that is made by adding boiling water and continuing to add more heat to the mixture is called a *decoction* and is usually reserved for making water extracts of heavy, dense plant materials, such as roots, barks, and sometimes seeds.[18]

Extensive toxicology investigations confirm that the main ingredient in bilberry, anthocyanoside, is devoid of toxic effects. Rats given doses as high as 400 mg per kg demonstrated no side effects, with excess anthocyanoside excreted through the urine and bile.[99,100] The German

Commission E Monograph lists no side effects, contraindications, or known drug interactions.[18]

In using the dried fruit version, users may want to consider where the berries were grown. Ascorbic acid content of *Vaccinium* berries grown in urban or industrial sites has been lower than those grown in rural areas, and a correlation was found between herbicide dose rate and residue levels in berries for herbicides 2,4,D, 2,4,5,T, and 4-chlor-2-methylphenoxyacetic acid.[37]

■ Cranberry

Description and History

Cranberry is a North American shrub having broad clusters of white flowers and scarlet fruit (Figure 14-2). Cranberries and the juice of cranberries have been recommended in American folk medicine for the treatment of urinary tract infections and for dissolving kidney and gallstones.[173]

Recommended Key Uses

Cranberries are recommended for the prevention and treatment of urinary tract infections.

Pharmacology and Actions

Cranberry's chemical constituents are anthocyanins (also found in bilberry), catechin, and triterpernoids. Cranberry's beneficial effects have been attributed to its hippuric acid content. In 1914, it was demonstrated that most of the various organic acids present in fruits are completely oxidized in the body and do not exhibit any acidic effect in urine. However, the acids in cranberries, prunes, and plums proved the exception. In the

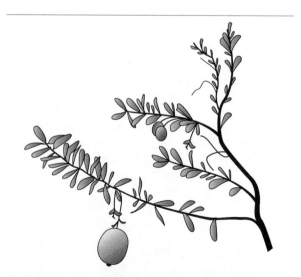

■ **Figure 14-2. Cranberry.** Treatment for urinary trace infections.

same year, it was reported that cranberries contained 0.06% benzoic acid. Approximately 9 years later, it was found that 24 hours after the ingestion of 305 g of cranberries, noticeable increases in both titratable and organic acids and a decrease in pH of the urine were produced. In 1933 it was shown that the ingestion of 100 g to 300 g of cranberries increased titratable acidity, organic acids, hippuric acid, hydrogen ion concentration, and ammonia, whereas the uric acid and urea nitrogen of urine were decreased slightly.[134]

A number of studies suggest that cranberry's effects are the result of antiadhesive agents. Adhesion of *Escherichia coli* (the most common bacteria causing urinary tract infections) to cells in the urinary and alimentary tracts enables the bacteria to withstand cleansing mechanisms and to overcome nutrient deprivation, resulting in a growth advantage and enhanced toxicity.

Cranberry juice contains two compounds that inhibit the *E. coli* adhesins that support urinary tract infections. One is fructose, which is in all fruit juices; it inhibits the MS fibrial adhesin. The other inhibitor is a polymeric compound of unknown nature that inhibits the MR adhesins associated with *E. coli.* The antiadhesive agents in juices from *Vaccinium* berries may act in the gut (the source of most uropathogens), in the bladder, or in both by preventing colonization of these sites.[127]

Researchers in Israel tested blueberry, cranberry, grapefruit, guava, mango, orange, and pineapple to see whether they could inhibit cell adhesive ability of *E. coli.* Only cranberry and blueberry juice, both of the *Vaccinium* genus, were effective. Cranberry juice inhibited adhesion activity of all 30 urinary isolates tested, but in only 4 of the 20 fecal isolates tested.[127]

Clinically Controlled Trials

Effects on Urinary Tract Infections

Although many have debated the effectiveness of cranberries as medical intervention, studies have supported the folk-medicine claims. Women are more prone to urinary tract infections than men and are sometimes placed on daily (or precoital) doses of antibiotics. Cranberry juice may work as a natural adjunctive or preventative therapy to urinary tract infection. This is important, since overuse of antibiotics can lead to resistance to their effectiveness.

In controlled trials, 77 *E. coli* isolates with significant bacteriuria were exposed to cranberry juice. Bacterial adherence to epithelial cells was inhibited 75%+ in 60% of the isolates. Juice was

given to 15 mice in place of water for 14 days. Urine from these mice, but not the urine from the control mice, inhibited *E. coli* adherence to uroepithelial cells by 80%. When similar tests were run with human subjects, significant antiadherence activity was reported in the urine of 15 of 22 volunteers 1 to 3 hours after drinking 15 ounces of juice. Urine samples taken before administering the juice served as control samples.[155] When it became clear that cranberry juice could inhibit adherence, both fructose and vitamin C were also tested for their adherence-inhibitory capacity. Adding extra fructose to cranberry juice showed no added effect. When concentration of cranberry juice was reduced to 10%, a small additive effect could be seen. No observable effect of vitamin C was found.

In a randomized, placebo-controlled, double-blind trial, 153 older women drank 300 ml of cranberry juice or a placebo drink (matched for taste and vitamin C content) each day for 6 months. Probability of infection recovery or development over 1-month intervals was estimated, based on the probabilities of transition into or out of bacteriuria with pyuria. Treated subjects were found to produce only 42% of the urine bacteria produced by those in the control group. Odds of remaining infected, since the subjects were infected in the previous month, were estimated to be 27% of those in the control group.[4]

Bacteriuria is common among older women. Although much bacteriuria in this age group is asymptomatic and does not require treatment, a large proportion of women older than 65 years experience at least one urinary tract infection per year.

In an uncontrolled trial, cranberry juice was administered to 60 patients with clinical diagnoses of acute urinary tract infection. After 21 days of treatment with 16 ounces of cranberry juice a day, 53% of patients had positive clinical responses. Moderate improvement was found in 20% of patients. Infection persisted or recurred during the 6 weeks after treatment in 27 patients; 8 of the 27 patients were asymptomatic. Negative urine cultures and absence of clinical complaints were found in 17 patients at the 6-week posttherapy follow-up.[134]

Dosage, Toxicity, and Side Effects

Cranberry juice has not been found to elicit side effects even in large doses. Dosage recommendations are 8 ounces of unsweetened cranberry juice, two to three times a day.

Based on the findings, cranberry juice may be a good preventative strategy for female patients prone to urinary tract infections.[173]

■ Echinacea

Description and History

Echinacea is a perennial herb found in the eastern and central United States and southern Canada (Figure 14-3). There are nine species of echinacea, but *Echinacea augustifolia*, *Echinacea purpurea,* and *Echinacea pallida* are the most commonly used.[111] Historically, echinacea has been the most used herb for treatment of illness and injury among Native Americans. It has been used topically for wound healing, burns, abscesses, and insect bites and has been taken internally for infections, toothache, joint pain, and as an antidote for rattlesnake bites.[166]

Around 1980, echinacea was "rediscovered" in the United States because of consumer interest in treating immune system disorders such as candidiasis, chronic fatigue syndrome, acquired immunodeficiency syndrome (AIDS), and cancer.

Recommended Key Uses

The German Commission E recommends *E. pallida* root as supportive therapy for influenza-like infections. *E. purpurea* is recommended for supportive therapy for colds and chronic infections of the respiratory tract and lower urinary tract. It is also recommended for external use with poorly healing wounds and chronic ulcerations.[18]

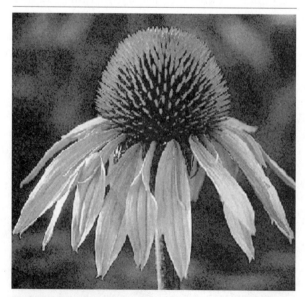

■ *Figure 14-3.* **Echinacea.** Treatment for influenza, colds, and infections of the respiratory tract.

Pharmacology and Actions

More than 350 studies have been performed on the pharmacologic applications of echinacea. The review of these studies is beyond the scope of this chapter; the combined outcomes are summarized.

Echinacea has been found to:
1. Support tissue regeneration
2. Produce antiinflammatory and immunostimulatory properties (i.e., affect the alternate complement pathway [enhancing transport of WBCs into infected areas])
3. Elevate WBC counts when low, and promote nonspecific T-cell activation, including T-cell replication, macrophage, and natural killer (NK) cell activity
4. Increase neutrophil numbers
5. Demonstrate antiviral, antibacterial, and anticancer properties

Bone argued cogently that the ability of echinacea to act as a T-cell activator has not been demonstrated. He notes that inappropriate conclusions have been drawn from in vitro research on polysaccharide isolates potentially contaminated with nitrogenous impurities. Recent studies that used purified polysaccharides found lower mitogenic action on T-lymphocytes. The relevance of the polysaccharide research to normal clinical use of echinacea extracts is questionable.[21]

These findings do not mean that echinacea does not stimulate T-cell function; rather, it means that polysaccharides are probably not responsible for the majority of this effect. Bauer and Wagner determined that the immunologic investigations conducted to date permit the following conclusions:

1. Lipophilic alkylamides and the polar caffeic acid derivative, cichoric acid, probably make a considerable contribution to the immunostimulatory action or activity of alcoholic echinacea extracts.
2. Apart from these two compounds, polysaccharides are also implicated in the activity of expressed echinacea juice.[10]

Phagocytic Properties

The most consistently proven effect of echinacea is its stimulation of phagocytosis (i.e., the "eating" of invading organisms by WBCs and lymphocytes). Two standard tests of phagocytic ability are used to compare immune stimulation:

1. Human WBCs are incubated with yeast and with echinacea. At a set time, blood cells are examined microscopically and a count is made of the numbers of yeast cells that have been gobbled up by the blood cells. In this test, var-

ious extracts of echinacea have increased phagocytosis by 20% to 40%.

2. The "carbon clearance test" measures the speed with which injected carbon particles are removed from the bloodstream of a mouse or rabbit. The quicker an animal can remove the foreign particles from its blood, the more the immune system has been stimulated. Echinacea excelled here, removing foreign particles more rapidly.

Other Actions

Echinacea has been demonstrated to cause proliferation of cells, enhancing overall immune system activity; it also stimulates production of interferon (IFN) and other important products of the immune system, including tumor necrosis factor (TNF). Echinacea inhibits the action of the enzyme hyaluronisase, which is secreted by bacteria, helping them gain access to healthy cells. Echinacea, in high concentrations, can counteract this enzyme. Echinacea also has fungicidal and bacteriostatic properties and an antiinflammatory effect.[9,12,79,119,161,169]

Antiinflammatory Effects

In 1957 it was found that *E. purpurea* caused a 22% reduction in inflammation among arthritis sufferers. Although echinacea is only half as effective as steroids, steroids have side effects, toxicity, and contraindications including suppressing immune function. Echinacea is nontoxic and adds immune stimulating properties.[165]

As with most herbs, we do not fully understand how they work. There are too many combinations of elements in each herb to identify precisely which components are bringing about reported effects. Further, extracts and preparation processes differ in strength and even in components, one from another. It has been repeatedly suggested that it may be unknown combinations of components resulting in the reported outcomes, not necessarily the biochemical "marker" assumed to be the major producer of the effect.

Produce-Purchasing Issues

It has been estimated that more than 50% and as much as 90% of the echinacea sold in the United States between 1908 and 1991 was actually *Parthenium integrifolium* (Missouri snakeroot). The user should be certain of which species of echinacea he or she has purchased and ask for quality-control documentation of supplier product. *E. augustifolia* was once considered the most

effective herbal species, but *E. purpurea* has out performed it in studies.

Clinically Controlled Trials

Effects on Healthy Subjects

Leukocytosis is defined as an initial drop in leukocyte numbers, mostly neutrophils. In human volunteers with no history of allergy, autoimmune disease, or severe illness, a state of leukocytosis was triggered 30 to 60 minutes after intravenous injection of 5 mg of echinacea. This was followed by a sudden and large increase of leukocytes 2 to 8 hours later and then normalization at 12 to 24 hours. A high number of juvenile stab cells then appeared, indicating migration of cells from bone marrow to peripheral blood. In essence, echinacea induced an acute phase immune reaction similar to what would occur in response to an infection. Adherence of neutrophils to blood vessels and migration of neutrophils and monocytes from the bone marrow into the peripheral blood was elicited. C-reactive protein (CRP) rose, being comparable with that of a viral infection with moderate symptoms. Those in the control group received a placebo injection with no effect on immunity.[138]

Since the dose was small (5 mg polysaccharides purified), side effects in humans demand special attention. The acute phase of CRP was induced, probably because of an activation of monocytes and macrophages to produce interleukins (IL)-6.

Effects on Cancer Patients

The levels of cytokines IL-1-alpha, IL-1-beta, IL-2, IL-6, TNF-alpha, and IFN-gamma were assessed in culture supernatants of stimulated whole blood cells derived from 23 patients undergoing a 4-week oral treatment with an extract from echinacea complex. All patients had curative surgery for a localized solid malignant tumor. Blood was taken before treatment and at 2 and 4 weeks of therapy. Twelve matched, untreated patients with tumors served as the control group.

After therapy with echinacea complex, no significant alteration in the production of cytokines could be seen, compared with those in the control group, and the leukocyte population remained constant. The authors concluded that the dosage used had no effect on the patients' lymphocyte activity as measured by their cytokine production.[46] This study used mixed tumors (breast=8, colorectal=8, lung=1, renal=2, prostate=2, corpus=1, melanoma=1).

The reason for no effect is possibly twofold: too low a concentration of the active substance in the extract or a wrong route of application. The authors did not use standardized dosages and did not use the most potent form of echinacea; rather, a mixture of three different kinds was used.[9]

Effects on Colds and Influenza

In an 8-week, double-blind, placebo-controlled study, patients with colds (N=108) received either 4 ml of *Echinacin* (a brand name for the stabilized juice of *E. purpurea*) or placebo twice daily. Echinacin resulted in a decreased frequency and severity of infections; 35.2% of Echinacin patients remained free of infection compared with 25.9% of those receiving placebos; the length of time between infection was 40 days for echinacea versus 25 days for placebo group; and infections were less severe in 78.6% of those taking echinacea.[148] Patients showing evidence of a weakened immune system benefited the most from echinacea.

In a double-blind, placebo-controlled study of 10 days duration, 180 patients (18- to 60-years-old) with influenza received either *E. purpurea* herb extract (90 drops, the 450 mg dose, or 180 drops, the 900 mg dose) or placebo drops. The 450 mg dose was no more effective than placebo, but the 900 mg dose produced significantly more relief of symptoms (e.g., weakness, low energy, chills, sweating, sore throat, muscle and joint aches, headaches).[25] This study demonstrated the importance of using an adequate dose of echinacea for the treatment of influenza and infection.

Effects on Chronic Fatigue Syndrome and Acquired Immunodeficiency Syndrome

Extracts of *E. purpurea* and *Panax ginseng* were evaluated for their capacity to stimulate cellular immune function by peripheral blood mononuclear cells (PBMC) from (1) normal patients, (2) patients with chronic fatigue syndrome, and (3) patients with AIDS. PBMC was tested in the absence and presence of concentrations of each extract.

NK cell function of all groups was significantly enhanced with both echinacea and ginseng, at concentrations of ≥ 0.1 ug/kg or 10 ug/kg, respectively. Similarly, the addition of either herb significantly increased antibody-dependent cellular cytotoxicity (ADCC) or PBMC from all subject groups. Thus both extracts enhanced cellular immune function of PBMC of normal individuals and patients with depressed cellular immunity.[152]

An exception to using echinacea for infection may be the treatment of AIDS. Stimulation of T cell replication and the increase of TNF levels may also stimulate replication of the virus.[123] Although there are anecdotal stories of it helping human immunodeficiency viral (HIV) infected individuals, additional research is needed before it can be recommended for the treatment of this disease. If Bone's assertions were accurate, however, echinacea may prove beneficial to patients with AIDS without this risk.

Effects on Candida Infections

In a 10-week, clinically controlled trial, the effect of Echinacin was studied on 203 women with recurrent vaginal *Candida* infections. Econazole nitrate cream was applied locally for 6 days to all patients. The subjects were assigned to one of five groups: (1) no additional treatment, (2) Echinacin administered intravenously, (3) intramuscularly, (4) subcutaneously, or (5) orally. Outcomes were assessed at 2 and 10 weeks. Recurrence for the econazole-only group was 60.5%. In the Echinacin groups, the recurrence rate was 15% for the intravenous group, 5% for the intramuscular group, 15% for the subcutaneous group, and 16.7% for the oral group.[32]

Reviews of Multiple Clinically Controlled Trials

Review of 26 controlled clinical trials (18 randomized, 11 double blind) looked at groups treated with pure echinacea extracts or mixtures containing the herb. Nineteen trials studied whether the preparation prevented or cured infections (e.g., colds or influenza); four studied reduction of side effects of cancer therapies, and three studied whether echinacea affected indicators of immune function. The authors found positive results for 30 of the 34 groups. Evidence clearly points to echinacea as having a positive effect on immunity, but some trials were poor in quality and failed to provide enough information to make clear recommendations about **how much** of which preparation to use under different conditions.[112]

Dosage, Toxicity, and Side Effects

Echinacea is indicated for viral and bacterial infections, chronic respiratory infections, wounds, chronic ulcerations, colds, and influenza. It is contraindicated for progressive systemic diseases, such as tuberculosis, leucosis, collagenosis, multiple scleroses, AIDS, HIV infection, and other auto-immune diseases in which the immune system, itself, causes disease disturbances in the body.[17,163]

The majority of clinical trials on echinacea used an extract of juice of the above-ground portion of *E. purpurea*. There is an important point here—there are nine difference species of echinacea, and different species produce different biochemical effects. *E. purpurea* is the one that seems to work best.

In laboratory studies that test the ability of echinacea to ward off colds or influenza, it has been found that an effective method of dosing is 3 days on and 3 days off. This regimen is because healthy immune systems can be stimulated only briefly before returning to normal. After several days without echinacea, immunostimulation can again be elicited. Other writers have suggested several weeks on and off with existing illness. The better method has not been determined. Recent studies have suggested patients with impaired immune function benefit from a regimen of 8 weeks on and 1 week off.[25,148]

The types of echinacea preparations most used and most reported in the research include the following:

1. Stabilized juice of *E. purpurea* tops, which is often sold under the trade name Echinacin
2. Fresh or dried whole plant preparations of *E. purpurea*, *E. augustifolia*, or *E. pallida*
3. Fresh or dried preparations of the roots of the three forms of echinacea

Category 1 is often administered by intramuscular injection. Most practitioners do not use *E. purpurea* stabilized juice by injection, but the research on this product and dosage make up the bulk of clinical work on echinacea. Category 2 and 3 are given in tablets, liquids, capsules, and powders.

Although ground, powdered, freeze-dried, and tinctures are considered effective, experts believe the fresh-pressed juice of *E. purpurea* to be the best preparation because it gives the greatest range of active compounds and has the greatest level of clinical support.[17]

Recommended dose is 6 ml to 9 ml expressed juice (*E. Purpurea*) or tincture (1:5) with native dry extract, corresponding to 900 mg herb (7:1 to 11:1) (*E. pallida* root).[17]

Echinacea is not toxic when taken at recommended doses, and no studies were found reporting acute or chronic toxicity reactions. Given intravenously, the fresh pressed juice of *E. purpurea* has, on occasion, caused fever (0.5° to 1.0° C). The secretion of IF and IL-1 by activated macrophages is presumed to be the cause of this reaction.[9] Side effects of nausea and vomiting have been reported.

■ Feverfew

Description and History

Feverfew is a member of the sunflower family. It has round, leafy branching stems with green leaflets (Figure 14-4). The flowers are small, favor-

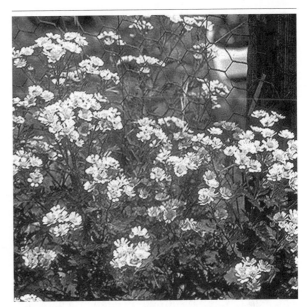

■ **Figure 14-4. Feverfew.** Treatment for migraine headache.

ing the daisy family, with yellow disks. It has 10 to 20 white rays. This plant is cultivated in flower gardens throughout Europe and the United States.

Historically, feverfew has been used as a febrifuge (fever reducer) and as a treatment for migraines and arthritis, as well as for anemia, earache, dysmenorrhea (menstrual pain), dyspepsia (upset stomach), trauma, and intestinal parasites.

Feverfew as medical treatment dates back to Dioscorides, a first century Greek physician who recommended it for headaches, menstrual irregularities, stomach pain, and fevers. In 1633, Gerarde's *Herball* suggests the plant as a treatment for headache pain. It is used in South America for colic, morning sickness, and kidney pain; in Costa Rica it is used as a digestive aid.[54]

Recommended Key Uses

Feverfew is recommended for treatment of migraine headaches, fever, and inflammation.[123]

Pharmacology and Actions

The major active chemicals in feverfew are sesquiterpene lactones, principally parthenolide.[43] Extracts of feverfew behave like NSAIDs or aspirin. Extracts of feverfew inhibit the agents that promote inflammation, including the prostaglandins, leukotrienes, and thromboxanes. Unlike aspirin, however, feverfew inhibits inflammation in its initial stages, much like cortisone.[107]

Feverfew inhibits platelet aggregation and enhances secretion of the allergic and inflammatory agents histamine and serotonin. It also has a tonic effect on vascular smooth muscle.[8,69] Feverfew evokes changes in the metabolism of arachidonic acid; it inhibits both the uptake and the liberation of arachidonic acid into and from platelet membrane phospholipids.[70,103]

Clinically Controlled Trials

Effects on Migraine Headache Pain

In a double-blind, placebo-controlled study, 17 subjects were selected who suffered from classical migraine headache pain for 2 or more years and who had ingested one to four feverfew leaves daily for 3 or more months to prevent the onset of migraine pain. These subjects were then randomly given either dried feverfew or a placebo. The placebo group had a significant increase in pain frequency and severity, nausea, and vomiting. The feverfew group showed no change. This study demonstrated the effects of withdrawing feverfew, not its first-use effects, and it identified that response to feverfew intake was not a placebo response.[83]

In a randomized, double-blind, placebo-controlled, cross-over study, 60 patients who suffered with migraine pain took either a capsule of dried feverfew or placebo for 4 months, then crossed over for 4 more months. In each 2-month period, feverfew reduced the mean number and severity of attacks and the degree of vomiting, although the duration of individual attacks remained the same.[122] There was a 24% reduction in the number of attacks during feverfew treatment, but there was no significant alternation in the duration of individual attacks. There was a trend (p=0.06) toward milder headaches with feverfew and a significant reduction (p<0.02) in nausea and vomiting accompanying the attacks. In this study, 68 working days were lost during the feverfew phases compared with 76 lost days during the placebo phase. Of all the feverfew periods, 36% were graded as "much better" for migraine pain and only one patient was graded as much worse compared with placebo values (21% and 10%, respectively). Mouth ulceration was more common during treatment than with the placebo.

Effects on Rheumatoid Arthritis

The release of inflammatory agents was found to be inhibited more effectively by feverfew than by NSAIDS or aspirin. This finding led many to believe that feverfew would be effective in the treatment of rheumatoid arthritis. To test this theory, a double-blind, placebo-controlled study of 41

female patients with symptomatic rheumatoid arthritis were given either dried chopped feverfew (70 mg to 86 mg) or placebo capsules once daily for 6 weeks. Outcomes demonstrated no benefit to those receiving feverfew compared with placebo. The dose used in this study may have been too small to prove beneficial (70 mg versus the 100 mg to 125 mg used in other studies), and the parthenolide level was not standardized. Because of these flaws, no definitive conclusions could be drawn from the outcomes.[130]

Dosage, Toxicity, and Side Effects

Effectiveness depends on the levels of parthenolide in the herb compound. An analysis of parthenolide content of more than 35 different commercial preparations showed a wide variation in the amount of parthenolide, with the majority containing no parthenolide or only traces.[71]

In the migraine studies where outcomes were positive, the dose was roughly 0.25 mg to 0.5 mg. These doses prevented attack. If an attack was already occurring, a higher dose of 1 g to 2 g was required to eliminate the ongoing pain. It is suggested the sufferer chew two fresh (or frozen) leaves per day, or take capsules containing approximately 85 mg of leaf material.

Feverfew in the form of an infusion is said to lower BP, serve as a digestive aid, and bring on menstruation. For infusion, $1/2$ to 1 teaspoon per cup of boiling water, steeped 5 to 10 minutes is suggested. Two cups a day is recommended.

No toxic reactions have been reported in the studies. However, as mentioned, chewing the leaves can result in ulcerations and the development of dermatitis from external contact in some sensitive persons.[6]

As listed in the Nottingham clinical trial, reported side effects included mouth ulceration, indigestion, heartburn, and dizziness. No changes were reported in hematologic and biochemical tests, including urea, creatinine, electrolytes, blood sugar, and liver function. In the London study, 11.3% of feverfew users developed mouth ulceration. Migraine sufferers who eat the leaves every day can develop mouth ulcers, loss of taste, and swelling of mouth, lips, or tongue. Although capsules reduce these side effects, they are not completely eliminated.[6]

Feverfew is contraindicated for children younger than 2 years old. Pregnant women should err on the side of caution and not use it because of its purported ability to elicit menstruation. Individuals who have blood-clotting disorders or who are taking anticoagulant medications should consult a physician before using.

■ Ginkgo Biloba

Description and History

Ginkgo biloba is the only member of its family and genus. It is a magnificent tree that lives as long as 1000 years. It can grow to a height of 122 feet and to a diameter of 4 feet (Figure 14-5). Its branches bear fan-shaped leaves 5 cm to 10 cm in width. Ginkgo has been evolutionally unchanged for over 200 million years and is referred to as a "living fossil."[123]

After the ice age, the Ginkgo tree survived only in China, where it later became cultivated as a sacred tree and was found decorating Buddhist temples throughout Asia.

The medicinal use of Ginkgo can be traced to Chinese *Materia Medica* of 2800 BC. Traditional Chinese physicians use Ginkgo to treat asthma and chilblains (i.e., extreme cold exposure causing itching, burning, and lesions) and swelling of hands and feet. Ancient Chinese and Japanese traditions called for the roasting of Ginkgo seeds as a digestive aid and to prevent drunkenness. In the Ayurvedic tradition, Ginkgo is associated with long life and is used in longevity elixirs.[123]

Recommended Key Uses

The main indications for Ginkgo are peripheral vascular diseases such as intermittent claudication and, more importantly, cerebral insufficiency. Cerebral insufficiency is an imprecise term describing a collection of symptoms including difficulties concentrating, loss of memory, absent-mindedness, confusion, lack of energy, tiredness, decreased physical performance, depressive mood, anxiety, dizziness, tinnitus, and headache. These symptoms have been associated with impaired cerebral circulation and are thought to be early indications of dementia of degenerative or multiple infarct type.

Because of a degeneration with neuronal loss and impaired neurotransmission with dementia, cerebral insufficiency is associated with disturbances in oxygen and glucose supply. Release of free radicals and lipid peroxidation may occur in these circumstances with harmful consequences.

Key suggested uses for Ginkgo include cerebral vascular insufficiency (insufficient blood to the brain), vascular insufficiency (intermittent claudication, Raynaud's disease), retinopathy (macular degeneration, diabetic retinopathy), neuralgia and neuropathy, depression, dementia, inner ear dysfunction (vertigo, tinnitus), multiple sclerosis, premenstrual syndrome, and impotence.[17]

Pharmacology and Actions

The female Ginkgo bears both an inedible fruit and an edible nut that is often used in oriental cuisine. A highly technical extract from the leaves, called Ginkgo biloba extract (GBE), is used for medicinal purposes. The leaves are harvested in the summer because this is when the highest level of active compounds exists. GBE is concentrated and standardized to a consistent level of its most active component, ginkogolides. GBE was originally developed in Germany by the Schwab Company, which also sponsored most of the research on Ginkgo.

GBE entered the market in Germany in 1982, is now used by more than 10 million Europeans annually, is government approved, and is covered by insurance and the German national health care system. GBE is now one of the most widely used medicines in Europe and is considered the best researched herb in the world today. Nonstandardized Ginkgo products are also available, although they are not recommended.

When properly prepared, Ginkgo seems to have an effect on blood vessels, increasing blood flow without changing BP. It is widely used for a variety of circulatory problems, including those related to eye disorders. Ginkgo has several active components including the Ginkgo flavone glycosides or Ginkgo heterosides, several terpene molecules, and organic acids.

The standardized concentrated GBE is 24% Ginkgo heteroside. The total extract has been

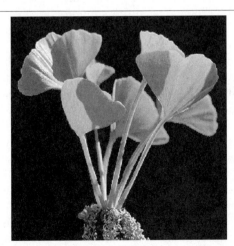

■ **Figure 14-5. Ginkgo biloba.** Treatment for cerebral insufficiency and intermittent claudication.

found to be more active than any single isolated component, which suggests a synergism among the various components.[40,92,93]

Ginkgo provides health benefits in the following ways:

1. Tissue effects include membrane stabilization, as well as antioxidant and free radical–scavenging actions.
2. Use of oxygen and glucose is improved; most especially, it clears toxic metabolites that accumulate during ischemia.
3. Nerve cells, including brain cells, are protected.
4. Vascular effects exerted on the lining of the arteries, capillaries, and veins are the regulation of blood vessel tone and vasodilation and increased blood flow.
5. Platelet aggregation, platelet adhesion, and degranulation are inhibited (i.e., allergic and inflammatory components are released). Specifically, the platelet-activating factor (PAF) is potently inhibited.
6. Neuron metabolism and neurotransmitter disturbances are beneficially influenced.[40,88,93,95]

Four different Ginkgo preparations are typically used in controlled trials: Tebonin, Tanakan, Rokan, and Kaveri. The first three are different names for the same extract, Egb 761, and the amount of Ginkgo flavone glycosides (24%) and terpenoids (6%) is standardized. Kaveri, LI 1370, is standardized on the same ingredients in similar doses (25% Ginkgo flavone glycosides and 6% terpenoids).

Clinically Controlled Trials

Effects on Tinnitus
Permanent severe tinnitus is difficult to treat, and the results from the use of Ginkgo for this disorder are conflicting. A study by Meyer found Ginkgo improved tinnitus for all patients; Coles' study received mixed results. The difference may be that Meyer's patients had recent-onset tinnitus, whereas Coles' patients had tinnitus for 3 years or longer.[33,114]

Effects on Impotence
In a study of 60 men with impotence caused by arterial flow problems and who had not responded to papaverine injections of 50 mg, Ginkgo improved blood flow within 8 weeks, as assessed by duplex sonography. After 6 months, half of the men regained potency. Twenty-five percent of patients showed improved arterial inflow, but they did not regain potency. In 20% of treated patients, a new trial of papaverine injection was then successful. This trial was interesting because conventional treatment had failed with these men.[154]

Effects on Cerebral Insufficiency
As noted, cerebral insufficiency is an imprecise term used to describe a collection of symptoms that include: (1) difficulties concentrating, (2) loss of memory, (3) absentmindedness, (4) confusion, (5) lack of energy, (6) tiredness, (7) decreased physical performance, (8) depressive mood, (9) anxiety, (10) dizziness, (11) tinnitus, and (12) headache. These symptoms have been associated with impaired cerebral circulation and are thought to be early indications of dementia from a degenerative condition or from multiple infarctions.

In a randomized, double-blind, placebo-controlled study of patients with early Alzheimer's disease (N=40), participants received 240 mg Ginkgo or placebo daily and were assessed at baseline and at 1, 2, and 3 months. Memory, attention, psychopathologic rating, psychomotor performance, functional dynamics, and neurophysiologic performance (i.e., electroencephalogram [EEG]) improved significantly compared with those in the control group.[75] In the EEG theta-alpha quotient, Ginkgo significantly reduced the theta wave component at 1 month and even more so after 3 months of treatment. This demonstrated that patients were more alert and able to concentrate more effectively with Ginkgo therapy.

In a randomized, placebo-controlled, double-blind trial, 40 patients (mean age 68 years old) with moderate dementia received infusions of Egb 761 or placebo for 4 days a week for 4 weeks. Ginkgo patients scored significantly better for all outcome measurements (e.g., daily living, illness symptoms, depression) than did those in the placebo group. The authors found Ginkgo superior to placebo for behavioral, psychopathologic, and psychometric planes.[64]

In a randomized, double-blind, placebo-controlled, multicenter study, 156 patients with mild-to-moderate multiple infarction or primary degenerative dementia of an Alzheimer's type received 240 mg Ginkgo extract or placebo for 24 weeks. Psychopathologic, attention, memory, and assessment of daily life activities significantly demonstrated the clinical efficacy of Ginkgo extract in the treatment of Alzheimer's disease and multiple infarction dementia.[87]

There was a trend toward improvement for mild depression. Subjects in the Egb group reported 63 adverse reactions, but only 5 were severe. Subjects in the placebo group reported 59 adverse reactions.

Overall, studies suggest that Ginkgo is most effective in delaying mental deterioration of Alzheimer's disease rather than in reversing the process. Therefore it is most effective in the early stages. If mental deficiency is caused by vascular insufficiency or depression, it is usually effective in reversing the process.

In a randomized, placebo-controlled, double-blind study, 31 patients, age 50+ with mild-to-moderate memory impairment received 40 mg of Ginkgo extract or placebo three times daily. Ginkgo significantly improved cognitive function at both 12 and 24 weeks as assessed by the Kendrick battery. At 24 weeks, response speed on a classification task was significantly superior to those in the placebo group.[137]

In a multicenter, randomized, placebo-controlled study, 72 outpatients with cerebral insufficiency received Ginkgo or placebo for 24 weeks. Statistically significant improvement in short-term memory was found at 6 weeks and significant learning rate improvement was observed at 24 weeks in those who received Ginkgo, but no improvements were observed in the placebo group. The authors concluded Ginkgo significantly improves mental performance by 24 weeks.[59]

In a metaanalysis of 40 studies, with the 8 best placebo-controlled trials being assessed, it was found that Ginkgo was more effective than placebo for a variety of patient complaints, including memory and concentration problems, headaches, depression, confusion, dizziness, and tiredness. When compared with published trials of a pharmaceutical treatment (codergocrine) for cerebral insufficiency, the authors found that Ginkgo was equally as effective.[92] The dose for most trials was 120 mg to 160 mg.

A metaanalysis was performed of 11 randomized, placebo-controlled, double-blind studies of Ginkgo biloba for treatment of cerebrovascular insufficiency in geriatric subjects. For individual symptoms, Ginkgo biloba was found significantly superior to placebo. The analysis of total scores of clinical symptoms from all relevant studies indicated that seven studies confirmed the effectiveness of Ginkgo compared with placebo, whereas one study was inconclusive. Outcomes confirmed the therapeutic effectiveness of Ginkgo regarding the clinical symptom complex.[78]

Effects in Combination with Antidepressants

In a randomized, placebo-controlled, double-blind study, 40 patients (aged 51 to 78 years) with mild-to-moderate cerebral dysfunction combined with depressive episodes were studied. These patients had demonstrated insufficient response to treatment with tricyclates and tetracyclic antidepressants for at least 3 months. During the study, patients continued on antidepressant therapy and were randomized to receive either Egb 761 (240 mg/day) or placebo. Patients treated with Egb 761 demonstrated declines in the Hamilton Depression Scale (HAMD) from 14 to 7. This decline occurred within 4 weeks. At 8 weeks, scores declined to 4.5.[151] These differences were highly significant (p=0.001 at 4 weeks and 0.01 at 8 weeks). Placebo scores remained virtually identical over time. This study suggested Ginkgo might be effective in combination with tricyclates, when the medication alone is not effective. A significant improvement in cognitive function was also noted.

Intervention for Reperfusion Injury

This matching, placebo-controlled study evaluated 15 patients undergoing aortic valve replacement to determine whether reperfusion-induced lipid peroxidation, ascorbate depletion, tissue necrosis, and cardiac damage is reduced by orally administering Ginkgo biloba for 5 days before cardiopulmonary bypass surgery.

Plasma samples were taken from peripheral circulation and the coronary sinus (1) before incision, (2) during ischemia, (3) within the first 30 minutes after unclamping, and (4) up to 8 days after surgery. Upon aortic unclamping, Ginkgo inhibited the transcardiac release of thiobarcituric acid-reactive species and attenuated the early decrease in dimethylsulfoxide ascorbyl free radical levels. It significantly delayed leakage of myoglobin and had a significant effect on ventricular myosin leakage. In summary, Ginkgo was successful in limiting oxidative stress in response to cardiovascular surgery.[132]

Effects on Acute Ischemic Stroke

Ischemic stroke is the death of brain tissue (cerebral infarction) resulting from a lack of blood flow caused by the blocking of a blood vessel and insufficient oxygen to the brain. In a double-blind, placebo-controlled study, patients of acute ischemic stroke received either 40 mg of Ginkgo extract (N=21) or placebo (N=26), both at 6-hour intervals. Computerized tomographic scanning confirmed acute ischemic infarction. At 2 and 4 weeks, both groups showed significant improvement in Mathew's scale score. In comparing outcomes with other studies, the authors concluded that Ginkgo was given too late and in too small a dose to be effective.[57] Essentially, there is a window of opportunity for the beneficial effect of Ginkgo administration after a stroke event.

In the previous study, Ginkgo had been administered more than 48 hours after stroke. The authors noted that 40 other trials of Ginkgo and chronic cerebral ischemia had demonstrated clinical differences between the treated and placebo groups, but Ginkgo was given less than 6 hours after stroke in those cases and in larger doses.

Effects on Intermittent Claudication

Intermittent claudication (IC) refers to tightening and fatiguing pain in the leg muscles, particularly the calves, in response to exercise; it is caused by a blockage of adequate blood flow.

In a critical review of the literature, the author retrieved 17 placebo-controlled trials of pentoxifylline, a popular drug used for the treatment of IC. The majority confirmed that pentoxifylline significantly prolonged walking distance.[48] Pentoxifylline is thought to work by reducing blood viscosity, increasing the flexibility and distensibility of red blood cells (RBCs) and preventing RBC and platelet aggregation. It must be used with extreme caution in patients with coronary artery disease or cerebrovascular insufficiency because it may lessen oxygen delivery to the heart and brain. Thus Ginkgo may be a safer method of the treatment for IC.

In a review of nine double-blind, randomized clinical trials of GBE versus controls, GBE was found superior to placebo (eight studies) and equal to pentoxifylline (one study). Measurements of pain-free walking distance (75% to 110%) and maximum walking distance (52.6% to 119%) dramatically increased, and plethysmographic and Doppler ultrasound measurements demonstrated increased blood flow through the affected limb. Blood lactate levels also dropped. The authors judged Ginkgo superior to pentoxifylline as a treatment for IC both on outcome and safety measures. He noted that longer GBE use provided the greatest benefit. Most studies suggested 120 mg to 160 mg per day of GBE given over three dosage periods.

In a randomized, double-blind, placebo-controlled trial, 61 patients received either Ginkgo or placebo for 24 weeks. Thereafter, Ginkgo patients were given the option of continuing treatment on an open basis for 65 weeks total. Ginkgo provided significantly greater pain relief and walking tolerance than placebo at 24 weeks, and improvement continued through the duration of the study.[11]

Not all studies of Ginkgo have produced positive outcomes. In a randomized, double-blind, cross-over study, 18 older female patients with stable IC received 120 mg GBE-8 twice a day, followed by placebo twice a day, for 3 months each. Differences in peripheral BP, walking tolerance, and leg pain severity were insignificant. Systemic BP was reduced by both placebo and Ginkgo. With Ginkgo, concentration and inability to remember were reduced, compared with placebo. Short-term memory did not change significantly. The authors concluded Ginkgo improved cognitive function in older patients with moderate arterial insufficiency, but it did not change signs and symptoms of vascular disease.[41]

Review of Metaanalyses of Controlled Trials

Fifteen controlled trials demonstrate that Ginkgo can help with IC, although only two trials were deemed acceptable in quality.[93]

In a metaanalysis of five placebo-controlled trials of GBE for the treatment of peripheral arterial disease, improvement was assessed by increased walking distance, measured by treadmill exercise. The global effect size of increased walking distance was 0.75; that is, the increase is 0.75 a standard deviation higher than attributable to placebo. This value is highly significant from zero, demonstrating GBE is a highly therapeutic treatment of peripheral arterial disease.[146]

Dosage, Toxicity, and Side Effects

Ginkgo must be taken consistently for 12 weeks to be most effective. Some positive benefit is observed at the 2- to 3-week point, with optimal benefits at 12 weeks. Side effects from the extracts are uncommon. In 44 double-blind studies involving almost 10,000 subjects, reported side effects were extremely rare. The most common side effects are gastrointestinal discomfort (21 cases), headaches (7 cases), and dizziness (6 cases). Allergic skin reaction, burning eyes, and breathlessness have been reported. There are no known drug interactions.[18]

■ Goldenseal

Description and History

Goldenseal is native to North America and is cultivated in Oregon and Washington (Figure 14-6). The perennial herb has a knotty yellow rhizome from which arise one single leaf and an erect hairy stem. In the spring, it bears two 5- to 9-lobed leaves that terminate in a single greenish-white flower.

The parts used for medicinal purposes are the dried rhizome and roots. The American Indians used goldenseal as both an herbal medicine and a

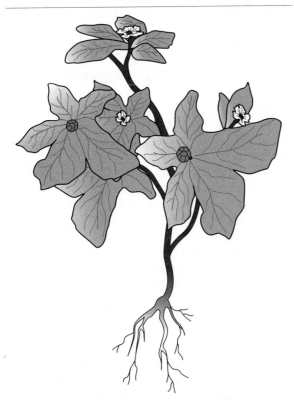

■ **Figure 14-6. Goldenseal.** Treatment of infection and congestion of mucous membranes.

clothing dye. Goldenseal was used medicinally to sooth the mucous membranes lining the respiratory, digestive, and genital and urinary tracts in conditions induced by allergy or infection.[43]

Cherokee Indians used goldenseal to treat cancer and dyspepsia, to improve appetite, and as a wash for local inflammatory conditions. Comanche Indians used it for an eye wash, stimulant, diuretic, laxative, and astringent. The Iroquois made infusions or decoctions of the roots for diarrhea, liver troubles, fever, sour stomach, gas, and pneumonia, and they used it as a stimulant for heart trouble or a run-down system.[110,123]

In the nineteenth century, American settlers considered goldenseal a cure-all. It remains an official pharmaceutical medicine in 11 countries, although it has virtually disappeared from orthodox use in American conventional medicine. Herbalists value goldenseal for treating cold and influenza symptoms and sore throats. Its astringency and antiseptic properties are responsible for its popularity as a throat treatment.

For more than 3000 years, extracts of goldenseal have been used as an antidiarrheal medication in the practice of both Ayurvedic medicine in India and traditional Chinese medicine. As one of several indigenous antidiarrheal plant extracts studied in India by Dutta and colleagues approximately 40 years ago, it alone was found to reduce the severity of *Vibrio cholerae* infection in rabbit models.[44]

Recommended Key Uses

Goldenseal is recommended for treatment of infection and congestion of the mucous membranes, digestive disorders, gastritis, peptic ulcers, colitis, anorexia, and painful menstruation.

Pharmacology and Actions

The benefits of goldenseal are produced by its content of isoquinoline alkaloids, one of which is berberine, the most widely studied alkaloid. Berberine exhibits a broad spectrum of antibiotic activity, including action against bacteria, protozoa, and fungi, specifically *Staphylococcus*.[3,65,106] One of Goldenseal's components, berberine, is used for treating wounds and open ulcerations because its astringency helps stop bleeding and forms a protective barrier, while the antiseptic properties help prevent infection.

In animal studies, Sack and Froehlich found that berberine inhibited the secretory responses of *Vibrio cholerae* and *E. coli* by 70% in a rabbit ligated intestinal loop model. The drug was effective when given either before or after toxin binding and when given intratubally or by stomach injection. It also inhibited secretory response of *E. coli* in infant mouse models.[140]

Researchers tested whether berberine sulphate had in vitro antiprotozoal (antiparasitic) activity when added to *Entamoeba histolytica*, *Giardia lamblia*, and *Trichomonas vaginalis*. Morphologic changes were monitored in the parasites by light and electron microscope. In all three, inhibition of growth was dose-dependent. Morphologic degeneration included trophozoite swelling, autophagic vaculoes, and increased autophagic vacuole number.[86]

Clinically Controlled Trials

Effects on Gastroenteritis

A randomized, controlled assessment of goldenseal's efficacy against diarrhea in acute gastroenteritis was held in Bombay, India, in 1964. Goldenseal (50 mg three times daily) was added to a routine line of treatment in the cases of 100 patients (the extra-treatment group), whereas subjects receiving full treatment but without golden seal served as the control group (N=100). Intravenous fluids corrected fluid and electrolyte imbalances. Groups were matched for signs and symptoms. Clinical responses were assessed every 6 hours. Patients were classified as mild, moderate, or severe according to the number of stools, level of dehydration, and whether collapse occurred (i.e., pulse is imperceptible and BP could not be recorded).

Berberine patients with severe abdominal pain (40%) recovered from pain in less than 24 hours, whereas those in the control group required antispasmodics for pain relief. Patient recovery time—assessed as less than two semisolid stools in 24 hours—was statistically significant for the berberine groups as compared with regular treatment (0.05). Five patients in the control group died, but all berberine patients survived. The authors concluded that goldenseal is an excellent antidiarrheal agent.[85]

In a follow-on trial that occurred at completion of the aforementioned study, 30 male patients with gastroenteritis received only goldenseal and fluids, without the standard treatment. Diarrhea was controlled in less than 24 hours for 15 of the patients, with more than 90% recovering in less than 48 hours. Two patients took 5 days to fully recover.[85]

Effects on Escherichia Coli and Cholera

In randomized controlled trials, 165 patients with acute diarrhea because of enterotoxigenic *E. coli* or *Vibrio cholerae* received 400 mg of berberine in a single dose. Mean stool volumes of patients in the treatment group were significantly less than those in the control group during three consecutive 8-hour periods. At 24 hours, more patients with *E. coli* diarrhea no longer suffered from the disorder (42% versus 20%, $p<0.05$). In patients with *Vibrio cholerae* diarrhea who received 400 mg berberine, the mean 8-hour stool volume at 16 hours declined significantly more than those in the control group. However, patients with *Vibrio cholerae* who received 1200 mg berberine **plus** tetracycline did not have significant reductions in stools compared with patients who received tetracycline alone. No side effects of berberine were noted. Results indicated that berberine is effective and safe as an antisecretory drug for *E. coli* diarrhea, but activity against *Vibrio cholerae* is slight and not additive to tetracycline.[136]

Effects on Trachoma

Worldwide, trachoma is one of the most widespread of all eye diseases, affecting approximately 500 million people in the world. It is estimated that this disease blinds 2 million people. In India,

trachoma and its associated infections are responsible for 20% of blindness caused by the fact that, economically, the country or individual or both cannot afford proper care. In rural areas of Delhi, 190 children with trachoma, stage IIa or IIb, aged 9 to 11 years, were given one of the following treatments:

1. 0.2% berberine drops and ointment
2. 0.12% berberine with 0.5% neomycin and ointment
3. 20% sodium sulfacetamide drops and 6% sodium sulfacetamide ointment
4. Placebo drops (normal saline) and placebo ointment (paraffin base)
   The patients were followed for 3 months.

Patients were assessed as either cured clinically or microbiologically negative. With berberine alone, 83.3% of patients were cured clinically and 50% were found microbiologically negative. When berberine and neomycin were used as treatment, 86% of patients were cured clinically and 58.83% were found microbiologically negative. With sulfacetemide, 72.72% were clinically cured and 40.90% were found microbiologically negative. This trial was the first blinded study to demonstrate berberine as effective against trachoma.[116]

Timing of Treatment

Bergner argued that goldenseal's wide reputation as an "herbal antibiotic" is most accurate when it is administered in one of the following ways:

1. Topically or applied directly to an infected wound or ulcer
2. In the mouth or pharynx
3. To stimulate the natural mucus in the gut, which kills bacteria in gastrointestinal illnesses with its **own** immunoglobulin A (IgA)

The use of goldenseal for "curing" a cold or influenza is ineffective, he argued.

Well-trained herbalists use goldenseal in subacute and chronic mucous membrane conditions, but it is not recommended for acute inflammations of the same. *Acute inflammation* of the mucous membranes is defined by antibody-laden mucus that flows freely, mechanically washing away invaders or tagging them for IgA antibody destruction. Inflammation and swelling of the tissues prevent penetration by invaders and flood the area with immune cells. In this state, healing occurs. *Subacute inflammation* of the mucous membranes occurs after the initial fever or inflammation subsides. The area may then become congested with the boggy by-products of the immune battle; the process that initially walled off the area in a protective way now blocks the influx of immune components. Ulceration, scarring, and other lesions develop. Secondary infections may set in. Although the body has begun accumulating high levels of antibodies to the infectious agent, they cannot get to the congested tissues. *Chronic inflammation* of mucous membranes is marked by ulceration and scarring of the membranes. They become dry and cracked as mucous secretions are blocked or deranged. Bleeding may occur, and secondary infections may be present because of the weakened circulation of immune components.

Taken too early in the healing process, especially in higher than traditional doses, goldenseal can actually have the following negative effects:

1. Exhausting the mucous glands by over stimulating them, resulting in dry membranes (i.e., two to three goldenseal capsules can have a distinct drying effect on the membranes)
2. Inhibiting the healthy inflammatory reaction, weakening the immune response, and prolonging the illness
3. Weakening the digestive system[14]

Bergner asserts that directly killing the germs does not cause the antibiotic effect against diarrheal infections; rather, the antibiotic effect is the result of increasing the flow of healthy mucus, which contains its own innate antibiotic factors—IgA antibodies. This effect is unnecessary in the early stages of a cold or influenza when mucus is already flowing freely.

Essentially, a cold may seem to be getting better because of the drying effect, but goldenseal taken in the early stages of a cold may actually inhibit the natural defenses against whatever "bug" has infected the patient. It may be appropriate to use goldenseal on the third or fourth day of the cold or influenza when there is a fear of an antibacterial infection. At this later stage, goldenseal will restore a healthy flow of mucus to the stagnant membranes.

Dosage, Toxicity, and Side Effects

Berberine-containing plants are generally nontoxic at recommended doses. They are not recommended, however, during pregnancy or in extremely high doses, which can interfere with vitamin B metabolism.[73]

There has been a belief (based on rumor) that goldenseal ingested in large quantities can mask drug tests, including marijuana, heroin, cocaine, and amphetamines. This is myth, with no demonstrated foundation in truth.

■ Kava Kava

Description and History

Kava, a slow growing perennial that reaches a height as tall as 3 meters, is a member of the pepper family (Figure 14-7). The plant has few leaves, and those are thin and heart shaped. Although Kava flowers, it cannot reproduce; it is dependent on human effort to guarantee its continuance. Its roots, which can reach 3 meters in length, are the parts of the plant used for medicinal purposes. The island communities of the Pacific, including Micronesia, Melanesia, and Polynesia, are the areas where Kava has historically been grown. Its origins predate written history in that part of the world, and Captain James Cook first described it during his 1768 voyage to the South Seas. Numerous legends of its creation abound.[123]

Kava was and still is valued for its "magical" properties when served as a ceremonial drink. Originally, village women made the drink by chewing the roots, spitting them out with saliva into a bowl, and then adding coconut milk. The mixture was then strained, and great quantities of the liquid swallowed as quickly as possible. In 1992, Hilary Clinton participated in a kava ceremony conducted by the Samoan community on Oahu.

Kava drinkers describe a sense of tranquility, relaxation, sociability, well being, and contentment after drinking the liquid; fatigue and anxiety are also lessened. If taken in excess, drinkers

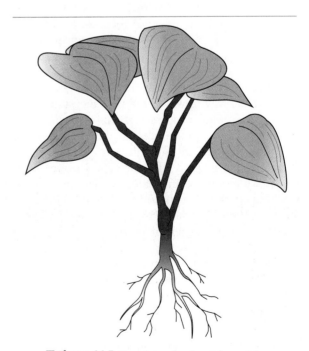

■ **Figure 14-7. Kava kava.** Treatment for anxiety.

become tired, muscle action becomes unsteady, and the partaker usually falls asleep. One researcher described the effect as euphoric, moving one's thinking processes from a linear state to one of a greater sense of "being" and contentment with "being." The senses (sight, smell, sound) are heightened. Drinking approximately 150 mm of certain varieties of Kava is sufficient to put most persons into a deep, dreamless sleep within 30 minutes.

Kava does not produce morning-after effects. Some drinkers have described it as a positive substitute for alcohol, producing happy rather than sullen moods with no hangovers and no side effects.

Recommended Key Uses

Kava is recommended for the treatment of nervous anxiety, stress, and restlessness.[18,123]

Pharmacology and Actions

Generally, kava kava is considered a safe, nonaddictive anxiety-reducing agent, comparable with benzodiazepines such as Valium. In animal studies, kava has demonstrated its ability as a sedative, analgesic, anticonvulsant, and muscle relaxant.

Kava kava rhizoma consists of the dried rhizomes of *Piper methysticum.* The drug contains kavapyrones (kawain). The component responsible for kava's effects is called *kavalactone,* and this component exerts its effects by atypical mechanisms. For example, most sedative drugs work by binding specific receptors, whereas kavalactones somehow modify receptor domains. Further, kava seems to act primarily on the limbic system—the ancient, emotional part of the brain. It is thought that kava may also promote sleep by altering the way in which the limbic system modulates emotional processes. It appears many of our laboratory models are not designed nor are they sophisticated enough to evaluate how kavalactones produce their effects. In one study on kava's pain relieving effects, researchers could not demonstrate any binding to opioid receptors. Further, they determined that the muscle-relaxing effects were not responsible for the pain-relieving effects. They also used models in which nonopiate analgesics like aspirin and NSAIDs were ineffective. These outcomes mean that kava reduces pain in a manner unlike morphine, aspirin, or any other pain reliever.[81]

In an important German study, researchers investigated the effects of kavain and kava extract on EEG patterns. It was found that the limbic structures of the brain and, in particular, the amygdalar complex are the preferential site of action for both kavain and the kava extract. The EEG changes for kava were more extensive than for kavain alone. The limbic system effect is important since this portion of the brain is implicated in modulating emotional processes.

Kava demonstrated no significant interaction with γ-aminobutyric acid (GABA) or with benzodiazepine binding sites in the brain.[38,76]

This is important because drugs such as Xanax and Valium act by specifically binding GABA receptors. Valerian root, another herbal sedative, weakly binds to similar receptors. Kava is less selective. Kava does not reduce pain by the same pathway as that used by opiate analgesics; it creates EEG changes similar to antianxiety drugs but without their sedative or hypnotic effects. It also does not impair cognitive activity, whereas patients taking oxazepam lose cognitive ability.

Another interesting effect is that kava does not lose effectiveness with time, even when consumed in huge amounts. It also has been demonstrated to protect against brain damage caused by ischemia because of the kavalactone's ability to limit the infarction area to a mild anticonvulsant effect.[7,42]

Clinically Controlled Trials

Effects on Anxiety

In a placebo-controlled, double-blind study of 38 patients with anxiety associated with neurotic disturbances, effects of kavain were compared with oxazepam, a benzodiazepine acting on GABA in the limbic system. Outcomes demonstrated the substances were equivalent in their anxiety-reducing effects.[102]

In a double-blind, placebo-controlled study (4-week duration), 58 patients with an anxiety syndrome of nonpsychotic origin received kava extract WS 1490 or a placebo. The Hamilton Anxiety Scale (HAMA), Adjectives List, and Clinical Global Impression Scale demonstrated from week 1 that kava produced significantly superior outcomes compared with placebo. Improvements continued progressively for 4 weeks. No side effects were noted.[91]

In a multicenter, double-blind, placebo-controlled study, 101 outpatients suffering from anxiety of nonpsychotic origin (e.g., agoraphobia, specific phobia, generalized anxiety disorder, adjustment disorder) participated in a 25-week trial using an extract of kava kava. From week 8, the treatment group demonstrated significantly superior outcomes compared with placebo, as assessed by HAMA, Self-Report Symptom Inventory, and Adjective Mood Scale. Adverse events were rare and evenly distributed between placebo and treatment. Outcomes suggest kava may be beneficial as a treatment alternative to tricyclic antidepressants and benzodiazepines in anxiety disorders. Kava had none of the tolerance problems or potential addictive qualities associated with the other medications.[167]

Many women face the emotional challenges of the climacteric period of life (i.e., endocrinal, somatic, and transitory psychologic changes occurring in the transition to menopause). In a randomized, placebo-controlled, double-blind study, 40 patients with climacteric-related symptoms were treated for 8 weeks with kava WS 1490 extract or placebo. From 1 week of treatment, the kava group demonstrated significantly superior outcomes compared with placebo. HAMA, patient diaries, Depressive Symptom Index, Clinical Global Impression Scale, and climacteric symptom indexes (e.g., Kuppermann Index and Schneider Scale) assessed the outcomes. Outcomes demonstrated a high level of efficacy of kava extract in treating psychosomatic dysfunctions in the climacteric period.[170]

Effects on Cognitive Functioning

Within the neurophysiologic domain, the effects of psychotropic drugs can be evaluated with a quantitative evaluation of the spontaneous EEG. More recently, the recording of the *event-related brain potentials* (ERPs) has been introduced into pharmacopsychology. ERPs are scale-recorded electrical potentials generated by neural activity and associated with specific sensory, cognitive, and motor processes. Unlike behavioral measurements, they reflect the continuum of processes between stimulus and response, thereby providing information about their time course, neuronal strength, and cerebral localization. The main advantage of the use of ERPs is that their different components can be related to certain steps in the processing of information and can identify possible effects of drugs on memory performance.

In a double-blind, cross-over study, the effects of oxazepam and an extract of kava roots were tested with 12 volunteers. Behavior and ERPs in a recognition-memory task were assessed. Within a list of visually presented words, the subjects identified those words that were shown for the first time as opposed to those that had been repeated. Oxazepam produced a reduction of a negative component in the 250-500 ms range for both old and new words and a reduction of old and new differences in the ERP (a significantly worse recog-

nition rate). Kava, on the other hand, showed a slightly increased recognition rate and a larger ERP difference between old and new words. In summary, Kava produced memory effects as good and, in some cases, slightly better than placebo, whereas oxazepam degraded memory quality by producing an insufficient or rudimentary code for the words, leading to a decreased familiarization and recognition of the words.[121]

In a placebo-controlled, double-blind study of 84 patients with anxiety symptoms, kavain improved vigilance, memory, and reaction time.[147]

In summary, kava did not alter behavior as compared with placebo; oxazepam, on the other hand, slowed reaction, reduced correct answers, and did not enhance memory as compared with placebo.

Dosage, Toxicity and Side Effects

Dosage depends on the amount of kavalactones. When pure kavalactones are used, as in clinical studies, the recommended dosage is 45 mg to 70 mg of kavalactones three times daily. For sedative treatment, 180 mg to 210 mg of kavalactones can be taken 1 hour before bedtime.

Although Samoans were known to ingest several bowls containing 250 mg of kavalactones each at one sitting, this is not recommended if consciousness is desired. Recent studies have used well-defined kava extracts, but evidence suggests that the whole complex of kavalactones taken together in their natural form provides the greatest pharmacologic activity. Further, kavalactones are more rapidly absorbed when given orally as an extract of the root rather than as isolated kavalactones. The bioavailability of lactones is three to five times higher from extract than from isolated substances.[89]

Although side effects have not been noted when kava is ingested in recommended quantities, high doses consumed over periods of a few months to years can lead to "kava dermopathy," a condition in which a generalized scaly eruption of skin takes place. The palms of the hands, soles of the feet, forearms, back, and shins are especially affected.

The only treatment is to discontinue the kava for a period. Subjects taking extremely high doses (310 g or more per week) for prolonged periods demonstrated biochemical abnormalities (e.g., low levels of serum albumin, protein, urea, bilirubin), blood in the urine, increased RBC volume, decreased platelet and lymphocyte counts, and shortness of breath. As subjects also reported heavy alcohol and tobacco use, it is difficult to sort out whether either of these or the kava contributed to the effects. However, large doses should be discouraged in any case.[109,139]

The German Commission E monograph notes that when taking kava, potentiation of effect is possible for other substances acting on the central nervous system, such as alcohol, barbiturates, and psychopharmacologic agents. The German Commission E has ruled kava kava contraindicated during pregnancy, while nursing, or for endogenous depression. Duration of administration should be limited to 3 months or less, unless under medical supervision. Even when administered within prescribed doses, this herb may adversely affect motor reflexes and judgment when driving and operating heavy equipment.[18]

■ Milk Thistle

Description and History

Milk thistle is found in dry rock soils in southern and western Europe and in some parts of the United States (Figure 14-8). Stems reach 1 to 3 feet high, bearing dark green shiny leaves with spiny, scalloped edges and white-streaked veins. Flowers are reddish purple, ending with sharp spines. Seeds, fruit, and leaves are used for medicinal purposes. Historically, milk thistle has been used to assist nursing mothers in producing milk. It has also been used in Germany for the treatment of jaundice.

Recommended Key Uses

Key uses for milk thistle include psoriasis, gallstones, hepatitis, and liver disorders.[19,149,150,171]

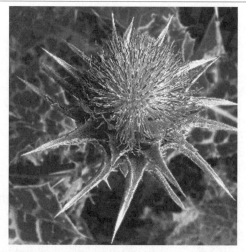

■ *Figure 14-8. Milk thistle. Treatment of liver disorders.*

Pharmacology and Actions

Effective treatment of liver disorders led to the pharmacologic discovery that *silymarin* (the active component in milk thistle) is one of the most potent liver-protecting substances known. Milk thistle's ability to prevent liver destruction is because of silymarin's ability to:

1. Inhibit free radicals by acting as an antioxidant. (It is 10 times as potent as vitamin E.)
2. Increase glutathione content in the liver by 35% in healthy subjects. (Glutathione increases the liver's ability to detoxify.)
3. Act as a potent inhibitor of the enzyme lipoxygenase, thereby inhibiting the formation of leukotrienes.[1,5,52,53,72,124,164]

Researchers often use an increase in the enzyme PDE (e.g., cyclic adenosine monophasphate [cAMP] phosphodiesterase) as a marker of increased inflammatory processes. Therefore PDE inhibition is a parameter used to test the potency of antiinflammatory drugs. Silymarin, the active principle of milk thistle, is a potent inhibitor of PDE. Its main constituents, silybin, silydianin, and silychristin, are 12 to 52 times more active than theophylline and 1 to 3 times more active than papaverine in inhibiting PDE.[94]

The inhibition of PDE by plant phenolics and the eventual increase of the cellular concentration of cAMP and guanosine monophasphate (GMP) offer a good explanation for properties of the milk thistle compounds, particularly their spasmolytic and antiinflammatory activities.[13,39,105]

Clinically Controlled Trials

Effects on Biliary Lipid Composition
In a placebo-controlled study, four patients with gallstones and six patients who had undergone a cholecystectomy (surgical removal of gallbladder) were given 420 mg of silymarin daily for 30 days (treatment group). Nine surgical patients received placebo. Bile specimens were analyzed before and after treatment. After 1 month, surgical patients taking silymarin showed significantly decreased cholesterol concentration compared with pretreatment level. Phospholipids and total bile salts were slightly but not significantly increased for treatment subjects. Similar results were found in the four patients with gallstones, whereas the nine control subjects did not demonstrate significant change. The results suggest that silymarin treatment influences biliary lipid composition, mainly by reducing biliary cholesterol concentration without altering biliary bile salt excretion.

In vitro, silymarin showed a dose-dependent inhibitory effect on hydroxy-methyl-glutaryl co-enzyme A (HMG-CoA) reductase activity, suggesting that reduced cholesterol excretion might be related to a reduction of cholesterol neosynthesis.[125]

Protection from Poisonous Substances

In a randomized, controlled study, 84 rats were given lethal doses of the deadliest mushroom, *Amanita phalloides,* the "poison deathcap." Half of the animals (treatment group) received silybin 1 hour before the toxin was given. Within 5 hours, 90% of untreated animals died, with hemorrhaging of the liver observed with light and electron microscopy. The rats treated with silybin all survived.[162]

Pretreatment with a single dose of silybin completely abolished the morphologic changes induced by the toxin and significantly decreased the activities of serum enzymes. Silybin when given alone did not result in changes of serum enzymes activities or hepatocytic ultra structure.

Effects on Liver Disease

In a 4-week, randomized, double-blind, placebo-controlled study, 97 patients with liver disease received either a daily dosage of 420 mg of silymarin (treatment group) or placebo. The patients were selected on the basis of elevated serum transaminase levels. In general, the series represented a relatively slight acute and subacute liver disease, mostly induced by alcohol abuse. Treated patients had a greater decrease in liver enzyme tests than controls. Patients having liver biopsies before and after treatment (N=29) showed more improvement than those in the placebo group.[142]

Only one selection criterion was used in this study—the increase in the serum level transaminases. Because patients suffered from alcoholism, the outcomes cannot be generalized to liver disease in general. The results refer only to acute and subacute alcohol-induced liver disease of a relatively slight degree.

In a double-blind, placebo-controlled trial (mean illness of 41 months, N=170), silymarin (200 mg three times daily) was assessed on mortality of patients with cirrhosis (70% histologically confirmed). For those given silymarin, the 2-year mortality rate was 23%; for placebo group, the rate was 33%. By life table analysis, cumulative 2-year survival rate was 82% and 68%, respectively. At 4 years, rates were 58% with silymarin and 38% with placebo. Patients with less severe scarring and with alcohol-induced cirrhosis performed best.[51]

Dosage, Toxicity and Side Effects

The recommended dosage of milk thistle is based on its silymarin content, which is 70 mg to 210 mg three times daily. Standardized extracts are preferred, and the best results are achieved at higher dosages (140 mg three times daily).

Dosage of silymarin bound to phosphatidylcholine (the most active combination) is recommended at 100 mg to 200 mg two times daily. The German Commission Monograph E notes that the average daily dose of drug is 12 g to 15g or formulations equivalent to 200 mg to 400 mg of silymarin, calculated as silybin.[18]

Silymarin is low in toxicity. At high doses when taken for short periods, silymarin showed no toxicity. Even long-term use resulted in little difficulty. Long-term use at high doses resulted in loose stools as a result and, in some cases, increased bile flow and secretion.[5,18]

■ St. John's Wort

Description and History

St. John's wort is a member of the genus *Hypericum* of which there are 400 species worldwide (Figure 14-9). This shrub plant is covered with bright yellow flowers. It grows best in dry gravel soils and in sunny places. St. John's wort is found in many parts of the world, including Europe and the United States. Both Pliny and

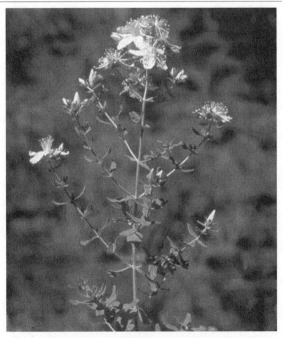

■ **Figure 14-9. St. John's wort.** Treatment for mild-to-moderate depression.

Hippocrates were reported to prescribe St. John's wort to treat illness.

Its Latin name, *hypericum performatum* is Greek, meaning "over an apparition." It was believed that one whiff of this herb could drive away evil spirits. The name "St. John's wort" came from a folk legend claiming that red spots, symbolic of St. John's blood, appeared on the leaves of the plant on the anniversary of St. John's beheading. Another tale claims that if a person sleeps with a piece of the plant under his or her pillow on St. John's Eve, the saint will appear in a dream, bless them, and prevent them from dying during the next year.[123]

In the Middle Ages, people believed St. John's wort had magical powers. Historically, the herb has been used medically for the purposes of treating wounds, kidney and lung ailments, and depression.[74]

Recommended Key Uses

St. John's wort is approved by the German Commission E for treatment of psychovegetative disturbances, depressive moods, anxiety, or nervous unrest. Oily hypericum preparations are recommended for dyspeptic complaints. St. John's wort is approved for external use (oily hypericum) for treatment and after therapy of acute and contused injuries, myalgia, and first-degree burns.[18]

Pharmacology and Actions

Some of the pharmacologic properties of St. John's wort include psychotropic, antidepressant, antiviral, and antibiotic effects, as well as increased healing of wounds and burns. Its psychoactive ingredients are hypericin and pseudohypericin.

Effects on Mood State

A common theory hypothesizes that depression is caused by deficiency or decreased effectiveness of norepinephrine and serotonin, which act as nerve impulse transmitting substances (neurotransmitters) in particular nerve pathways. One method for treating depression is the use of monoamine oxidase (MAO) inhibitors that retard one of the enzymes responsible for monoamine breakdown. MAO inhibitors then increase the concentration of neurotransmitters in the central nervous system. MAO inhibitors are currently used to treat mild-to-moderate depression.

Although previous studies have reported that hypericin inhibit MAO, other studies have failed to confirm this effect. In a study by Suzuki, the extract used in the study was only about 80% pure;

the other 20% of the extract could have led to a weak enzyme inhibition. The MAO inhibition shown for hypericum may not be pharmacologically relevant, since it has not been confirmed in vivo. Studies on the serotonin reuptake inhibition (SSRI) effects of St. John's wort also are mixed.[77] If the effects of St. John's wort are not caused exclusively by MAO inhibition or SSRI effects, then how, pharmacologically, does St. John's wort work? The study that follows sought to answer this question.

Testing the Actions

To determine how St. John's wort elicits its mood-evaluating effects, both a pure and a crude extract of hypericum was tested with a battery of 39 in vitro receptor assays and 2 enzyme assays. Hypericin alone had an affinity for N-methyl-D-aspartate (NMDA) receptors, whereas the crude extract had significant receptor affinity for adenosine, GABA A, GABA B, benzodiazepine, inositol triphosphate, and monamine oxidase A and B. However, with the exception of GABA A and B, the concentrations of hypericum extract required for the other identified in vitro activities are unlikely to be attained after oral administration in animals or humans. These data are consistent with recent pharmacologic evidence that suggests other unknown constituents of the plant may be of greater importance for its reported psychotherapeutic activity. The possible importance of GABA-receptor binding in the pharmacology of hypericum is being further evaluated.

In animal studies, the extract of St. John's wort was found to enhance exploratory activity in mice, extend narcotic sleeping time in a dose-dependent fashion, antagonize reserpine effects, and decrease aggressive behavior in socially isolated male mice.[128] (Reserpine is a drug that inhibits norepinephrine release, depleting norepinephrine from the adrenergic nerve endings). In animal studies, these are the types of behavior expected from an antidepressant drug.

Effects on Antiviral Activity

In an animal study of mice infected with retroviruses, hypericin and pseudohypericin displayed an extremely effective antiviral activity when administered to infected mice. Two mechanisms were later described. The first concerned inhibition of assembly or processing of intact virions from infected cells. The virions released contained no detectable reverse transcriptase activity. These compounds also directly inactivated mature and assembled retroviruses.[98,113,120,144,145]

Clinically Controlled Trials

In a multicenter, double-blind, placebo-controlled trial, 105 outpatients with neurotic depressions of short duration received 300 mg hypericum extract or placebo three times a day. In this study, 67% of the treated patients and 28% of placebo patients were identified as "responders," with demonstrated significant differences at week 2 (0.05) and week 4 (0.01). Most significant were improvements for feelings of sadness, hopelessness, helplessness, uselessness, difficulty falling asleep, and emotional fear. No improvements for feelings of guilt or somatic fear were found.[67]

In a double-blind, random-order trial, 12 subjects received three single intravenous doses of 300, 900, or 1800 mg of hypericum extract. Each dose was separated by a 10-day waiting period. After a 4-week washout period, patients took 300 mg of hypericum every 5 hours for 14 days. Hypericum was still measurable 72 hours after the lowest dose and 120 hours after the two higher doses. Pseudohypericin was undetectable in most cases at 72 hours.

In oral doses, hypericum reached steady-state level in the blood within 6 to 7 days. Median half-life for absorption distribution and elimination were 0.6, 6.0, and 43.1 hours for hypericin. Single and steady-state doses were well tolerated. Headache and fatigue occurred sporadically, irrespective of dose. No abnormality of any laboratory parameter and no skin reactions were observed with any dose.[90]

In a 6-week, controlled, randomized, clinical trial (N=135), patients with a diagnosis of major depression (single or recurrent episode), neurotic depression, or adjustment disorder with depressed mood received either hypericum extract (300 mg three times a day) or imipramine (25 mg three times a day). Significant reductions in the HAMD, depression scales according to von Zerssen and the Clinical Global Impressions (CGI) scale in both groups. No significant improvement differences were found between groups; hypericin was as effective as imipramine.

There was a trend of greater improvement on the CGI for patients taking hypericum. When HAMD scores greater than 20 were considered, there was significantly greater improvement after 6 weeks for patients taking St. John's wort. There were no serious side effects for hypericum, but three severe adverse reactions occurred in patients taking imipramine.[168]

In a randomized, clinically controlled trial (N=86) of 4 weeks in duration, male and female patients with depression and a HAMD score greater than 15 were randomized to receive 300 mg three times daily of hypericum or 25 mg maprotiline three times daily. Both groups significantly improved with no measurable differences between groups. Based on a ratio of 50% improvement of original score or a score less than 11, 67% of those given maprotiline and 61% of those taking St. John's wort made clinically significant improvements.

In general, maprotiline caused more rapid change than St. John's wort; however, at 4 weeks, results were of similar magnitude in both groups. At 4 weeks, more patients taking St. John's wort were rated "cured" than patients taking maprotiline. Mild-to-moderate side effects were reported in 35% of those taking maprotiline and 25% of those taking St. John's wort.[66]

In a single-blind, controlled trial (N=20), patients with seasonal affective disorder (SAD) participated in a 4-week trial. All were treated with 300 mg hypericum three times daily. Group 1 received bright light therapy (3000 lux) and group 2 received dim light (300 lux, a placebo light treatment), for 2 hours daily. The HAMD, Profile of Mood State, and von Zerssen self-rating scores were significantly and equally improved over baseline for both groups. The authors concluded hypericum is as effective as bright light in treatment of SAD.[108]

Reviews and Metaanalyses

In a metaanalysis of randomized clinical trials of St. John's wort for treatment of depression, 23 randomized, controlled trials, 1757 outpatients with mild-to-moderate severe depression were evaluated. Hypericum was compared with antidepressant drugs in 80 trials, and 14 were placebo controlled. Side effects occurred in 19.8% of patients on hypericum and 52.8% of patients on antidepressants. The authors concluded that hypericum is more effective than placebo, and it is as effective an antidepressant for the treatment of mild-to-moderate severe but not severe depression.[101]

In a systematic review (902 patients, 12 studies, 11 double blind, and 4- to 8-week duration), the author evaluated eight trials of St. John's wort compared with placebo, and three trials compared with standard medication. Eight trails found St. John's wort superior to placebo; three trials found St. John's wort as effective as tricyclic antidepressants but with no significant side effects. It was noted that ingestion of St. John's wort can cause subjects to sunburn more easily, however.[49]

Although St. John's wort seems to work with a variety of depressive forms, additional trials are needed to compare hypericum with other anti-depressants in well-defined groups of patients, investigate long-term side effects, and evaluate the relative efficacy of different preparations and doses.

Dosage, Toxicity, and Side Effects

St. John's wort extract standardized to 0.3% hypericin is considered most effective for the treatment of depression. The recommended dosage of this extract as antidepressant is 30 mg three times daily taken with meals.[123] The German Commission E suggests an average daily dose of 2 g to 4 g of drug or 0.2 mg to 1 mg of total hypericin in other forms of drug application.[18]

One side effect of St. John's wort is that it can cause severe photosensitivity. This has been reported only in a few cases, and typically where persons were taking extreme amounts for the treatment of HIV infections (St. John's wort has antiviral and antibacterial properties). Although initially promising, trials on St. John's Wort as treatment for HIV and AIDS proved disappointing, because significant blood levels of hypericin could not be achieved with oral or intravenous extracts. Additional trials with synthetic hypericin were undertaken and are in progress.[34,55,63,157]

Slight in vitro uterotonic effects in animal models suggest that caution should be taken in using St. John's wort during pregnancy, and therapeutic ultraviolet treatment should be avoided while taking hypericum because of its photosensitizing effect.

Duke University was awarded a 3-year, $4.3 million contract to conduct the first U.S. study of St. John's wort for the treatment of patients with major depression. In this study, patients (N=336) were randomized to one of three groups: (1) uniform dose of St. John's wort, (2) placebo, or (3) SSRI. Enrollment for the 8-week trial began in mid 1998. Study participants who responded positively to St. John's wort were followed for 18 weeks. For additional information on this study or to follow the results, OAM's web site at www.altmed.od.nih.gov is suggested.

■ Saw Palmetto

Description and History

Saw palmetto is a small palm tree that grows in the West Indies and from South Carolina to Florida in the United States (Figure 14-10). It grows 6 to 10 feet high, with 2 to 4 feet of spiny-toothed leaves that form a fan shape. The berries are used for medicinal purposes. The American Indians used saw palmetto berries to treat genital and urinary tract problems. Men took it to decrease irritation in the mucous membranes of the urinary and prostate tract, and women took it for disorders of the mammary glands. It was believed saw palmetto would eventually cause the breasts to enlarge as well. Many herbalists have recommended it for its aphrodisiac qualities.[123]

Recommended Key Uses

The prostate is a hormone-dependent gland under the control of the hormone dihydrotestosterone (DHT) acting at the level of the prostatic androgen receptor.[29] Saw palmetto is recommended as treatment of *benign prostatic hyperplasia* (BPH) stages I and II. Stage I is characterized by increase in frequency of urination, abnormally frequent urination, night urination, delayed onset of urination, and weak urinary stream. Stage II is characterized by the beginning of the decompensation of the bladder function accompanied by formation of residual urine and urge to urinate.[18]

BPH is caused by an accumulation of testosterone in the prostate. Once testosterone is in the prostate, it can become converted to the more potent DHT, which stimulates cells to multiply excessively, causing prostate enlargement. Between 50% and 60% of men between the ages of 40 and 59 years have BPH, and the disorder is characterized by increased urinary frequency, night-time awakening to empty the bladder, and reduced force and caliber of urination.

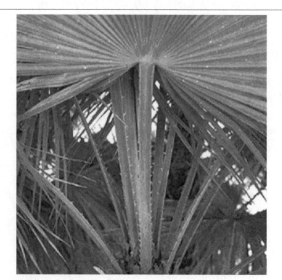

■ **Figure 14-10. Saw palmetto.** Treatment for benign prostatic hyperplasia.

Pharmacology and Actions

Saw palmetto inhibits the intraprostatic conversion of testosterone to DHT and inhibits DHT's intracellular binding and transport. It also has an antiestrogenic effect. Estrogen contributes to BPH in men.[20,27,30,36,47,159]

Clinically Controlled Trials

Effects on Benign Prostatic Hyperplasia

Uncontrolled Trials. In an uncontrolled, 3-month study, 305 patients with mild-to-moderate symptoms of BPH received 160 mg of saw palmetto extract twice daily. After 45 days of treatment, significant improvement was found in urinary flow rates, residual urinary volume, prostate size, and quality of life, as assessed by the International Prostate Symptom Score. At 90 days, 88% of patients and 88% of physicians reported that the therapy was effective.[24]

Placebo-Controlled Trials. In a double-blind, placebo-controlled trial, 50 patients received Permixon (PA 109), a form of saw palmetto and 44 patients received a placebo pill. The urinary rate of flow for those in the PA 109 group improved by 50%, and the number of nighttime trips to the bathroom decreased significantly. Further, patient- and physician-rated improvement was significantly greater than placebo (all outcomes p>0.001).[29] PA 109 was tolerated well with less reported side effects during the study by those receiving the drug (5 reports) than those receiving the placebo (11 reports). All side effects were minor (e.g., headache), and standard blood chemistry measurements showed no alterations.

Drug Comparison Trials. In a double-blind, comparative, parallel-group study (3-week duration), 63 patients received either 2.5 mg of alfuzosin twice a day or 160 mg of *serenoa repens* (saw palmetto) twice a day. Alfuzosin was found superior to serenoa repens on clinical symptom scales (e.g., Boyarsky's scale, visual analog scale, clinical global impression), urinary flow rates (uroflowmetry), and residual urinary volume (transabdominal ultrasound). Significant side effects were absent for both groups.[60]

Because the drug finasteride is accompanied by significant decreases in prostate-specific antigen (PSA) levels (50% with a 5 mg dose), this treatment carries the risk of masking the development of prostate cancer during treatment. Therefore saw palmetto may be a safer treatment for prostate dysfunction.

In a randomized, placebo-controlled, 1-week study (N=32) comparing finasteride (Proscar) with serenoa repens (Permixon), the effect of single and multiple doses of the drugs on the inhibition of 5-alpha reductase were assessed by serum DHT levels. (Group 1=finasteride 5 mg once a day [N=10]; group 2=serenoa repens 80 mg twice a day [N=11]; and group 3=placebo once a day [N=11] for 7 days). The single dose of finasteride reduced serum DHT levels 65% in 12 hours and 52% to 60% with multiple doses in 7 days. Neither Permixon nor the placebo-reduced serum DHT, demonstrating the efficacy of finasteride, but not serenoa repens, as an inhibitor of 5-alpha reductase. Therefore this study did not support the hypothesis of a prostatic mechanism of action through the inhibition of 5-alpha reductase.[158]

Review of Therapeutic Efficacy

In a review of saw palmetto's therapeutic efficacy to treat BPH, it was determined that serenoa repens, 160 mg twice daily for 1 to 3 months, was significantly superior to placebo in improving objective and subjective symptoms. Nocturia was reduced by 33% to 74% (placebo by 13% to 39%); urinary frequency during the day decreased between 11% and 43% (placebo 1% and 29%); peak urinary flow rate increased 26% to 50% (placebo 2% to 35%). In a comparative trial of 1000+ men, 160 mg of serenoa repens twice daily was compared with 5 mg of finasteride once daily for 6 months. The two drugs were comparable in outcomes. In smaller comparative trials, some differences were demonstrated between serenoa repens and alpha 1-receptor antagonists. The most reported adverse event with serenoa repens was mild nausea or abdominal pain. The author concluded that serenoa repens is a useful alternative to alpha receptors and finasteride in the treatment of BPH.[133]

Dosages, Toxicity, and Side Effects

Fat-soluble saw palmetto extracts standardized to contain 85% to 95% fatty acids and sterols should be used at the recommended dosage of 160 mg twice daily. Crude berries or tinctures cannot achieve the dose required to treat prostate difficulties effectively.

Finasteride caused impotence or loss of libido in some men and can cause birth defects in children of women who handle the pills or are exposed to semen of men using the drug. Saw palmetto has fewer side effects. No significant side effects were reported in clinical trials testing the saw palmetto berry or its extract with human subjects.

An Expert Speaks: Dr. Andrew Weil

Andrew Weil, M.D., has degrees in biology and medicine from Harvard University. He has traveled all over the world, studying healers and healing systems. Recognized as an international expert on alternative therapies, Dr. Weil is Associate Director of the Division of Social Perspectives in Medicine and Director of the Program in Integrative Medicine at the University of Arizona in Tucson. He has authored several books including *The Natural Mind, Health and Healing, Spontaneous Healing, Eight Weeks to Optimal Health, Ask Dr. Weil,* and *Natural Health and Natural Healing.* In the following interview, he shares his views on the medical acceptance of alternative therapies and herbal remedies.

Question. How do you explain the current interest in alternative therapies in the medical community?

Answer. The interest in alternative therapies now qualifies as a genuine sociocultural trend that is bringing all sorts of ideas and practices— from natural foods to Chinese medicine—from the fringes of society into the mainstream. Consumer interest has helped create a long-over-due openness in the medical profession.

Question. How did you become interested in herbs for medicinal use?

Answer. Well, I always had a life-long interest in plants, and I was originally a student in biology. So it was a very natural process to get back in touch with botany and its use in medicine. As a physician with a passion and desire to understand the interactions of mind and body, broad experiences with healing traditions of other cultures, and with a great concern for the widening gulf between what the consumer expects from physicians and what medical schools produce, the study of herbs was [for me] an integral part of the picture.

Question. Would you say that your experience with the plant medicines as you wrote about in your book, *The Marriage of the Sun and Moon,* inspired your interest?

Answer. That [book] follows my botany studies more. Yes, but this was just the beginning of my interest.

Question. What do you think of the current acceptance and applications of herbs in medicine?

Answer. This is the beginning of a huge realm of Western medicine, and there is more and more acceptance of this aspect of medicine. Plant medicine has been such a deep resource for the health of humans the world over, and it would be unnatural to ignore them [herbs]. Since we became so involved with science after the Second World War, we in Western medicine began to focus on the hope of a "better life through chemistry." But, plants have been our natural resources since life began, and we are now realizing this. This is part of the current revolution, but it has been a part of healing since the beginning of humankind.

Question. How do you respond to critics who are concerned about the potential toxicity of herbs?

Answer. I think that toxicity is a relative insignificant issue in comparison to drugs. The much greater issue is the efficacy of herbs. I readily agree that there is potential toxicity in herbs, but it is nowhere near the toxicity potentials of modern pharmaceuticals. The dangers reach critical levels very quickly. In a recent study, the researchers found that the death rate for women was three times higher from properly prescribed drugs than from breast cancer. Now we could relate that to toxicity of drugs, which is an obvious concern to us all. I think that the quality of herbs is a greater concern.

Question. In terms of herbal use, there is concern over quality assurance since herbals are not monitored as pharmaceuticals are by the FDA. Would you favor FDA supervision of herbals?

Answer. I think there should be regulation. I would like to see the FDA set up a division that would focus on dietary supplements, such as herbs and vitamins. It would have to be based on appropriate models of efficacy and [prescribed dosage] levels that are to be provided to the public.

Question. What do you see as the future of herbs in medicine?

Answer. I see the future very well. I can envision centers that do research on these [herbal] elements and that serve to develop protocols of special treatments for disease. I see physicians being trained in these medicines that complement other medical tools. I hope that the future of herbs will not meet the same end as other processes we have used. For example, many times we have used plants as a basis for treating some problem. When we discover such a cure, we run to the laboratories and synthesize it down to its basic ingredients and sell it as a drug. Willow bark, for instance, is the basis for aspirin. But, we have come to appreciate and understand that the complexity of the plant has to be honored in its wholeness, and there are different effects from how it is administered [as plant or drug].

Question. Do you have any special message for the new medical student or nursing student as he or she begins their lessons in healing?

Answer. I would like to tell them to learn as much as they can. This medical evolution is essential if our institutions are to survive. The doctors of the future will have the benefit of integrated medicine—the integration of alternative into conventional medicine. This will be the next major leap in evolution of medical care, not only here in the United States but throughout the world.

■ Chapter Review

Herbal medications can offer tremendous benefit to overall health when quality-controlled products are used, the appropriate herbal is chosen, and dosage and method of use are carefully considered. On the other hand, the patient or user must always be aware that "natural" is not synonymous with "safe"—the risks and potential side effects of herbals must also be evaluated carefully. In the hands of a responsible and well-educated user, herbals can be an important additive to traditional medical care. The advice of a professional and accredited herbalist is always beneficial in evaluating the wise choice of an herbal medicine.

CRITICAL THINKING AND CLINICAL APPLICATION EXERCISES

1. Discuss whether herbal preparations containing the whole herb or herbal preparations synthesized from the major active ingredient in the herb will be more effective. Defend your choice.
2. Discuss the problems of quality control of herbal products in the United States. What can a patient do, when purchasing an herb, to guarantee the quality and dosage of the herbal product?
3. How important is it that the major active ingredient in an herb be standardized? Why or why not?

Matching Terms and Definitions

Match each numbered definition with the correct term. Place the corresponding letter in the space provided.

a. Cranberry
b. Echinacea
c. Feverfew
d. Bilberry
e. Ginkgo biloba
f. Goldenseal
g. Kava
h. Milk thistle
i. Saw palmetto
j. St. John's wort

_____ 1. Treatment of psoriasis, gallstones, hepatitis, and liver disorders

_____ 2. Treatment of infection and congestion of the mucous membranes, digestive disorders, gastritis, peptic ulcers, colitis, anorexia, and painful menstruation

_____ 3. Treatment of psychovegetative disturbances, depressive moods, anxiety, and nervous unrest

_____ 4. Treatment of BPH18

_____ 5. Supportive therapy for influenza-like infections, colds, and chronic infections of the respiratory tract and lower urinary tract, and poorly healing wounds and chronic ulcerations

_____ 6. Treatment of cerebral vascular insufficiency, vascular insufficiency (IC, Raynaud's disease), retinopathy (macular degeneration, diabetic retinopathy), neuralgia and neuropathy, depression, dementia, inner ear dysfunction (vertigo, tinnitus), multiple sclerosis, premenstrual syndrome, and impotence

_____ 7. Prevention and treatment of urinary tract infections

_____ 8. Treatment of nonspecific, acute diarrhea; local therapy of mild inflammation of the mucous membranes of mouth and throat

_____ 9. Treatment of migraine headaches, fever, and inflammation

_____ 10. Treatment of nervous anxiety, stress, and restlessness

References

1. Adzet T: Polyphenolic compounds with biological and pharmacological activity, *Herbs Spices Med Plants* 1:167, 1986.
2. Amella M et al: Inhibition of mast cell histamine release by flavonoids and bioflavonoids, *Plants Med* 51:16, 1985.
3. Amin AH, Subbaiah TV, Abbasi KM: Berberine sulfate: antimicrobial activity, bioassay, and mode of action, *Can J Microbiol* 15:1067, 1969.
4. Avorn J et al: Reduction of bacteriuria and pyuria after ingestion of cranberry juice, *JAMA* 271(10):751, 1994.
5. Awang DV: Milk thistle, *Can Pharmacol J* 422:403, 1993.
6. Awang DV: Herbal medicine: feverfew, *Can Pharmacol J* 122:266, 1989.
7. Backhauss C, Krieglstein J: Extract of kava (Piper methysticum) and its methysticum constituents protect brain tissue against ischemic damage in rodents, *Eur J Pharmacol* 14:265, 1992.
8. Barsby RWJ et al: Feverfew and vascular smooth muscle: extracts from fresh and dried plants show opposing pharmacological profiles, dependent upon sesquiterpene lactone content, *Planta Med* 59:20, 1993.
9. Bauer R, Wagner H: Echinacea species as potential immunostimulatory drugs, *Econ Med Plant Res* 5:253, 1991.
10. Bauer R, Wagner H: In Wagner H, Farnsworth NR, editors, *Economic and medicinal plant research,* London, 1991, Academic Press.
11. Bauer U: Ginkgo biloba extract in the treatment of arteriopathy of the lower limbs. Sixty-five week study, *Presse Med* 15:1546, 1986.
12. Bau R et al: Immunological in vivo and in vitro examinations of Echinacea extracts, *Arzneimittelforschung* 38:276, 1988.
13. Berenguer J, Carrasco D: Double-blind trial of silymarin versus placebo in the treatment of chronic hepatitis, *Muench Med Wochenschr* 119:240, 1977.
14. Bergner P: Goldenseal and the common cold: the antibiotic myth, *Med Herbalism* 8(4):3, 1997.
15. Bertuglia S, Malandrino S, Colantuoni A: Effect of Vacinnium myrtillus anthocyanosides on ischemia reperfusion injury in hamster cheek pouch microcirculation, *Pharm Res* 31(3/4):183, 1995.
16. Bever B, Zahnd G: Plants with oral hypoglycemic action, *Q J Crude Drug Res* 17:139, 1979.
17. Blumenthal M et al: *German commission E monographs: therapeutic monographs for medicinal plants for human use,* Austin, TX, 1998, American Botanical Council.
18. Blumenthal M: *The complete German commission E monographs: therapeutic guide to herbal medicines,* Boston, 1998, Integrative Medicine.
19. Boari C et al: Toxic occupational liver diseases. Therapeutic effects of silymarin, *Minerva Med* 72:2679, 1981.
20. Boccafoschi, Annoscia S: Comparison of serenoa repens extract with placebo by controlled clinical trial in patients with prostatic adenomatosis, *Urologia* 50:1257, 1983.
21. Bone K: Echinacea: what makes it work? *Med Herb* 3(2):19, 1997.
22. Bottecchia D et al: Preliminary report on the inhibitory effect of *Vaccinium myrtillus* anthocyanosides on platelet aggregation and clot retraction, *Fitoterapia* 48:3, 1987.
23. Bower B: Herbal medicine: Rx for chimps? *Science News* 129:138, 1986.
24. Braeckman J: The extract of serenoa repens in the treatment of benign prostatic hyperplasia: a multi-center open study, *Curr Ther Res* 55:776, 1994.
25. Braunig B et al: Echinacea purpurea radix for strengthening the immune response in flu-like infections, *Z Phytother* 13:7, 1992.
26. Bravetti G: Preventive medical treatment of senile cataract with vitamin E and anthocyanosides: clinical evaluation, *Ann Ottalmolecular Clin Ocularity* 115:109, 1989.
27. Carilla E et al: Binding of Permixon, a new treatment for prostatic benign hyperplasia to the cytosolic androgen receptor in the rate prostate, *J Steroid Biochem* 20:521, 1984.
28. Caselli L: Clinical and electroretinographic study on activity of anthocyanosides, *Arch Med Intern* 37:29, 1985.
29. Champault G, Patel JC, Bonnard AM: A double-blind trial of an extract of the plant Serenoa repens in benign prostatic hyperplasia, *Br J Clin Pharmacol* 18:461, 1984.
30. Champault G et al: Medical treatment of prostatic adenoma. Controlled trial: PA 109 vs placebo in 110 patients, *Ann Urol (Paris)* 18:407, 1984.
31. Cignarella A, Nastasi M, Cavalli E, Puglisi L: Novel lipid-lowering properties of *Vaccinium myrtillus L.* leaves, a traditional antidiabetic treatment, in several models of a rat dyslipidemia: a comparison with ciprofibrate, *Thromb Res* 84(5):311, 1996.
32. Coeugniet E, Kuhnast R: Recurrent candidiasis: adjuvant immunotherapy with different formulations of Echinacea, *Therapiewoche* 36:3352, 1986.
33. Coles RRA: Trial of an extract of Ginkgo biloba (EGB) for tinnitus and hearing loss, *Clin Otolaryngol* 13:501,1988.
34. Cooper WC, James J: An observational study of the safety and efficacy of hypericin in HIV+ subjects, *Int Conf AIDS* (abstract) 6:369, 1990.
35. Criston A, Magistretti MJ: Antiulcer and healing activity of *Vaccinium myrtillus* anthocyanosides, *Farmaco (Roma)* 42(2):29, 1986.
36. Cukier et al: Permixon versus placebo, *CR Ther Pharmacol Clin* 4(25):15, 1985.
37. Cunio L: Vaccinium myrtillus, Medicinal plant review, *Aust J Med Herbalism* 5(4):81, 1993.
38. Davies LP, Drew CA, Duffield P, Johnston GA, Jamieson DD: Kava pyrones and resin: studies on GABA and benzodiazepine binding sites in rodent brain, *Pharmacol Toxicol* 71:120, 1992.
39. Deak G et al: Immunomodulator effect of silymarin therapy in chronic alcoholic liver diseases, *Orv Hetil* 131:1291, 1990.
40. DeFeudis FV: *Ginkgo biloba extract (Egb 761), pharmaceutical activities and clinical applications,* Paris, 1991, Reed Elsevier.
41. Drabaek H, Petersen JR, Winberg N, Hansen KF, Mehlsen J: The effects of Ginkgo biloba extract in patients with intermittent claudication, *Ugeskr Laeger* 158(27):3928, 1996.
42. Duffield PH, Jamieson D: Development of tolerance to kava in mice, *Clin Exp Pharmacol Physiol* 18:571, 1991.
43. Duke JA: *Handbook of medicinal herbs,* Boca Raton, 1985, CRC Press.
44. Dutta NK, Panse MV: Usefulness of berberine in the treatment of cholera (experimental), *Indian J Med Res* 50:732, 1962.
45. Eisenberg DM et al: Trends in alternative medicine use in the United States, 1990-1997. Results of a follow-up survey, *JAMA* 1569, 1998.
46. Elasser-Beila U, Willenbacher W et al: Cytokine production in leukocyte cultures during therapy with Echinacea Extract, *J Clin Lab Analysis* 10:441, 1996.
47. Emili E, Lo Cigno M, Petrone U: Clinical trial of a new drug for treating hypertrophy of the prostate (Permixon), *Urologia* 50:1042, 1983.
48. Ernst E: Pentoxifylline for intermittent claudication. A critical review, *Angiology* 45:339, 1994.
49. Ernst E: St. John's wort, an antidepressant? A systematic, criteria-based review, *Phytomedicine* 2(1):67, 1995.
50. Farnsworth NR, Akerele O, Bingel AS et al: Medicinal plants in therapy, *Bull World Health Organ* 63(6):965, 1985.

51. Ferenci P et al: Randomized controlled trial of silymarin treatment in patients with cirrhosis of the liver, *J Hepatol* 9:105, 1989.

52. Fiebrich F, Koch H: Silymarin, an inhibitor of lipoxygenase, *Experientia* 35(12):1548, 1979.

53. Fiebrich F, Koch H: Silymarin, an inhibitor of prostaglandin synthetase, *Experientia* 35(12):1550, 1979.

54. Foster S: Feverfew: when the head hurts, *Alternative Complement Ther* 9:335, 1995.

55. Furner V, Bek M, Gold J: A phase I/II unblinded dose ranging study of hypericin in HIV positive subjects, *Int Conf AIDS* (abstract WB 2071) 7:199, 1991.

56. Gabor M: Pharmacologic effects of flavonoids on blood vessels, *Angiologica* 9:355, 1972.

57. Garg RK, Nag D, Agrawal A: A double-blind, placebo-controlled trial of ginkgo biloba extract in acute cerebral ischemia, *J Assoc Physicians India* 43(11):760, 1995.

58. Gloria E, Peria A: Effect of anthocyanosides on the absolute visual threshold, *Ann Opthalmol Clin Ocul* 92:595, 1966.

59. Grassel E: Effect of Ginkgo-biloba extract on mental performance. Double-blind study using computerized measurement conditions in patients with cerebral insufficiency, *Fortschr Med* 110(5):73, 1992.

60. Grasso M, Montesano A et al: Comparative effects of alfuzosin vs. serenoa repens in the treatment of symptomatic benign prostatic hyperplasia, *Arch Esp Urol* 48(1):97, 1995.

61. Grieve M: *A modern herbal,* New York, 1971, Dover Publications.

62. Griggs B: *Green pharmacy: a history of herbal medicine,* London, 1981, Robert Hale.

63. Gulick R et al: Human hypericism: a photosensitivity reaction to hypericin (St. John's wort), *Int Conf AIDS* 8:B90, 1992.

64. Haase J, Halama P, Horr R: Effectiveness of brief infusions with Ginkgo biloba Special Extract Egb 761 in dementia of the vascular and Alzheimer's type, *Z Gerontol Geriatr* 29(4):302, 1996.

65. Hahn FE, Ciak J: Berberine, *Antibiot* 3:577, 1976.

66. Harrer G, Hubner WD, Podzuweit H: Effectiveness and tolerance of the hypericum extract LI 160 compared to maprotiline: a multicentre double-blind study, *J Ger Psychiatry* Neurol 7(suppl 1):S24, 194.

67. Harrer G, Sommer H: Treatment of mild/moderate depressions with hypericum, *Phytomedicine* 1:3, 1994.

68. Havsteen B: Flavonoids, a class of natural products of high pharmacological potency, *Biochem Pharmacol* 32:1141, 1983.

69. Heptinstall S et al: Extracts of feverfew inhibit granule secretion in blood platelets and polmorphonuclear leukocytes, *Lancet* 1(8437):1071, 1985.

70. Heptinstall S et al: Extracts of feverfew may inhibit platelet behavior via neutralization of sulphydryl groups, *J Pharm Pharmacol* 39(6):459, 1987.

71. Heptinstall S et al: Parthenolide content and bioactivity of feverfew (*Tanacetum Parthenium L*). Estimation of commercial and authenticated feverfew products, *J Pharm Pharmacol* 44:391, 1992.

72. Hikino H et al: Antihepatoxic actions of flavonolignans from silybum marianum fruits, *Planta Med* 50:248, 1984.

73. Hladon B: Toxicity of berberine sulfate, *Acta Pol Pharm* 32:113, 1975.

74. Hobbs C: St. John's wort, hypericum perforatum L, *Herbal Gram* 50:272, 1984.

75. Hofferberth B: The efficacy of Egb 761 in patients with senile dementia of the Alzheimer's type: a double-blind, placebo-controlled study on different levels of investigation, *Hum Psychopharmacol* 9:215, 1994.

76. Holm E, Staedt U, Heep J, Kortsik C, Behne F, Kaske A, Mennicke I, Untersuchungen zum Wirkungspofil von D: The action profile of D,L-kavain. Cerebral sites and sleep-wakefulness—rhythm in animals, *Arzneimittelforschung* 41:673, 1991.

77. Holzl J, Demisch L, Gollnik B: Investigations about anti-depressive and mood changing effects of hypericum perforatum, *Planta Med* 55:643, 1989.

78. Hopfenmuller W: Evidence for a therapeutic effect of Ginkgo biloba special extract. Meta-analysis of 11 clinical studies in patients with cerebrovascular insufficiency in old age, *Arzneimittelforschung* 44(9):1005, 1994.

79. Hopp E, Burn H: Ground substance in the nose in health and infection, *Ann Otol Rhinol Laryngol* 65:480, 1956.

80. IRI scanner data: Food, drug, mass market combined, total US, 52 weeks ending December 28, 1997.

81. Jamieson DD, Duffield PH: The antiniciceptive action of kava components in mice, *Clin Exp Pharmacol Physiol* 17:495, 1990.

82. Jayle GE, Aubert L: Action des glucosides d'anthocyanes sur la vision scotopique et mesopique du sujet normal, *Therapie* 19:171, 1964.

83. Johnson ES et al: Efficacy of feverfew as prophylactic treatment of migraine, *BMJ* 291:569, 1985.

84. Jonadet M et al: Anthocyanosides extracted from Vitis vinifera, Vaccinium myrtillus and Pinus martinnus I. Elastase-inhibiting activities in vitro II. Compared angio-protective activities in vivo, *J Pharm Belgenique* 38, 1983.

85. Kamat SA: Clinical trial with bererine hydrochloride for the control of diarrhea in acute gastroenteritis, *J Assoc Physicians India* 15:525, 1967.

86. Kaneda Y et al: In vitro effects of berberine sulfate on the growth of entamoeba histolytica, giardia lamblia and tricomonas vaginalis, *Ann Trop Med Parasitol* 85:417, 1991.

87. Kanowski S, Herrmann WM, Stephan K, Wierich W, Horr R: Proof of efficacy of the ginkgo biloba special extract Egb 761 in outpatients suffering from mild to moderate primary degenerative dementia of the Alzheimer's type or multi-infarct dementia, *Pharmacopsychiatry* 29(2):47, 1996.

88. Karchar L, Zagerman P, Krieglstein J: Effect of an extract on Ginkgo biloba on rat brain energy metabolism in hypoxia, *Naunyn-Schmiedeberg's Arch Pharmacol* 327:31, 1984.

89. Keledjian J et al: Uptake into mouserain of four compounds present in the psychoactive behavage kava, *J Pharm Sci* 77:1003, 1988.

90. Kerb R et al: Single-dose and steady-state pharmacokinetics of hypericin and pseudohypericin, *Antimicrob Agents Chemother* 40(9):2087, 1996.

91. Kinzler E, Kromer J, Lehmann E: Effect of a special extract in patients with anxiety, tension, and excitation states of non-psychotic genesis. Double blind study with placebos over 4 weeks, *Arzneimittelforschung* 41:584, 1991.

92. Kleijnen J, Knipschild P: Ginkgo biloba for cerebral insufficiency, *Br J Clin Pharmacol* 34:352, 1992.

93. Kleijnen J, Knipschild P: Ginkgo biloba, *Lancet* 340:1136, 1992.

94. Kock HP, Bachner J, Loffler E: Silymarin: potent inhibitor of cyclic AMP phosphodiesterase, *Methods Find Exp Clin Pharmacol* 7:409, 1985.

95. Koltai M et al: Platelet activating factor (PAF). A review of its effects, antagonists and possible future clinical implications (part II), *Drugs* 42(2):174, 1991.

96. Kuhnau J: The flavonoids, a class of semi-essential food components: their role in human nutrition, *World Rev Nutr Diet* 24:117, 1976.

97. Laplaud PM, Lelubre A, Chapman MJ: Antioxidant action of *Vacinnium myrtillus* extract on human low density lipoproteins in vitro: initial observations, *Fundam Clin Pharmacol* 11:35, 1997.

98. Lavie G et al: Studies of the mechanism of action of the antiretroviral agents hypericin and pseudohypericin, *Proc Natl Acad Sci U S A* 86:5963, 1989.

99. Lietti A, Forni G: Studies on Vaccinium myrtillus anthocyanosides I. *Arzneimittelforschung* 26:829, 1976.

100. Lietti A, Forni G: Studies on Vaccinium myrtillus antho-cyanosides II. *Arzneimittelforschung* 26:832, 1976.

101. Linde K, Ramirez G, Mulrow CD et al: St. John's wort for depression—an overview and meta-analysis of ran-domised clinical trials, *BMJ* 313(7052):253, 1996.

102. Lindenberg D, Pitule-Schodel H: D,L-Kavain in compari-son with oxazepam in anxiety disorders. A double-blind study of clinical effectiveness, *Fortschr Med* 108:49, 1990.

103. Loesche W, Groenewegen WA et al: Effects of an extract of feverfew *(Tanacetum parthenium)* on arachidonic acid metabolism in human blood platelets, *Biomed Biochim Acta* 47:10, 1988.

104. Magistretti MJ, Conti M, Cristoni A: Antiulcer activity of an anthocyanidin from Vaccinium myrtillus, *Arzneimittel-forschung* 38(5):686,1988.

105. Magliulo E, Gagliardi B, Fiori GP: Results of a double blind study on the effect of silymarin in the treatment of acute viral hepatitis, carried out at two medical centres, *Med Klin* 73:1060, 1978.

106. Majahan VM, Sharma A, Rattan A: Antimycotic activity of berberine sulphate: an alkaloid from an Indian medicinal herb, *Sabouraudia* 20:79, 1982.

107. Makheja AM, Bailey JM: A platelet phospholipase inhibitor from the medicinal herb feverfew, *Prostaglan-dins Leukot Med* 8:653, 1982.

108. Martinez B, Kasper S, Ruhrman S, Moller HJ: Hypericum in the treatment of seasonal affective disorders, *J Geriatr Psychiatry Neurol* 7(supp 1):S29, 1994.

109. Mathews JD et al: Effects of the heave usage of kava on physical health: summary of a pilot survey in an aborigi-nal community, *Med J Aust* 148:548, 1988.

110. McCaleb R: Goldenseal: medicinal herb, *Better Nutr Today Living* 8:52, 1993.

111. McGregor RL: The taxonomy of the genus Echinacea, *Univ Kans Sci Bull* 48:113, 1968.

112. Melchart D, Linde K, Wku F et al: Immunomodulation with Echinacea—a systematic review of controlled clini-cal trials, *Phytomedicine* 1:245, 1994.

113. Meruelo D, Lavie G, Lavie D: Therapeutic agents with dramatic antiretroviral activity and little toxicity at effec-tive doses: aromatic polycyclic diones hypericin and pseudohypericin, *Proc Natl Acad Sci U S A* 85:5230, 1988.

114. Meyer B: A multicenter randomized double-blind study of Ginkgo biloba extract versus placebo in the treatment of tinnitus. In Rokan, Funfgeld EW, editor: *Ginkgo biloba. Recent results in pharmacology and clinic,* New York, 1988, Springer-Verlag.

115. Middleton E: The flavonoids, *Trends Pharm Sci* 5:335, 1984.

116. Mohan M et al: Berberine in trachoma, *Indian J Opthalmolmic Sci* 30:69, 1982.

117. Monbiosse JC, Braquet P, Borel JP: Oxygen-free radicals as mediators of collagen breakage, *Agents Actions* 15:49, 1984.

118. Morazzoni P, Magistretti MJ: Effects of *Vaccinium myr-tillus* anthocyanosides on prostacyclin like activity in rat arterial tissue, *Fitoterapia* 57:11, 1986.

119. Mose J: Effect of echinacin on phagocytosis and natural killer cells, *Med Klin* 34:1463, 1983.

120. Muldner VH, Zoller M: Antidepressive effect of a hyper-icum extract standardized to the active hypericine com-plex, *Arzneimittelforschung* 34:918, 1984.

121. Munte TF et al: Effects of oxazepam and an extract of kava roots (Piper methysticum) on event-related poten-tials in a word recognition task, *Neuropyschobiology* 27:46, 1993.

122. Murphy JJ, Heptinstall S, Mitchell JRA: Randomised double-blind placebo-controlled trial of feverfew in migraine prevention, *Lancet* 2189, 1988.

123. Murray MT: *The healing power of herbs,* Rocklin, CA, 1995, Prima Publishing.

124. Muzes G et al: Effect of the bioflavonoid silymarin on the in vitro activity and expression of super oxide dismutase (SOD) enzyme, *Acta Physiol Hung* 78:3, 1991.

125. Nassauto G et al: Effect of silibinin on bilary lipid compo-sition. Experimental and clinical study, *J Hepatol* 12:290, 1991.

126. National Institutes of Health, Office of Alternative Medicine: *Alternative medicine: expanding medical horizons,* Bethesda, MD, 1992, NIH.

127. Ofek I et al: Anti-Escherichia Coli adhesion activity of cranberry and blueberry juices, *N Engl J Med* 324(22):1599, 1991.

128. Okpanyi VSN, Weicher ML: Animal experiments on the psychotropic action of a Hypericum extract, *Arzneimittel-forschung* 37:10, 1987.

129. 103rd Congress, Public Law 103-417 (Oct 25, 1994): *Dietary supplement health and education act of 1994.*

130. Patrick M et al: Feverfew in rheumatoid arthritis: a dou-ble blind, placebo controlled study, *Ann Rheum Dis* 48:547, 1989.

131. Pharmaceutical Research and Manufacturers of America: Information from www.http://www.phrma.org/.

132. Pietri S, Seguin JR, d'Arbigny P et al: Ginkgo biloba extract (Egb 761) pretreatment limits free radical-induced oxidative stress in patients undergoing coronary bypass surgery, *Cardiovasc Drugs Ther* 11(2):121, 1997.

133. Plosker GL, Brogden RN: Serenoa repens (Permixon). A review of its pharmacology and therapeutic efficacy in benign prostatic hyperplasia, *Drugs Aging* 9(5):379, 1996.

134. Prodromos PN et al: Cranberry juice in the treatment of urinary tract infections, *Southwestern Med* 47:17, 1968.

135. Pulliero G, Montin S et al: Ex vivo study of the inhibitory effects of V myrtillus anthocyanosides on human platelet aggregation, *Fitoterapia* 60(1):69, 1989.

136. Rabbani GH et al: Randomized controlled trial of berber-ine sulfate therapy for diarrhea due to enterotoxigenic *Escherichia coli* and *Vibrio cholerae, J Infect Dis* 155:979, 1987.

137. Rai GS, Shovlin C, Wesnes KA: A double-blind, placebo controlled study of Ginkgo biloba extract (tanakan) in elderly outpatients with mild to moderate memory impairment, *Curr Med Res Opin* 12(6):350, 1991.

138. Roesler J, Emmendorffer A, Steinmuller C et al: Application of purified polysaccharides from cell cultures of the plant echinacea purpurea to test subjects mediates activation of the phagocyte system, *Int J Immunophar-macol* 13(7):931, 1991.

139. Ruze P: Kava-induced dermopathy: a niacin deficiency, *Lancet* 335:1442, 1990.

140. Sack RB, Froehlich JL: Berberine inhibits intestinal secretory response of vibrio cholerae toxins and escherichia coli enterotoxins, *Infect Immun* 35:471, 1982.

141. Salaa D, Rolando M, Rossi PL, Pissarello L: Effect of anthocyanosides on visual performances at low illumina-tion, *Minerva Oftalmoigal* 21:283, 1979.

142. Salmi HA, Sarna S: Effect of silymarin on chemical, functional, and morphological alteration of the liver. A double-blind controlled study, *Scand J Gastroenterol* 17:417, 1982.

143. Scharrer A, Ober M: Anthocyanosides in the treatment of retinopathies, *Klin Monatsbl Augenheilkd* 178:386, 1981.

144. Schlich D, Brauchmann F, Schenk N: Treatment of depressive conditions with hypericum, *Psychology* 13:440, 1987.

145. Schmidt U, Sommer H: St. John's wort extract in the ambulatory therapy of depression. Attention and reaction ability are preserved, *Forschr Med* 111:339, 1993.

146. Schneider B: Ginkgo biloba extract in peripheral arterial diseases. Meta-analysis of controlled clinical studies, *Arzneimittelforschung* 42:428, 1992.

147. Scholing WE, Clausen HD: On the effect of D,L-kavain in comparison with oxazepam in anxiety disorders. A double-blind study of clinical effectiveness, *Arzneimittelforschung* 41:54, 1991 and 1993; 27:46, 1993.

148. Schoneberger D: The influence of immune-stimulating effects of pressed juice from echinacea purpurea on the course and severity of colds. Results of a double-blind study, *Forum Immunol* 8:2, 1992.

149. Schopen RD et al: Searching for a new therapeutic principle. Experience with hepatic therapeutic agent Legalon, *Med Welt* 20:888, 1969.

150. Schopen RD, Lange OK: Therapy of hepatoses. Therapeutic use of Silymarin, *Med Welt* 21:691, 1970.

151. Schubert H, Halam P: Depressive episode primarily unresponsive to therapy in elderly patients: efficacy of ginkgo biloba (Egb 761) in combination with antidepressants, *Geriatr Forsch* 3:45, 1993.

152. See DM, Broumand N, Sahl L, Tilles JG: In vitro effects of echinacea and ginseng on natural killer and antibody-dependent cytotoxicity in healthy subjects and chronic fatigue syndrome or acquired immunodeficiency syndrome patients, *Immunopharmacol* 35:229, 1997.

153. Siegel RK: Ginseng abuse syndrome, *JAMA* 241:1614, 1979.

154. Sikora R, Sohn M, Deutz F-J et al: Ginkgo biloba extract in the therapy of erectile dysfunction, *J Urology* 141:188A, 1989.

155. Sobata AE: Inhibition of bacterial adherence by cranberry juice: potential use for the treatment of urinary tract infections, *J Urology* 131:1013, 1984.

156. Solecki RS, Shanidar IV: A Neanderthal flower burial of northern Iraq, *Science* 190:880, 1975.

157. Steinbeck-Klose A, Wernet P: Successful long term treatment over 40 months of HIV patients with intravenous hypericin, *Int Conf AIDS* (abstract PO-B26-2012) 9(1):470, 1993.

158. Strauch G, Perles P, Vergult G et al: Comparison of finasteride (Proscar) and serenoa repens (Permixon) in the inhibition of 5-alpha reductase in healthy male volunteers, *Eur Urol* 26(3):247, 1994.

159. Sultan C et al: Inhibition of androgen metabolism and binding by a liposteroic extract of seronoa repens B in human foreskin fibroblasts, *J Steroid Biochem* 20:515, 1984.

160. Terrasse J, Moinade S: Premiers resultats obtenus avec un nouveau facteur vitamininque "P" less anthocyanosides extraits du Vaccinium myrtillus, *Presse Med* 72:397, 1964.

161. Tragni E et al: Evidence from two classic irritation tests for an anti-inflammatory action of a natural extract, echinacina B, *Food Chem Toxicol* 23:317, 1985.

162. Tuchweber B, Sieck R, Trost W: Prevention by silybin of phalloidin-induced acute hepatoxicity, *Toxicol Appl Pharmacol* 51:265, 1979.

163. Tyler VE: *Herbs of choice: the therapeutic use of phytomedicinals,* Binghampton, NY, 1994, Pharmaceutical Products Press.

164. Valenzuela A et al: Selectivity of silymarin on the increase of the glutathione content in different tissues of the rat, *Plant Med* 55:420, 1989.

165. Voaden D, Jacobson M: Tumor inhibitors. 3. Identification and synthesis of an oncolytic hydrocarbon from American coneflower roots, *J Med Chem* 15:619, 1972.

166. Vogel VJ: *American Indian medicine,* Norman, OK, 1970, University of Oklahoma Press.

167. Volz HP, Kieser M: Kava-kava extract WS 1490 versus placebo in anxiety disorders—a randomized placebo-controlled 25-week outpatient trial, *Pharmacopsychiatry* 1:1, 1997.

168. Vorbach EU, Hubner WD, Arnoldt KH: Effectiveness and tolerance of the hypericum extract LI 160 in comparison with imipramine: randomized double-blind study with 135 outpatients, *J Geriatr Psychiatry Neurol* 7(suppl 1):S19, 1994.

169. Wagner H et al: In vitro inhibition of arachidonate metabolism by some alkylamides and phenylated phenols, *Planta Med* 55:566, 1989.

170. Warnecke G: Psychosomatic dysfunctions in the female climacteric. Clinical effectiveness and tolerance of kava extract WS 1490, *Fortschr Med* 109(4):119, 1991.

171. Weber G, Galle K: The liver, a therapeutic target in dermatoses, *Med Welt* 34(4):108, 1983.

172. Wegman R, Maeda K, Tronche P, Bastide P: Effects of anthocyanosides on photoreceptors. Cytoenzymatic aspects, *Ann Histochim* 14:237, 1969.

173. Weiner MA, Weiner JA: *Herbs that heal,* Mill Valley, CA, 1994, Quantum.

174. Zaragoza F, Iglesias I, Benedi J: Comparative study of the anti-aggregation effects of anthocyanosides and other agents, *Arch Farmacol Toxicol* 11:183, 1985.

15

Exercise as an Alternative Therapy

Lyn W. Freeman

G. Frank Lawlis

WHY READ THIS CHAPTER?

This chapter addresses the use of exercise as complementary treatment for the conditions of cardiovascular and pulmonary disease and emotional dysfunction.

There is evidence supporting aerobic exercise as a primary treatment for these conditions. Too often, unhealthy lifestyle habits are significant contributors to disease progression. Recognition of this fact, applied as a simple lifestyle adjustment, can in many cases reverse or improve disease effects.

There are known physiologic pathways that explain the health effects of exercise, and health benefits have been empirically demonstrated in controlled experiments. From these experiments, specific exercise protocols have been developed for addressing symptoms of disease. The integration of appropriate, well-researched exercise protocols with the approaches of conventional medical can result in the optimal treatment of cardiovascular, pulmonary, and depressive disorders.

CHAPTER AT A GLANCE

This chapter focuses on three primary conditions that are significantly improved by exercise: cardiovascular disease, pulmonary dysfunction, and depression.

An overview is provided of the function of the cardiovascular and pulmonary systems. Clinical research on outcomes of exercise as treatment for cardiovascular disease and pulmonary dysfunction are examined. Evidence that exercise modulates mood state is also explored. Indications and contraindications for exercise therapy are presented as road maps for prescriptions and recommendations of exercise for optimal health outcomes. Effects of exercise on immune function and other disease states are discussed.

Implications for exercise as primary medical treatment are briefly examined. No explicit recommendations are made for preventive medicine, outside of the fact that moderate exercise appears to extend life.

Use it or lose it.

ANONYMOUS

CHAPTER OBJECTIVES

After completing this chapter, you should be able to:

1. Describe the physiologic and psychologic effects of exercise.
2. Explore the use of exercise rehabilitation protocols for the treatment of cardiovascular and pulmonary diseases.
3. Explain the relevance of exercise for stress management.
4. Compare and contrast the implications of exercise for depression and anxiety disorders.
5. Discuss the use of exercise as a therapy for other health concerns, such as diabetes, cancer, aging, menopause, urinary incontinence, and human immunodeficiency virus (HIV), and acquired immunodeficiency syndrome (AIDS).
6. Define the major indications and contraindications for the prescription of exercise therapy for disease states.

■ 425 ■

It has always been understood that exercise is a requirement for increased strength, endurance, vigor, and health. Hippocrates, the father of modern medicine, argued strongly that exercise was a necessity for maintaining optimal quality of life. He stated:

> "All parts of the body which have a function, if used in moderation and exercised in labours in which each is accustomed, become thereby healthy, well-developed and age more slowly, but if unused and left idle, they become liable to disease, defective in growth, and age quickly."

In today's society, exercise also serves as complementary therapy for certain chronic diseases.

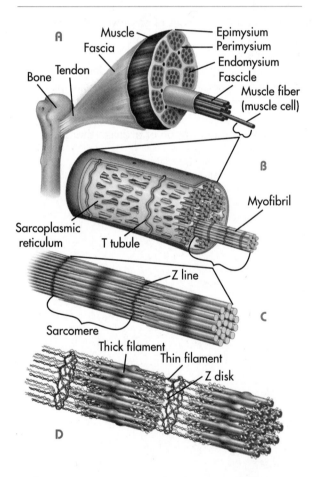

■ **Figure 15-1. Structure of skeletal muscle. A,** Skeletal muscle organ, composed of bundles of contractile muscle fibers held together by connective tissue. **B,** Greater magnification of single fiber showing smaller fibers—myofibrils—in the sarcoplasm. Note sarcoplasmic reticulum and T tubules forming a three-part structure called a triad. **C,** Myofibril magnified further to show sarcomere between successive Z lines. Cross striae are visible. **D,** Molecular structure of myofibral showing thick myofilaments and thin myofilaments. *Modified from Thibodeau GA, Patton KT:* Anatomy & physiology, *St Louis, 1999, Mosby.*

Exercise has been demonstrated to strengthen the cardiovascular and immune systems, (the bodily systems most effected by chronic disease) and to improve mood state (an effector of biochemical responses).

To understand how exercise produces these outcomes, a basic knowledge of muscle functioning is required.

■ Mechanisms Underlying Exercise Physiology

Physiologic and Biochemical Reactions Leading to Muscle Contraction

Muscles perform their work by contracting muscle fibers at the microscopic level within many myofibrils of a single muscle fiber. Muscle tissues that perform contractions are made up of two different types of rodlike protein filaments, or myofilaments, called *actin* and *myosin.* Together, these two myofilaments form the protein framework of the muscle fiber called the *sarcomere* (Figure 15-1).

The energy required for muscles to contract is obtained by hydrolysis of a nucleotide called *adenosine triphosphate* (ATP). Two of three phosphate groups in ATP are attached by high-energy bonds that, when broken, produce the energy required to pull the thin myofilaments during a muscle contraction. Muscle contractions work somewhat like a loaded slingshot. Before a muscle contracts, each myosin cross bridge moves into a resting position when an ATP molecule binds to it. The ATP molecule then breaks its high-energy bond, releasing the inorganic phosphate (P_1) and transferring the energy to the myosin cross bridge. The resting muscle, like a slingshot, is now ready to "spring." When myosin binds to actin, the energy is released and the cross bridge springs back to its original position. Essentially, ATP provides the energy necessary to perform the work of pulling the thin filaments during contraction. Another ATP molecule then binds to the myosin cross bridge, which again releases actin and moves into a resting cycle, available for the next muscle contraction. As long as ATP is available and actin sites are unblocked, this cycle will continue (Figure 15-2). The available stores of ATP are limited, and the effects of ATP are transient; consequently, ATP must be constantly resynthesized in working skeletal muscles for the muscles to perform (i.e., to contract) continuously. To sustain exercise, ATP is synthesized aerobically, primarily from carbohydrates and fats (Figure 15-3).

Aerobic and Anaerobic Respiration

Aerobic respiration is a catabolic process that produces the maximum amount of energy available from each glucose molecule. When sufficient oxygen is available, it combines with hydrogen ions to form water and carbon dioxide and, thus, a higher yield of ATP. By contrast, when sufficient oxygen is not available, hydrogen accumulates and blocks the aerobic cycle, so that the cells must rely on anaerobic respiration for energy. *Anaerobic respiration* does not require oxygen to produce ATP and has the added advantage of being a very rapid process. Muscle fibers having difficulty getting oxygen, (i.e., fibers generating a great deal of force very quickly) must rely on anaerobic respiration to resynthesize ATP molecules.[72]

Exercise and Protein Synthesis

Because muscle is composed largely of protein, there is evidence that exercise strongly affects protein synthesis. Indeed, exercise has been reported to activate the entire protein synthesizing machinery. Exercise activates the transport of amino acids—the building blocks of proteins—into the exercising fiber; it increases levels of both ribonucleic acid (RNA)-polymerase and messenger-RNA (mRNA); and finally, it increases protein synthesis itself.

Exercise is such a powerful stimulator of protein synthesis that even in the absence of growth hormone, insulin, or adequate food intake, it will cause muscle strengthening, or hypertrophy, in an animal that is otherwise in negative nitrogen bal-

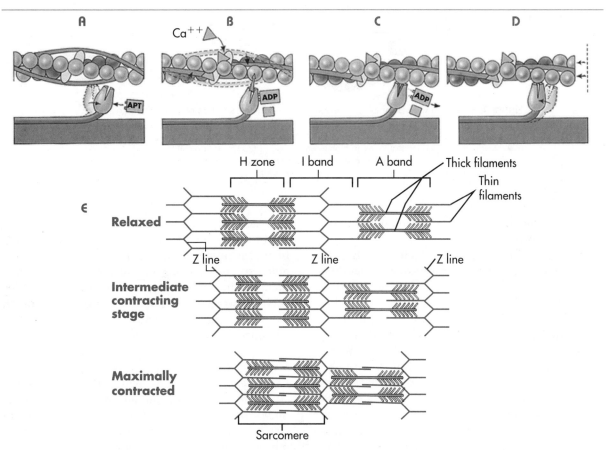

■ *Figure 15-2.* **The molecular basis of muscle contraction. A,** Each myosin cross bridge in the thick filament moves into a resting position after an ATP binds and transfers its energy. **B,** Calcium ions released from the SR bind to troponin in the thin filament, allowing tropomyosin to shift from its position blocking the active sites of actin molecules. **C,** Each myosin cross bridge then binds to an active site on a thin filament, displacing the remnants of ATP hydrolsis—adenosine diphosphate (ADP) and inorganic phosphate (Pi). **D,** The release of stored energy from step A provides the force needed for each cross bridge to move back to its original position, pulling actin along with it. Each cross bridge will remain bound to actin until another ATP binds to it and pulls it back into its resting position (A). **E, Sliding filament theory.** During contraction, myosin cross bridge pull the thin filaments toward the center of each sarcomere, thus shortening the myofibril and the entire muscle fiber. *Modified from Thibodeau GA, Patton KT:* Anatomy & physiology, *St Louis, 1999, Mosby.*

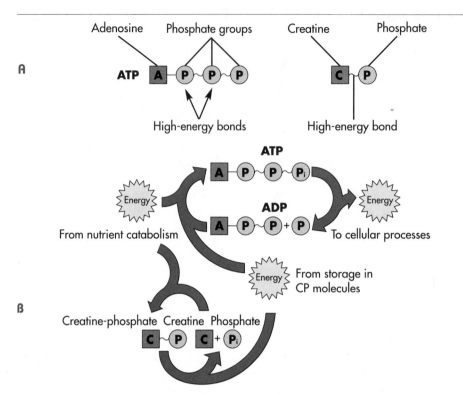

■ **Figure 15-3. Energy sources for muscle contraction. A,** The basic structure of two high-energy molecules in the sarcoplasm: adenosine trihosphate (ATP) and creatine phosphate. **B,** This diagram shows how energy released during the catabolism of nutrients can be transferred to the high-energy bonds of ATP directly or stored temporarily in the high-energy bond of the CP. During contraction, ATP is hydrolyzed, and the energy of the broken bond is transferred to a myosin cross bridge. *Modified from Thibodeau GA, Patton KT:* Anatomy and physiology, *ed 4, St Louis, 1999, Mosby.*

ance. Even the muscle wasting action of cortisone is offset by exercise.

Research findings have led some scientists to hypothesize that strenuous exercise can affect the genetic system—the basic map of life. Dog hearts were exercised by constricting the ascending aorta so that the hearts had to beat harder to pump sufficient blood. Extracts were then prepared from the hypertrophying dog hearts. When the extract was perfused, or pumped, into the hearts of other dogs and even rats, the extract caused increased synthesis of mRNA and protein.[33] In other words, when the cardiac muscle was exercised, some substance activated the muscle genes to increase protein synthesis. It has been suggested that if exercise can modify the genetic structure of the heart, perhaps it can affect the architectural map of other systems (e.g., immune and nervous) as well.

■ Types of Exercise

Aerobic and Anaerobic Exercise

Aerobic exercise refers to the repetitive movement of large muscle groups in which energy is derived from aerobic metabolism, which can only occur in the presence of oxygen. Activities such as walking, biking, swimming, and jogging are considered aerobic exercises. *Anaerobic exercise* uses anaerobic metabolism for energy, and includes activities such as weight lifting and sprinting. The quick fiber recruitment activities of anaerobic exercise can occur in the absence of oxygen.

Exercise Strategies

Exercise protocols are divided into two general strategies; *resistance* and *endurance*. The *resistance strategy*, often delivered with the use of weights or torsion, emphasizes intense, forced muscle contraction. When performed with greater resistance (e.g., heavy weights), increased muscle fiber creates bulk and enhances power. The *endurance strategy* prolongs muscle activity but with less resistance. This strategy creates broader fiber participation, and muscles become long and thin rather than bulky. Long distance runners are usually good examples of the effective use of an endurance strategy.

Although there are controversies as to what amount, type, and intensity of exercise is most beneficial, it is clear that the musculoskeletal system demands a certain amount of exercise to remain vital. For example, when a person is on complete bed rest and all exercise is limited, muscle strength atrophies at approximately 3% per day. Without some demand, muscles quickly weaken and become inadequate to perform even the most basic functions. Exercise can reverse this trend. Exercise programs for nursing home residents of advanced age and frailty have consistently demonstrated significant improvement in mood and strength.[22,23,57]

∎ Exercise and Cardiovascular Disease

Heart attack resulting from cardiovascular disease is the leading cause of death in the industrialized world and one of the most common causes of disabilities.[1] Its three clinical manifestations are *angina* (chest pain because of a lack of oxygen), *myocardial infarction* (heart attack or death of heart muscle because of a lack of oxygen), and sudden cardiac death. These outcomes now seem almost inevitable accompaniments of modern lifestyles.

Cardiovascular Disease Defined

Cardiovascular disease is a progressive, chronic disease process closely aligned to certain epidemiologically documented risk factors. Patients with this disease are suffering from a progressive process known as atherosclerosis. *Atherosclerosis* refers to the accumulation of fatty materials that accumulate under the inner lining of the arterial wall. Atherosclerosis can affect the arteries of the brain, heart, kidneys, other vital organs and even the arteries of the arms and legs. When atherosclerosis develops in the carotid arteries that supply the brain, a stroke may occur; when it develops in the coronary arteries that supply the heart, a heart attack may occur.[6]

Causes of Cardiovascular Disease

Atherosclerosis begins when white blood cells (WBCs), called monocytes, migrate from the bloodstream into the wall of the artery and transform into cells that accumulate fatty materials. As this process continues, a thickening, called *plaque,* develops in the inner lining of the artery. Each area of thickening, called an *atheroma,* consists of various fatty materials, principally *cholesterol.* Arteries affected by atherosclerosis lose their elasticity, and as the plaques grow, the arteries narrow (Figure 15-4). With time, atheromas collect calcium, become brittle, and may rupture. A ruptured atheroma spills its fatty contents and may

trigger a blood clot, or *thrombus,* leading to myocardial infarction or stroke. Symptoms include angina, leg cramps, or *intermittent claudication* brought on because of a lack of oxygen to the heart or legs.

Theoretical Explanations for Cardiovascular Disease

The mechanisms underlying cardiovascular disease are still complex and not resolved to a central link. The two most common theoretical explanations for cardiovascular disease have recently been combined into the *Unified Hypothesis of Atherogenesis,* which proposes that there are two primary components of atherosclerosis: (1) endothelial cell injury, or (2) damage and lipid infiltration (insudation).[17,29,44,77] Figure 15-5 summarizes the steps involved in the Unified Hypothesis of Atherogenesis—the formation of atheromas.

One research perspective is that chronic exercise significantly increases coronary artery diameter and myocardial capillarization, improving or reversing atherosclerosis.[12,18,34,47,51]

In animal studies, Macaque monkeys were fed a controlled diet that was designed to create atherosclerotic conditions. The exercised group developed no atherosclerosis, whereas the control group did.[45]

Risk Factors for Cardiovascular Disease and Cardiac Death

In 1949 a study was initiated in Framingham, Massachusetts, to determine the relationship between lifestyle and personal attributes and the development of cardiovascular disease (atherosclerosis). This prospective epidemiologic study of 5209 men and women, aged 30 to 62 years old, produced significant findings. In this study, only 2% of the population were lost to follow-up and 80% of the subjects completed all biennial examinations.[13] Gordon and Kannel updated the findings of the Framingham study and more precisely identified the major risk factors for the development of atherosclerosis.[31,42]

The risk factors that predict the occurrence of cardiovascular disease, as identified in Framingham and in more current studies, are:

∎ Male gender[27]
∎ Family history of coronary disease[27]
∎ Elevated serum cholesterol[24,26]
∎ Hypertension[26]
∎ Cigarette smoking[24,26]
∎ Diabetes mellitus[27]
∎ Obesity[27]
∎ Psychologic stress[40,65]
∎ Physical inactivity[27]

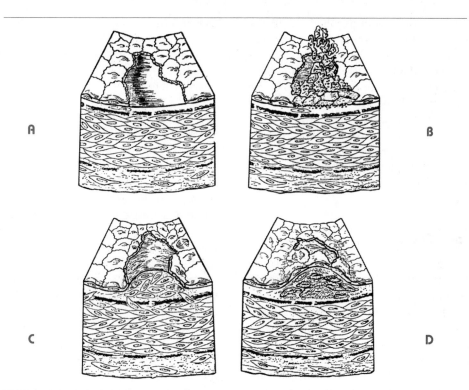

■ **Figure 15-4. A,** Diagram of area of endothelial damage or injury, the major initial phase of atherogenesis. **B,** Secondary phase of atherogenesis involving platelet aggregation, a phase that probably precedes smooth muscle cell proliferations. **C,** Diagram of smooth muscle cell proliferation and migration from the media to the intima. **D,** Insudation of low-density lipoprotein cholesterol within the inner layers of the arterial wall. *Modified from Ross R, Glosmet JA: The pathogenesis of atherosclerosis,* N Engl J Med 295:420, 1976.

Of these risk factors, the statistically strongest and most predictive were smoking, elevated cholesterol, and hypertension. Of the risk factors for cardiovascular disease, elevated serum cholesterol, obesity, psychologic stress, and physical inactivity were most modifiable by exercise.

Elevated Cholesterol and Physical Inactivity

The two major classes of lipoproteins responsible for the transport of endogenous cholesterol are low-density lipoproteins (LDLs) and high-density lipoproteins (HDLs).[79] There is ample scientific evidence that elevated serum levels of LDL and low serum levels of HDL or both increase the risk for the development of cardiovascular disease. A high total LDL to HDL ratio, such as 10, indicates that only a small portion of the total cholesterol is HDLs, which places the person at double the normal risk for experiencing a future cardiac event.[30,58,69]

The role of genetics in cardiovascular disease is not clearly understood. Some experts, most notably Kannel, believe that a family history of coronary disease may be a risk because of shared family habits, such as smoking, poor diet, and, most important, a sedentary life style.[48]

■ Effects of Cardiac Rehabilitation Exercise Training

Multiple epidemiologic studies have concluded that some form of exercise is associated with significant reductions in cardiovascular disease and related deaths (Table 15-1). Clinically controlled trials have also found that exercise prescriptions provide health benefits to patients who are diagnosed with cardiovascular disease. Cardiac rehabilitation exercise training has been consistently demonstrated to improve objective measures of exercise tolerance without significant cardiovascular complications or other adverse outcomes. The National Heart, Lung, and Blood Institute (NHLBI) recommends appropriately prescribed exercise training as an integral component of cardiac rehabilitation services, particularly for patients with decreased exercise tolerance. Exercise is required on a continual basis if improved exercise tolerance is to be sustained.[73]

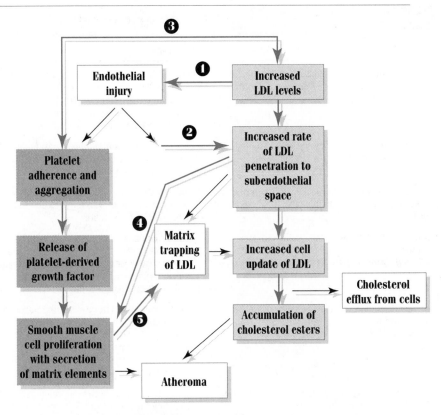

■ **Figure 15-5.** A summary of the various steps involved with the Unified Hypothesis of atherogenesis. *Modified from Steinberg D, Olefsky JM, editors:* Hypercholesterolemia and atherosclerosis: pathogenesis and prevention, *New York, 1987, Churchill Livingstone.*

Clinically Controlled Trials

NHLBI identified more than 114 scientific studies addressing the effects of cardiac rehabilitation exercise training on measures of exercise tolerance. Of these, 46 were randomized controlled trials. Cardiac rehabilitation exercise training was compared with a no-exercise control group in 35 of the 46 trials. The 11 remaining studies evaluated issues pertaining to exercise training, such as comparison of various intensities of training and exercise as a sole intervention compared with multifactorial cardiac rehabilitation (e.g., effects of dietary, educational, psychosocial, and other behavioral factors). Trials using 30 or more subjects are described in Table 15-2. Of the 35 randomized trials that compared exercise training with no exercise, 30 reported statistically significant improvement in exercise tolerance in patients in the exercise group versus the control group. The most consistent benefit of training appeared to occur when exercise was performed at least three times a week for 12 or more weeks. Sessions of 20 to 40 minutes at an intensity approximating 70% to 85% of each patient's maxi-

mal exercise heart rate provided beneficial outcomes. No statistically significant increase in cardiovascular complications or other adverse outcomes were reported in any of the randomized controlled trials.

Five controlled trials evaluated the effects of lower versus higher intensity exercise. Three trials documented significantly greater improvement in exercise tolerance with high-intensity as compared with low-intensity exercise, although in one study, there was no significant difference in tolerance at the 1-year follow-up.[28,63,80] Two reports found no significant differences in exercise tolerance between low- and high-intensity training.[7,8] Essentially, the regular and continual practice of exercise was the beneficial factor.

Exercise Tolerance

The scientific data clearly established that improvements in objectively measured exercise tolerance result from cardiac rehabilitation exercise training. Therefore appropriately prescribed and conducted exercise should be a key component of cardiac rehabilitation services for the

TABLE 15-1	**Summary of Epidemiologic Studies Relating the Benefits of Exercise for Cardiovascular Disease**
STUDY	**RESULTS**
Leon AS et al: Leisure time physical activity levels and risk of coronary heart disease and death: the multiple risk factor intervention trial, *JAMA* 258:2388, 1987.	In a multiple risk factor intervention trial, 12,138 middle-aged men at high risk of coronary heart disease were followed for 7 years Moderate leisure time activities were associated with 63% as many fatal coronary heart disease and sudden deaths and 70% as many total deaths as low leisure-time activity
Slattery ML et al: Leisure time physical activity and coronary heart disease death, *Circulation* 79:304, 1989.	17-20 yrs of mortality follow-up of male railroad workers (N=3043) found those who were sedentary died from coronary heart disease 40% more often than workers who were active
Salonen JT et al: Leisure time and occupational physical activity: risk of death from ischemic heart disease, *Am J Epidemiol* 127:87, 1988.	In a cohort study of 15,088 persons aged 30-59 yrs in Finland, those who were sedentary in leisure time and at work had an excess of ischemic disease death
Hambrecht R et al: Various intensities of leisure time physical activity in patients with coronary artery disease, *J Am Coll Cardiol* 22:468, 1993.	In a randomized controlled study, with 62 patients with coronary artery disease; improvement in cardiac fitness occurred with 1400 kcal/wk exercise; 1533 kcal/wk was required to halt progression of coronary atherosclerotic lesions; regression of coronary lesions required 2200 kcal/wk physical activity (6 hrs/wk)
Willich SN et al: Physical exertion as a trigger of acute myocardial infarction, *N Engl J Med* 329:1684, 1993.	In 1194 patients with myocardial infarction, 7.1% had engaged in physical exertion at the onset, only 3.9% of controls had engaged in physical exertion during that period Strenuous activity was associated with an increase of risk, particularly among patients who exercise infrequently, with a three-fold risk when strenuous exercise occurred 3 hrs after waking
Lakka TA et al: Relation of leisure-time physical activity and cardiorespiratory fitness to the risk of acute myocardial infarction in men, *N Engl J Med* 330:154, 1994.	Men with no heart disease or cancer (N=1453, aged 42-60 yrs) were followed for 5 yrs With 17 confounding variables controlled, those who reported the highest level of weekly activity (conditioning 2+ hrs) and who had maximal oxygen uptake had 60% fewer heart attacks than inactive men
Berlin JA, Colditz G: A meta-analysis of physical activity in the prevention of coronary heart disease, *Am J Epidemiol* 132:612, 1990.	Metaanalysis of 27 randomized controlled trials on exercise and heart attack demonstrated being sedentary doubled the risk of heart disease, the stronger methodologically the study, exercise resulted protection against heart attacks
Kiely DK et al: Physical activity and stroke: the Framingham study, *Am J Epidemiol* 140(7):608, 1990.	In the Framingham study, two separate analyses were performed, one during midlife (N=4196 men and women, mean age=49.8) another when cohort was older (mean age=63.0) Outcomes suggest medium and high levels of physical activity protected against stroke in men, especially older men No significant protective effect for women was found

patient with angina pectoris, myocardial infarction, coronary artery bypass grafting (CABG), and percutaneous transluminal coronary angioplasty (PICA), as well as for patients with compensated heart failure or decreased ventricular ejection fraction.

The angiographic evidence of the beneficial effects of aerobic exercise on cardiovascular disease progression is by no means extensive. However, Kramsch and others have published evidence that moderate exercise, when carried out over a period of 3 or more years and when associated with improvements in HDL, LDL, and triglyceride levels, resulted in (1) decreased degrees of atherosclerosis; (2) decreased lesion size and collagen accumulation; and (3) increased vessel lumen (space in the interior of the artery). The authors concluded that regular aerobic exercise may prevent, retard, and reverse the development of coronary atherosclerosis.[46]

Case study: Frank

Frank (55 years old) had always been involved in some form of physical activity in his life, but during the past 10 years, he had ceased to participate in any regular exercise program. During the last 5 years, he had experienced significant stres-

Text continued on page 436

TABLE 15-2 | **Clinically Controlled Trials of Cardiac Rehabilitation Exercise Training**

AUTHOR(S)	PATIENTS	INTERVENTION	OUTCOME
DeBusk RF et al: A case-management system for coronary risk factor modification after acute myocardial infarction, *Ann Intern Med* 120:721, 1994.	N=585 men and women 293 trained 292 control	Multifactorial home exercise 60%-85% maximal baseline exercise test heart rate 30 min, 5 times/wk for 4 wks, 100% thereafter Transtelephonic ECG and portable heart rate monitor plus self-monitoring logs	Significant increase in functional capacity with training vs usual care (p<0.001 group differences) 20 minutes, 5 times/wk, for 6 months plus step diet (both coronary heart groups)
Flether BJ et al: Exercise testing and training in physically disabled men with clinical evidence of coronary artery disease, *Am J Cardiol* 73:170, 1994.	N=88 men 41 trained 47 control with catheritized, documented stable disease	Home exercise training with transtelephonic ECG monitor, arm exercise specially adapted wheelchair cranking	Significant decrease in resting heart rate and mean peak rate pressure product vs baseline, for trained group only (p<0.03) No difference between groups in exercise duration, maximal oxygen consumption, or rate of perceived exertion
Haskell et al: Effects of intensive multiple risk factor reduction on coronary artherosclerosis and clinical cardiac events in men and women with coronary artery disease: the Stanford Coronary Risk Intervention Project (SCRIP), *Circulation* 89:975,1994.	300 men and women (88% men) Catherization-documented CHD, 145 medically treated, 139 PTCA and 16 CABG patients	Home rehabilitation including lipid lowering meds, diet, behavioral management, smoking cessation, and individual exercise training and transtelephonic ECG monitoring 4-year follow-up	Increased exercise tolerance intervention vs usual care (p=0.001)
Hambrecht R et al: Various intensities of leisure time physical activity in patients with coronary artery disease: effects on cardiorespiratory fitness and progression of coronary atherosclerotic lesions, *J Am Coll Cardiol* 22:468, 1993.	N=88 men and women 45 trained 43 control Stable angina catheterized documented CHD	Cycle ergometry training 6 times/day for 10-min sessions 75% baseline exercise test maximal oxygen consumption, then home exercise 30 min/day 75% intensity plus 2 group training sessions 60 min/wk Follow-up at 1 year	Significantly increased exercise tolerance (maximal oxygen consumption) trained vs control (p<0.05) Significantly increased maximal exercise duration, trained vs control (p<0.001)
Guinnuzzi P et al: Long-term physical training and left ventricular remodeling after anterior myocardial infarction: results of the exercise in anterior myocardial infarction (EAMI) trial, *J Am Coll Cardiol* 22:1821, 1993.	N=103 men 51 trained 52 control	Supervised ergometry (cycle), 30 min 3 times/wk for 2 mos 80% maximal baseline exercise test heart rate followed by 4 mos home exercise 3 times/week at 80% intensity plus 30 min walking per day	Significant increases in maximal work capacity; increased anaerobic (lactate) threshold for trained group only (p<0.001 vs baseline) At maximal workload, significant reduction in heart rate, rate-pressure product and venous lactate concentration, training vs controls (p<0.01)
Engblom E et al: Exercise habits and physical performance during comprehensive rehabilitation after coronary artery bypass surgery, *Eur Heart J* 13:1053, 1992.	N=171 men 93 trained 78 control	21 hrs supervised aerobic exercise for 3 wks, 70% maximal baseline exercise test heart rate	Significantly increased physical work capacity in trained vs control groups (p>0.05) Follow-up at 6 and 12 mos
Giannuzzi P et al: EAMI-exercise training in anterior myocardial infarction: an ongoing multicenter randomized study; preliminary results on left ventricular function and remodeling, *Chest* 101(5 suppl):315S, 1992.	N=49 men 25 trained 24 control 4-8 wks post Q-wave MI	Supervised cycle ergometry 30 mins, 3 times/wk, 80% maximal baseline exercise test heart rate for 2 mos Next 4 mos, home exercise Follow-up at 6 mos	Physical work capacity increased significantly for trained vs control group (p<0.05) Significantly increased maximal exercise duration for trained vs control group (p<0.001)

CABG, Coronary artery bypass grafting; *CHD,* congenital heart disease; *ECG,* electroencephalographic; *MI,* myocardial infarction; *PTCA,* percutaneous transluminal coronary angioplasty.

Continued

TABLE 15-2	Clinically Controlled Trials of Cardiac Rehabilitation Exercise Training—cont'd		
AUTHOR(S)	**PATIENTS**	**INTERVENTION**	**OUTCOME**
Schuler G et al: Regular physician exercise and low-fat diet: effects on progression of coronary artery disease, *Circulation* 86:1, 1992.	N=113 men 56 trained 57 usual care Catheritized, documented stable CHD	2-hr/wk exercise training 75%-85% maximal baseline exercise test heart rate at 1 yr plus strict diet	Significantly better exercise tolerance (work capacity and oxygen consumption) for trained vs control group (p<0.05)
Oldridge NB et al: Effects on quality of life with comprehensive rehabilitation after acute myocardial infarction, *Am J Cardiol* 67:1984, 1991.	N=201 men and women 99 trained 102 usual care	Counseling and supervised aerobic exercise 50 mins 2 times/wk for 8 wks at 65% maximal baseline exercise test heart rate Follow-up at 1 yr	Significantly improved exercise tolerance in trained vs control group at 8 wks (p<0.05) but not at 1 yr
Hamalainen H et al: (1989). Long-term reduction in sudden deaths after a multifactorial intervention programme in patients with myocardial infarction: 10-year results of a controlled investigation, *Eur Heart J* 10:55, 1989.	N=375 men 188 trained 187 control Consecutive MI patients	Exercise tailored to individual capacity, also antismoking, diet advice, and counseling provided	No significant group differences at maximal exercise testing at 10 yrs
Grodzinski E et al: Effects of a four-week training program on left ventricular function as assessed by radionuclide ventriculography. *J Cardiopulmon Rehabil* 7:518, 1987.	N=99 men and women 53 trained 46 controls Exercise began 5-8 wks post-MI	Aerobic exercise twice/daily, 5 times/wk, 30-min sessions; 80% maximal baseline exercise test heart rate Follow-up at 5 wk	Significantly greater increase in exercise tolerance in training vs controls (p<0.05) Equivalent improvement among patients with low-ejection fraction
Sebrechts CP et al: Myocardial perfusion changes following 1 year of exercise training assessed by thallium-201 circumferential count profiles, *Am Heart J* 112:1217, 1986.	N=56 men 27 trained 29 control Stable CHD (77% before MI)	Supervised aerobic exercise 1 hr 3 times/week at 75%-80% maximal oxygen uptake at baseline (1-yr duration)	Significant increase in maximal estimated oxygen consumption (p<0.001) and exercise duration (p<0.01) for trained group only
Taylor CB et al: The effects of exercise training programs on psychosocial improvement in uncomplicated postmyocardial infarction patients, *J Psychosom Res* 30: 581, 1986.	N=143 24 exercise test only 48 home exercise and exercise test 45 exercise test and supervised exercise 26 control Within 3 wks of uncomplicated MI	Exercise training, similar intensity. Follow-up at 26 wks	Increase in functional capacity significantly greater in exercise vs no-exercise groups (p<0.05) No significant differences between home and gymnasium exercise group
DeBusk RF et al: Medically directed at-home rehabilitation soon after uncomplicated acute myocardial infarction: a new model for patient care, *Am J Cardiol* 55:251, 1985.	N=100 men 30 gymnasium exercised 33 telephonic ECG monitored Home exercise 37 controls	Exercise training both groups at 70%-85% maximal baseline exercise test heart rate, 5 times/wk for 30 mins Follow-up at 26 wks	Significantly greater increase in exercise tolerance for both exercise groups vs control (p<0.05) No significant difference between home and gym exercise groups
Marra S et al: Long-term follow-up after a controlled randomized post-myocardial infarction rehabilitation programme: effects on morbidity and mortality, *Eur Heart J* 6:656, 1985.	N=161 81 trained 80 control Exercise began 45 days after MI	Supervised monitored exercise 1 hr 4 times/wk at 80%-90% maximal baseline exercise test heart rate, 8-9 wks Control group was home exercise of cycling, walking, and calisthenics Follow-up at 4 yrs 6 mos	Physical work capacity and maximal double product significantly greater supervised exercise vs home exercise control (p<0.001) 55 months after completion of exercise training

CABG, Coronary artery bypass grafting; *CHD*, congenital heart disease; *ECG*, electroencephalographic; *MI*, myocardial infarction; *PTCA*, percutaneous transluminal coronary angioplasty.

TABLE 15-2 Clinically Controlled Trials of Cardiac Rehabilitation Exercise Training—cont'd

AUTHOR(S)	PATIENTS	INTERVENTION	OUTCOME
May GA, Nagle FJ: Changes in rate-pressure product with physical training of individuals with coronary artery disease, *Phys Ther* 64:1361, 1984.	N=121 71 trained 50 coronary controls, 24 controls (no coronary disease) Catheritized document-ed, stable CHD	Supervised aerobic exercise 2-3 times/wk for 50- to 75-min sessions at 70%-80% maximal baseline exercise test heart rate for 10-12 mos Follow-up at 10-12 mos	Significant increase in maximal oxygen consumption for trained vs control group (p<0.01) Significant decrease submaximal rate-pressure product, signifi-cant increase in maximal rate pressure product in trained vs control group (p<0.01)
Froelicher V et al: A randomized trial of exercise training in patients with coronary heart disease, *JAMA* 252, 1291, 1984.	N=146 men 72 trained 74 controls Stable CHD	Supervised aerobic exercise 45 mins 3 times/wk at 60%-85% estimated maximal oxygen con-sumption at baseline exercise test for initial 8 wks This was followed by 46 weeks gymnasium or walk/run program Follow-up at 1 yr	Significant increase in submaxi-mal and maximal exercise tol-erance for trained vs control (p<0.05) Oxygen consumption increased significantly at rest and sub-maximal heart rate decreased significantly in trained vs con-trols (p,0.05)
Hung J et al: Changes in rest and exercise myocardial perfusion and left ventricular function 3 to 26 weeks after clinically uncom-plicated acute myocardial infarction: effects of exercise training, *Am J Cardiol* 54:943, 1984.	N=53 23 men trained 30 control Uncomplicated MI	Cycle ergometry exercise with transtelephonic ECG Monitoring at home 30-min sessions 5 times/wk for 11 wks at 70%-85% maximal baseline exercise test heart rate Follow-up at 26 wks	Significant increases in exercise tolerance for the trained vs control group (p<0.01)
Bengtsson K: Rehabilitation after myocardial infarction: a con-trolled study, *Scand J Rehabil Med* 15:1, 1983.	N=126 (mixed) 62 trained 64 control MI patients	Supervised aerobic exercise, 30 mins, 2 times/wk for 3 mos at 90% baseline exercise test heart rate plus individual group and family counseling Follow-up at 14 mos	Significantly lower systolic blood pressure, rest and submaximal exercise in trained vs control patients (p<0.005) No difference between groups at maximal work load at 1 yr
Roman O et al: Cardiac rehabilita-tion after acute myocardial infarction: 9-year controlled fol-low-up study, *Cardiology* 70:223,1983.	N=193 men 93 trained 100 control MI patients	Supervised aerobic exercise, 30 mins, 3 times/wk at 70% maxi-mal baseline exercise test heart rate for 42 mos mean training duration 12-mo follow-up	Significant increase in peak oxy-gen consumption compared with baseline for trained patients at 6 mos No significant improvement at 12 months No improvement for controls Significant difference between trained and control group at 12 mos
Stern MJ et al: The group coun-seling vs exercise therapy: a controlled intervention with sub-jects following myocardial infarction, *Arch Intern Med* 143:1719,1983.	N=91 (mixed) 31 counseling 38 exercise 22 control MI patients	Supervised exercise 3 times/wk for 12 wks at 85% maximal baseline exercise test heart rate Group counseling once a week for 12 wks, 60-75 mins Follow-up at 3, 6, and 12 mos	Significant increase exercise tol-erance for the exercised group, but not for controls or counsel-ing group at 3 and 6 mos (p<0.001) There were no group differences at 12 mos
Carson P et al: Exercise after myocardial infarction: a con-trolled trial, *J Royal Coll Phys London* 16:147, 1982.	N=303 151 trained 152 control MI patients	Supervised aerobic exercise 2 times/wk for 12 wks Isometric exercise prescribed	Significantly higher functional capacity for trained vs control patients at 5 mos, 1 and 2 yrs but not 3 yrs (p<0.001)

Continued

TABLE 15-2	Clinically Controlled Trials of Cardiac Rehabilitation Exercise Training—cont'd		
AUTHOR(S)	**PATIENTS**	**INTERVENTION**	**OUTCOME**
Sivarajan ES et al: Treadmill test responses to an early exercise program after myocardial infarction: a randomized study, *Circulation* 65.1420, 1982.	N=258 men and women 88 exercise only 86 exercise plus teaching or counseling 84 controls Uncomplicated MI	Home exercise prescribed and updated weekly Exercise twice a day until work return; then once daily, for 3 mo Education/counseling, eight 1-hr sessions weekly Follow-up at 3 and 6 mos	No differences among groups in hemodynamic response to low-level exercise testing at 3 or 6 mos
Mayou R et al: Early rehabilitation after myocardial infarction, *Lancet* 2:1399, 1982.	N=115 men 43 exercise 35 advice only 37 controls MI patients of 4 wks	Eight aerobic exercise sessions, (2 times a wk for 4 wks) Follow-up at 3 mos	Submaximal exercise tolerance exercise improved significantly as compared with other 2 groups (p<0.001)
Kallio V et al: Reduction in sudden deaths by a multifactorial intervention programme after acute myocardial infarction, *Lancet* 2(8152):1091, 1979.	N=375 men 187 training 188 control MI patients 2 wks after release	Supervised cycle ergometry exercise training Exercise most intense first 3 mos; plus health education and psychosocial advice Follow-up at 2 yrs	Cycle ergometry physical work capacity at 1, 2, and 3 yrs was not significantly different between groups
Wilhelmsen L et al: A controlled trial of physical training after myocardial infarction: effects on risk factors, nonfatal reinfarction, and death, *Prev Med* 4:491, 1975.	N=315 men 158 trained 157 controls 3 mos after MI	Supervised aerobic exercise 3.5 hours/wk at 80% baseline maximal exercise test heart rate plus supplemental home-cycle ergometry 9-mos duration	Significant decrease in submaximal heart rate vs baseline for trained patients only

CABG, Coronary artery bypass grafting; *CHD*, congenital heart disease; *ECG*, electroencephalographic; *MI*, myocardial infarction; *PTCA*, percutaneous transluminal coronary angioplasty.

sors—moving his home to another state, changing jobs with the move, and being demoted a year later. He was experiencing sexual difficulties and was constantly exposed to environmental contaminants (petroleum). While making a presentation, he passed out and was admitted to the emergency room. After a thorough evaluation, it was determined that Frank had suffered a heart attack—a blood clot in the right posterior artery. Angioplasty procedures were successful in opening the vessel, but caution was called for because a partial closure of the anterior artery was also noted. Prognosis was guarded because of the concern of disease progression.

Frank's resting blood pressure was 100 systolic, 65 diastolic, and his heart rate was 46 beats per minute. These numbers were low because the blood clot was slowing his cardiac output. He carried 265 pounds on his 74-inch frame. No other health factors appeared significant. No family history and no significant medical measures would have predicted the heart attack.

Frank was placed on a treatment regimen of moderate exercise (walking at least 30 minutes each day), a low-fat diet, and a biofeedback-assisted relaxation program twice a day for 6 weeks. At 6 weeks, Frank's stress test demonstrated that he could safely increase his exercise output. Frank then began to exercise on a treadmill (2 miles) four times a week, and he swam a quarter of a mile the remaining days. Both strengthening and stretching exercises and meditation stress management were added to his routine, and the diet program was maintained. Over a 9-month period, he lost 65 pounds.

Although Frank changed more than his exercise program (e.g., new job, new location, counseling for his intimacy issues, stress management), his yearly checkups demonstrated excellent health indices. Frank reduced his exercise program to a treadmill workout and modified his nonfat diet to include fish oils. His blood pressure stabilized at 128 systolic, 92 diastolic and his pulse rate to 50 beats per minute. No other symptoms emerged.

Exercise is beneficial to the cardiovascular system. There is also evidence that exercise is an effective intervention for pulmonary disease. Before discussing the pulmonary research, the mechanisms related to pulmonary function are reviewed.

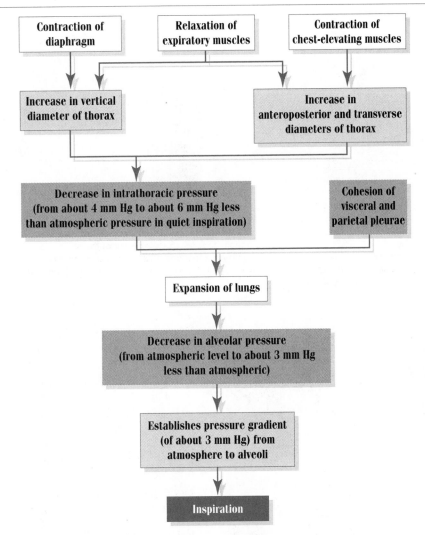

■ **Figure 15-6. Mechanics of inspiration.** *Modified from Thibodeau GA, Patton KT:* Anatomy and physiology, *ed 4, St Louis, 1999, Mosby.*

■ Exercise and Mechanisms of Pulmonary Function

A properly functioning pulmonary system ensures that tissues receive an adequate supply of oxygen and that carbon dioxide is promptly removed from the body. To accomplish this, the pulmonary system performs two basic functions: ventilation and respiration.

Pulmonary Ventilation

Pulmonary ventilation is a technical term for what most of us call "breathing." In phase I (inspiration), air moves into the lungs; in phase II (expiration), air moves out of the lungs. Contraction of the diaphragm alone, or of the diaphragm and the external intercostal muscles, produces quiet inspi-

ration (Figure 15-6). As the diaphragm contracts, it descends, making the thoracic cavity longer. Contraction of the external intercostal muscles then pulls the anterior end of each rib up and out, elevating the attached sternum and enlarging the thorax from front to back and side to side (Figure 15-7). In short, the ventilation process performs the work of getting the air into and out of the lungs.

The volume of air normally exhaled after a typical inspiration is called *tidal volume*. At maximal exercise, the ventilatory pump appears to be limited to a maximum of 50 breaths per minute and a tidal volume of approximately 50% of the lung's vital capacity.[14,15,41,52] The consensus among researchers is that the mechanics of the system limit the pump's efficiency.

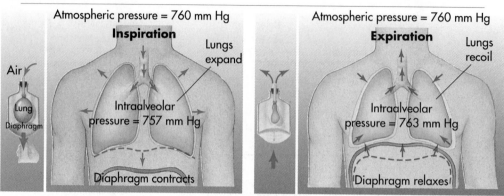

Atmospheric pressure = 760 mm Hg

Inspiration

Lungs expand

Air

Lung

Diaphragm

Intraalveolar pressure = 757 mm Hg

Diaphragm contracts

Atmospheric pressure = 760 mm Hg

Expiration

Lungs recoil

Intraalveolar pressure = 763 mm Hg

Diaphragm relaxes

■ **Figure 15-7. Mechanics of ventilation.** During inspiration, the diaphragm contracts, increasing the volume of the thoracic cavity. This increase in volume results in a decrease in pressure, which causes air to rush into the lungs. During expiration, the diaphragm returns to an upward position, reducing the volume in the thoracic cavity. Air pressure then increases, forcing air out of the lungs. Insets show the classic model in which a jar represents the rib cage, a rubber sheet represents the diaphragm, and a balloon represents the lungs. *Modified from Thibodeau GA, Patton KT:* Anatomy and physiology, *ed 4, St Louis, 1999, Mosby.*

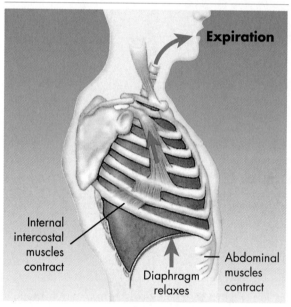

Expiration

Internal intercostal muscles contract

Diaphragm relaxes

Abdominal muscles contract

■ **Figure 15-8. Mechanics of expiration.** *Modified from Thibodeau GA, Patton KT:* Anatomy & physiology, *St Louis, 1999, Mosby.*

Pulmonary Respiration

Pulmonary respiration refers to the process of bringing oxygen into the lungs, transferring oxygen to the blood, and expelling the waste product called carbon dioxide. The exchange of oxygen and carbon dioxide takes place between the millions of alveoli in the lungs and the capillaries that surround them. In short, inhaled oxygen moves from the alveoli to the blood in the capillaries, and carbon dioxide moves from the blood in the capillaries to the alveoli (Figure 15-8).

The anatomic structure of the lung is particularly suited to its gas exchange responsibilities. The structure of the lung compartments (alveoli) incorporates a massive surface area (over 80 square meters). The pulmonary circulation covers nearly 90% of the alveolar surface, creating a potential blood gas interface of over 70 square meters of available gas exchange (Figure 15-9).

Exercise and the Pulmonary System

An overview of the pulmonary system helps us comprehend some of the benefits of physical exercise. The results of exercise are: (1) the development of a more efficient exchange of gas (respiration), (2) increased and broader activities of the ventilation process, and (3) a more efficient elimination of toxins and carbon dioxide.

Development of More Efficient Exchange of Gases

As tolerance for physical exertion increases, physiologic reaction becomes more adaptable and habitual. In response to an ongoing exercise program, blood cells increase their capacity to react to gas transfer. Athletes often refer to this effect as "getting a second wind." The body's tolerance for exertion is extended and endurance is increased.

Effectiveness under stress is also increased, and exercised individuals are less vulnerable to mental and physical exhaustion. Body strength

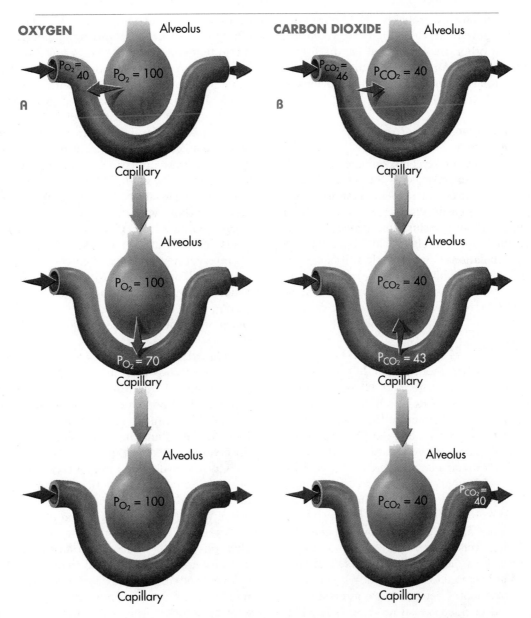

OXYGEN

Alveolus

$P_{O_2} = 40$ $P_{O_2} = 100$

A

Capillary

Alveolus

$P_{O_2} = 100$

$P_{O_2} = 70$

Capillary

Alveolus

$P_{O_2} = 100$

Capillary

CARBON DIOXIDE

Alveolus

$P_{CO_2} = 46$ $P_{CO_2} = 40$

B

Capillary

Alveolus

$P_{CO_2} = 40$

$P_{CO_2} = 43$

Capillary

Alveolus

$P_{CO_2} = 40$

$P_{CO_2} = 40$

Capillary

∎ **Figure 15-9. Pulmonary gas exchange, A,** As blood enters a pulmonary capillary, oxygen diffuses down its pressure gradient (into the blood). Oxygen continues diffusing into the blood until equilibration has occurred (or until the blood leaves the capillary). **B,** As blood enters a pulmonary capillary, carbon dioxide diffuses down its pressure gradient (out of the blood). As with oxygen, carbon dioxide continues diffusing as long as there is a pressure gradient. *Modified from Thibodeau GA, Patton KT:* Anatomy and physiology, *ed 4, St Louis, 1999, Mosby.*

increases and problem solving and emotional stability are enhanced because of increased oxygen to the brain.

Increased and Broader Activities of the Ventilation Process

As one begins an exercise program and the physical challenge to lung vital capacity occurs, a natural increase in lobe utilization takes place. Too

often, a relatively small lobe capacity is used in day-to-day activities. Under use can lead to atrophy and poorly developed lung processes. Lack of lung activity is highly associated with vulnerability to colds, influenza, and other respiratory diseases. The reduction of oxygen intake can restrict physical abilities, reduce the capacity for problem solving, and interfere with emotional stability.

Lifestyle habits are probably the greatest contributor to pulmonary dysfunction. Cigarette smoking and other environmental factors create obstacles to healthy functioning of the pulmonary system—a situation that becomes most obvious in crisis and high-stress situations.

More Efficient Elimination of Toxins and Carbon Dioxide

Just as the transfer of oxygen is enhanced through more disciplined exercise, so is the release of carbon dioxide and toxic waste. With exercise, toxic elements can be easily discharged through both the ventilation and respiration processes. For example, the lungs can release old tobacco smoke by heavy exhalation. Often, people will cough up congestive phlegm while exercising, relieving the load of infection. Stress caused by toxic accumulation can also be released.

An Expert Speaks: Dr. Steven Blair

Since 1980, Dr. Steven Blair has served as Director of Epidemiology and Clinical Applications and Director of Research at The Cooper Institute of Aerobics Research. He is responsible for the Aerobics Center Longitudinal Study and has authored or co-authored more than 200 publications on the effects of exercise of health, longevity, and human performance. In the following interview, he describes his findings on the effects of exercise on health.

Question. Can you describe how you became involved in exercise research?

Answer. I was active in sports in school and thought that I wanted to be a coach. When I went to graduate school, I became more interested in research and decided on an academic career. I started my academic work at the University of South Carolina where I founded and directed the Human Performance Laboratory. For the first few years, I focused on exercise physiology, but gradually my interest shifted to preventive cardiology and epidemiology. For the past 20 years, I have worked primarily in these areas.

Question. What, in your opinion, are some of the most profound findings resulting from your research?

Answer. Our research has shown that a low level of cardiorespiratory fitness is a strong predictor of incidence of chronic diseases or conditions such as hypertension, coronary heart disease, type 2 diabetes, and functional limitations.

Low-fit men and women are more than twice as likely to die during follow-up as compared with fit individuals. In our study, low fitness is as strong a predictor of mortality as is cigarette smoking. Furthermore, improving from low to moderate fitness is associated with as big a decrease in subsequent mortality risk as is stopping smoking. Cardiorespiratory fitness appears to protect against early mortality in various subgroups in the population, including the fat and thin, men and women, old and middle aged, and those with elevated blood pressure or cholesterol and those with normal values of these variables. Our work on physical activity interventions demonstrates that lifestyle physical activity interventions are as effective as traditional structured approaches to exercise in helping sedentary men and women increase participation in regular physical activity, improving aerobic power, and reducing risk of coronary heart disease.

Question. Tell me about the research you are currently working on.

Answer. We continue to follow the Cooper Clinic patient population in the Aerobics Center Longitudinal Study. Current areas of interest include: describing more completely the specific dose-response relationship between physical activity or cardiorespiratory fitness and various health outcomes, the relation of fitness to mortality in various body composition groups, and the interrelationships of diet and physical activity in relation to development of chronic disease. Our physical activity intervention research includes randomized clinical trials on promoting physical activity by mail and telephone interventions and the dose-response relation of physical activity in the treatment of patients with mild-to-moderate depressive disorders.

Question. How do you think exercise should be integrated into health care settings, hospitals, and HMOs [health maintenance organizations] in the future?

Answer. All primary care physicians should include physical activity as one of the "vital signs" and routinely inquire about the patients' activity patterns. They should provide advice, counseling, and encouragement to their patients to increase and maintain appropriate physical activity levels. Physical activity is as important to good health as not smoking, eating a healthful diet, managing stress, getting proper rest, and obtaining quality medical care.

■ Exercise and Chronic Obstructive Pulmonary Disease

Chronic obstructive pulmonary disease (COPD) is the persistent obstruction of the airways caused by emphysema or chronic bronchitis. *Emphysema* is an enlargement of the tiny air sacs of the lungs (alveoli) and the destruction of their walls. *Chronic bronchitis* is a persistent chronic cough that produces sputum that is not the result of a medically discernible cause. The bronchial glands are also enlarged, causing excess secretion of mucus.[6] The overall prevalence of COPD in the United States is 4% to 6% in men and 1% to 3% in women. In persons older than 55 years of age, COPD is confirmed in approximately 10% to 15% of the population. Asthma is a serious chronic condition currently affecting more than 17 million Americans. Between 1982 and 1995, the overall prevalence rate for asthma increased by 63.2%. In 1995, an estimated 16.4 million Americans suffered from COPD, representing a 60% increase since 1982. By 1996, COPD was ranked fourth among leading causes of death. COPD encompasses many conditions, the most prominent of which are chronic bronchitis and emphysema.[81]

Exercise for patients with pulmonary disease, although controversial, has substantial support. Findings demonstrate increased work performed on exercise tests, a decrease in the number of hospitalizations, and an improved sense of well being among patients.[36,49,76] These positive findings have led to an increased interest in exercise as treatment for pulmonary disorders. The primary goal of rehabilitation is to restore the patient to the highest possible level of independent function. This goal is accomplished by helping patients increase their activity through exercise training and by reducing or gaining control of symptoms— most specifically, dyspnea (breathlessness).

Clinically Controlled Trials of Exercise Interventions

A recent review of the literature identified 14 controlled trials of exercise as intervention for COPD.[64] In all but three studies, average forced expiratory volume per second (FEV_1) was in the range of 0.8 L to 1.2 L or 33% to 39% predicted, indicating severe airflow limitation. Most studies administered exercise programs predominantly in an outpatient, supervised setting; three examined the use of unsupervised home exercise programs, and two other programs were conducted in an inpatient rehabilitation center. The studies since 1980, evaluating 20 or more subjects, are described in Table 15-3.

A variety of lower extremity exercise forms were used, with walking the predominant exercise (3 studies), followed by treadmill, stationary bike, stair climbing, and, in one study, a combination of all of these. The duration of the exercise programs ranged from 4 to 46 weeks, with the majority of programs lasting 6 to 8 weeks (five studies) or 12 to 24 weeks (six studies). Session frequency was typically three per week. Outcome measures in these studies included timed walking tests, incremental treadmill and stationary bicycle protocols, and constant work rate treadmill and cycle studies. In the nine studies that used timed walking tests, all but one reported significant and clinically valuable increases. A review of these studies failed to provide the data necessary to recommend an optimal specific training regimen for patients with COPD.

Although the literature confirmed that appropriate exercise protocols are beneficial as treatment for COPD, less research is available on exercise programs for patients with other diseases, such as asthma, cystic fibrosis, and restrictive lung diseases.[3,11,60-62] The relatively sparse literature regarding the effectiveness of non-COPD exercise protocols makes it impossible to extrapolate the same benefits to exercise as treatment of other lung diseases. Available literature suggests benefit, but more research is needed to confirm improvements and to define the most effective exercise protocols for individual conditions.

In summary, there is substantial evidence that lower extremity exercise training is a beneficial intervention for patients with COPD. Benefits may be both physiologic (e.g., improved activity levels and reduced dyspnea) and psychologic (e.g., elevated mood state). However, the optimal specific exercise prescription guidelines for the muscles of ambulation cannot currently be defined with certainty.

■ Aerobic Exercise and Mood State Modulation

The psychophysiologic model for how exercise affects emotional states is derived from many implied variables. The most current biological model is based on the logic that depression and anxiety are characterized by a depletion of monoamine neurotransmitters, such as norepinephrine and serotonin, and that exercise increas-

| TABLE 15-3 | **Clinically Controlled Trials of Pulmonary Rehabilitation Exercise Training** |

AUTHOR(S)	PATIENTS	INTERVENTION	OUTCOME
Berry MJ et al: Inspiratory muscle training and whole-body reconditioning in chronic obstructive pulmonary disease: a controlled randomized trial, *Am J Respir Crit Care Med* 153:1812, 1996.	N=17 9 trained 8 controls FEV_1 mean 1.47 L (46% predicted)	12-wk supervised outpatient walking exercise program, 3 times/wk, 20 mins/session Intensity at 50%-75% of heart rate reserve Follow-up at 12 wks	Trained group demonstrated increased distance in 12-min walk There was no significant increase in treadmill time or dyspnea ratings Controls experienced no change
Strijbos JH et al: A comparison between an outpatient hospital-based pulmonary rehabilitation program and a home-care pulmonary rehabilitation program in patients with COPD: a follow-up of 18 months, *Chest* 109:366, 1996.	N=45 15 outpatient rehabilitation 15 home rehabilitation, 15 controls FEV_1 mean 1.23 L (43% predicted)	12-wk outpatient program (24 1-hr exercise sessions plus 3 nurse education and 3 physician visits) vs home rehabilitation (24 1-hr sessions plus 3 nurse and 3 physician visits) vs controls Exercise included walking, stair climbing and cycle exercise Follow-up at 18 mos	Both rehabilitation groups experienced improvements in 4-min walk distance and peak work rate in cycle ergometer tests and dyspnea scores At 18 mos, the home-trained group maintained better Control group had no significant changes
O'Donnell DE et al: The impact of exercise reconditioning on breathlessness in severe chronic airflow limitation, *Am J Crit Care Med* 152:2005, 1995.	N=60 (72% male) 30 trained 30 controls FEV_1, mean 0.96 L (38% predicted)	6-wk outpatient exercise program (18 1.5-hr sessions) with multimodality upper and lower extremity training with some education); vs waitlist controls 6-wk follow-up	Trained group produced 18% increase in 6-min walk distance; in incremental cycle ergometer test, 33% in peak work rate, but no increase in peak VO_2 Decrease in breathlessness ratings No change in control group
Ries AL et al. Effects of pulmonary rehabilitation on physiologic and psychosocial outcomes in patients with chronic obstructive pulmonary disease, *Ann Intern Med* 122:823, 1995.	N=119 57 trained 62 education controls FEV_1 mean 1.23 L	8-wk outpatient rehabilitation program (12 4-hour sessions of treadmill, walking, education, and psychosocial support) plus monthly visits for 1 yr Educational control program was 4 2-hr education sessions Follow-up at 6 yrs	At 8 wks, trained group improved treadmill test by 9% increase in peak VO_2, 33% increase in maximum treadmill workload, 85% increase in treadmill duration Breathlessness decreased No significant changes occurred for controls

FEV_1, Forced expiratory volume per second; VO_2, oxygen uptake.

es levels of metabolites for these transmitters. The nervous system, especially its emotional centers, is coordinated by neurotransmitters. Although there are numerous types and names for these substances, they all serve as synaptic modulators, often increasing or decreasing other chemical messengers by their presence. For example, the substance serotonin is a precursor to tryptophane, which is a pain reducer and modifier of emotion. Several drugs for depression management inhibit the uptake of serotonin to reduce depression symptoms.

The most appealing theory suggests that exercise releases endogenous opioid peptides, increasing the levels of endorphins. This, some researchers believe, explains the emotional "high" an athlete feels when he or she exercises intensely. Struder, Hollmann, and others evaluated the ratio of free tryptophane to branched-chain amino acids and plasma prolactin during exercise for eight male athletes.[71] They concluded that predictable changes in peripheral acid concentrations occurred and served to modify serotonergic levels.

A third psychophysiologic model suggests that an increased level of oxygen to the brain and other systems induce a sense of euphoria for the participant. A fourth explanation is that with muscular exertion, the body releases stored stress associated with accumulated emotional demands. Some health theories assert that specific kinds of exercise promote these releases (e.g., yoga, bioenergetics and tai chi).

A psychologic theory used to explain improvement suggests that individuals find satisfaction in achieving physical goals. The accomplishment of a difficult task, such as maintaining an exercise ritual as a personal goal, increases the individual's sense of personal control.

TABLE 15-3	Clinically Controlled Trials of Pulmonary Rehabilitation Exercise Training—cont'd		
AUTHOR(S)	**PATIENTS**	**INTERVENTION**	**OUTCOME**
Goldstein RS et al: Randomized controlled trial of respiratory rehabilitation, *Lancet* 344:1394, 1994.	N=89 45 trained 44 controls FEV_1 mean by 35% predicted	8 wks of upper/lower exercise plus education plus 16-wk outpatient program Control was conventional care Exercise included treadmill, 20 mins/day, 3 times/wk Follow-up at 24 wks	Significant differences in improvement between trained and control group in 6-min walk, tolerance of cycle ergometer work rate Controls decreased peak work rate (9%) and decreased in peak VO_2
Reardon J et al: The effect of comprehensive outpatient pulmonary rehabilitation on dyspnea, *Chest* 105:1046, 1994.	N=20 10 trained 10 controls FEV_1 mean 0.87 L	6-wk outpatient rehabilitation program (12 3-hr sessions with education and upper/lower body exercise plus inspiratory resistance) Controls received no training Exercise included stair climbing, treadmill, and cycle Exercise 3 times/wk Heart rate maximum 70%-85% Follow-up at 6 wks	40% increase, treadmill duration but no change in VO_2 or other variables for trained group Dyspnea ratings decreased No significant changes for controls
Wijkstra PJ et al: Quality of life in patients with chronic obstructive pulmonary disease improves after rehabilitation at home, *Eur Respir J* 7:269, 1994.	N=43 28 trained 15 controls) FEV_1 mean 1.33 L (44% predicted)	12-wk outpatient program, 24 sessions of cycle, upper extremities, and inspiratory exercise; also monthly nurse/physician visits Follow-up at 12 wks	10% increase in incremental cycle peak work rate and significant increase in peak VO_2 Controls experienced a 9% decrease in peak work rate and a decrease in peak VO_2
Weiner P et al: Inspiratory muscle train combined with general exercise reconditioning in patients with COPD, *Chest* 102:1351, 1992.	N=24 12 trained 12 controls FEV_1 mean 36% predicted	6-mo supervised outpatient cycle ergometer Exercise program, 3 times/wk for 20 mins each session, reaching 50% of peak work rate Follow-up at 6 mos	No change in 12-minute walk distance; 102% increase in endurance time in constant work rate ergometer test Controls demonstrated no significant changes
Cockcroft AE et al: Randomized controlled trial of rehabilitation in chronic respiratory disability, *Thorax* 36:200, 1981.	N=34 18 trained 16 controls FEV_1 mean 1.43 L	5-wk program at center followed by unsupervised home exercise for 6 mos Daily exercise with cycle, walking, and other exercises Follow-up at 8 mos	At 6 wks, 12-min walk distance increased by 3% but no significant increase in VO_2 No significant change in control group
Sinclair DJ, Ingram CG: Controlled trial of supervised exercise training in chronic bronchitis, *BMJ* 280:519, 1980.	N=33 17 trained 16 controls) FEV_1 mean 1.06 L	Daily home exercise program; supervised weekly, 12-min plus stair climbing; average duration 14 mins Follow-up mean, 11 mos	Trained group increased 12-min walk distance by 22% Control group made no improvement

■ Research on Empirical Psychologic Response

Effects on Stress and Anxiety

Several studies have examined differences in stress responses among subjects who differ in physical fitness. Holmes and Roth assessed aerobic fitness of 72 women by means of a submaximal cycle ergometer test.[38] The authors then compared the heart rate and subjective arousal responses with a memory test of the 10 least-fit and 10 most-fit subjects. It was found that the most-fit subjects showed a smaller increase in heart rate during the memory test as compared with least-fit subjects, but the fitness had no effect on subjective response. Another study demonstrated that diastolic blood pressure changes in response to a cognitive task were smaller for most subjects over 40 years of age and compared with a same-aged unfit population. Light and colleagues and Van Doornen and de Geus also reported similar results.[39,50,74]

Although much of the early research in this area has been correlational, recent research has used longitudinal designs with subjects randomly assigned to exercise training programs. Table 15-4 summarizes the designs and results of these studies.

RESEARCH STUDY Effect of Aerobic Exercise on Self-Esteem and Depression and Anxiety Symptoms Among Breast Cancer Survivors

Purpose
To evaluate the effects of 10 weeks of aerobic exercise on depression, anxiety, and self-esteem in survivors of breast cancer

Design
Experimental, cross-over design

Setting
Midwestern University town

Sample
Twenty-four survivors of breast cancer (mean time after surgery was 41.8 months; ranging from 1 to 99 months) were recruited via mail and cancer support groups. The mean age of the sample was 48.9 years.

Methods
Subjects were randomly assigned into exercise (group 1), exercise plus behavior modification (group 2), and control (group 3). Groups 1 and 2 exercised aerobically 4 days a week at greater than or equal to 60% of age-predicted maximal heart rate for 10 weeks. Data were collected pretest, posttest, and cross-over (12 weeks after posttest). Because pretest or posttest scores showed no statistical differences between groups 1 and 2, the data were combined to form one group.

Main Research Variables
Aerobic exercise (4 days per week; 30 to 40 minutes per session), depression, (Beck Depression Inventory [BDI]), anxiety (Speilberger State-Trait Anxiety Inventory), and self-esteem (Rosenberg Self-Esteem Inventory)

Findings
Pretest to posttest analyses revealed that women who exercised had significantly less depression and state and trait anxiety over time compared with those in the control group. After the cross-over, the control group demonstrated comparable improvements in both depressive and state anxiety scores. Self-esteem did not change significantly. Subjects who received exercise recommendations from their physicians exercised significantly more than subjects that received no recommendation.

Conclusions
Mild-to-moderate aerobic exercise may have therapeutic value to survivors of breast cancer with respect to depressive and anxiety symptoms, but not to self-esteem. A physician's recommendation to exercise appears to be an important factor in a patient's exercise adherence.

Although these summarized studies examined psychophysiologic responses to laboratory stress, several studies focused on responsiveness to real-life events. In a correlational study, high-stress college students who participated in an exercise program reported greater decreases in depression than those who participated in a relaxation program or no treatment.[66]

Several investigators have reported that single bouts of physical exercise produce anxiolytic (anxiety-reducing) effects. Bahrke and Morgan reported decreases in anxiety for subjects in an exercise group, although the control subjects showed comparable changes.[4] In another study, psychologic tension was significantly reduced by moderate and intense exercise, but not mild exercise.[20] By contrast, Steptoe and Cox found increases in tension and fatigue following high-intensity exercise and positive mood changes after low-intensity exercise.[70] Swimmers showed decreases in anger, tension, depression, and confusion and an increase in vigor after exercise, whereas control subjects showed no differences.[5] Boutcher and Landers found a decrease in anxiety after running exercise in subjects who were regular runners, but they found no decrease in anxiety in nonrunners.[9]

> **Points to Ponder** Running with meditation relaxation has been found more effective than group therapy for subjects with unipolar depression.[43]

Effects on Depression

Some studies have found exercise to be as effective as psychotherapy in reducing depression scores. In the Greist study, 12 weeks of running and individual psychotherapy, both significantly reduced minor depression in 28 subjects.[32] Freemont and Craighead studied 49 patients with elevated BDI scores who were randomly assigned to cognitive therapy, aerobic exercise, or a combination of the two.[25] After 10 weeks, similar and significant improvements were noted in all treatments.

Several studies have tried to compare effects of specific kinds of exercise on depression. One such study reported by Doyne and others compared the effectiveness of aerobic and nonaerobic exercises in the treatment of 40 depressed women.[16] The subjects were randomly assigned to an 8-week running program, a weight-lifting program, or a wait-list control group. Both exercise conditions significantly reduced depression compared with the control condition. In another study, Martinsen and associates compared walking and jogging programs to a nonaerobic protocol of muscle strengthening, endurance, and flexibility.[54] Although aerobic capacity increased significantly more for the walking and jogging group, both treatments significantly reduced depression

TABLE 15-4	Studies of the Modulatory Effects of Exercise on Stress Response			
STUDY	**SUBJECTS**	**CONTROL CONDITION**	**EXERCISE TRAINING**	**STRESSORS**
Blumenthal JA et al: Exercise training in healthy type A middle-aged men: effects on behavioral and cardiovascular responses, *Psychosom Med* 50:418, 1988.	36 Type A men (age 44.4)	Strength training	Aerobic exercise 3 times/wk, 12 wks	MAT
Blumenthal JA et al: Aerobic exercise reduces levels of cardiovascular and sympathoadrenal responses to mental stress in subjects without prior evidence of myocardial ischemia, *Am J Cardiol* 65:93, 1990.	37 Type A men (aged 42)	Strength training	Aerobic exercise 3 times/wk, 12 wks	MAT
Blumenthal JA et al: Stress reactivity and exercise training in pre and post menopausal women, *Health Psychol* 10:384, 1991.	46 women (aged 50)	Strength training	Aerobic exercise 3 times/wk	Speech, cold-pressor task
De Geus EJC et al: Existing and training induced differences in aerobic fitness: their relationship to psychological response patterns during different types of stress, *Psychophysiology* 27:457, 1990.	26 men (aged 18-28)	Waiting list	Aerobic exercise 4 times/wk	Variety of tasks to increased BP
Holmes DS, McGilley BM: Influence of a brief aerobic training program on heart rate and subjective response to a psychologic stressor, *Psychosom Med* 49:366, 1987.	67 women (aged 17-20)	Psychology class	Aerobic exercise 2 times/wk, 13 wks	Digits backward
Holmes DS, Roth DL: Effects of aerobic exercise training and relaxation training on cardiovascular activity during psychological stress, *J Psychosom Res* 32:469, 1987.	49 students (ages unknown)	Relaxation; no treatment	Aerobic exercise 3 times/wk, 11 wks	Digits backward

MAT, Mental arithmetic task.

scores. These studies suggest that physical conditioning can serve as treatment intervention for depression.

Two studies have examined the combined effects of exercise and antidepressive medication on depression symptoms. Martinsen and colleagues studied the effects of exercise with 49 hospitalized patients diagnosed with major depression and randomly assigned them to either a walking and jogging group or a control group participating in occupational therapy.[55] Approximately half of the patients received medication. The combination of exercise and tricyclic antidepressants was no more effective than exercise alone. The second study compared 8 weeks of aerobic versus nonaerobic exercise in a group of 99 inpatients with DSM-IIIR (Diagnostic and Statistical Manual of Mental Disorders, level III) diagnoses of major depression, dysthymia, or atypical depression.[10] In each group, 14 patients received tricyclic antidepressants. The combined regimen of exercise and antidepressant pharmacotherapy was, in this case, found to be superior to exercise alone. The summary of exercise programs for mood state management is presented in Table 15-5.

Effects on Immune Function

There is a small but emerging subset of research on the effects of exercise on immune function. Oxygen efficiency may empower immune cells to become more active; hormonal balance to become more stabilized; and negative effects of depression on immune function to be modulated by exercise.

Hoffman-Goetz, Simpson, and associates studied lymphocyte responsivity to submaximal exercise in 18 men and noted a noticeable increase in natural killer (NK) cells after 1 day of activity.[37] Perhaps more remarkable was that the total number of NK cells in the mononuclear leukocyte fraction of blood increased significantly after exercise. Venge and others found that neutrophil chemotactic activity increased for exercised patients with asthma.[75] Severs, Brenner, and colleagues related increased counts of immune cell components (CD#, CD4, CD8, and CD19) to the heat generated at core temperature by exercise.[68] It has been implied that exercise may benefit patients suffering from immune compromised diseases such as cancer. One should, nonetheless, be cautious in prescribing exercise for persons

| TABLE 15-5 | Clinically Controlled Trials of Exercise and Depressed Adults |

AUTHOR(S)	SUBJECTS	INTERVENTION GROUPS	LENGTH OF PROGRAM	DEPRESSION MEASURES	FITNESS MEASURES	IMPROVED MOOD	IMPROVED FITNESS
Brown RS et al: The prescription of exercise for depression, *Phys Sports Med* 35, 1978.	101 college students	Jogging 3 times/wk Jogging 5 times/wk Control	10 wk	MMPI ZSDRS>50	12-min fitness rest	Yes, only in jogging groups	Not described
Doyne EJ et al: Aerobic exercise as a treatment for depression, *Behav Ther* 14:434, 1983.	4 female patients, 19-24 yrs	Bicycle Attention-placebo (within subjects)	6 wk	Research diagnostic criteria Depression adjective list BDI	Treadmill test	Yes	Yes
Doyne EJ et al: Running versus weight lifting in the treatment of depression, *J Consult Clin Psychol* 55:748, 1987.	40 females, 18-35 yrs	Running Weight lifting Wait list	8 wk	Research diagnostic criteria Depression adjective list BDI HRS-D	Treadmill test	Yes, only in 2 exercise groups	Yes, only in 2 exercise groups
Freemont J, Craighead LW: Aerobic exercise and cognitive therapy in the treatment of dysphoric moods, *Cogn Ther Res* 2:241, 1987.	49 subjects, 19-62 yrs	Running CBT Running and CBT	10 wk	BDI>9 <30	Recovery heart rate	Yes, all 3 groups	No
Greist JH: Exercise intervention with depressed outpatients. In Morgan WP, Goldston SE, editors: *Exercise and mental health*, New York, 1987, Hemisphere Publishing.	60 outpatients	Running Therapy Relaxation	12 wk	SCL-90>50	Treadmill test	Yes, all 3 groups	Yes, only in running group

suffering from these kinds of illnesses. Too much exercise may serve to further deplete the immune reserves.

Case study: Judy

Judy had recently been diagnosed with stage I breast cancer, and although she was given a very positive prognosis, she was depressed and anxious. When she was asked about her cancer, she immediately replied that it was a consequence of her depression. The depression was apparently related to her husband's affair 5 years earlier.

Judy had gone to psychotherapy for 3 years and was taking antidepressive medication, which made her drowsy and withdrawn at times. The tumor in her breast had been surgically removed, and with chemotherapy she had become free of disease. However, she felt that if her depression continued, the disease would soon reappear.

Judy was put on a moderate exercise program, which consisted of treadmill endurance of 4 miles or 30 minutes (whichever came first). She was also placed on a stress diet of low sugar and low fat (although her weight was very appropriate for her size and frame). A counseling program was started in which she participated in an individual session once a week. She focused on imagery and stress management in her therapy. She also participated in a cancer support group twice a month.

Within 3 weeks, Judy's moods were elevated to the point that she discarded her antidepressive drugs. Approximately 3 weeks later, she felt no further need for her counseling sessions. At 10-year follow-up, her checkups for cancer demonstrated no recurrence, and her depression continued to be controlled by her exercise protocol. Her present exercise program is a brisk walk for 45 minutes with strengthening exercises for her indi-

TABLE 15-5	Experimental Studies of Exercise and Depressed Adults—cont'd						
AUTHOR(S)	SUBJECTS	INTERVENTION GROUPS	LENGTH OF PROGRAM	DEPRESSION MEASURES	FITNESS MEASURES	IMPROVED MOOD	IMPROVED FITNESS
Klein MH et al: A comparative outcome study of group psychotherapy vs exercise treatment for depression, *Int J Ment Health* 13:148, 1985.	28 outpatients, 18-30 yrs	Running Therapy (time-limit) Therapy (time-unlimited)	10 wk	Research diagnostic criteria SCL-90	None	Yes, all 3 groups	NA
Hannaford CP et al: Psychophysiological effects of a running program on depression and anxiety in a psychiatric population, *Psychol Rec* 38:37, 1988.	35 male inpatients, 25-60 yrs	Running Corrective therapy Wait list	8 wk	ZSDRS	1.5 mile test	Yes, in running and corrective therapy groups	Yes, only in running group
Kavanagh T et al: Depression following myocardial infarction: the effects of distance running, *Ann N Y Acad Sci* 301:1029, 1977.	44 post-MI male patients	Jogging	2-4 yrs	MMPI>70	Bicycle test	Yes	Yes
Klein MH et al: A comparative outcome study of group psychotherapy vs exercise treatment for depression, *Int J Ment Health* 13:148, 1985.	74 outpatients mean=29 yrs	Running Relaxation therapy	12 wk	Research diagnostic criteria SCL-90 HRS-D	None	Yes, all 3 groups	NA
Martinsen EW et al: Comparing aerobic with nonaerobic forms of exercise in the treatment of clinical depression: a randomized trial, *Comp Psychiatry* 30:324, 1989.	43 inpatients, 17-60 yrs	Aerobic occupational therapy	9 wk	BDI Depressive analogue scale	Bicycle test	Yes, only in aerobic group with>15% fitness improvement	Yes, only in aerobic group with>15% improvement

Continued

vidual muscle groups. To avoid boredom, she changes her program from time to time, switching back and forth between jogging, swimming, group exercise, and tennis. She faithfully continues a level of moderate exercise on a daily basis.

■ Summaries of Other Beneficial Aspects of Exercise

A combination of epidemiologic and clinically controlled trials suggest positive benefits from exercise for the conditions of diabetes, cancer, aging, menopause, urinary incontinence, impotence, and HIV and AIDS. Although the studies are few, they suggest benefits that include the following:

1. Reduced risk of disease or improved control of disease
2. Increased strength and functionality
3. Improved mood states
4. Improved immune function

Outcomes from these studies are described in Table 15-6.

■ Indications and Contraindications

Indications

In summary, exercise is recommended for the following:

1. Individuals capable of viewing physical activity in a positive way
2. Health problems that can benefit from exercise prescriptions, especially cardiovascular disease; diabetes; COPD; asthma; cancer (especially breast and prostate); back pain; AIDS and HIV; depression, anxiety, and emotional stress; incontinence and bed wetting; impotence; and health issues related to aging (e.g., osteoporosis)
3. Treatment of disease as a preventive medicine (see interview with Dr. Steven Blair)

TABLE 15-5	Experimental Studies of Exercise and Depressed Adults—cont'd						
AUTHOR(S)	**SUBJECTS**	**INTERVENTION GROUPS**	**LENGTH OF PROGRAM**	**DEPRESSION MEASURES**	**FITNESS MEASURES**	**IMPROVED MOOD**	**IMPROVED FITNESS**
Martinsen EW et al: Effects of aerobic exercise on depression: a controlled study, *BMJ* 291:109, 1985.	98 inpatients x=41 yrs	Running Weight lifting	8 wk	MADRS BDI	Bicycle test	Yes, in both groups	Yes, only in running group
McCann IL, Holmes DS: Influence of aerobic exercise on depression, *J Pers Soc Psychol* 46:1142, 1984.	43 female students	Aerobic Relaxation No treatment	10 wk	BDI>11	12-minute run	Yes, only in aerobic group	Yes, only in aerobic group
McNeil JK et al: The effect of exercise on depressive symptoms in the moderately depressed elderly, *Psychol Aging* 6:487, 1991.	30 older adults x=73 yrs 52 subjects 20-60 yrs	Walking Social contact Wait list	6 wk	BDI>12<24	12-minute walk	Yes, only in walking and social group	Yes, only in walking group
Sexton H et al: Exercise intensity and reduction in neurotic symptoms: a controlled follow-up study, *Acta Psychiatr Scand* 80:231, 1989.	15 subjects 25-53 yrs	Walking Jogging	8 wk	SCL-90	Bicycle test	Yes, in both groups	Yes, only in jogging group
Sime WE: Exercise in the prevention and treatment of depression. In Morgan WP, Goldston SE, editors: *Exercise and mental health*. New York, 1987, Hemisphere Publishing.	53 subjects 20-60 yrs	Aerobic exercise	10 wk	BDI	Bicycle test	Yes	No
Steptoe A et al: The effects of exercise training on mood and perceived coping ability in anxious adults from the general population, *J Psychosom Res* 33:537, 1989.	124 subjects 19-58 yrs	Walking/ jogging strength/ Flexibility	10 wk	POMS	Predicted VO₂ max	Yes, in both groups	Yes
Veale D et al: Aerobic exercise in the adjunctive treatment of depression: a randomized clinical trial, *Res Soc Med* 3:20, 1992.	41 college men	Jogging Relaxation/ yoga control	12 wk	Clinical interview schedule BDI	Bicycle test	Yes, in jogging and yoga groups	Yes, in jogging and yoga groups
Williams JIM, Getty D: Effect of levels of psychological mood states, physical fitness, and plasma beta-endorphins, *Percept Mot Skills* 63:1099, 1986.		Jogging/ aerobic dance Nonaerobic Control	10 wk	ZSRDS POMS	Recovery heart rate	Yes, for all groups	Yes, only for aerobic group

Contraindications

Exercise is not recommended for individuals who cannot positively embrace exercise as an important feature of his or her health plan; otherwise, it may become a source of stress, thereby becoming a negative health factor. Working under stress or duress has the same detrimental effects as other destructive lifestyles, defeating the positive aspects of exercise itself. The patient's response to an exercise prescription must be evaluated to ensure that feelings of guilt, punishment, or physical self-abuse (doing too much too soon) do not sabotage the intended positive effects of exercise.

Persons with very poor physical conditioning are prone to accidental injury. A supervised toning and strengthening regimen may be required before the person begins a home-based exercise protocol.

TABLE 15-6	Summaries of Benefits of Exercise and Other Health Issues

STUDY	RESULTS
DIABETES	
Helmrich SP et al: Physical activity and reduced occurrence of non-insulin-dependent diabetes mellitus, *N Engl J Med* 325:147, 1991.	Physical activity in 5990 male alumni at the University of Pennsylvania was tracked from 1962-1976 The number of calories burned in weekly activity were inversely related to the development of non–insulin-dependent diabetes, with the risk dropping 6% for each 500 calories burned per wk
Manson JE et al: A prospective study of exercise and incidence of diabetes among US male physicians, *JAMA* 268:63, 1992.	Medical researchers found diabetes decreased with increasing frequency exercise With 1.0=normal population, 0.77 once weekly, 0.62 at 2-4 times/wk, and 0.58 for 5+/wk Reduction persisted after adjustment for age and body mass; a 42% difference existed in those exercising most and least
CANCER	
Albanes D et al: Physical activity and risk of cancer in NHANES 1 population, *Am J Public Health* 79:744, 1989.	In a retrospective study (N=12,548 men and women) of the role of recreational and nonrecreational physical activity, inactive men developed cancer at 1.8 times the rate of active men; the rate of active women was about 1.3 times that of active women
Bernstein L et al: Physical exercise and reduced risk of breast cancer in young women, *J Natl Can Instit* 86(18):1403, 1994.	545 women with breast cancer before age 40 was matched with women without breast cancer Women who exercised 1-3 hrs/wk since puberty reduced breast cancer by 30% compared with inactive women; those who exercised 4+/wk reduced risk by 50% or more compared with inactive women
AGING	
Fiatarone MA et al: High-intensity strength training in nonagenarians: effects on skeletal muscle, *JAMA* 263:3029, 1990.	10 volunteers 90+ years of age took 8 wks high-intensity resistance training Strength gains averaged 174% in 9 participants completing the training Mid-thigh muscle area increased 9%, gait speed 48% High-resistance training led to significant gains in muscle strength, size, and functional mobility in frail persons up to 96 years of age
Fiatarone MA et al: Exercise training & nutritional supplementation for physical frailty in very elderly people, *N Engl J Med* 330:1769, 1994.	In a randomized, placebo-controlled trial of 100 frail residents: Group 1 received high-intensity resistance training Group 2 received multinutrient supplements Group 3 received both Group 4 received neither At 10 wks, strength +113% in Groups 1 and 3, 3% in Group 4; gait +12% in Groups 1 and 3, −1% in Group 4; stair climbing +29% in Groups 1 and 3, +3.6 in Groups 2 and 4; thigh muscle +2.7 in Groups 1 and 3, −1.8% in Groups 2 and 4
Ettinger WH et al: A randomized trial comparing aerobic exercise and resistance exercise with a health education program in older adults with knee osteoarthritis: the fitness arthritis and seniors trial (FAST), *JAMA* 277(1):25, 1997.	In a randomized, single-blind trial (18-mo duration) at two medical centers, 385 (60+) years with radiographically evident knee osteoarthritis, pain, and physical disability completed aerobic exercise (Group 1), resistance exercise (Group 2), or health education program (Group 3) Groups 1 and 2 had significant reductions in physical disability, knee pain, improved 6-min walk, stair climb and descent, time to lift and carry 10 lbs and get in and out of car compared with Group 3
Blumenthal JA et al: Effects of exercise training on bone density in older men and women, *J Am Geriatr Soc* 39(11):1065, 1991.	In a randomized controlled cross-over trial, 101 (age=60+) subjects performed aerobic exercises (1 hr, 3 times/wk), nonaerobic yoga (1 hr, 2 times/wk), or control VO_2 at 4 mos was +10%-15% with 1%-6% improvement with 10+ mos Aerobic fitness was associated with significant increases in bone density for men

AIDS, Acquired immunodeficiency syndrome; *HIV*, human immunodeficiency virus; *NK*, natural killer; VO_2, oxygen uptake.

Continued

TABLE 15-6	Summaries of Benefits of Exercise and Other Health Issues—cont'd

STUDY	RESULTS
AGING—CONT'D	
Preisinger E et al: Exercise therapy for osteoporosis: results of a randomized controlled trial, *Br J Sports Med* 30:3 209, 1996.	A randomized exercise on bone and back complaints on 92 postmenopausal women were allocated to Group 1 (compliant to exercise), Group 2 (noncompliant to exercise) or Group 3 (no exercise) The results showed significant decrease in bone density in Groups 2 and 3; no loss in Group 1
EXERCISE AND MENOPAUSE	
Chow R et al: Effect of two randomized exercise programs on bone mass of healthy postmenopausal women, *BMJ* 295:1441,1987.	48 postmenopausal women randomized into performing aerobic exercise (Group 1), aerobics plus low-intensity isotonic and isometric strength exercises (Group 2), and control (Group 3) At 1 yr, women in Groups 1 and 2 gained bone mass and had higher levels of fitness than Group 3, who lost bone mass
Slaven L, Lee C: Exercise and menopausal status, *Health Psychol* 16(3):203, 1997.	Two studies examined exercise effects on 220 premenopausal, perimenopausal, postmenopausal women Regular exercisers' moods were significantly more positive than sedentary women's regardless of menopausal status Given the disproportionately high levels of depression and psychologic distress experienced by women, use of exercise as a treatment was recommended
URINARY INCONTINENCE AND IMPOTENCE	
Klarskov P et al: Pelvic floor exercise vs surgery for female urinary stress incontinence, *Urol Int* 41:129, 1986.	50 female stress-incontinent patients were randomized to either surgery or to Kegel exercises Surgical outcomes were superior, but 42% of the Kegel patients improved to the point of declining surgery
Elia G, Bergman A: Pelvic muscle exercises: when do they work? *Obstetr Gynecol* 81(2):283, 1993.	Of 36 women taught Kegel exercises, 20 (56%) were cured or substantially improved after 3 mos of training. 16 severe patients were unchanged An 80% pressure transmission ratio between the abdomen and urethra was an indicator of success with Kegel training
Schneider MS et al: Kegel exercises and childhood incontinence: a new role for an old treatment, *J Pediatr* 124:91, 1994.	In an uncontrolled study of 79 children with daytime incontinence, two thirds were also bedwetters After 2 hrs of training, 60% were cured, and 14% had significant reductions of symptoms Night wetting was also eliminated or improved in 70% of the patients
Claes H, Baert L: Pelvic floor exercise vs surgery in the treatment of impotence, *Br J Urol* 71:52, 1993.	In a randomized, controlled study, 150 men with erectile dysfunction and venous leakage were assigned to surgery or to a pelvic floor training program Surgery was not found superior in restoring erections at 4 mos 42% of patients who finished the exercise program were cured, 31% improved, 58% of patients who finished pelvic training were sufficiently satisfied to refuse surgery

AIDS, Acquired immunodeficiency syndrome; *HIV,* human immunodeficiency virus; *NK,* natural killer; VO_2, oxygen uptake.

The exercise protocol needs to be designed and supervised by someone with the experience and education necessary to benefit the patient. Programs need to be designed for the individual, especially in the cases of the older adult and those recovering from illness. Moderation is the critical factor.

■ Chapter Review

In summary, moderate exercise is definitely a safe and positive prescription for many health issues. Because solid research in this field is just emerging, there is still a tremendous need for clinical judgment. There is no doubt that a sedentary lifestyle is predictably bad for one's health, and some recommendation for moderate activity should be a mandatory component of any health plan. The amount and type of exercise must be carefully considered. The research is clear that some form of exercise serves as prevention or treatment for a number of disease categories, including cardiovascular and pulmonary disease, cancer, skeletal problems (e.g., back pain, osteoporosis), depression, and diabetes.

TABLE 15-6	Summaries of Benefits of Exercise and Other Health Issues—cont'd

STUDY	RESULTS
HIV/AIDS—CONT'D	
LaPierriere A et al: Exercise intervention attenuates emotional distress and natural killer cell decrements following notification of positive serologic status for HIV-1, *Biofeedback Self-Regul* 15:229, 1990.	Untested homosexual subjects were randomly assigned to 45 mins stationary biking (80% max, 3 times/wk) for 10 wks or to control group Subjects were tested and given results at 5 wks HIV and control subjects demonstrated significantly more anxiety, depression, and declines in NK cell function
Spence DW et al: Progressive resistance exercise: effects of muscle function and anthropometry of a select AIDS population, *Arch Phys Med Rehabil* 71:644, 1990.	Exercised HIV and subjects showed no increase in distress and no decrease in NK function Randomized, controlled study of 24 HIV subjects and subjects recently recovered from one episode of *P. carinii* pneumonia, compared 6 wks of resistance training 3 times/wk to a control Results demonstrated increases in 13 of 15 variables of body dimensions, body mass, and strength for the exercised group, whereas the control group declined in all areas
Rigsby LW et al: Effects of exercise training on men seropositive for the human immunodeficiency virus-1, *Med Sci Sports* 24:6, 1992.	A double-blind, placebo-controlled 12-wk study of 37 HIV and health-status matched men compared strength training, flexibility, and aerobic condition with health counseling, including relaxation imagery There were significant improvements for exercise group in strength and fitness, but not for serum lymphocytes
Schlenzig C et al: Supervised physical exercise leads to psychological and immunological improvements in pre-AIDS patients. Proceedings of 5th International Conference on AIDS, Montreal, 1989.	28 HIV-infected individuals with advanced disease status exercised in 1-hr sports games, 2 times/wk for 8 wks Results included reductions in anxiety, depression, increased CD4 cell counts, and improved CD4/CD8 ratio
Keyes C et al: *Effect of cardiovascular conditioning in HIV infection.* Proceedings of 5th International Conference on AIDS, Montreal, 1989.	Using a standardized 8-week aerobic exercise program, CD4 and CD4/CD8 ratio established healthier levels

It is important to include some form of evaluation of lifestyle as part of a medical examination. Special programs directed by qualified specialists, trained in the use of exercise as therapy, should be common medical practice.

RESEARCH STUDY **Exercise Program in the Treatment of Fibromyalgia[53]**

Objective
To assess the utility of an exercise program, which included aerobic, flexibility, and strengthening elements, in the treatment of fibromyalgia (FM). FM is a chronic musculoskeletal condition characterized by diffuse musculoskeletal pain and aching. It has been suggested that aerobic exercise is helpful in its treatment.

Methods
Sixty patients, who met the American College of Rheumatology criteria for FM and who had no significant co-morbidities, participated in the study. Measurements performed on each patient at the prestudy and poststudy assessments included the number of tender points (TPs), total myalgic scores (TMS), aerobic fitness (AF), and flexibility and isokinetic strength. After the initial evaluation, the patients were randomly assigned to either an exercise or a relaxation group. Each group met three times a week for 6 weeks for 1 hour of supervised exercise or relaxation. All patient data were stored in a computerized database, and statistical analysis was performed on all prestudy and poststudy assessments.

Results
Thirty-eight patients (18 and 20 patients in the exercise and relaxation groups, respectively) completed the study. Analysis of data showed no significant difference between the groups in their prestudy assessment. Poststudy assessments, however, showed a significant improvement between the exercise and relaxation groups in TPs ($p<0.05$), TMS ($p<0.05$), and AF ($p<0.05$). Similar improvements were also found when the prestudy and poststudy assessments of the exercise group were compared.

Conclusion
Exercise is helpful in the management of FM in the short term. It also shows the patients with FM can undertake an exercise program that includes aerobic, flexibility, and strength-training exercises without adverse effects. The long-term utility of this type of exercise requires further evaluation.

■ Review Questions

1. Describe at least one theory that promotes exercise as beneficial for cardiovascular problems.
2. Describe how exercise affects pulmonary function.

3. Explain at least four reasons for using exercise as part of a treatment plan for depression.
4. Discuss the pros and cons of exercise for problems of aging.

CRITICAL THINKING AND CLINICAL APPLICATION EXERCISES

1. Discuss the research related to depression states and exercise from the perspective of biochemical changes. Provide the most feasible explanation for these outcomes.
2. Discuss the problems of sending patients to a general spa or gym in prescribing an exercise regimen. What are some issues of personalities and health myths that may compromise positive outcomes?
3. Relate the findings of the exercise literature to the fields of relaxation and imagery. How do these outcomes appear to support each other?

References

1. American Heart Association: *1992 heart and stroke facts,* Dallas, 1992, American Heart Association.
2. Reference deleted.
3. Bach JR: Pulmonary rehabilitation in musculoskeletal disorders. In Fishman AP, editor: *Pulmonary rehabilitation: lung biology in health disease,* New York, 1996, Marcel Dekker.
4. Bahrke MS, Morgan WP: Anxiety reduction following exercise and meditation, *Cognitive Ther Res* 2:323, 1978.
5. Berger BG, Owen DR: Mood alteration with swimming: swimmers really do "feel better," *Psychosom Med* 45:425, 1983.
6. Berkow R, Beers MH, Fletcher AJ, editors: *The Merck manual of medical information,* Whitehouse Station, NJ, 1997, Merck.
7. Blumenthal JA, Emergy CF, Rejeski WJ: The effects of exercise training on psychosocial functioning after myocardial infarction, *J Cardiopul Rehab* 8:183, 1988.
8. Blumenthal JA, Rejeski WJ, Walsh-Riddle M, Emergy CF, Miller H, Roard S, Ribisl PM, Morris B, Brubaker P, Williams RS: Comparison of high and low intensity exercise training early after acute myocardial infarction, *Am J Cardiol* 61:26, 1988.
9. Boutcher SH, Landers DM: The effects of vigorous exercise on anxiety, heart rate, and alpha activity of runners and nonrunners, *Psychophysiology* 25:696, 1988.
10. Brown RS, Ramirez DE, Taub JM: The prescription of exercise for depression, *Physician Sports Med* 35, 1978.
11. Clark CJ: The role of physical training in asthma. In Casaburi R, Petty TL, editors: *Principles and practice of pulmonary rehabilitation,* Philadelphia, 1993, WB Saunders.
12. Cohen MV, Yipintsoi T, Scheuer J: Coronary collateral stimulation by exercise in dogs with stenotic coronary arteries, *J Appl Physiol* 52:664, 1982.
13. Dawber et al: An approach to longitudinal studies in a community: the Framington Study, *Ann N Y Acad Sci* 107:539, 1963.
14. Dempsey JA, Gladhill N, Reddan W et al: Pulmonary adaptation to exercise: effects of exercise type and duration, chronic hypoxia and physical training, *Ann N Y Acad Sci* 301:243, 1976.
15. Dempsey JA, Vidruk EH, Mastenbrook SM: Pulmonary controlled systems in exercise, *Federal Proc* 39:1498, 1980.
16. Doyne EJ, Ossip-Klein DJ, Bowman ED, Osborn KM, McDougall-Wilson IB, Neimeyer RA: Running versus weight lifting in the treatment of depression, *J Consult Clin Psychol* 55:748, 1987.
17. Duguid JD: *The dynamics of atherosclerosis,* Aberdeen, Scotland, 1976, Aberdeen University Press.
18. Eckstein RW: Effect of exercise and coronary artery narrowing on coronary collateral circulation, *Circ Res* 5:230, 1957.
19. Fairweather MM, Sidaway B: Ideokinetic imagery as a postural development technique, *Res Q Exerc Sport* 64:385, 1993.
20. Farrell PA, Gustafson AB, Morgan WP, Pert CB: Enkephalins, catecholamines, and psychological mood alterations: effects of prolonged exercise, *Med Sci Sports Exerc* 19:347, 1987.
21. Reference deleted.
22. Fiatarone MA et al: Exercise training and nutritional supplementation for physical frailty in very elderly people, *N Engl J Med* 330:1769, 1994.
23. Fiatarone MA, Marks EC, Ryan ND et al: High intensity strength training in nonagenarians: effects on skeletal muscle, *JAMA* 263:3029, 1990.
24. Forbiszewski R, Worowski K: Enhancement of platelet aggregation and adhesiveness by beta lipoproteins, *J Atherosclerosis* Res 8:988, 1968.
25. Freemont J, Craighead LW: Aerobic exercise and cognitive therapy in the treatment of dysphoric moods, *Cognitive Ther Res* 2:241, 1987.
26. French JK et al: Association of angiographically detected coronary artery disease with low levels of high-density lipoprotein, cholesterol, and systemic hypertension, *Am J Cardiol* 71:505, 1993.
27. Genest JJ et al: Prevalence of risk factors in men with premature coronary artery disease, *Am J Cardiol* 67:1185, 1991.
28. Goble AJ, Hare DL, Macdonald PS, Oliver RG, Reid MA, Worcester MC: Effect of early programmes of high and low intensity exercise on physical performance after transmural acute myocardial infarction, *Br Heart J* 65:126, 1991.

29. Goldstein JL, Brown MS: Atherosclerosis: the low-density lipoprotein receptor hypothesis, *Metabolism* 26:1257, 1977.
30. Gordon T et al: High density lipoproteins as a protective factor against CHD, *Am J Med* 62:707, 1977.
31. Gordon T, Kannel WB: Predisposition to atherosclerosis in the head, heart, and legs: the Framingham Study, *JAMA* 221:661, 1972.
32. Greist JH: Exercise intervention with depressed outpatients. In Morgan WP, Goldston SE, editors: *Exercise and mental health,* New York, 1987, Hemisphere Publishing.
33. Hammond GL, Lai Y-K: The molecules that initiate cardiac hypertrophy are not species specific, *Science* 216:529, 1982.
34. Heaton WH, Marr KC, Capurro NL et al: Beneficial effect of physical training on blood flow to myocardium perfused by chronic collaterals in the exercising dog, *Circulation* 57:575, 1978.
35. Reference deleted.
36. Hodgkin JE, editor: *Chronic pulmonary disease: current concepts in diagnosis and comprehensive care,* Park Ridge, IL, 1979, American College of Chest Physicians.
37. Hoffman-Goetz L, Simpson JR, Cipp N, Arumugam Y, Houston ME: Lymphocyte subset responses to repeated submaximal exercise in men, *J Appl Physiol* 68(3):1069, 1990.
38. Holmes DS, Roth DL: Association of aerobic fitness with pulse rate and subjective responses to psychological stress, *Psychophysiology* 22:525, 1985.
39. Hull EM, Young SH, Ziegler MG: Aerobic fitness affects cardiovascular and catecholamine responses to stressors, *Psychophysiology* 21:353, 1984.
40. Jenkins CD et al: Prediction of clinical coronary heart disease by a test for the coronary-prone behavior pattern, *N Engl J Med* 290:1271, 1974.
41. Jensen JJ, Lyager S, Redersen OF: The relationship between maximal ventilation, breathing pattern and mechanical limitation of ventilation, *J Physiol* 390:521, 1980.
42. Kannel WB: Some lessons in cardiovascular epidemiology from Framingham, *Am J Cardiol* 37:269, 1976.
43. Klein MH, Greist JH, Gurman AS et al: A comparative outcome study of group psychotherapy vs exercise treatments for depression, *Int J Mental Health* 13(3-4):148, 1985.
44. Kottke BA: Current understanding of the mechanisms of atherogenesis, *Am J Cardiol* 72:48, 1993.
45. Kramsch DM, Aspen AJ, Abramowitz BM et al: Reduction of coronary atherosclerosis by moderate conditioning exercise in monkeys on an atherogenic diet, *N Engl J Med* 305:1483, 1981.
46. Kramash DM et al: Reduction of coronary atherosclerosis by moderate conditioning exercise in monkeys on an atherogenic diet, *N Engl J Med* 305:1483, 1981.
47. Leon AS, Bloor CM: The effect of complete and partial deconditioning on exercise induced cardiovascular changes in the rat. In Manninen V, Holenen P, editors: *Physical activity and coronary artery disease. Advances in Cardiology,* 1976, Karger, Basel.
48. Leon AS, Connett J, Jacobs DR Jr, Rauramaa R: Leisure time physical activity levels and risk of coronary heart disease and death: the Multiple Risk Factor Intervention Trial, *JAMA* 258:2388, 1987.
49. Lertzman MM, Cherniack RM: Rehabilitation of patients with chronic obstructive pulmonary disease, *Am Rev Respir Dis* 114:1145, 1976.
50. Light KC, Obrist PA, James SA, Strogatz DS: Cardiovascular responses to stress: II. Relationships to aerobic exercise patterns, *Psychophysiology* 24:79, 1987.
51. Ljungqvist A, Unge G: The proliferative activity of the myocardial tissue in various forms of experimental cardiac hypertrophy, *Acta Pathol Microbiol Scand* 81: 233, 1973.
52. Luce JM, Culver BH: Respiratory muscle function in health and disease, *Chest* 81:82, 1982.
53. Martin L, Nutting A, MacIntosh BR, Edworthy SM, Butterwick D, Cook J: An exercise program in the treatment of fibromyalgia, *J Rheumatol* 23(6):1050, 1996.
54. Martinsen EW, Hoffart A, Solberg O: Comparing aerobic with nonaerobic forms of exercise in the treatment of clinical depression: a randomized trial, *Comp Psychiatry* 30:324, 1989.
55. Martinsen EW, Medhus A, Sandvik L: Effects of aerobic exercise on depression: a controlled study, *BMJ* 291:109, 1985.
56. Reference deleted.
57. McMurdo MET, Renine L: A controlled trial of exercise by residents of old people's homes, *Age Aging* 22:11, 1993.
58. Miller GJ et al: Plasma high-density lipoprotein concentration and development of ischemic heart disease, *Lancet* 1:16, 1975.
59. Reference deleted.
60. Novitch RS, Thomas HM III: Pulmonary rehabilitation in chronic pulmonary interstitial disease. In Fishman AP, editor: *Pulmonary rehabilitation: lung biology in health and disease,* New York, 1996, Marcel Dekker.
61. Novitch RS, Thomas HM: Rehabilitation of patients with chronic ventilatory limitation from nonobstructive lung disease. In Casaburi R, Petty RL, editors: *Principles and practice of pulmonary rehabilitation,* Philadelphia, 1993, WB Saunders.
62. Orenstein DM, Noyes BE: Cystic fibrosis. In Casaburi R, Petty TL, editors: *Principles and practice of pulmonary rehabilitation,* Philadelphia, 1993, WB Saunders.
63. Rechnitzer PA et al: Ontario exercise-heart collaborative study: relation of exercise to the recurrence rate of myocardial infarction in men, *Am J Cardiol* 51:65, 1983.
64. Reis et al: Pulmonary rehabilitation. Joint ACCP/AACPR evidence-based guidelines, *Chest* 112:127, 1997.
65. Rosenman RH et al: Coronary heart disease in the Western Collaborative Group Study: final follow-up experience of 8½ years, *JAMA* 233(8):872, 1975.
66. Roth DL, Holmes DS: Influence of aerobic exercise training and relaxation training on physical and psychological health following stressful life events, *Psychosom Med* 49:355, 1987.
67. Segar ML, Katch VL, Roth RS, Garcia AW, Portner TI, Glickman SG, Haslanger S, Wilkins EG: The effect of aerobic exercise on self-esteem and depressive and anxiety symptoms among breast cancer survivors, *Oncol Nurs Forum* 25(1):107, 1998.
68. Severs Y, Brenner I, Shek PN, Shephard RJ: Effects of heat and intermittent exercise on leukocyte and sub-population cell counts, *Eur J Appl Physiol* 74(3):234, 1996.
69. Solymoss BC et al: Relation of coronary artery disease in women <60 years of age to the combined elevation of serum lipoprotein and total cholesterol to high-density cholesterol ratio. *Am J Cardiol* 72:1215, 1993.
70. Steptoe A, Cox S: Acute effects of aerobic exercise on mood, *Health Psychol* 7:329, 1988.
71. Struder HK, Hollmann W, Platen P, Wostmann R, Ferrauti A, Weber K: Effect of exercise intensity on free tryptophan to branched chain amino acids ratio and plasma prolactin during endurance exercise, *Can J Appl Physiol* 3:280, 1997.
72. Thibodeau GA, Patton KT: *Anatomy and physiology,* ed 3, St Louis, 1996, Mosby.
73. US Department of Health and Human Services: Cardiac rehabilitation: clinical practice guidelines 17, 1995, National Heart, Lung, and Blood Institute.
74. Van Doornen LJP, De Geus EJC: Aerobic fitness and the cardiovascular response to stress, *Psychophysiology* 26:17, 1989.
75. Venge P, Henriksen J, Dahl R, Hakansson L: Exercise-induced asthma and the generation of neutrophil chemotactic activity, *J Allergy Clin Immunol* 85(2):498, 1990.

76. Vyas MN, Bannister EW, Morton JW et al: Response to exercise in patients with chronic airway obstruction, *Am Rev Respir Dis* 103:390, 1971.

77. Walton KW: Pathogenetic mechanism in atherosclerosis, *Am J Cardiol* 35:542, 1975.

78. Wang Y, Morgan WP: The effect of imagery on the psychophysiological responses to imagined exercises, *Behav Brain Res* 52(2):167, 1992.

79. Wilson PWF: High-density lipoprotein, low-density lipoprotein and coronary artery disease, *Am J Cardiol* 66:7-A, 1990.

80. Worcester MC, Hare DL, Oliver RG, Reid MA, Goble AJ: Early programmes of high and low intensity exercise and quality of life after acute myocardial infarction, *BMJ* 307:1244, 1993.

81. American Lung Association: *Trends in asthma morbidity and mortality. Trends in chronic bronchitis and emphysema: morbidity and mortality,* www.lungusa.org/data.

Energetics and Spirituality

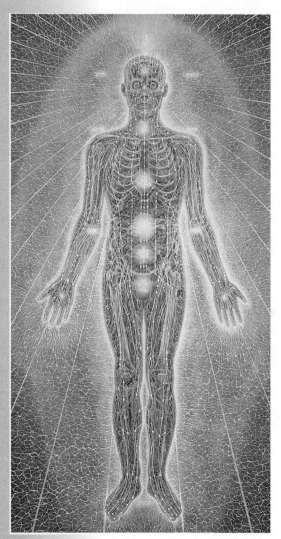

16

Electromagnetic Medicine

G. Frank Lawlis

WHY READ THIS CHAPTER?

Tales of electromagnetic effects have entertained us for generations. The fascinating antics of Mesmer and his "animal magnetism" and the tales of Frankenstein restored to life by electricity have provided fodder for movie scripts and books. These tales also fueled unbridled enthusiastic belief in electromagnetic effects as the hidden key to health and life. Early supporters' attempts to demonstrate that electromagnetic effects alter health outcomes were inconclusive. Although broad-reaching claims were made for electromagnetic effects, proponents failed to demonstrate scientifically validated health benefits. As a result, a tremendous outcry grew in the medical and scientific communities concerning the elaborate claims made for electromagnetic therapies.

Today, claims are still being made as to the wonders of electromagnetic medicine. In this chapter we explore the aspects of electromagnetic effects that are worthy of consideration.

The chapter presents a brief history of discoveries related to electromagnetic approaches since the eighteenth century. A review is provided of the electromagnetic approaches that have applied scientific methodology to the treatment or diagnosis of disease states. There are exciting medical possibilities for the use of electromagnetic effects, including bone repair, soft-tissue wound healing, treatment of autoimmune diseases, pain management, immune restoration, and neurology. Certainly, the student needs to understand the current controversies that exist.

Although there are historical accounts of medical uses of electromagnetic forces, bioelectromagnetics as a field began to emerge with the development of computers and other technology. Today, a few courageous scientists are leading the way in the development of this new field, and this text highlights a fascinating new chapter in medical history.

CHAPTER AT A GLANCE

This text on electromagnetic forces is intended to familiarize the reader with the history of electromagnetic medical approaches. The chapter includes a brief history and general information of the mechanics of electromagnetic forces and fields. The terminology used in the field, such as gauss and volts, is explained. Research on clinical applications for disease categories is reviewed. There are relatively few studies to confirm medical benefits from electromagnetic applications; however, these few are of substantial quality and serve to create more interest in the field. Medical and scientific researchers are, nonetheless, justified in questioning the unproven use of electromagnetic devices as treatment for illness and disease. These concerns are profiled for the reader.

$$E = MC^2$$

ALBERT EINSTEIN

CHAPTER OBJECTIVES

After completing this chapter, you should be able to:

1. Discuss the history of electromagnetic approaches to medicine.
2. Define the terminology related to bioelectromagnetics and electromagnetic medicine.
3. Describe the research methodology used in electromagnetic medicine and the outcomes from electromagnetic research. These areas include bone repair, neurology, soft-tissue repair, autoimmune mechanisms, pain, and immune restoration.
4. Discuss, compare, and contrast the current medical and scientific controversies that exist in relation to the uses of electromagnetic approaches.
5. Evaluate the current knowledge and the potential of bioelectromagnetic medicine.

■ Brief History of the Research in Electromagnetic Medicine

Except for the last 100 years, electromagnetic (EM) forces have been primarily the domains of nature, and humans were generally unaware or did not care that these invisible powers affected their lives. This was soon altered when, in 1882, Thomas Edison set up the first commercial electric power system in New York City. In 1888, Heinrich Hertz discovered radio waves; and by 1893, Nikola Tesla used the first *alternating current* (AC) power system to light up the Chicago World's Fair. Approximately 2 years later, Tesla began harnessing the energy of Niagara Falls; soon after, Guglielmo Marconi sent a radiotelegraph message across the Atlantic Ocean. The invention of the vacuum tube in 1907 led to radio transmission by voice in 1915. The development of appliances, cell telephones, and computers all emerged as a giant explosion of the use of this exciting but still poorly understood energy.

For generations, bioelectromagnetic (BEM) medicine has received a great deal of attention. Many EM devices have been touted as the answer to human suffering. Most are displayed at the *Electric Museum of Medicine* in Minneapolis, an exhibition made possible in part by Earl Bakken, the patent holder of the external pacemaker that is still used throughout traditional medicine today.

Like many alternative therapies, the techniques of EM medicine date back to ancient times. The Romans used electric eels to deal with such problems as prolapsed rectums. Many early uses of EM devices as treatment for pathologic dysfunctions in the human body have withstood scientific scrutiny, eventually becoming integrated into standard care. For example, no one questions the use of the pacemaker, electrocardiogram (ECG), electroencephalogram (EEG), electromylogram (EMG), and magnetic resonance imaging (MRI). The gist of the controversy is not that BEM approaches are unworthy of consideration. The problem is that we still have little understanding of the health applications for BEM approaches and that many individuals are representing its medical benefits far beyond what has been scientifically validated.

Historically Opposing Principles: Vitalistic and Mechanistic Schools of Thought

Belief in electricity as the body's life force was an issue of discord between scientific factions of the 1700s. Principles of opposing scientific schools of thought (mechanism versus vitalism of life) were bitterly contested. Simply put, the *mechanism* school supported the concept that the life process

was simply a complex mechanical response to the world, and disease was a dysfunction of one of the laws of biology and physics. The *vitalism* school of thought held that the life process was a unique internal force with its own power and flow. Disease was defined as a disruption of that flow.

Enthusiasm for the magic of invisible EM forces was exploited by many leading scientists of the times. Mesmer considered this force inherent in the human psyche, and he called it "animal magnetism." Mesmer demonstrated the emotional impact of this force by sitting men and women across from each other with their legs interspaced between each other. Within minutes, the participants would begin to swoon and many fainted from the powerful experience. *Mesmerism*—the surrendering of one's will to the practitioner—was also accomplished by the magnetic power of eye contact.

Current of Injury

Lungi Galvani, an anatomy professor in the medical school at the University of Bologna, is given credit for discovering the *current of injury* in 1794. Galvani noticed that frogs' legs (intended for his dinner), which he hung in a row on copper hooks on his balcony, twitched whenever the breeze blew them against the ironwork. Galvani's wife, Lucia, also noticed that the muscles of a frog's leg contracted when a laboratory assistant touched the main nerve with a steel scalpel at the same instant a spark leaped from one of the electrical machines across the room. Galvani believed that the metal railing and scalpel had somehow drawn forth electricity hidden in the nerves. He experimented for years with nerves from frogs' legs and reported to the Bologna Academy of Science in 1791 that the vital spirit in living things was the energy of electricity.

Within 2 years, Alesandro Volta, a physicist at the University of Padua (after whom the measurement of electricity, *volts,* was named), proved that Galvani had, in fact, discovered a new kind of electricity—but a steady current rather than mere sparks. Volta proved this by generating a bimetallic *direct current* (DC)—a flow of electrons between two metals connected by a conducting medium. This, Volta surmised, was what had actually occurred on Galvoni's balcony; the metals in the copper hooks and iron railing created a DC connection. However, what had served as the conducting medium? The frogs' legs, more or less bags of weak solution, provided the electrolytes. This discovery challenged the conclusion that there was a "life force" rather than an electrical process.

Galvani then responded by demonstrating that frogs' legs could be made to twitch with no metal in the circuit. In one procedure, the experimenter touched one leg nerve with the frog's dissected naked spinal cord, while holding the other leg to complete the circuit. Here, the current was true animal electricity, coming from the amputation wound at the base of the leg.

In 1797, Baron Alexander von Humboldt, the explorer-naturalist who founded geology, demonstrated that both Volta and Galvani were correct. Bimetallic currents were real, but so was spontaneous electricity from injured flesh. However, since Volta had declared that the force was electricity—a detectable, measurable entity—the accepted argument became that electricity was mechanism based. Galvani died penniless, his home and property confiscated by the invading French. Volta, by contrast, grew famous, developing his storage batteries with Napoleon's support.

Action Potential

Emil Du Bois-Reymond, a physiology student of physics professor Carlo Matteucci, demonstrated that when a nerve was stimulated, an impulse traveled along the nerve fiber. In the 1840s, Du Bois-Reymond measured the impulse electrically and concluded that the impulse was a mass of electronic particles, like the current in a wire. In 1868 his student, Julius Bernstein, clarified the nature of this activity with the hypothesis of the *action potential*. This hypothesis stated that the nerve impulse was not a current; rather, it was a disturbance in the ionic properties of the membrane, and this perturbation traveled along the nerve fiber or axon.

Bernstein postulated that the membrane of a nerve fiber could sort out the negative ions on the outside of the cell from the negative ions on the inside of the cell. This was the stable state. If this stable state became depolarized, the ions would cross the membrane and reverse the potential. The effect could be measured electrically, although the effect did not fit the definition of an electrical impulse (electron flux). Although today we accept this hypothesis, no one has clearly identified what gives the membrane the energy to pump these ions back and forth.

Electrical versus Chemical Forces

Otto Loewi, a research professor at the New York University School of Medicine, is credited with the discovery of neurotransmitters and the development of the biological basis for EM measurement in the body. At that time, it was thought that only an electric charge, not a chemical one, could jump across the synaptic cleft. Thus the vital force could only be explained as an electrical field. This belief was based on the phenomenon that a frog heart will continue to beat for several days when removed from its nerves and that stimulating one of its nerves will slow the heartbeat.

In a follow-up experiment, a heart was placed in a solution and a nerve stimulated to slow its beat. The heart was then withdrawn from the solution and another heart was placed in the same solution, but a nerve in the heart was not stimulated. This second unstimulated heart, like the one stimulated before it, slowed as well. It was concluded that a chemical, which had leached into the solution from the first heart, produced this outcome. That chemical was identified as acetylcholine, a neurotransmitter, and in 1936, Otto Loewi was awarded the Nobel Prize for this discovery. With a chemical explanation for the transmission for neurologic impulses, EM as the only source of the vital essence of life was seriously challenged.

While Loewi and others were researching other neurotransmitters, in 1875, Richard Caton detected an electric field around the heads of animals. However, it was not until 1924 that a German psychiatrist created the first version of an EEG by inserting platinum wires into his son's scalp.

It was hypothesized that there was only one brain frequency, but current scientific thought assigned four basic frequencies to states of consciousness. Delta waves (0.5 hertz [Hz] to 3 Hz) designates sleep; theta frequencies of 4 Hz to 8 Hz indicates trance; 9 Hz to 12 Hz implies alpha state, the meditation level of calmness; and any frequency greater than 12 Hz is generally related to wakefulness and problem solving or the Beta state.

Consciousness and the Computer

As computer technology became more available, the metaphor of "information processing" was applied to neurologic firing mechanisms and to thought. For example, John von Neumann elaborated on this concept by comparing how changes in information in computers are expressed in the magnitude or polarity of a current. Computers generally break down information into bits by a binary code—yes or no. Hence, the binary numbering system consists of 1s and 0s. Although the binary system is clumsy for individual computation of even simple arithmetic, the sheer power and speed of the computer overcomes this handicap. Since neurons always fire as an all-or-nothing phenomenon, the metaphor of the brain as a hybrid, 3-pound meat computer extended the mathematical model of human functioning.

Problems with the Electrical versus the Chemical Approach

Although the electrical and chemical models were considered reasonable explanations for how the neurologic system functions, there were still problems with these theories. First, if the biochemical model were correct, an impulse created by nerve stimulation would be as likely to travel in either direction; yet, it traveled in only one direction. Second, although nerve impulses were essential for regeneration, the action potentials were silent during this process. No impulses have been found that are related to regrowth, and neurotransmitters such as acetylcholine have been ruled out as growth stimulators.

Contributions of Robert Becker

Robert O. Becker is the man most responsible for bringing EM medicine into its modern form and for clarifying some of these issues. In 1956, Dr. Becker began his medical career as an orthopedic surgeon at the Veteran's Administration Hospital in Syracuse, New York, while simultaneously teaching at the Upstate Medical Center. Dr. Becker's interest in the regeneration of tissue began as an undergraduate when he researched the properties of limb regrowth with salamanders. A detailed account of his many innovations in understanding the electrical basis of regeneration is in his book, *The Body Electric,* but a synopsis of his contributions is briefly described in this text.[10]

Using salamanders and frogs as his subjects, Becker and his colleagues began the difficult task of measuring the tiny amount of current required to regenerate their limbs. One of his first conclusions was that he could measure a consistent current pathway from the central nervous system to the peripheral regions as a positive to negative DC direction (Figure 16-1). One of the functions of this phenomenon was to energize the mending broken bones. Moreover, they found that brain function could be modified by electrical and magnetic stimulation, which in turn affected the healing processes. For example, when the salamander's limb was injured, the repair process appeared to require a constant negative current through the injury so that the rehabilitation process could be successful and limb could be regenerated in proper proportion and function. In other words, the electrical field served as an architectural plan for repair. He also discovered that anesthesia could be achieved for the salamander by passing a DC or magnetic field through the organism.

Becker went on to show how bone pressures could be measured through electrical means and how they serve as rectifiers of the EM field. He developed a well-articulated process of bone healing via the use of EM stimulation. For example, he explained how the apatite crystal located around the collagen fiber acts as a semiconductor and, in essence, as a transducer, creating a device that converts other forces into electricity.

Becker went on to hypothesize how genes could be unlocked through electrical stimulation, although this and other applications to human injury have yet to be studied and confirmed. One of the findings that holds a great deal of interest for practitioners of other healing therapies is that even the regrowth and healing capabilities of

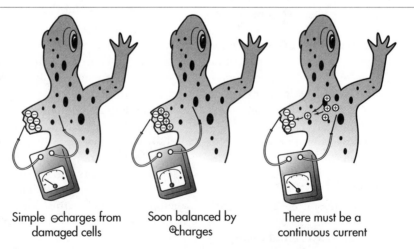

Simple ⊖charges from damaged cells

Soon balanced by ⊕charges

There must be a continuous current

■ **Figure 16-1.** Using salamanders and frogs as his subjects, Becker and his colleagues began the difficult task of measuring the tiny amount of current required to regenerate their limbs. *Modified from Becker R: The body electric, New York, 1985, William Morrow.*

lower animals appear to come from the animal's consciousness. If the brain activity is subdued or confused, the rehabilitation is not successful. This phenomenon may be an explanation for how a healer may empower a patient to overcome systemic disease through imagery or persuasion. (See Chapters 8 and 9 on hypnosis and imagery.)

The history of the research in this field is not clearly delineated, and interested researchers have made intuitive leaps that far exceed their knowledge and understanding of EM fields. Numerous EM gadgets have been marketed for a variety of aliments and are still sold through self-help magazines and anti-aging journals. Pioneering researchers continue to seek methods to harness this powerful force in a way that can be validated scientifically and clinically controlled. However, EM medicine is currently more of an art than a science—an art form that is without a substantive basis.

> **Points to Ponder** Weak EM fields helped reverse the symptoms of Gilles de la Tourette's syndrome in a 6-year-old child. Tourette's syndrome is a severe neuropsychiatric disorder with abnormalities such as tics, hyperactivity, self-multilatory behavior, obsessive-compulsive tendencies, and conduct disorders.[60] ■

■ Mechanics of Electromagnetic Approaches

Everything electrical comes from the phenomenon of *charge.* The fundamental event of charge exists in two opposite forms or *polarities.* One polarity is designated *positive* and the other is *negative. Protons* have a positive charge and make up a part of the nucleus of an atom. *Neutrons* are so named because they have no charge, yet they make up the rest of the nucleus of the atom. The negative charged elements of the atom are labeled *electrons,* and they vibrate around the outside of the atom. To maintain stability, there must be the same number of protons and electrons, each carrying the same amount of charge. Electrons are much smaller than protons and can be dislodged more easily from one atomic family to another; hence, they are the primary carriers of electric charge. When there is a surplus of electrons, the atom has a negative charge; when there is a surplus of protons, it has a positive charge.

A flow or flux of electrons is called a *current.* The speed of the electrons are measured in units called *amperes,* and the power behind the flow is measured in *volts.* When the consistent flow of electrons is in one direction, usually in polarity of positive to negative, the system is DC; when the current is alternating in one direction and then the other, the system is referred to as AC. The latter type of current is used for our electric appliances.

A current flows when a source of electrons (negative charge) is connected to something that has fewer free electrons (positive charge). The path by which electrons flow is called a *conductor.* If there is no conductor, there is no flow; however, there can be a potential for flow called the *electric potential.* If power continues to build so that the energy finally leaps the space, a spark is created. An electric field forms around the electric charge, and this field is measured in volts per unit of area.

■ Electric Fields versus Magnetic Fields

Electrical fields must be distinguished from magnetic fields. *Magnetism* is less understood, but it is observed in the behavior of an object that has two polarities demonstrating attraction or repulsion in a predictable fashion. In essence, magnetism is a set of lines of force that has direction and shape. The measurement used for strength of the magnetic force is in *gauss units* (named after the discoverer, Karl Friedrich Gauss). Any flow of electrons sets up a combined electric and magnetic field around the current. Just as a current produces a magnetic field orthogonal (90%) to its direction, a magnetic field moving across a conductor will produce an electric current (Figure 16-2). In fact, the electric generator is merely a conductor rotating through magnetic fields.

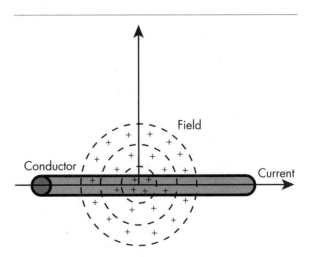

■ *Figure* 16-2. Just as a current produces a magnetic field orthogonally to its direction, a magnetic field moving across a conductor will produce an electric current.

In summary, EM forces are identified only by observation. Scientists have no known mechanism for the actual process of how EM works or how it interacts with life. The inference is that we can generate EM forces in reliable ways when we disturb charged particles and when these particles have polarities. The development of computer and appliance technology has certainly affected our current lifestyles, but we have yet to determine the impact on our health.

■ Electromagnetic Fields

A generated EM field theoretically extends out in space to infinity, decreasing in strength with distance and ultimately becoming lost in the jumble of other electrical and magnetic fields that fill space. Since the field fluctuates at a certain frequency, it also has a wave motion (Figure 16-3). The wave moves outward at the speed of light (roughly 186,000 miles per second). As a result, it has a wavelength (i.e., the distance between crests of the wave) that is inversely related to its frequency. For example, a 1-Hz frequency (one cycle per second) has a wavelength of 186,000 miles; a 1-million-Hz or 1-megahertz (MHz), frequency

has a wavelength of several hundred feet; and a 100-MHz frequency has a wavelength of about 6 feet.

All of the known frequencies of EM waves or fields are represented in a spectrum, ranging from DC (zero frequency) to the highest frequencies, such as gamma and cosmic rays. The EM spectrum includes x-rays, visible light, microwaves, and television and radio frequencies, among many others. Moreover, all the fields are force fields that carry energy through space and are capable of producing an effect at a distance.

Since the *photon* is a tiny packet of energy that has no measurable mass, the greater the energy of the photon, the greater the frequency associated with its waveform. The human eye detects only a narrow band of frequencies within the EM spectrum. A photon stimulates the retina in the back of the eye, resulting in a signal that is electrically measurable in the nervous system, producing the sensation of light.

Table 16-1 shows the usual classification of EM fields in terms of their frequency of oscillation, ranging from zero through extremely low frequency (ELF), low frequency (LF), radio frequency (RF), microwave and radar, infrared, visible light, ultraviolet, x-rays, and gamma rays. For oscillating fields, the higher the frequency, the greater the energy.

Endogenous fields (fields produced within the body) are to be distinguished from *exogenous fields* (fields produced by sources outside the body).[52] Exogenous fields can be classified as either natural, such as the earth's geomagnetic

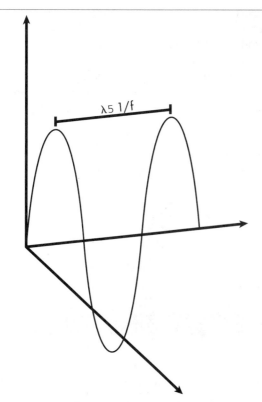

■ *Figure 16-3.* The field fluctuates at a certain frequency, producing a wave motion.

TABLE 16-1	Electromagnetic Spectrum	
FREQUENCY RANGE (Hz)	**CLASSIFICATION**	**BIOLOGICAL EFFECT**
0	Direct current	Nonionizing
0–300	Extremely-low frequency	Nonionizing
300–10^4	Low frequency	Nonionizing
10^4–10^9	Radio frequency	Nonionizing
10^9–10^{12}	Microwave and radar bands	Nonionizing
10^{12}–4×10^{14}	Infrared band	Nonionizing
4×10^{14}–7×10^{14}	Visible light	Weakly ionizing
7×10^{14}–10^{18}	Ultraviolet band	Weakly ionizing
10^{18}–10^{20}	X-rays	Strongly ionizing
Over 10^{20}	Gamma rays	Strongly ionizing

field, or artificial, such as power lines, transformers, appliances, radio transmitters, and medical devices. The term *electropollution* refers to EM fields that may be associated with health risks.

In radiation biophysics, an EM field is classified as *ionizing* when its energy is high enough to dislodge electrons from an atom or molecule. High-energy, high-frequency forms of radiation, such as gamma rays and x-rays, are **strongly** ionizing in biological matter. For this reason, prolonged exposure to such rays is harmful. Radiation in the middle portion of the frequency and energy spectrum, such as visible, especially ultraviolet light—is **weakly** ionizing (i.e., it can be ionizing, depending on the target molecules).

Exogenous Fields and Health Effects

Although it has long been known that exposure to strongly ionizing radiation can cause extreme damage in biological tissues, only recently have epidemiologic studies and other evidence implicated long-term exposure to nonionizing, exogenous EM fields (e.g., those emitted by power lines) as an increased health hazard. This hazard may increase the risk of developing leukemia in children.[6,43,71]

It also has been discovered that oscillating nonionizing fields in the ELF range can have vigorous biological effects that may be beneficial and thus not harmful.[8,15] This discovery is a cornerstone in the foundation of BEM medicine research and application.

Specific changes in the field configuration and exposure pattern of low-level fields can produce highly specific biological responses. Specific frequencies have highly specific effects on tissues in the body, just as drugs have their specific effects on target tissues. Actual mechanisms by which fields produce biological effects have yet to be clearly determined; however, evidence suggests that the cell membrane may be one of the primary locations of positive intervention. EM forces at the membrane's outer surface may modify ligand-receptor interactions (i.e., the binding of messenger chemicals, such as hormones and growth factors, to specialized cell membrane molecules, called receptors), which in turn may alter the state of large membrane molecules that play a role in controlling the cell's internal processes.[66]

Endogenous Fields as Medically Useful Information

Another line of study focuses on the endogenous EM fields. At the level of body tissues and organs, electrical activity is known to exhibit patterns that contain medically useful information. For example, the diagnostic procedures of EEG and ECG are based on detection of endogenous fields produced in the central nervous system and heart muscle. Taking the observation in these two systems a step further, current research is exploring the possibility that weak fields associated with nerve activity in other tissues and organs may also carry information of diagnostic value. New technologies for constructing extremely sensitive EM transducers (e.g., magnetometers and electrometers) and for signal processing have recently made this line of research feasible.

Recent BEM research has uncovered a form of endogenous radiation in the visible region of the spectrum that is emitted by most living organisms, ranging from plant seeds to humans.[18,40,49-51] Some evidence indicates that this extremely low-level light, known as *biophoton emission,* may be important in bioregulation, membrane transport, and gene expression. The beneficial and harmful effects of exogenous fields may be mediated by alterations in endogenous fields. Thus externally applied fields from medical devices may act to correct abnormalities in endogenous fields characteristic of disease states. Furthermore, the energy of the biophotons and processes involving their emission, as well as other endogenous fields of the body, may prove to be involved in energetic therapies, such as healer interactions.

At the cutting edge of BEM medicine research lies the question of how endogenous fields may alter because of changes in consciousness. The recent formation and rapid growth of the International Society for the Study of Subtle Energies and Energy Medicine is indicative of the growing interest in this field.

> **Points to Ponder** In a randomized, double-blind study, nonthermal pulsed EM energy significantly increased the healing rate of pressure ulcers in patients with spinal cord injuries.[57]

Medical Applications of Bioelectromagnetics

Most of today's medical devices use relatively high levels of EM energy.[52] The main topic of this chapter, however, is the use of the nonionizing portion of the EM spectrum, particularly at low levels.

Nonionizing medical applications may be classified according to whether they are *thermal* (heat producing in biologic tissue) or *nonthermal.* Thermal applications of nonionizing radiation (e.g., application of heat) include hyperthermia laser, surgery, and diathermy. The most important EM modalities in alternative medicine are the nonthermal applications of nonionizing radiation. The term nonthermal is used with two different meanings in the medical and scientific literature. *Biologically* or medically, nonthermal means that the application "causes no significant gross tissue heating." *Physically* or scientifically, nonthermal means that the application is "below the thermal noise limit at physiologic temperatures." The energy level of thermal noise is much lower than that required to heat tissue; thus any physically nonthermal application is automatically biologically nonthermal.

■ New and Unconventional Electromagnetic Approaches

The eight major new and unconventional applications of nonthermal, nonionizing EM fields are:
1. Bone repair
2. Stimulation and measurement of nerve activity
3. Soft-tissue wound healing
4. Autoimmune mechanisms
5. Pain management
6. Regeneration
7. Immune system restoration
8. Microwave resonance therapy

Bone Repair

Three types of applied EM fields are known to promote healing of nonunion bone fractures, that is, those that fail to heal spontaneously. They are (1) pulsed EM fields (PEMFs) and sinusoidal EM fields (AC fields); (2) DC fields, and (3) combined AC-DC magnetic fields tuned to ion-resonant frequencies. (These fields are extremely low intensity and physically nonthermal.)[70]

Approval of the U.S. Food and Drug Administration (FDA) has been obtained on PEMF and DC applications and is pending for the AC-DC application. In PEMF and AC applications, the repetition frequencies used are in the ELF range. In DC applications, magnetic field intensities range from 100 microgauss to 100 gauss, and electric currents range from less than 0.1 microampere to milliamperes.[2] FDA approval of these therapies covers only their use to promote healing of nonunion bone fractures, not to accelerate routine healing of uncomplicated fractures.

Efficacy of EM bone repair treatment has been confirmed in double-blind clinical trials.[3,62] Since 1985 it is conservatively estimated that more than 100,000 people had been treated with such devices.[4,5,13,14,27,31,34,42]

Stimulation and Measurement of Nerve Activity

Applications for the stimulation and measurement of nerve activity fall into the following seven categories:
1. Transcutaneous electrical nerve stimulation
2. Transcranial electrostimulation
3. Neuromagnetic stimulation
4. Electromyography
5. Electroencephalography
6. Electroretinography
7. Low-energy emission therapy

Transcutaneous Electrical Nerve Stimulation

In transcutaneous electrical nerve stimulation (TENS), two electrodes are applied to the skin via wires attached to a portable electrical generating device, which may be clipped to the patient's belt. More than 100 types of FDA-approved TENS devices are currently available and used for pain relief in physical therapy. Although each device usually offers some variances as to wave form and frequencies, they either interrupt the neurologic communication of pain pathways by the distraction of conscious attention or by shifting the activity of neurotransmitters, which releases endorphins.

Transcranial Electrostimulation

Transcranial electrostimulation (TCES) devices are similar to the TENS units. They apply extremely low currents—below the nerve excitation threshold—to the brain via two electrodes applied to the head and are used for behavioral and psychologic modification, such as the reduction of symptoms of depression, anxiety, and insomnia.[63] A recent metaanalysis covering at least 12 clinical trials selected from more than 100 published reports found that TCES alleviates anxiety.[36] With support from the National Institutes of Health (NIH), TCES is under evaluation for alleviating drug dependence.

Neuromagnetic Stimulation

In the application of neuromagnetic stimulation, which has both diagnostic and therapeutic uses, a magnetic pulse is noninvasively applied to a part of the patient's body to stimulate nerve activity. In diagnostic use, a pulse is applied to the cerebral cortex, and the patient's physiologic responses are monitored to obtain a dynamic picture of the brain-body interface.[29] As a treatment modality, it is being used in lieu of electroshock therapy to treat seizures and certain types of affective disorders, such as major depression.[1] Neuromagnetic stimulation also is used in nerve conduction studies for conditions such as carpal tunnel syndrome.

Points to Ponder Sandyk applied AC-pulsed EM applications in the treatment of multiple sclerosis (MS) and the management of Parkinson's disease.[59,61] Patients with MS demonstrated improvement in mobility, vision, bladder function, mood, heat tolerance, sleep, and clarity of thinking. Patients with Parkinson's disease improved mobility and significantly reduced symptoms of freezing, falling, and tremors. ■

Electromyography

EMG is a diagnostic application that detects electrical potentials associated with muscle contraction. Specific electrical patterns have been associated with certain abnormal states (e.g., denervated muscle). This method, along with EMG biofeedback, is being used to treat carpal tunnel syndrome and other movement disorders.

Electroencephalography

EEG is a neurodiagnostic application that detects brainwaves. Coupled with EEG biofeedback, it is used to treat a variety of conditions, such as learning disabilities, attention deficit and hyperactivity disorders, chronic alcoholism, and stroke.

Electroretinography

Electroretinography is a diagnostic application that monitors electrical potentials across the retina to assess eye movements. Electroretinography is one of the few methods available for noninvasive monitoring of rapid–eye movement sleep.

Low-Energy Emission Therapy

Low-energy emission therapy uses an antenna positioned in the patient's mouth to administer amplitude-modulated EM fields. It has been shown to affect the central nervous system, and pilot clinical studies show efficacy in treating insomnia and hypertension.[36,47,59]

Soft-Tissue Wound Healing

The following studies have demonstrated accelerated healing of soft-tissue wounds using DC, PEMF, and electrochemical modalities:

- Several reports indicate that EM applications may trigger healing when wound healing is abnormal (retarded or arrested).[37,69]
- PEMFs have been used clinically to treat venous skin ulcers. Results of several double-blind studies show that PEMF stimulation promotes cell activation and cell proliferation through an effect on the cell membrane, particularly on endothelial cells.[33,65]

- ELF and RF fields are applied to accelerate wound healing. Since skin wounds have unique electrical potentials and currents, stimulation of these electrical factors by a variety of exogenous EM fields can aid in the healing process by causing dedifferentiation (i.e., conversion to a more primitive form) of nearby cells, followed by accelerated cell proliferation.[44]
- An electrochemical treatment that provides regenerative wound healing uses electricity solely to introduce active metallic ions, such as silver, into the tissue. The electric field plays no role itself.[6,7,11]
- PEMF increases the rate of formation of epithelial (skin) cells in partially healed wounds.[41]
- AC EM fields promote the repair of injured vascular networks.[30]
- Electromagnetic devices have been patented for treating atherosclerotic lesions (i.e., small blood clots that build up on the walls of arteries and cause cardiovascular disease) and for controlling tissue growth.[28,39]

Autoimmune Mechanisms

In a recent clinical trial using a double-blind, randomized protocol with placebo control, patients with osteoarthritis (primarily of the knee) were treated noninvasively by pulsed 30-Hz, 60-gauss PEMFs. The treatment group improved substantially more than the placebo group.[67] It is believed that applied magnetic fields act to suppress inflammatory responses at the cell membrane level.[45]

Pain Management

Electrical stimulation for pain was introduced with TENS and received a great deal of attention for the treatment of back pain. Using the "gate theory" of neurologic pathways, electrical stimulation is purported to distract the pain signals along C fibers, which denote a more exquisite sensation at the conscious level, to the A fibers, which denotes a less emphatic sensation. Since patient responsiveness to this model is inconsistent, it was theorized that the stimulation might also affect neurotransmission, stimulating endorphins or other neurotransmitters that influence states of consciousness and awareness of physical or mental sensations.

Electrical current applied to inserted acupuncture needles is often used to enhance or replace manual needling. Clinical benefit has also been demonstrated for electrical stimulation applied directly to acupoints without the use of the needles. In a controlled study, electrostimulation as a replacement for acupuncture was applied to acupuncture points by a TENS unit. This method was also found effective in inducing uterine contractions in postterm pregnant women.[23] In one of the few double-blind studies with static magnetic fields, Vallbona applied active (300- to 500-gauss) and placebo magnets over trigger points on 50 patients with postpoliomyelitis pain symptoms. Vallbona found significant reductions in pain (76% for the treatment group versus 19% for control group).[68]

In a randomized trial, Colbert and others used tectonic magnetic mattress pads with 25 female patients with fibromyalgia.[19] Using magnets of 3950-gauss rating and approximately 1100 gauss on the surface of the magnets, the patients slept on the pads nightly. Compared with a control group, patients receiving treatment showed (1) significant improvement in physical functioning (30% compared with 3%), (2) decreased pain (38% compared with 8%), and (3) improvement in sleep (37% compared with 6%).

Regeneration

Animal research in the area of regeneration indicates that the body's endogenous EM fields are involved in growth processes and that modifications of these fields can lead to modest regeneration of severed limbs.[9,11] The studies indicate that low-intensity microwaves stimulate the division of bone marrow stem cells. Low-intensity microwaves may also be useful in enhancing the effects of chemotherapy by maintaining the formation and development, or hematopoiesis, of various types of blood cells.[22] Further, research with rats has shown that electrostimulation at certain points can enhance peripheral motor nerve regeneration and sensory nerve sprouting.[48]

The following studies are also relevant in the use of electrostimulation:

- PEMF applications for peripheral nerve regeneration[46,64]
- Pulsed, high-frequency EM fields for human wrist nerve regeneration[73]
- DC applications for rat spinal cord regeneration[25,32]
- BEM for rat sciatic nerve regeneration[35,53-55]

Immune System Restoration

During the last 2 decades, the effects of EM exposure on the immune system and its components have been extensively studied. Although early studies indicated that long-term exposure to EM fields might negatively affect the immune system, there is promising new research showing that applied EM fields may beneficially modulate immune responses. For example, studies with human lymphocytes show that exogenous EM or magnetic fields can produce changes in calcium transport and cause mediation of the mitogenic response. In other words, exogenous EM or magnetic fields can stimulate the division of cellular nuclei or cause certain types of immune cells to divide and reproduce rapidly in response to certain stimuli or mitogens. These findings have led researchers to investigate the possible augmentation of natural killer (NK) cells by applied EM fields. NK cells are important in helping the body fight cancer and viruses.[16,17,20,21] Salvatore and others showed improvements in the neoplastic cell kill rate of antineoplastic chemotherapy when the chemotherapy was coupled with LF magnetic fields.[56]

Low-level PEMFs have been shown to suppress levels of melatonin, which is secreted by the pineal gland and is believed to regulate the body's inner clock.[38,72] Melatonin as a hormone is oncostatic; that is, it stops cancer growth. Thus if melatonin can be suppressed by certain magnetic fields, it may be possible to use magnetic fields with different characteristics to stimulate melatonin secretion for the treatment of cancer. Other applications may include the use of EM fields to affect melatonin secretion, thereby normalizing circadian rhythms in people with jet lag and sleep-cycle disturbances.

Microwave Resonance Therapy

A variety of alternative medical practices developed outside the United States use nonionizing fields at nonthermal intensities, such as *microwave resonance therapy* (MRT). Used primarily in Russia, MRT employs low-intensity (either continuous or pulse-modulated), sinusoidal microwave radiation to treat a variety of conditions, including arthritis, ulcers, esophagitis, hypertension, chronic pain, cerebral palsy, neurologic disorders, and side effects of chemotherapy.[22]

The mechanism of action of MRT is thought to involve modifications in cell membrane transportation or production of chemical mediators or both. Although a sizable body of Russian literature exists on this technique, independent validation studies have not been conducted in the West. However, if such treatments prove to be effective, we may need to revise the current theories on the nature of how biological information is stored in molecular structures. It may be that such information is stored at the level of the whole organism in the endogenous energy field, which may be used in biological regulation and cellular communication. If exogenous, extremely low-level nonionizing fields with energy contents below the thermal noise limit produce biological effects, they may be acting on the body in such a way that they alter the body's own field. In other words, the exogenous EM fields may alter biological information.

■ Medical Issues

A number of uncharacterized "black box" medical treatment and diagnostic devices—some legal and some illegal—have been associated with EM medical treatment. It is unknown whether these devices operate on the basis of the principles of BEM medicine. Among these devices are (1) adionics devices, (2) Lakhovsky multiple-wave oscillators, (3) Priore's machines, (4) Rife's inert gas discharge tubes, (5) violet ray tubes, (6) Reich's orgone energy devices, (7) galvanic skin response machines, and (8) biocircuit devices.

There are at least six alternative explanations for how these and other such devices operate:

1. They are ineffectual and are based on erroneous application of physical principles.
2. They may be operating on sound principles of EM medicine, but no clear mechanisms have been explained.
3. They may operate on other principles, such as acoustic principles (sound or ultrasound waves) rather than those of EM.
4. In the case of diagnostic devices, they may work by focusing the intuitive capacity of the practitioner.
5. In the case of long-distance applications, they may operate by means of properties of consciousness of patient and practitioner.
6. They may operate on the energy of some domain that is uncharacterized at present.

A 1990 survey showed that approximately 1% of the U.S. population used energy healing techniques that included a variety of EM devices.[24] Indeed, the respondents in this survey more often used energy healing techniques than homeopathy and acupuncture in the treatment of either serious or chronic disease. In addition to the use of devices by practitioners, a plethora of consumer medical products that use magnetic energy are purported to promote relaxation or to treat a variety of illnesses. For example, there are mattress pads with magnets for beds; there are magnets that attach to the site of an athletic injury; and there are small pelletlike magnets to place over specific points on the body.

Some of these medical modalities, although presently accepted medically or legally in the United States, have not necessarily passed the most recent requirements of safety or effectiveness. FDA approval of a significant number of devices, primarily those used in bone repair and neurostimulation, were "grandfathered." In other words, medical devices that were sold in the United States before the Medical Device Law automatically received FDA approval for use in the same manner and for the same medical conditions for which they were used before the law's enactment in the late 1970s. The FDA approved the devices on the basis of "presumption," but they usually remain incompletely studied. Grandfathering by the FDA applies not only to EM devices, but it applies to all devices covered by the Medical Device Law. However, neither the safety nor effectiveness of grandfathered devices is established. Reexamination of devices in use may be warranted.

■ Scientific Controversy

Some physicists claim that low-intensity, nonionizing EM fields have no bioeffects other than resistive heating of tissue. One such argument is based on a physical model in which power density is the only EM field parameter considered relevant to biological systems. The argument asserts that measurable nonthermal bioeffects of EM fields are "impossible" because they contradict known physical laws or require a "new physics" to explain them.

However, numerous independent experiments reported in the refereed journal research literature conclusively established that nonthermal bioeffects of low-intensity EM fields do indeed exist. Moreover, the experimental results lend support to certain new approaches in theoretical modeling of the interactions between EM fields and biological matter. Most researchers now believe that the bioeffects will become comprehensible, not by forsaking physics but by developing more sophisticated, detailed models based on known physical laws in which additional parameters (e.g., frequency, intensity, waveform, field directionality) are taken into account.

> **Points to Ponder**   In Japan, pulsed EM fields are used in spinal fusion to minimize vertebral bone mineral loss.[34]

An Expert Speaks: Dr. Beverly Rubik

Dr. Beverly Rubik received her PhD in biophysics from University of California, Berkeley, in 1979. She has published numerous articles related to BEM approaches and was editorial consultant and contributor for several publications including: *Biophoton Emission and Beyond; Microbial Mysteries: The Evolution and Implications of Pleomorphism; Alternative Medicine: Expanding Medical Horizons; The Heart of Healing;* and *The Interrelationship Between Mind and Matter.* She serves as an advisory board member to numerous organizations, journals, and groups including the NIH, Office of Complementary and Alternative Medicine; the *Journal of Complementary Therapies in Medicine,* and *Alternative Therapies in Health and Medicine.* She is founder and president of the Institute for Frontier Science.

Question. Dr. Rubik, most of us are confused by the term "bioelectromagnetics." Can you explain this scientific discipline in a way that will help us grasp what it is all about?

Answer. Bioelectromagnetics is an interdisciplinary science at the interface of physics, biology, and medicine that deals with the effects of low-level electricity, magnetism, and electromagnetic fields on life. Only a few decades ago, it was discovered that organisms are exquisitely sensitive to extremely low-level fields. Of course, life evolved in a sea of such energies that were naturally emanating from the earth and cosmos, so it makes sense that organisms have adapted to using them as part of their normal physiologic functions. Moreover, organisms are fundamentally bioelectric and emit similar low-level fields, which is the basis of the electroencephalogram and electrocardiogram used in medical diagnostics.

Question. How did you become interested in this field of study?

Answer. I was intrigued with some of the unexplained features of life, such as consciousness and the capacity for self-healing. I studied biophysics, including bioelectromagnetics back at the time when this field was just being "born." I also explored more unconventional topics such as "subtle energies" in living systems. Going between the cracks of disciplines where few have gone before, one can ask novel questions about the nature of life and healing. I knew from the history of science and medicine that this [electromagnetics] had great potential for future breakthroughs that have often come from outside the beaten path. Today, I consider myself a "frontier scientist," working on research questions that fall outside the dominant scientific paradigm but, nonetheless, are captivating a growing number of researchers.

Over 20 years ago, I wondered whether electromagnetic energies might someday be controlled and used for healing or even become the basis of a completely new medicine. Robert Becker's experiments in the 1960s intrigued me—demonstrating particular electrical signals in the regenerating salamander that were not present in the frog or the mouse. The salamander can regrow an amputated leg or tail all by itself, but the frog or mouse can not. Becker further showed that the frog and mouse could be induced to regrow a severed limb by applying external electricity with characteristics similar to those in the regenerating salamander.

Question. Is it possible to stimulate regrowth of amputated limbs in humans?

Answer. Such regeneration effects on whole limbs have never been shown in humans. Nonetheless, bioelectromagnetic medicine was launched with the first regeneration device that stimulated bone growth in nonunion bone fractures. Today, these devices consist of external coils that are placed around broken limbs and emit pulses of magnetic energy. They induce electric currents deep in the tissues that promote bone tissue growth. Although these devices have been FDA approved for more than 20 years, the fact is that they are not used very often when indicated. Instead, invasive and expensive surgeries are typically done by orthopedists who plant steel pins or plates to help such recalcitrant fractures mend. Clearly, medicine is slow to change, especially where big business economics governs hospital practices.

Question. I assume there is considerable research being done now to explore the possibilities of bioelectromagnetics for medical interventions.

Answer. Unfortunately, funding for such research is not easy to obtain. One reason is that the worldview of life as a biochemical machine dominates conventional biology and medicine, rendering novel biophysical discoveries incomprehensible unless there are molecular mechanisms elucidated. The fact is that we do not understand how certain very weak fields can interact with the organism and promote healing. Moreover, the public is more concerned over the potential hazards of electromagnetic fields in the environment and tends to think—wrongly so—

that all such fields may be harmful to life. Unfortunately, the federal government has been slow to recognize the importance of this frontier area for future medicine, so very little support is available for research on the therapeutic effects of low-level fields.

Question. What research projects are you currently working on?

Answer. Presently, I am developing clinical trials to study a new bandage from Japan containing semiconductors that shows great promise in reducing inflammation and in accelerating wound healing. We hope to show that this novel device can prevent the typical swelling and bruising following facial plastic surgery. Because beauty has high social value, this work may have significant [influence] on medical acceptance and stimulate greater interest in this area. I am also working on scientific theory. Is bioelectromagnetics possibly more fundamental than biochemistry? Can bioinformation, carried by exceedingly weak and possibly highly organized complex electromagnetic signals, be one of the salient features of life that has been missed by modern biology, which is entirely focused on biomolecules? Will we someday be able to decipher the meaning of biophoton emission—very weak natural light emitted from the body—to give us information about the status of our health?

Question. What do you see as the future of bioelectromagnetics?

Answer. Bioelectromagnetics may eventually provide a scientific foundation, if not an explanation, for "energy medicine," including acupuncture, homeopathy, and other medical modalities in which very small energy nudges are delivered to the body. Such a scientific framework may be essential to the integration of these complementary medicine modalities into our medical system. I am indeed curious about "subtle energies" such as qi, prana, the vital force of Hahnemann's homeopathy, and energy that may be exchanged during certain types of healer interventions. I have done sufficient research on such phenomena to be convinced of them. An important question is whether these phenomena are essentially manifestations of bioelectromagnetics or whether there might be other, more subtle fields or energies in life. "Subtle energies" or "subtle interactions" in healing processes takes us to the frontier where mind and matter interact. These areas may also offer clues toward a deeper understanding of mind-body medicine and distant healing.

■ Chapter Review

Clinical trials of BEM-based treatments may yield useful results for the following conditions: (a) arthritis, (b) psychophysiologic states (including drug dependence and epilepsy), (c) wound healing and regeneration, (d) intractable pain, (e) MS and Parkinson's disease, (f) spinal cord injury, (g) closed head injury, (h) cerebral palsy (spasticity reduction), (i) learning disabilities, (j) headache, (k) degenerative conditions associated with aging, (l) cancer, and (m) acquired immunodeficiency syndrome (AIDS).

EM fields may be applied clinically as the primary therapy or as complementary therapy along with other treatments in the conditions listed. Effectiveness can be measured via the following clinical markers:

- **Arthritis.** The usual clinical criteria, including decrease of pain, less swelling, and thus a greater potential for mobility
- **Psychophysiologic problems.** Relief from symptoms of drug withdrawal and alleviation of depressive anxiety and its symptoms
- **Epilepsy.** Return to greater normality in EEG, more normal sleep patterns, and reduction in required drug dosages
- **Wound healing and regeneration.** Repair of soft tissue and reduction of collagenous tissue in scar formation; regrowth via blastemal primitive cell formation and increase in tensile strength of surgical wounds; alleviation of decubitus chronic ulcers (bedsores); increased angiogenesis (regrowth of vascular tissue, such as blood vessels); and healing of recalcitrant (unresponsive to treatment) chronic venous ulcers

Just as exposure to high-energy radiation has unquestioned hazards, radiation has long been a key weapon in the fight against many types of disease. Likewise, although there are indications that some EM fields may be hazardous, there is now increasing evidence that there are beneficial bioeffects of certain low-intensity, nonthermal EM fields.

In clinical practice, BEM applications offer the possibility of more economical and more effective diagnostics and new noninvasive therapies for medical problems, including those considered intractable or recalcitrant to conventional treatments. In biomedical research, EM medicine can provide a better understanding of the fundamental mechanisms of communication and regulation at levels ranging from intracellular to organismic. Improved knowledge of fundamental mechanisms of EM field interactions could directly lead to major advances in diagnostic and treatment methods.

For the following reasons, BEM medicine may be the most important next step in medical care since antibiotics:

1. BEM fields invoke an integrated response in the body and mind—a generalized field. Because of this, all bodily systems, including consciousness, would need to be considered as part of the patient's total experience in the healing process. In essence, the schizophrenic approach of medical care as specializations would evolve toward a broader regard for the individual, thus providing a more holistic framework of health.

2. Drugs often require time to build to sufficient levels for beneficial effects. BEM approaches would respond more quickly, and adjustment of effective (and less destructive) doses could be determined.

3. Specific patterns of EM stimuli may be identified for optimal regenerational growth of specific bodily structures, and damaged tissues may be regenerated, eventually leading to the regeneration of injured spinal cords.

4. Benefits may be realized for those diseases with episodic properties, such as MS and depression.

■ Review Questions

1. What individuals have been most instrumental in introducing EM approaches to medical science?
2. What are the elements of an atom that have electric charge?
3. What necessary process takes place to have an electric current?
4. What is the relationship between an electric current and a magnetic field?
5. What is the difference between an endogenous field and an exogenous field?
6. Define ionizing.
7. Define ELF.
8. Define nonthermal, as it relates to medical care.
9. Describe at least four areas of EM applications that warrant consideration in medical care.
10. Discuss some of the medical controversy over BEM medicine.

CRITICAL THINKING AND CLINICAL APPLICATION EXERCISES

1. Since EM approaches have been shown to have harmful effects on body tissue, what would you recommend as safeguards for patient care?
2. What are the actual mechanics of how EM fields interact with physical dynamics?
3. Suppose a patient has strong anxiety attacks with severe back pain, and the typical approaches, such as psychotropic drugs, psychotherapy, and educational programs, have not worked. Under what circumstances would you suggest BEM medicine?

References

1. Anninos PA, Tsagas N. Magnetic stimulation in the treatment of partial seizures, *Int J Neurosci* 60:141, 1991.
2. Baranowski TJ, Black J: Stimulation of osteogenesis. In Blank M, Findl E, editors: *Mechanistic approaches to interactions of electric and electromagnetic fields with living systems,* New York, 1987, Plenum Press.
3. Barker AT, Dixon RA, Sharrard WJW, Sutcliffe ML: Pulsed magnetic field therapy for tibial nonunion: interim results of a double-blind trial, *Lancet* 1(8384):994, 1984.
4. Bassett CAL, Mitchell SN, Gaston SR: Pulsing electromagnetic field treatment in ununited fractures and failed arthrodoses, *JAMA* 247:623, 1982.
5. Bassett CAL, Pawluk RD, Pilla AA: Augmentation of bone repair by inductively coupled electromagnetic fields, *Science* 184:575, 1974.
6. Becker RO: A technique for producing regenerative healing in humans, *Frontier Perspectives* 1(2):1, 1990.
7. Becker RO: Effect of anodally generated silver ions on fibrosarcoma cells, *Electro Magnetobiol* 11:57, 1992.
8. Becker RO, Marino AA: *Electromagnetism and life,* Albany, NY, 1982, State University of New York Press.
9. Becker RO, Spadero JA: Electrical stimulation of partial limb regeneration in mammals, *Bull N Y Acad Med* 48:627, 1972.

10. Becker R: *The body electric,* New York, 1985, William Morrow.

11. Becker RO: *The effect of electrically generated silver ions on human cells,* Bethesda, MD, 1987, Proceedings of 1st International Conference on Gold and Silver in Medicine.

12. Bierbaum PJ, Peters JM, editors: *Proceedings of the scientific workshop on the health effects of electric and magnetic fields on workers,* Cincinnati, OH, NIOSH Rep No. 91-111, 1991, National Technical Information Service.

13. Brighton CT, Black J, Friedenberg ZB, Esterhai JL, Day L, Connally JF: A multicenter study of the treatment of nonunion with constant direct current, *J Bone Joint Surg* 63A:2, 1981.

14. Brighton CT, Black J, Pollack SR, editors: Electrical properties of bone and cartilage: experimental effects, 1979.

15. Brighton CT, Pollack SR, editors: *Electromagnetics in medicine and biology,* San Francisco, 1991, San Francisco Press.

16. Cadossi R, Emilia G, Torelli G: Lymphocytes and pulsing magnetic fields. In Marino AA, editor: *Modern bioelectricity,* New York, 1988, Marcel Dekker.

17. Cadossi R, Iverson R, Hentz VR, Zucchini P, Emilia G, Torelli G: Effect of low-frequency low-energy pulsing electromagnetic fields on mice undergoing bone marrow transplantation, *Int J Immunopathol Pharmacol* 1:57, 1988.

18. Chwirot WB: Ultraweak photon emission and another meiotic cycle in Larix europaea (experimental investigation of Nagl and Popp's electromagnetic model of differentiation), *Experientia* 44:594, 1988.

19. Colbert AP, Baker E, Markov MS: *Use of tectonic magnetic mattress pad in patient with fibromyalgia,* Twentieth Annual Meeting, St. Petersburg Beach, FL, 1998, Bioelectromagnetic Society.

20. Cossarizza A, Monti D, Bersani F et al: Extremely low-frequency pulsed electromagnetic fields increase interleukin-2 (IL-2) utilization and IL-2 receptor expression in mitogen-stimulated human lymphocytes from old subjects, *FEBS Lett* 248:141, 1989.

21. Cossarizza A, Monti D, Sola P et al: DNA repair after irradiation in lymphocytes exposed to low-frequency, *Radiation Res* 118:161, 1989.

22. Devyatkov ND, Gulyaev YV et al: *Digest of papers. International symposium on millimeter waves of nonthermal intensity in medicine,* Moscow, 1991, Research and Development Association and Research Institute of USSR Ministry of Electronic Industry.

23. Dunn PA, Rogers D: Transcutaneous electrical nerve stimulation at acupuncture points in the induction of uterine contractions, *Obstetr Gynecol* 73:286, 1989.

24. Eisenberg DM, Kessler RC, Foster C et al: Unconventional medicine in the United States: prevalence, costs, and patterns of use, *N Engl J Med* 328:246, 1993.

25. Fehlings MG, Hurlbert RJ, Tator CH: *An examination of direct current fields for the treatment of spinal cord injury.* Paper presented at the 1st World Congress for Electricity and Magnetism in Biology and Medicine, Orlando, 1992.

26. Foley-Nolan D, Moore K, Codd M, Barry C, O'Connor P, Coughlan RJ: Low energy, high frequency pulse electromagnetic theory for acute whiplash injuries, *Scand J Rehab Med* 24(1):51, 1992.

27. Goldenberg DM, Hansen HJ: Electric enhancement of bone healing, *Science* 175:1118, 1972.

28. Gordon RT: Process for the treatment of atherosclerotic lesions. U.S. Patent No. 4,622,953, November 18, 1986.

29. Hallett M, Cohen LG: Magnetism: a new method for stimulation of nerve and brain, *JAMA* 262(4):538, 1989.

30. Herbst E, Sisken BF, Wang HZ: *Assessment of vascular network in rat skin flaps subjected to sinusoidal EMFs using image analysis techniques.* Transactions of the 8th annual meeting of the bioelectrical repair and growth society, Washington, DC, 1988.

31. Hinsenkamp M, Ryaby J, Burny F: Treatment of nonunion by pulsing electromagnetic fields: European multicenter study of 308 cases, *Reconstr Surg Traumatol* 19:147, 1985.

32. Hurlbert RJ, Tator CH: *Effect of disc vs. cuff electrode configuration on tolerance of the rat spinal cord to DC stimulation.* Paper presented at the 1st World Congress for Electricity and Magnetism in Biology and Medicine, Orlando, 1992.

33. Ieran M, Zaffuto S, Bagnacani M, Annovi M, Moratti A, Cadossi R: Effect of low-frequency pulsing electromagnetic fields on skin ulcers of venous origin in humans: a double-blind study, *J Orthop Res* 8:276, 1990.

34. Ito M, Fay LA, Ito Y, Yuan MR, Edwards WT, Yuan HA: The effect of pulsed electromagnetic fields on instrumented posterolateral spinal fusion and device-related stress shielding, *Spine* 2 (2):4 382, 1997.

35. Kanje M, Rusovan A: *Reversal of the stimulation of magnetic field exposure on regeneration of the rat sciatic nerve by a Ca antagonist.* Paper presented at the 1st World Congress for Electricity and Magnetism in Biology and Medicine, Orlando, 1992.

36. Klawansky S, Yueng A, Berkey C, Shah N, Zachery C, Chalmers TC: *Meta-analysis of randomized control trials of the efficacy of cranial electrostimulation in treating psychological and physiological conditions.* Report of the Technology Assessment Group, Department of Health Policy and Management, Harvard University School of Public Health, 1992.

37. Lee RC, Canaday DJ, Doong H: A review of the biophysical basis for the clinical application of electric fields in soft tissue repair, *J Burn Care Rehab* 14:319, 1993.

38. Lerchl A, Nonaka KO, Stokkan KA, Reiter RJ: Marked rapid alterations in nocturnal pineal serotonin metabolism in mice and rats exposed to weak intermittent magnetic fields, *Biochem Biophys Res Commun* 169:102, 1990.

39. Liboff AR, McLeod BR, Smith SD: *Method and apparatus for controlling tissue growth with an applied fluctuating magnetic field,* US Patent No. 5,123,898, June 23, 1992.

40. Mathew R, Rumar S: The non-exponential decay pattern of the weak luminescence from seedlings in *Cicer arietinum L.* Stimulated by pulsating electric fields, *Experientia.* Manuscript submitted for publication, 1999.

41. Mertz PM, Davis SC, Eaglstein WH: *Pulsed electrical stimulation increases the rate of epithelialization in partial thickness wounds.* Transactions of the 8th annual meeting of the bioelectrical repair and growth society, Washington, DC, 1988.

42. Mooney V: A randomized double-blind prospective study of the efficacy of pulsed electromagnetic fields for interbody lumbar fusions, *Spine* 15(7):708, 1990.

43. Nair I, Morgan MG, Florig HK: *Biological effects of power frequency electric and magnetic fields (background paper),* Office of Technology Assessment, Report No OTA-BP-E-53, Washington, DC, 1989, US Government Printing Office.

44. O'Connor ME, Bentall RHC, Monahan JC, editors: *Emerging electromagnetic medicine conference proceedings,* New York, 1990, Springer-Verlag.

45. O'Connor ME, Lovely RH, editors: Electromagnetic fields, 1988.

46. Orgel MG, Zienowicz RJ, Thomas BA, and Kurtz WH: *Peripheral nerve transection injury: the role of electromagnetic field therapy.* Paper presented at the 1st World Congress for Electricity and Magnetism in Biology and Medicine, Orlando, 1992.

47. Pasche B, Lebet TP, Barbault A, Rossel C, Kuster N: *Electroencephalographic changes and blood pressure lowering effect of low energy emission therapy* (abstract), Bioelectromagnetics Society Proceedings, F-3-5, 1989.

48. Pomeranz B, Mullen M, Markus H: Effect of applied electrical fields on sprouting of intact saphenous nerve in adult rat, *Brain Res* 303:331, 1984.

49. Popp FA, Gurwitsch AA, Inaba H et al: Biophoton emission (multiauthor review), *Experientia* 44:543, 1988.

50. Popp FA, Li KH, Gu Q, editors: *Recent advances in biophoton research and its applications,* Singapore and New York, 1992, World Scientific Publishing.

51. Popp FA, Nagl W, Li KH et al: Biophoton emission: new evidence for coherence and DNA as source, *Cell Biophysics* 6:33, 1984.

52. Rubik B, Becker R, Flower R, Hazlewood C, Liboff A, Walleczek J: *Bioelectromagnetics applications in medicine,* Panel Discussion, 1995.

53. Rusovan A, Kanje M: D600, a Ca antagonist, prevents stimulation of nerve regeneration by magnetic fields, *Neuroreport* 3:813, 1992.

54. Rusovan A, Kanje M, Mild KH: The stimulatory effect of magnetic fields on regeneration of the rat sciatic nerve is frequency dependent, *Exp Neurol* 117:81, 1992.

55. Rusovan A, Kanje M: Stimulation of regeneration of the rat sciatic nerve by 50-Hz sinusoidal magnetic fields, *Exp Neurol* 112:312, 1991.

56. Salvatore JR, Blackinton D, Polk C, Mehta S: Nonionizing electromagnetic radiation: a study of carcinogenic and cancer treatment potential, *Rev Environ Health* 10(3-4):197, 1994.

57. Salzberg CA, Cooper-Vastola SA, Perez F, Viehveck MG, Byrne DW: The effects of non-thermal pulsed electromagnetic energy on wound healing of pressure ulcers in spinal cord-injured patients: a randomized, double-blind study, *Ostomy Wound Manage* 41(3):42, 1995.

58. Sandyk R: A drug naive parkinsonian patient successfully treated with weak electromagnetic fields, *Int J Neurosci* 79(1-2):99, 1994.

59. Sandyk, R: Brief communication: electromagnetic fields improve visuospatial performance and reverse agraphia in a parkinsonian patient, *Int J Neurosci* 87(3-4):209, 1996.

60. Sandyk R: Improvement of right hemispheric functions in a child with Gilles de la Tourette's Syndrome by weak electromagnetic fields, *Int J Neurosci* 81(3-4):199, 1995.

61. Sandyk, R: Resolution of sleep paralysis by weak electromagnetic fields in a patient with multiple sclerosis, *Int J Neurosci* 90(3-4):145, 1997.

62. Sharrard WJW: A double-blind trial of pulsed electromagnetic fields for delayed union of tibial fractures, *J Bone Joint Surg* 72B:347, 1990.

63. Shealy N, Cady R, Veehoff D et al: Neuro-chemistry of depression, *Am J Pain Manage* 2:31, 1992.

64. Sisken BF: *Nerve regeneration: implications for clinical applications of electrical stimulation.* Paper presented at the 1st World Congress for Electricity and Magnetism in Biology and Medicine, Orlando, 1992.

65. Stiller MJ, Pak GH, Shupack JL, Thaler S, Kenny C, Jondreau L: A portable pulsed electromagnetic field (PEMF) device to enhance healing of recalcitrant venous ulcers: a double-blind placebo-controlled clinical trial, *Br J Dermatol* 127:147, 1992.

66. Tenforde TS, Kaune WT: Interaction of extremely low frequency electric and magnetic fields with humans, *Health Phys* 53:585, 1987.

67. Trock DH, Bollet AJ, Dyer RH Jr, Fieldings LP, Miner WK, Markoll R: A double-blind trial of the clinical effects of pulsed electromagnetic fields in osteoarthritis, *J Rheumatol* 20:456, 1993.

68. Vallbona C, Hazlewoord CF, Jurida G: Response of pain to static magnetic fields in postpolio patients: double-blind pilot study, *Arch Phys Med Rehab* 87(11):1200, 1997.

69. Vodovnik L, Karba R: Treatment of chronic wounds by means of electric and electromagnetic fields. Part 1: literature review, *Med Biol Eng Comput* 30(3):257, 1992.

70. Weinstein AM, McLeod BR, Smith SD, Liboff AR: *Ion resonance-tuned electromagnetic fields increase healing rate in ostectomized rabbits.* Abstracts of 36th Annual Meeting of Orthopedic Research, New Orleans, 1990.

71. Wilson BW, Stevens RG, Anderson LE, editors: *Extremely low frequency electromagnetic fields: the question of cancer,* Columbus, OH, 1990, Battelle Press.

72. Wilson BW, Wright CW, Morris JE et al: Evidence for an effect of ELF electromagnetic fields on human pineal gland function, *J Pineal Res* 9:259, 1990.

73. Wilson DH, Jagdeesh P, Neswman PP, Harriman DGF: The effects of pulsed electromagnetic energy on peripheral nerve regeneration, *Ann N Y Acad Sci* 238:575, 1974.

17

Spiritual Medicine

G. Frank Lawlis

WHY READ THIS CHAPTER?

Over the past decade, there has been a renewed public interest and belief in the "true healing capacity" of faith, prayer, and spirituality. With this new interest comes the question, "What is the appropriate role of spirituality and religion in medicine?" There are many testimonies of miraculous cures as a result of spiritual intervention. Clinical trials of spiritual interventions are, however, very limited.

Most of the world's medical philosophies are tied to the spiritual beliefs and rituals of their respective cultures. Yet, in the last century, a dualism has grown between religion and the science of medicine, resulting in a sense of professional hostility between the two philosophies.

This chapter explores the research that supports the role of spirituality in medical care and evaluates the evidence suggesting that patients benefit medically from its inclusion. The evidence, consisting mostly of correlational data with some controlled trials, remains too scant to allow the development of a body-spirit model of medicine or the demonstration of a cause-and-effect relationship. Nonetheless, the data are suggestive enough to demand an appraisal of the powerful effects of spirituality and faith on health outcomes.

The evidence, consisting mostly of correlational data with some controlled trials, remains too scant to allow the development of a body-spirit model of medicine or to demonstrate a cause-and-effect relationship. The evidence, consisting mostly of correlational data with some controlled trials, remains too scant to allow the development of a body-spirit model of medicine or to demonstrate a cause-and-effect relationship.

The student is invited to draw his or her own conclusions as to how religion may, once again, become an important component of medical care. This chapter may also serve as a stimulus for the reader to examine his or her own spiritual beliefs as they relate to health. The author hopes that this chapter will also encourage future research in this area.

CHAPTER AT A GLANCE

This chapter explores the relevance of religion and spiritual belief to health care, religion as a factor in recovery from illness, and illness prevention effects of spirituality and religion. The effects of religion and spirituality on health outcomes are referred to as "spiritual medicine."

The effects of religious commitment on heart disease, blood pressure, substance abuse prevention, suicide, and longevity are discussed. Prayer as a spiritual intervention is evaluated. The effects of prayer on human patients with leukemia and rheumatoid arthritis, on human tissue, and in critical care settings are described. The effects of prayer on fungi, yeast, bacteria, simple organisms, plants, and animals are explained. Finally, ritual—including shamanic traditional healing ritual—and its effects on health are examined. Indications and contraindications for religious and spiritual practices, as they relate to health care outcomes, are defined.

> In the future it will be considered unethical for a physician not to pray for his or her patient as part of quality health care.

LARRY DOSSEY, MD

CHAPTER OBJECTIVES

After completing this chapter, you should be able to:

1. Understand the relevance of a person's religious beliefs and practice as they apply to health and healing.
2. Discuss the effects of religious faith on the health dimensions from a preventive perspective.
3. Describe intervention factors that may influence medical outcomes.
4. Define the aspects of prayer and ritual as features of spirituality and health care.
5. Describe the underlying principles of religion, such as lifestyle and community support.

Since the beginning of recorded history, the healing arts have been at the core of spiritual practices. Perhaps the initial reason for this association was the cultural belief that the forces of illness have demonic motivations and that divine intervention is responsible for miraculous healing. Certainly, the Bible is an example of the philosophy that relates spiritual faith to healing.

Only in the last 100 years has medical science separated itself from religious ties. Rene Descartes has been credited for establishing separation between the soul and body, thus opening the door for the sciences to conduct autopsies of the human body and to explain other critical mechanisms of disease.

Wars between church and science have led to the branding of spirituality as "superstition and myth." Medical scientists are often ashamed to admit an interest in things spiritual. Freud defined mystical experience as "infantile helplessness" and a "regression to primary narcissism." Patients and physicians alike are often labeled in this manner, if they express belief in religion or spirituality as a factor in healing.

Since 1993, when Dr. Larry Dossey, a pioneer of modern scientific medicine, wrote about "prayer as good medicine," medical and research interest in the possibility that a person's religion or spirituality influences health and healing has exploded.[15] The idea that physicians should consider religion and spirituality as significant factors in dealing with disease and recovery remains controversial. Since the scientific era became supreme, the concept that religious involvement or spirituality could beneficially affect the health and clinical course of individual patients was deemed implausible. Even those more empathetic may think that little, if any, published research has either supported or refuted this concept.

A review published in 1987 uncovered more than 200 studies containing religious terminology published in the medical literature during the past century.[50] Subsequent reviews have examined cause-specific morbidity and mortality rates among Catholic, Protestant, Jewish, Hindu, Buddhist, Parsi, and Muslim patients.[36,51,76] Statistically significant associations between religious belief and health measures have been established. Morbidity or mortality differences have been found for the health categories of heart disease, hypertension, stroke, cancer, and gastrointestinal disease. Health status indicators (e.g., self-reported health, symptoms, disability, and longevity) have also differed, based on the strength of religious commitment. The consistency and robustness of findings have led to the emergence of a growing area of research that is generally referred to as "spiritual medicine."

Systematic reviews and metaanalyses quantitatively confirm that religious involvement is an epidemiologically protective factor.[43,49,79] There have been many underlying reasons that may explain these high associations. It may be beneficial to identify known or hypothesized biobehavioral or psychosocial pathways through which religious or spiritual practice may promote health or prevent disease.[35] For example, spiritual practice has been shown to promote health-related behavior and lifestyles, both of which lower disease risk and enhance well-being. Spiritual practices also provide social support, which buffers stress and enhances coping.[48]

■ Relevance of Religion to Health Care

The majority of the patient populations have always been committed in their religious beliefs (Figure 17-1). Ninety-five percent of the U.S. population expresses a belief in God, and more than two thirds of the people claim that they base their entire approach to life on their religious beliefs.[4,22] What some clinicians may not be aware of, however, is the important role that a patient's religious beliefs can play in the clinical realm. Patient religiousness has been found to have much relevance to clinical outcomes and care, with the religious cultures of patients influencing illness prevention, coping, and care, as well as how patients view and define their illnesses. For example, a recent study of older inpatients found that one third of those surveyed believed that sickness was a punishment from God, and nearly four fifths of this surveyed population believed that good health was a blessing from God.[3] Another study, conducted on a sample of hospitalized psychiatric patients, supported the hypothesis that patients' religious beliefs influenced their perceptions of illness, with nearly half of the surveyed patients believing that leading a moral life could protect against illness and almost three quarters attributing their illness to a transgression or sin against God.[70]

> **Points to Ponder** At any given level of chronic illness, those who are more religious perceive their ability to function as higher than those who are not religious.[33]

that over half of the patients viewed their religious beliefs as an important factor in adjusting to their chronic and life-threatening illnesses. This study found that the importance of religious beliefs in coping with illness increased over time. Nearly half of the hemodialysis patients resurveyed 3 years after their initial interviews reported that their religious beliefs had become even more important to them in coping with their illnesses since their initial assessments.[59]

Idler and Kasl established a beneficial relationship between religious commitment and coping with illness and disability in their study of an older population.[33] In their longitudinal study spanning 7 years, the researchers found that a subgroup of religiously committed men who became disabled during the study period experienced lower rates of depression as a result of their disability than those who were less religiously committed. In addition, religious commitment was found to play an important role in improving the functional status of the disabled.

> **Points to Ponder**   Religiousness is associated with lower rates of cigarette smoking.[77] ■

■ Religion as a Factor in the Recovery from Illness

Patients' religious beliefs may assist them not only in coping with illness but also in recovering from illness. The importance of an individual's religious beliefs as a factor in recovery from illness was evaluated in a study of older women with hip fractures. Patients who regarded God as a source of strength and comfort and who attended religious services were able to walk a greater number of meters at discharge.[66] Even when the severity of the fracture was controlled, religiously committed patients still were found to walk further at discharge.

Patients undergoing heart surgery revealed a similarly protective quality of religious commitment. The researchers followed 232 patients after their elective heart surgery and analyzed which factors contributed to their recovery and survival.[62] The most consistent indicator of survival was the amount of strength or comfort that patients said they derived from their religious faith. These findings led the researchers to conclude that, "Those without any strength or comfort from religion had almost three times the risk of death as those with at least some strength and comfort." The researchers also speculated that a physician "probably cannot convince a patient to

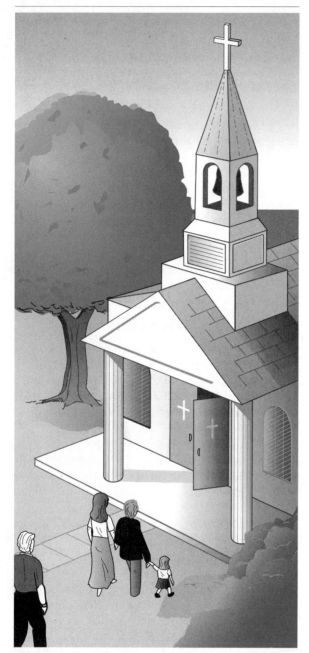

■ **Figure 17-1.** Persons who are committed to their religious beliefs cope better with illness and suffer less depression.

■ Adjustment to Illness

When a person experiences illness, their religious beliefs seem to take on greater importance. A study of a group of older inpatients suffering from a variety of clinical disorders found that more than 50% of the patients rated their religious beliefs as being a very important means of coping with their illness.[39] A similarly designed study of patients undergoing chronic hemodialysis found participate privately in religion...any more than he or she can successfully convince a patient to stop smoking." Yet, encouraging these activities "may improve quality of life and...alter their survival behaviors."

Religious commitment appears to be extremely important in the enhancement of recovery from mental illness. Andreasen was one of the first researchers to present data on the beneficial clinical role that a religious perspective can have in coping with and recovering from depression.[2] More recent studies have supported the finding that religion is associated with improved overall emotional functioning. For example, patients with schizophrenia who attended church or were given supportive aftercare by religious caregivers were found to have lower overall rates of rehospitalization.[11,38] In addition, after participating in religious worship, a significant reduction in the number of psychiatric symptoms was noted on patient self-report measures and in more objective physiologic measures.[18,20,28,56]

■ Illness Prevention and Health Enhancement

A number of recent studies have suggested that religious commitment could have a prophylactic or preventative effect on physical and mental health. Hannay, in an early study on the relationship between religious commitment and health status, reported that religious allegiance was inversely correlated with the frequency of physical, mental, and social symptoms found in an adult population in Scotland.[30] More recent studies reported similar results. For example, a recent cross-sectional survey of college students at a midwestern university found that religious commitment was positively associated with health-enhancing behaviors and attitudes. Further, religiously committed students reported fewer incidences of health-compromising behaviors and fewer personal injuries and illnesses.[60] Perhaps the critical factors were the implied lifestyles of the subjects. The more religious students avoided health-compromising behaviors, and they also were more likely to report frequent health-enhancing behaviors, such as health responsibility, self-actualization, exercise, nutrition, stress management, and interpersonal support.

These findings were replicated on a sample of students from a Canadian university in which the more religious students experienced fewer health care, dental care, and emergency visits than the less religious students.[21] In addition, the researchers discovered that the religiously committed students experienced less severe and less frequent stress than the students with less religious commitment; the more religious students also experienced higher levels of personal well-being and life satisfaction.

Religion has been identified as a potential buffer against stress, since the religiously committed individuals report much lower stress levels than those less committed. Research conducted on nonstudent populations has supported the idea that religious commitment is associated with an improved sense of well-being and decreased levels of stress. Several studies have found that the religiously committed adult enjoys a greater sense of overall life satisfaction and lower rates of depression than the nonreligious adult.[29,31,54,55,65] Even when the religiously committed person experiences levels of stress similar to those with less religious commitment, the more religious person experiences fewer adverse psychiatric consequences of stress, because his or her religious beliefs facilitate adjustment to stress and thus limit adverse clinical consequences.[52,74]

Preventing Heart Disease and High Blood Pressure

The beneficial effects of religion appear to serve as an important role in physical and psychologic stability. For example, religious commitment seems to have a potentially beneficial effect on heart disease and high blood pressure. Comstock and Partridge found that church-attending men and women had a decreased risk of arteriosclerotic disease as compared with non–church-attending individuals.[14] Among the female subjects, infrequent church attendees had approximately twice the risk of dying from heart disease as those who frequently attended church. Men who attended church at least weekly were also found to have much lower mortality rates from arteriosclerosis. Even after controlling for the effects of socioeconomic status and smoking, men who attended church regularly had nearly half the risk of dying from heart disease as compared with infrequent attendees.

In addition, a systematic review of 3 decades of research on the relationship between religious commitment and hypertension found that in nearly 90% of the reviewed studies, religious commitment was associated with low blood pressure. In addition, several religious groups had relatively low rates of hypertension-related morbidity and mortality.[51] These findings led the authors to conclude that, "Hypertension is a serious medical problem, which appears to be mitigated by religion."

These review findings were replicated and extended in a study that explored the relationship between religion and hypertension by comparing the blood pressure rates of church-attending smokers and nonsmokers with the blood pressure rates of non–church-attending smokers and nonsmokers.[42] Overall, those who rated religion as important and who frequently attended church had mean diastolic pressures almost 5 mm lower than those who found religion to be of little importance and who attended church infrequently—a finding that remained significant even after adjusting for other high blood pressure risk factors (e.g., age, socioeconomic status, weight). Most intriguingly, smokers who rated religion as being important to them were more than seven times less likely to have an abnormal diastolic pressure than smokers who gave a low rating for the personal importance of religion. Smokers who attended church at least once a week were four times less likely to have an abnormal diastolic pressure than smokers who seldom or never attended church. The finding that smokers enjoy a reduced risk of hypertension when they are committed in their religious faith runs contrary to the frequent assumption that religion may be clinically beneficial only because the religious are already avoiding unhealthy behaviors. Although the religiously committed population frequently avoids risk behaviors such as smoking, these findings for smokers suggest that the health benefits of religion may extend beyond the avoidance of health risk behaviors.

Preventing Substance Abuse

Research findings suggest that the presence of religion in an individual's life is linked with a decreased risk of drug abuse. In a review nearly 20 years old, Gorsuch and Butler first commented on the negative relationship between religious commitment and drug abuse, saying[24]:

> Whenever religion is used in an analysis, it predicts those who have not used an illicit drug, regardless of whether the religious variable is defined in terms of membership, active participation, religious upbringing, or meaningfulness of religion as viewed by the person.

Religion has been identified as a potential deterrent to self-destructive behaviors, such as drug and alcohol abuse. Indeed, those who abuse drugs have been found to have lower rates of religious practices and involvement than their nonabusing counterparts. Cancellaro and others observed that narcotic addicts were more than twice as unlikely to read their Bible as those in the control group in whose lives religion played a role.

The addicts were three times less likely to pray at meals and were more than five times less likely to talk to others about their religious beliefs.[10] In addition, whereas nearly 90% of addicts reported a reduction in their interest in religion during their adolescent years, only 20% of those in the control group reported a similar change during the same life stage.

Even when employing varying measures of religion, religious commitment is consistently associated with reduced drug abuse, as substantiated by more recent reviews.[23] Similarly, a national survey of 12,000 adolescents documented that the lowest rates of adolescent drug abuse were found among the more theologically conservative religious groups, and even the more theologically liberal groups still had slightly lower rates of drug abuse than those in the nonreligious group.[53] In addition, the researchers found that of all the various single-item measures of religious commitment used, the "importance of religion" was the best predictor of a lack of substance abuse. Thus these findings indicate that the lack of drug abuse by the religious can be attributable more to deeply internalized norms and values, rather than to the fear of drug use or peer pressure not to use drugs.

Just as religious commitment seems to be negatively correlated with drug abuse, similar results are found when examining the relationship between religious commitment and alcohol abuse. Paralleling the findings in the drug abuse literature, Koenig and others found that after controlling for predictive factors (e.g., age, sex, race, socioeconomic status, health status), religious practices including regular prayer, Bible study, and church attendance were inversely related to the risk of developing alcoholism.[40] These findings supported earlier work by Larson and Wilson, which revealed that those who abused alcohol rarely had a strong religious commitment.[44] Almost identical to the study by Cancellaro and associates on the religious lives of narcotic addicts, this study noted that nearly 90% of the chronic alcoholics surveyed had lost interest in religion during their teenage years, whereas among community control groups, only 20% had lost interest in religion during the same age period.[12] Further research has established a significant relationship between religious commitment and the nonuse or moderate use of alcohol. Most interestingly, whether or not a religion specifically proscribed, preached, or warned against alcohol use, those who were actively practicing in a religious congregation consumed substantially less alcohol than those who were not active.[1]

Preventing Suicide

Perhaps as a footnote to the association to substance abuse, religious commitment has been identified as enhancing well-being and limiting and handling stress. Religious commitment has been found to play an important role in the potential lowering of suicide rates. A recent systematic review of the relationship between religious commitment and the rate of suicide has found a negative relationship—that is, a lower suicide rate—between religious commitment and suicide in nearly every published study located.[23] Those who did not attend church have been found to be four times more likely to commit suicide than frequent church attendees, and the lack of church attendance has been identified as more accurately predicting higher suicide rates than any other factor including unemployment.[14,73] Ellis and Smith have found that spiritual well being is associated not only with moral objections to suicide but also with more reasons to live—an important deterrent to suicide.[19]

Enhancing Longevity

Although research has indicated that those with religious commitment enjoy better physical and mental health than those without commitment, do these health benefits translate into a longer life? Longevity is understandably one of the most revealing of all clinical outcomes and makes a striking case for the preventative and beneficial roles of religion in health. Gartner and others systematically reviewed the longevity research and found that in nearly every published study that included a religious variable, more religious individuals were found to live longer than nonreligious individuals.[23] For example, a 2-year longitudinal study of an older population living outside New Haven, Connecticut, assessed the relationship between religious commitment and life span.[81] Factors such as age, marital status, education, income, race, sex, health, and previous hospitalizations were all controlled. In addition, the researchers assessed (1) the frequency of attendance at religious services, (2) the level of personal religious commitment, and (3) the importance of religion as a source of strength. After the 2-year follow-up period, the less religious individuals were found to have mortality levels twice as high as the more religious group.

In an attempt to identify which social factors effectively reduced mortality rates, House and others conducted an even more extensive longitudinal study of 2700 people from the Tecumseh Community Health Study.[32] After controlling for appropriate mortality risk factors, only increased church attendance was found to decrease effectively the mortality level for women.

As previously discussed, Comstock and Partridge's landmark study on cardiovascular disease found that both men and women from Washington County, Maryland, who were religiously committed had a much lower rate of death from heart disease.[14] In addition, the researchers found that those with religious commitment were more protected from dying from a number of other diseases than those with a lower religious commitment. For example, death rates from pulmonary emphysema and suicide were more than twice as high for infrequent church attendees than for regular attendees, and death from cirrhosis of the liver was nearly four times as common among infrequent attendees when compared with regular attendees. These findings led the researchers to comment that, "Even if the mechanism of association of church attendance with disease is not discovered, this attribute, like that of smoking, could still prove useful in identifying groups at increased risk of suffering from a number of important diseases."

> **Points to Ponder** Certain religious groups have lower rates of cancer due to diet, lifestyle, and probably level of religious commitment; this protective effect appears to generalize to entire communities, affecting even those not of the same faith.[16]

■ Spiritual Intervention

Research in spiritual intervention for health has been addressed in two basic areas—prayer and shamanism. These two areas are addressed separately, but in many ways they share the general field of "transpersonal psychology."

Prayer

One of the earliest attempts in this century to study prayer scientifically was the Prayer Experiment begun at the University of Redlands in Redlands, California, in September 1951 (Figure 17-2). This experiment was popularized in a widely read book, *Prayer Can Change Your Life*, by Dr. William R. Parker and Elaine St. Johns.[63] The test group included 45 volunteers, aged 22 to 60 years of age. One third of the volunteers were university students and two thirds were homemakers, teachers, business persons, and others from the surrounding community. The volunteers brought a variety of problems to the study. These

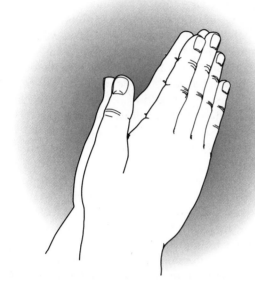

■ **Figure 17-2.** Prayer has been used in efforts to heal those in critical care, resolve emotional problems, and improve health in patients with chronic diseases, such as rheumatoid arthritis.

included depression and feeling "inactive and worn out" or "extinguished." Some had "exaggerated fears, lengthened shadows of the worry and depression that dog us all from time to time." Others belonged to the 50% to 75% "[majority] who seek medical treatment when there is nothing organically wrong."

The subjects were divided into three groups of 15 each. Group I was the "just-plain-psychology" group. No mention of religion was made during their therapy. Each person in this group professed a preference for this type of treatment or had been recommended for psychotherapy by their physicians.

Group II was the "just-plain-prayer" group. The subjects in this group prayed for themselves every night before retiring during the 9 months of the experiment. They were faithful, practicing Christians who expressed immense confidence in prayer and who believed psychologic counseling was unnecessary. They believed they knew how to pray, and no further techniques in prayer were offered. The object of their prayers was to eradicate the problems at hand, whether emotional or physical.

Group III was the "prayer-therapy" group. The subjects in this group met weekly for a 2-hour prayer session.

The three groups had no contact or communication with one another. They were given several psychologic tests before and after the experi-

ment. A skilled psychometrist with a degree in psychology, who was not directly involved in the experiment, administered all the tests. The tests included the Rorschach or "ink blot" test, which is designed to reveal something of the inner dynamics of the personality; the Szondi test, which offers further insight into certain personality syndromes; the Thematic Apperception test (TAT), which assesses a person's inner attitudes and feelings through free expression; and the Sentence Completion and Word Association tests, which assess the same.

The results of these tests were made available to the counselors in the psychotherapy group, who used them to guide patients through therapy. The "prayer-therapy" group (Group III) also used the test results. Each week each member received a sealed envelope containing a slip of paper on which was written a detrimental aspect of his or her personality that had been revealed on the tests. This allowed the person to focus on the negative trait and try to eliminate it by a specific prayer. As Group III continued to meet, the participants began to share the results of their tests and the barriers they encountered in dealing with them, as well as their successes. The psychologist and assistants who were conducting the overall experiment also knew the results of the tests.

After 9 months, an impartial psychologist administered the tests once again to all the subjects. Group I, the "just-plain-psychology" group, had a 65% improvement; group II, the "just-plain-prayer" group, had no improvement; group III, the "prayer-therapy" group, had a 72% improvement.

> **Points to Ponder**   Interventions for depression and anxiety disorder that integrate religion with psychotherapy induce recovery faster than secular techniques alone. ■

Prayer and Childhood Leukemia

Skeptics of prayer generally state that any proof that prayer is effective is only the result of poorly designed experiments and observations and is therefore an illusion. Skeptics believe that if the experiments are airtight, the effectiveness is eliminated. Since prayer violates the known laws governing physical reality, skeptics believe they know in advance that prayer cannot work.

A 1965 study, involving a prayer experiment performed on children with leukemia, is frequently cited by skeptics to prove these contentions.[13] A researcher randomly assigned 10 of 18 children with leukemia to be treated with prayer, administered by a church prayer group. All 18 children continued their routine medical treatments, but 10 of the 18 families were asked to pray at the church for the 10 children, and they received weekly reminders of their obligation to pray. Neither the children nor their treating physicians knew they were subjects of an experiment in prayer, nor did the praying families know that a controlled study was being conducted. The results of this study were inconclusive, with no significant differences between the two groups.

Prayer and Rheumatoid Arthritis

Another well-known study that attempted to assess the possible power of prayer in patients with rheumatoid arthritis was reported in 1965 from a London hospital. In this double-blind study, neither the patients nor the physicians knew for whom prayers were being said. Distant prayer groups offered prayers for 19 patients, whose course was compared with that of 19 control patients. Researchers matched the severity of the disease of the two groups, and medical therapy was continued as usual in both the control and experimental groups. The patients were carefully evaluated at the beginning of the study and again after 8 to 18 months. Only 6 of the 38 patients improved; 5 of these were in the prayer group. During the first half of the study, those in the prayer group improved more than those in the control group; in the last half of the study, the control group improved more than the prayer group. Although these results are encouraging for the positive effect of prayer, researchers found no statistical significance in this small study. Overall, this experiment contributes little to our scientific understanding of prayer.[37]

Prayer Involving Human Tissue

If our thoughts can affect "lower" biological systems, as reported in many of the studies that follow in this text, some researchers have suggested that living, human tissue might be more responsive to these effects. If so, what kind of human tissue would be most sensitive?

Nobel prize recipient neurophysiologist Sir John Eccles proposed that the human brain is exquisitely sensitive to thought. As he put it, the mind exerts continual "cognitive caresses" on the millions of neurons that make up the brain.[17] Does the brain's sensitivity to thought make it more likely to respond to not only our inner thoughts but to the mental efforts of other persons (i.e., healers) who may be at a distance?

Experimentally, it is difficult to use living brain tissue as a distant target for thought. We must obtain brain tissue surgically via biopsy, which involves risk. It is far easier to use other body tissues, such as various types of blood cells. Certain blood cells have a lot in common with brain tissue. For example, many white blood cells (WBCs) contain receptor sites for neurotransmitter molecules that are identical to those that exist in the brain. Similarly, WBCs manufacture some of the same neurotransmitters as those found in the brain. If mind "cognitively caresses" brain tissue, does it similarly affect blood cells that are functionally similar?

Dr. William G. Braud of the Mind Science Foundation in San Antonio, Texas, put this question to the test.[7] He wanted to know the answers to the following questions: (1) Can ordinary people mentally protect red blood cells (RBCs) from serious, stressful influences? (2) Can this protection be set from a distance? (3) Does this mentally protective effect work best on a subject's own RBCs, or does it equally protect the cells of others?

In Braud's experiment, 32 subjects—17 women and 15 men who were ranging in age from 23 to 53 years—mentally attempted to keep RBCs from dissolving when the samples were put in test tubes containing a dilute solution and then placed in a distant room. When put in a test tube, RBCs will gradually swell and burst, leaking their hemoglobin into the solution. This breakdown of cells, known as *hemolysis,* can be measured with extreme accuracy with a device known as a *spectrophotometer.*

Approximately half of Braud's subjects were instructed to try to protect their own blood cells mentally, and the other half were assigned to protect the blood cells of another person. It is important to note that the subjects were "blind"; that is, they did not know whether the blood came from their own or from someone else's body. During each session the subjects were placed in a quiet, comfortable room in one part of the building, and the tubes of blood were placed in a distant room in the same building. A session consisted of two control or rest periods of 15 minutes each and two 15-minute "protect" periods. As an aid to visualization and intention, the subjects looked at a color slide of healthy, intact RBCs. During the control periods, the subjects closed their eyes and thought about matters not connected with the experiment. The technician performing the hemolysis measurements on the RBCs in the distant room was also "blind"—ignorant as to whether the blood originated from the subject or someone else, and ignorant as to whether a control or a "protect" session was in progress.

Braud reached two important conclusions. First, the subjects could influence the rate of hemolysis of the distant RBCs to a degree unexplainable by chance. Second, the source of the blood was not significant in the group as a whole. However, when individual performances were examined, the five most skillful subjects in the entire experiment were those trying to influence their own blood.

Prayer in Critical Care

Cardiologist Randolph Byrd, a practicing Christian, designed his study as a scientific evaluation of the role of God in healing.[9] "After much prayer," he states, "the idea of what to do came to me." Over a 10-month period, a computer assigned 393 patients admitted to the coronary care unit at San Francisco General Hospital to either a group for whom home prayer groups offered prayers (192 patients) or to a group that was not remembered in prayer (201 patients). The study was designed according to rigid criteria, the kind usually used in clinical studies in medicine. It was a randomized, double-blind experiment in which the patients, nurses, and physicians did not know to which group the patients were assigned. Byrd recruited various religious groups to pray for members of the prayed-for group. The prayer groups were given the first names of their patients and a brief description of their diagnosis and condition. They were asked to pray each day, but they were given no instructions on how to pray. "Each person prayed for many different patients, but each patient in the experiment had between five and seven people praying for him or her," Byrd explained.

The prayed-for patients differed in several areas:

1. They were five times less likely than the not-prayed-for group to require antibiotics (3 patients compared with 16 patients).
2. They were three times less likely to develop pulmonary edema, a condition in which the lungs fill with fluid because of the failure of the heart to pump properly (6 patients compared with 18 patients).
3. None of the prayed-for group required endotracheal intubation, a procedure in which an artificial airway is inserted in the throat and attached to a mechanical ventilator. In the non-prayed-for group, 12 patients required mechanical ventilatory support.
4. Fewer patients in the prayed-for group died, although this difference was not statistically significant.

Sicher, Targ, Moore, and Smith conducted a controlled, randomized trial with 40 volunteer patients with advanced acquired immunodeficiency syndrome (AIDS).[71] Individuals from distant parts of the country with no contact and only a patient's name and photograph prayed for a patient. Those offering prayers were from a variety of spiritual practices (e.g., Christian, Jewish, Buddhist, Native American, and Shamanic), and they focused their attentions on their respective patients 6 days a week for 10 weeks. The patients were rotated from one practitioner to another each week. The "healing" group experienced fewer and less severe illnesses, fewer doctor visits, fewer hospitalizations, and improved moods as compared with those in the control group.

Case study: Sister Gertrude

Sister Gertrude of the Sisters of Charity in New Orleans was admitted as a patient to the Hotel-Dieu Hospital on December 27, 1934. She was jaundice and suffered from severe pain, nausea, chills, and a high fever. A preoperative diagnosis of cancer of the pancreas was made, and an exploratory laparotomy (incision into the loin) was performed on January 5, 1935. The head of the pancreas was found to be three times its normal size. Her condition appeared to be inoperable, and the prognosis was hopeless. Three pathologists diagnosed carcinoma (cancerous tumor) of the pancreas.

The sisters of the order interceded with Mother Seton, deceased founder of the order, in a series of novenas to spare the life of Sister Gertrude so that she might continue in service. Sister Gertrude began to improve and made a rapid recovery. She was discharged on February 1, and she returned to her duties on March 1, 1935.

After $7\frac{1}{2}$ years of continuous disease-free duty, Sister Gertrude suddenly died of a massive pulmonary embolism. The autopsy revealed no evidence of cancer of the pancreas.[61]

Effects of Spiritual Intervention on Human Beings

In another study performed at the Mind Science Foundation in San Antonio, Texas, researches William G. Braud and Marilyn Schlitz studied the ability of 62 people to influence the physiologic condition of 271 subjects.[8] The subjects were isolated from the influencers in distant rooms in the same building. Participants (influencers) ranged from 16 to 65 years of age and were selected from a pool of volunteers from the San Antonio community. They had learned about the experiments through local newspaper advertisements and articles, notices, lectures given by the foundation staff, and comments by other participants. An approximate equal number of men and women were involved.

Thirteen experiments were performed. The subjects were not selected on the basis of any special physical, physiologic, or psychologic characteristics; their interest in the research was the only criterion. In only one experiment were "special" subjects recruited—those in need of a "calming" influence on their physical condition. In other words, these subjects had evidence of greater-than-usual sympathetic autonomic activation as evidenced by stress-related complaints, excessive emotionality, excessive activity, tension headaches, high blood pressure, ulcers, or mental or physical hyperactivity. Before the experiment, these "special" subjects were screened by tests that confirmed they did indeed exhibit higher-than-average levels of arousal of the sympathetic nervous system.

The subjects, whose physical condition the influencers were attempting to change, were attached to instruments that measured their electrodermal activity—the ability of the skin to conduct an electrical current, which is an indicator of activity of the sympathetic part of the autonomic nervous system. At a given signal, the influencer would try to exert a calming or activating influence on the distant subject, who would be unaware when the attempt would be made. In each session, the influencer made 20 30-second attempts. During these "influence periods," the influencer used mental imagery and self-regulation techniques to induce the intended condition—either relaxation or activation, as demanded by the experimental protocol—in himself or herself and in the distant subject. The influencer would then imagine the desired outcomes of the polygraph pen tracings—a few small pen deflections for calming periods and many large pen deflections for activation periods.

The intentions seemed to "get through" to the subjects. The effect proved to be consistent, replicable, and robust. "Under certain conditions," the researchers noted, "the transpersonal imagery effect can compare favorably with an imagery effect upon one's own physiological activity."

Case study: Vittorio Micheli

Vittorio Micheli was inducted into the Italian Army in 1961 as physically fit. In April 1962, he reported to the Verona Military Hospital complaining of pains in the region of the left hip and haunch. Extensive examination and biopsies concluded a diagnosis of sarcoma (fleshy tumor) of the left pelvis.

By June the condition had worsened and, according to army records, the x-ray films showed "almost complete destruction of the left pelvis." Micheli was placed into a hip-to-toe cast. In August the army medical service concluded the case was not treatable by radiation. After 2 months of chemotherapy, no improvement was found and treatment was discontinued. In November, x-ray studies revealed a dislocation of the femoral head, and by January 1963 the femur had lost connection with the pelvis.

The following May, Micheli decided to go to Lourdes. Arriving at Lourdes still wearing his cast and suffering great pain, he plunged into the baths. Immediately the pain subsided and he had the feeling that his femur reattached itself to the pelvis. He felt well.

Returning to the hospital, the radiographic reports showed that the sarcoma was gone. He found a job in a factory, standing for 8 to 10 hours a day. The articulation (i.e., the union between two or more bones) was "normal" according to bureau records.

The medical bureau watched the case for 5 years, and in 1969 voted 12 to 0 that Micheli's case was inexplicable; it was declared a miracle. The records were sent to a large number of orthopedic surgeons and all replied that they had never encountered a case of a reconstruction of bone after a tumor of the bone.[61]

Effects of Spiritual Intervention on Fungi, Yeast, and Bacteria

A number of studies have researched the effects of healing on fungi, yeast, or bacteria. The following are some of the results.

■ Ten subjects tried to inhibit the growth of fungus cultures in the laboratory through conscious intent by concentrating on them for 15 minutes from a distance of approximately 1.5 yards. The cultures were then incubated for several more hours. Out of the 194 culture dishes, 151 showed retarded growth.[5]

- In a replication of the previous study, one group of subjects demonstrated the same effect (inhibiting the growth of fungus) in 16 out of 16 trials, while stationed from 1 to 15 miles away from the fungus cultures.[75]

- In another study, 60 subjects, not known to have healing abilities, were able to both impede and stimulate the growth of cultures of bacteria significantly.[57]

- In a similar experiment, two healers held a bottle of water in their hands for 30 minutes. Samples of the water were then added to solutions of yeast cells in test tubes. After incubation, the amount of carbon dioxide given off by the yeast cultures was measured, indicating the level of metabolic activity. Statistically significant increases in carbon dioxide production were observed by the yeast cultures given the "treated" water in four out of five tests.[25]

- Sixty university volunteers with no known healing abilities were asked to alter the genetic ability of a strain of the bacteria, *Escherichia coli,* which normally mutates from the inability to metabolize the sugar lactose (i.e., lactose negative) to the ability to use it (i.e., lactose positive) at a known rate. The subjects tried to influence six test tubes of bacterial cultures—three for increased mutation from lactose negative to lactose positive and three for decreased mutation of lactose negative to lactose positive. Three tubes were uninfluenced and served as controls. Results indicated that the bacteria mutated in the directions desired by the subjects.[58]

These experiments have implications for health and illness. Among them are the following:

1. There may be times when it would be helpful to inhibit the growth of pathogenic microorganisms, as in the case of infections. On the other hand, our bodies contain helpful, symbiotic microorganisms whose growth may need to be increased on certain occasions, such as after treatment with antibiotics, which kill "good" in addition to pathogenic bacteria. The ability to inhibit or increase the growth of bacterial or yeast populations could be a valuable health resource.

2. If genetic mutations can be influenced by the conscious efforts of others, as implied in one of the previous studies, then genes do not absolutely control our bodies. Biology therefore is not destiny.

   For most people, "mutation" has negative connotations, such as a normal gene mutating to a cancerous gene. Recent evidence shows the reverse can happen—abnormal genes can mutate to normal ones. This phenomenon, called "reverse mutation," has been discovered to occur in myotonic dystrophy, a disease that causes severe muscle weakness and strikes 1 in 80,000 people. Scientists do not know what causes "good" mutations. Is the mind involved? The previous research evidence suggests that we should not rule out the possibility.

3. Many believers in spiritual healing claim that for healing to occur, subjects must actively want it. These research studies suggest otherwise. We can assume that the microorganisms did not know they were subjects in an experiment. The observed effects do not depend on what the subject "thinks."

4. These experiments support the universal claim of healers that spiritual healing operates as powerfully at a distance as it does nearby.

5. Based on these studies, ordinary people have the ability to bring about biological changes in other living organisms. These outcomes suggest that everyone may possess innate healing abilities, at least to some degree.

6. Negative effects (inhibition of growth) and positive effects (promotion of growth) were observed in the previous experiments. These outcomes raise the possibility of the dark side to healing.

7. Although skeptics often criticize spiritual healing as simply a result of suggestion or an example of the placebo response, these experiments show that these explanations are not true, unless skeptics wish to attribute a high degree of consciousness to bacteria and yeast. These results suggest that the effects of spiritual healing can be completely independent of the psychology.

Effects of Spiritual Intervention on Cells

Cancer cells normally stick to the surface of the container in which they are cultured. Changes in their metabolism, injury, or death cause them to detach and slough off into the surrounding medium. Researchers can count the number of cells in the medium and thus judge the overall state of health of the cell culture.

British psychic Matthew Manning held his hands near flasks containing cancer cells and attempted to inhibit their growth. He was able to produce changes of 200% to 1200% in their growth characteristics when he was placed in a distant room that was shielded from electrical influences.[6]

Effects of Spiritual Intervention on the Movement of Simple Organisms

Several experiments have examined the ability of subjects to affect the movement of simple organisms. Intentionally, the motility and speed of motion of one-celled algae and paramecia and the movement characteristics of moth larvae have been significantly affected in a variety of experiments.[68]

Effects of Spiritual Intervention on Plants

In a well-known series of experiments, Dr. Bernard Grad of McGill University studied the healer, Oskar Estebany, who claimed he could transmit his healing through paper, water, and other materials. Grad damaged barley seeds by watering them with a 1% saline solution, which retards their normal growth rate. He found that the damaging effect of the saline could be inhibited when Estebany held the container of saline for 15 minutes.[27]

Healing Effects of Spiritual Intervention on Animals

Many studies have been performed to determine the effects of healing methods on animals. Some of the results are detailed in the following text:

- In an often-quoted classic study, Grad studied Estebany's ability to heal artificially created surgical wounds in 48 mice, compared with a control group who were wounded identically (the wounds were created by removing a $1/2$-inch $\times$ 1-inch piece of skin from their backs after anesthetizing them). Estebany held the cages of the experimental group 15 minutes twice daily for 14 days. This group healed significantly faster than the wounded mice whose cages were not held. This careful study once again tells us that healing works, and that the outcome is not only the result of suggestion.[26]

- In another experiment, Grad produced goiters in mice by giving them thiouracil, a goiter-producing drug, and a diet devoid of iodine. Estebany held the cages of one group of rats for 15 minutes twice daily, which seemed to protect the thyroid glands from enlarging. Compared with the rats in the control group, the glands of the treatment group grew significantly slower.[26,27]

- In a subsequent experiment, Grad tested Estebany's claim that secondary materials could transmit healing effects. In an experiment similar to the previous study, Estebany held some wool or cotton in his hands, which was then placed in the rats' cages for 1 hour every morning and evening for 6 days. The thyroid glands of the rats receiving this treatment grew significantly more slowly than the glands of the control rats. When the rats were returned to an iodine-containing diet, their thyroid glands returned to normal size more quickly than the glands of the control rats.

- In 21 experiments conducted over a period of several years, healers tried to awaken mice more quickly from general anesthesia. These experiments were increasingly refined. In one variation, only the image of the experimental mouse was projected on a television monitor in a distant room and then shown to the healer, who tried to intervene via the image. Out of the 21 studies, the "treated" mice in 19 studies showed significantly earlier recovery from anesthesia. The experimenters were able to identify a peculiar "lingering effect" in this series of studies. They found that when one side of a table was used by the healers, after the healers were dismissed and more anesthetized rats were placed immediately on the healer side of the table, the latter group of rats also recovered faster than the control rats placed on the table's other side.[78]

- In another experiment, a group of mice were injected with either a strain of malaria organisms or with sterile saline. The handlers of the mice were told that the injection contained either a high or low dose of microorganisms when, in fact, there were no high or low doses—the malaria injections were identical. The handlers were also told that a healer would try to heal some of the rats but not all, but no healer was employed. In one phase of the experiment, the results tended in the direction of the expectations of the handlers—the rats believed to have had low-dose injections did better. In addition, the mice coded for healing did better than those not designated to be healed, even though the information designating which groups were to be healed was unknown to the handlers. There should have been no differences between the high-dose and low-dose groups, since there was no difference in the strength of the injections. In addition, there should have been no difference between the healed and nonhealed groups, since there was no healer.[72]

This experiment raises profound questions about whether the double-blind experimental design used in medical research is as foolproof as believed. In double-blind situations, neither the experimenters nor the subjects know who is and is not receiving the treatment being studied (e.g., a new drug). Since the subjects do not know whether they are receiving the drug or placebo, they will not be as susceptible to the effects of suggestion. Since the experimenters are unaware of which subjects received the drug and which did not, they will be less prone to bias when assessing any effects they observe in the subjects. It is assumed that these precautions eliminate the effects of expectation and suggestion in both the researchers and subjects. In the previous study with malarial mice, however, the double-blind precautions were not sufficient. The outcome of the experiment mirrored the beliefs and expectations of the laboratory workers.

Similar findings have been observed in double-blind studies involving humans. Double-blind studies can, at times, be steered in directions that correspond to the thoughts and attitudes of the experimenters. This may shed light on why skeptical experimenters appear unable to replicate the findings of believers and why "true believers" seem more able to produce positive results. The validity of decades of experimental findings in medical research would need to be reevaluated, if it is found that the mind can "shove the data around."

> **Points to Ponder**   Frequent church attendance predicts lower levels of physical disability among older persons at one, two, and three years of follow-up.[34]
> ■

■ Shamanism and Spiritual Journeys

The term *shamanism* has been used to define a wide variety of practices and community roles. A similar term is that of "medicine man," an indigenous healer who uses various techniques to treat diseases. Medical anthropologists have studied many of these individuals, and unique talents and skills have been attributed to them. Some shamans use natural herbs from plants and earth substances for healing, and there is wide use of touching and massaging techniques. Singing and dancing rituals are very common.

The most academic definition of a shaman's discipline comes from Michael Harner's *The Way of a Shaman,* in which he examines how the shaman uses his or her skills to go to the spiritual realm to derive specific healing knowledge for an individual. Because of this spiritual perspective, shamanism rightfully belongs in a discussion of spiritual medicine. In the perspective of shamanic literature, "spiritual" refers to an extraordinary realm of consciousness and holds truth according to the parameters of the extraordinary realities. By this definition, Jesus Christ would be considered a shaman, since he apparently understood life and healed from an extraordinary frame of reference. This classification would be considered heresy in orthodox Christianity because of the imposition of Him into a pagan cult. Nevertheless, shamanism, as applied for this discussion, is defined in spiritual terms.

Even under the restriction of this definition, several unique shamanic approaches are used for healing. Some individuals travel to the spiritual realities under the influence of acoustical stimulation (e.g., drums, chanting, singing), some use psychotropic drugs (e.g., Ayayaska, muskin, mushrooms), some use pain induction and fasting, and some use a personal ritual involving breathing patterns and psychologic trance induction. Some Arabic cultures use the patterns on rugs in induce reality shifts (magic carpets?), and some use long journeys into the wilderness.

There is also variance as to the missions of the journeys. Many use the journeys to retrieve parts of the soul that escaped the body because of abuse or fear. Once an escaped part is replaced, healing can occur. Others focus on finding power sources or wisdom from which the right medicine for the ill person can be found. Other shamans seek protection from an evil force that may have caused the illness and they seek the power to neutralize it. These practices are common with voodooism and sorcerous spirituality. These attributions of illness may sound strange to us now, but they have been a component of Western medical historical beliefs. It was once believed that demons were responsible for community problems, and the reader is reminded of the Salem trials, during which thousands of "witches" were burned for their roles in bringing illness to their communities.

■ Shamanism and Transpersonal Medicine

In spite of the fact that modern scientific philosophy ridicules shamanistic concepts of medical care, the majority of people in the world still have belief in it, and it remains a primary source of health care. Whether it is the *culendaros* in the Mexican culture or the *singer* in Navaho tradition, these methods of healing seem to be embedded in the consciousness for healing or disease-provoking process. Several case studies are available that appear to document the healing skills of the shamans, even though the outcomes defy scientific understanding.[34] No studies of a scientific nature offers data on any disease other than preclinical findings; however, there is impressive documentation of individual experiences of shamanic healing skills.

Aspects of shamanic healing can be readily understood with the use of the term *transpersonal medicine,* a designation coined by Frank Lawlis to denote the influence of consciousness on the body from forces beyond sensorial stimulation or logical thought.[45] The term marries the prefix *trans,* which means *across, beyond,* or *through* and *personal,* which means *self* or *ego.* Since *medicine* refers to *healing,* transpersonal medicine is defined as healing from sources beyond or across the logical sources of ourselves, perhaps spiritual or magical sources.

Transpersonal medicine includes sources of healing that emerge from one's innermost unconsciousness; these sources may emerge from a genetic memory or instinctual image of survival as a symbol that the person understands. For example, the individual, dreaming of a bear, may interpret this symbol to mean a time of hibernation or quiet rejuvenation. Carl Jung wrote about such archetypes of healing that cross cultural boundaries.

Another feature of transpersonal influence may be the effect of another person's consciousness. The power of one individual's brain waves to influence another person, whether through persuasion or some other transpersonal force, is a well-documented phenomenon. Perhaps this is the feature of parapsychology related to the prayer studies. The field of transpersonal medicine is still in its scientific infancy. Nevertheless, belief in spiritual and magical powers of healing is not deterred.

■ Rituals

As in transpersonal medicine, ritual takes that which is experienced in the invisible, imagistic world of visions and feeling and reenacts it in the outer, visible world. Ritual enables people to transcend their self-imposed boundaries, connecting with the power of hope and the consciousness of sacred space. However, from a scientific perspective, what is known of ritual that supports the belief that it (ritual) can cause alteration of mental or physical conditions? Briefly, we discuss four areas of research that address the beneficial possibilities of ritual. From these studies, we can safely conclude that ritual reduces alienation, anxiety, and depression. In addition, the studies support

the concept that rituals help activate transformative realities for necessary change and engage the power of transpersonal influence through what may be termed "energy effects" from others.

Rituals Increase the Sense of Connectiveness

A recent article in *Science* cited 62 studies that reveal strong supportive documentation that the "lack of social support constitutes a major risk factor for mortality" and that social relationships protect health and enhance healing. Social support was defined in a variety of ways, including marital relationships, friendships, general family relationships, group memberships, and relationships with health care professionals. These social support networks were observed to have consistent positive effects on such variables as surgical recovery time, likelihood of birth complications, birth weight, and resistance to infectious diseases (e.g., tuberculosis, cardiovascular reactivity, ulcers, general stress responses). Documented biochemical changes included increased growth hormones, lower cholesterol levels, enhanced WBC activity, and reduced sympathetic nervous activity.

A study involving patients with chronic and intractable back pain was conducted in a clinic in northern Texas in which variables were measured before and during a 3-week inpatient hospital stay. Included in the variables was a set of measurable factors from the "Four Relationship Factor Questionnaire." These factors illustrated the power of the bond between the patients and the therapy group in which they participated during their hospital stay.[47] The factors measured were respect for the group's problem-solving abilities, identification with each other's problems, and ability to give affection when needed. Regardless of type of physical diagnosis, psychologic profile, or treatment, the strength of the bond with the group was consistently the variable most connected with whether the pain was reduced or remained the same.

These studies support one aspect of the power of ritual—social connectedness or universality. Ritual, as a formal process, provides at least a provision for the individual to receive the healing aspects of relationship in ways that have been experienced for generations. Thus ritual may influence the deep spheres of consciousness beyond the realms of our immediate memory and empower the body-mind spirit to harmony.

Rituals Encourage Hope

Inherent in reduced alienation is also a reduced sense of hopelessness. A broad array of research has demonstrated the correlated influence of hopelessness on a variety of psychologic and physical dysfunctions, including cancer growth and gastrointestinal conditions. Prolonged stress has long been thought to impede healing through the sustained arousal of biochemical factors (e.g., certain hormones), setting the stage for the diagnoses of cardiovascular and immunity deficient diseases that are the result of a compromised resistance to invasion. More important for chronic conditions, stress has been listed as a probable agent in the decrease of damaged cell recovery through a mechanism of the deoxyribonucleic acid (DNA) repair process. The argument that stress has a negative influence on both psychologic and physical processes has been articulated and incorporated into the general context of health care.

Conversely, the role of stress reduction in health care is more indirect in terms of evidence. We can extrapolate from the biochemistry of stress the assumption that the reduction of stress enhances health, at least to the point of negating the destruction created by anxiety and depression. If ritual can help create self-esteem and relaxation, it follows that the corticosteroids and vasoconstriction related to both catecholamines and muscular tension will decrease. As stress is reduced, the hyperactive hormones and body tension is restored to balance. Because biofeedback treatment focuses on the patient's ability to relax the body and mind, many diseases and symptoms (e.g., hypertension and tension headaches) resolve themselves through training. These methods are considered treatments of choice for many stress-induced disorders because these treatments teach the patient to control his or her symptoms.

One of the pioneering studies in this field, conducted by Peavey, Lawlis, and Govern, tested the hypothesis of enhanced health through a stress-management process.[64] The study divided a group of college students into high- and low-stressed subgroups and evaluated their respective immunity factors, principally the neutrophils' response. (Neutrophils are WBCs that constantly patrol our bloodstream for toxins and other "enemies.") As expected, the results (later replicated in several studies) revealed that the high-stressed participants were significantly more impaired in terms of immunity factors than the low-stressed group. The next step for these highly stressed subjects was participation in a stress management program. An evaluation after the stress management program revealed that the high-stress participants' immune responses had changed to approximate that of the low-stress participants.

In an article published in the *Clinical Psychology Review*, which evaluated the implications of stress management specifically for postsurgical issues, 168 references were cited.[69] The conclusion of the article was that the most fruitful approach was to target the ritualistic features of the hospital ward for positive attribution in surgical procedures. More specifically, it suggested social support and opportunities for active coping for direct enhancement of physiologic features.

Lawlis, Selby, Hinnant, and McCoy conducted a well-controlled retrospective study in which specific ritual-related features (e.g., anxiety-reduction skills, consciousness-altering techniques, and family support instructions) were administered to patients undergoing back surgery.[46] The results were indicative of improved healing processes by significantly shorter hospital stays and fewer pain indicators and complications. The most consistent finding was that psychologic approaches, regardless of orientation, help patients increase hopefulness and reduce anxiety or depression.

> **Points to Ponder**   A large segment of the American population (as high as 20% to 40%) revealed that religion is one of the most important factors that enable them to cope with stressful life circumstances.[41]

■ Contraindications and Indications

For some valid reasons, the medical community has viewed religious and spiritual practices with suspicion. Most relevant among the concerns is not whether they "work"; rather, the time invested in spiritual practices do not allow for other efforts to be in effect at the same time. For example, time can be critical in the treatment of some diseases such as infections and cancers, especially childhood cancers. By not providing immediate care to the child, he or she is placed in danger of rapid deterioration of body defenses and exploitation of disease.

Another critical issue is that many of the protocols of some spiritual practices are dangerous. For example, one approach to the childbirthing care in Africa is to instruct the mother to begin "pushing" immediately into the first phase. The shaman consider this practice important. However, by doing so, the mother is usually exhausted by the time of birth and the frequency of epilepsy in these villages is extremely high.

An overzealous dependency on religious faith may interfere with the important decision making required during the treatment of a catastrophic illness. Important judgments and plans have to be made as they relate to the management of life situations and care. In addition, money may be spent on irresponsible schemes and "gurus" who make life-extending claims on the basis of false hope.

An Expert Speaks: Larry Dossey, MD

Dr. Larry Dossey is a physician of internal medicine. Dossey is past president of The Isthmus Institute of Dallas, an organization dedicated to exploring the possible convergence of science and religious thought. He lectures widely in the United States and abroad, and in 1988 he delivered the annual Mahatma Gandhi Memorial Lecture in New Delhi, India—the only physician ever invited to do so. Dr. Dossey has published numerous articles and is the author of seven books, including: *Space, Time, & Medicine* (1982), *Beyond Illness* (1984), *Recovering the Soul: A Scientific and Spiritual Search* (1989), *Meaning and Medicine* (1991), *Prayer is Good Medicine* (1996), and *Be Careful What You Pray For—You Just Might Get It* (1997).

Dr. Dossey is the former co-chair of the Panel on Mind/Body Interventions, Office of Alternative Medicine, National Institutes of Health. He is also the executive editor of the journal *Alternative Therapies in Health and Medicine*. In the following interview, he shares his thoughts on spirituality and prayer in healing.

Question. How did you get interested in the concept of spiritual medicine?

Answer. I was initially influenced by personal illness. Since childhood, I was afflicted with severe, classical migraine headaches—profound pain, incapacitation, and blindness. None of the conventional treatments worked. After medical school, I discovered biofeedback, which is a way of altering one's thoughts and emotional responses to quiet one's body. This was a godsend for the migraine, and it opened my awareness of the role of perceived meanings, including spirituality, in health.

I continued to pursue the role of the mind in health and wrote several books about this area. I began to pay special attention to the role of spiritual meanings in health in the mid-1980s, when I discovered actual scientific studies supporting the effects of distant intercessory prayer in healing. This clearly went beyond anything I'd encountered in mind-body medicine, whose basic tenet is that **your own** thoughts could affect **your** body. In intercessory prayer, my thoughts affect **someone else's** body—at a distance, even when they are unaware that I'm praying for them.

I have always been fascinated by the relationship of the mind and the brain, and this data clearly suggested that some aspect of human consciousness is not limited to the physical body.

The more I pursued this evidence, the more impressed I became. The database is huge—more than 150 studies, in both humans and animals—that one's thoughts can make a difference in others, at a distance. So, there really was no epiphany or single, dramatic event that captured my attention. Those two experiences—my own illness and the scientific evidence—did it for me.

Question. How do you see prayer and spirituality used in today's medicine?

Answer. First, there's no excuse not to use it. Why? The evidence is overwhelming that people who follow some spiritual practice or religion in their life—it really doesn't seem to matter which one—live longer and are healthier in the process. If something affects longevity and health, it is automatically the responsibility of medicine to pay attention to it.

There are two ways that spirituality helps—as a form of prevention and as an intervention when disease occurs. Studies are emerging that show that prayer has a role in helping people recover from serious illness. Two of the diseases that have been studied are cardiovascular illness, such as heart attack, and AIDS. Surgical wounds have also been shown to heal faster with prayer or prayerlike healing intentions. Side effects from cardiovascular tests, such as heart catheters, and recovery following coronary bypass surgery have responded to prayer in careful studies. Interestingly, it isn't just the recipient of prayer who benefits. One study showed that the person doing the praying improved as much as the individual receiving the prayer.

People often regard prayer and spiritual interventions as a last-ditch effort, something to be tacked on if conventional methods fail. I believe these methods should be used as the initial intervention, and if we used them in daily life, fewer people would need medical and surgical interventions in the first place.

Question. How do you see the field of spiritual medicine evolving in the future?

Answer. Health care workers and institutions are faced with a challenge. In view of the evidence favoring the role of prayer and spiritual interventions in healing, how can they be justified in ignoring them? How can they **not** offer these interventions to their patients? To avoid doing so is an ethical and moral issue. It would be like withholding a potent drug or surgical procedure from someone who may benefit from it.

How we go about practicing "spiritual medicine" remains to be seen. Hospitals may emphasize a greater role for clergy, chaplains, and pastoral counselors; or physicians and nurses may pray for or with their patients; or the names of patients, with their permission, may be farmed out to prayer groups around the nation and world, as is being done in some hospitals already. How these interventions actually unfold remains to be seen. We can be creative and imaginative as we go forward. As we do so, we must avoid following some sort of formula that could be applied equally and identically to all institutions everywhere. A cookie-cutter approach will never work in this field. Each community, each hospital, each region of the country is different. These interventions must grow organically, out of the hearts and souls of individuals. These [interventions] must embody religious tolerance, and they must honor the tremendous variety of religious expression that exists in the United States.

We are well on our way. Four years ago, three medical schools in the United States had courses exploring the role of religious devotion and prayer in healing; currently, 50 medical schools have such courses. In addition, a majority of medical schools offer courses in alternative medicine, many of which emphasize the spiritual side of healing. There is no going back, because of the growing data that underlie this field. So, at long last, spirituality is reentering medicine—to which most people would probably say, "It's about time."

One point should be emphasized. We're going to see an **integration** of physical and spiritual interventions in healing, not a replacement of one by the other. This, I feel, is as it should be.

One final point, as we go forward, let's not fall into the trap of using prayer and religion as if it were the latest antibiotic or surgical procedure. To use prayer only as a practical tool is to ignore its most majestic function, which, I believe, is to connect us with the Absolute, however conceived.

■ Chapter Review

Spiritual medicine is certainly not new to the field of healing. In fact, one may speculate that it is the oldest and most widely used medical approach in the world. Humans tend to continue to do what has been accepted in the past. Therefore wisdom predicts that religion will have a permanent role in medicine as we know it. Yet, fear and hostility continue to flare on both sides of the controversy (scientific and religious) concerning the power of spirituality to heal.

Today, the trend toward more scientific inquiry into spiritual influence is extremely relevant. Trust in drugs and surgery has reached an all time low, as suffering from chronic diseases (e.g., autoimmune diseases, asthma) reach epidemic proportions. The time is quickly approaching when medicine will have to reintegrate certain important factors related to spirituality. Hopefully, scientists and theologians alike will continue to seek the seeds of truth concerning the healing potentials of spirituality and religion.

■ Review Questions

1. What are some important features of religious practice that reflect on disease prevention?
2. What are the underlying dimensions contained in a religious discipline that would account for better health?
3. What evidence supports the possibility that spiritual intervention, such as prayer or ritual, affects a person's health?
4. What are at least two features of ritual that would influence health outcomes regardless of the nature of the individual's religious beliefs?
5. What basis is there for the belief that the spiritual practice of the health care provider could influence outcomes of a health intervention?

C RITICAL THINKING AND CLINICAL APPLICATION EXERCISES

1. This chapter has made some assumptions that spirituality influences health. Formulate your own arguments for whether spirituality can or cannot influence health.
2. Since religious and spiritual variables appear to affect health outcomes, should this factor be considered in determining insurance premiums for health insurance? Why or why not?
3. Speculate on the underlying reasons for the sharp debate that exists between some scientists and religious groups.

References

1. Amoateng AY, Bahr SJ: Religion, family, and adolescent drug use, *Sociol Perspect* 29:53, 1986.
2. Andreasen NJ: The role of religion in depression, *J Religion Health* 11:153, 1972.
3. Bearon LB, Koenig HG: Religious cognitions and use of prayer in health and illness, *Gerontologist* 30(2):249, 1990.
4. Bergin AE, Jensen JP: Religiosity of psychotherapists: a national survey, *Psychother* 27(1):3, 1990.
5. Berry J: General and comparative study of the psychokinetic effect on a fungus culture, *J Parapsychol* 32:237, 1968.
6. Braud WG, Davis G, Wood R: Experiments with Matthew Manning, *J Am Soc Psychical Res* 50(782):199, 1979.
7. Braud WG: Distant mental influence of rate of hemolysis of human red blood cells, *J Am Soc Psychical Res* 84(1):1, 1990.
8. Braud WG: Using living targets in psi research, *Parapsychol Rev* 20(6):1, 1989.
9. Byrd R: Positive therapeutic effects of intercessory prayer: a coronary care unit population, *South Med J* 81(7):826, 1988.
10. Cancellaro LA, Larson DB, Wilson WP: Religious life of narcotics addicts, *South Med J* 75(10):1166, 1982.
11. Chu C, Klein HE: Psychological and environmental variables in outcome of black schizophrenics, *J Natl Med Assoc* 77:793, 1985.
12. Cochran JK, Begley L, Bock EW: Religiosity and alcohol behavior: an exploration of reference group therapy, *Sociol Forum* 3:256, 1988.
13. Collipp PJ: The efficacy of prayer: a triple blind study, *Med Times* 97(5):201, 1969.
14. Comstock GW, Partridge KB: Church attendance and health, *J Chron Dis* 25:665, 1972.
15. Dossey L: *Healing words,* San Francisco, 1993, Harper.
16. Dwyer JW, Clarke LL, Miller MK: The effect of religious concentration and affiliation on county cancer mortality rates, *J Health Soc Behav* 31:185, 1990.
17. Eccles J: The human person in its two-way relationship to the brain. In Morris JD, Roll WG, Morris RL, editors: *Research in parapsychology,* Metuchen, NJ, 1976, Scarecrow Press.
18. Elkins D, Anchor KN, Sandler HM: Relaxation training and prayer behavior as tension reduction techniques, *Behav Engl* 5:81, 1979.
19. Ellis JB, Smith PC: Spiritual well-being, social desirability, and reasons for living: is there a connection? *Int J Soc Psychiatry* 37(1):57, 1991.
20. Finney JR, Malony HN: An empirical study of contemplative prayer as an adjunct to psychotherapy, *J Psychol Theol* 13:284, 1985.
21. Frankel BG, Hewitt WE: Religion and well-being among Canadian university students: the role of faith groups on campus, *J Sci Study Religion* 33(1):62, 1994.
22. Gallup Organization: Gallup Report No. 236. *Religion in America,* Princeton, 1985, The Gallup Organization.
23. Gartner J, Larson DB, Allen GD et al: Religious commitment and mental health: a review of the empirical literature, *J Psychol Theol* 19:6, 1991.
24. Gorsuch RL, Butler MC: Initial drug abuse: a view of predisposing social psychological factors, *Psychol Bull* 3:120, 1976.
25. Grad B: *A telekinetic effect on plant growth. III. Stimulating and inhibiting effects.* Research brief presented to the Seventh Annual Convention of the Parapsychological Association, Oxford University, 1964.
26. Grad B, Cadoret RJ, Paul GI: The influence of an unorthodox method of treatment on wound healing in mice, *Int J Parapsychol* 3:5, 1961.
27. Grad B: Some biological effects of laying-on of hands: a review of experiments with animals and plants, *J Am Soc Psychical Res* 59:95, 1965.
28. Griffith EE, Mahy GE, Young JL: Psychological benefits of spiritual Baptist "mourning," II: an empirical assessment, *Am J Psychiatry* 143:226, 1986.
29. Hadaway CK, Roof WC: Religious commitment and the quality of life in American society, *Rev Religious Res* 19(3):295, 1978.
30. Hannay DR: Religion and health, *Soc Sci Med* 14A:683, 1980.
31. Hertsgaard D, Light H: Anxiety, depression, and hostility in rural women, *Psychol Rep* 55:673, 1984.
32. House JS, Robbins C, Metzner HL: The association of social relationships and activities with mortality: prospective evidence from the Tecumseh community health study, *Am J Epidemiol* 114, 1984.
33. Idler EL, Kasl SV: Religion, disability, depression, and the timing of death, *Am J Sociol* 97(4):1052, 1992.
34. Idler EL, Kasl SV: Religious involvement and the health of the elderly, *Soc Forces* 66:226, 1992.
35. Idler EL: Religious involvement and the health of the elderly: some hypotheses and an initial test, *Soc Forces* 66:226, 1987.
36. Jarvis GK, Northcutt HC: Religious differences in morbidity and mortality, *Soc Sci Med* 25:813, 1987.
37. Joyce CRB, Welldon MC: The objective efficacy of prayer: a double-blind clinical trial, *J Chron Dis* 18:367, 1965.
38. Katkin S, Zimmerman V, Rosenthal J, Ginsberg M: Using volunteer therapists to reduce hospital readmissions, *Hosp Community Psychiatry* 26:151, 1975.
39. Koenig HG, Cohen HJ, Blazer DG et al: Religious coping and depression among elderly hospitalized medically ill men, *Am J Psychiatry* 149(12):1693, 1992.
40. Koenig HG, George LK, Meador KG et al: Religious practices and alcoholism in a southern adult population, *Hosp Community Psychiatry* 45(3):225, 1994.
41. Koenig HG, Kvale JN, Ferrell C: Religion and well-being in later life, *Gerontologist* 28:18, 1988.
42. Larson DB, Koenig HG, Kaplan BH et al: The impact of religion on men's blood pressure, *J Religion Health* 28:265, 1989.
43. Larson DB, Pattison EM, Blazer DG, Omran AR, Kaplan BH: Systematic analysis of research on religious variables in four major psychiatric journals, 1978-1982, *Am J Psychiatry* 143:329, 1986.
44. Larson DB, Wilson WP: Religious life of alcoholics, *South Med J* 73:723, 1980.
45. Lawlis GF: *Transpersonal medicine,* Willitis, CA, 1996, Shambhala.
46. Lawlis GF, Selby D, Hinnant G, McCoy E: Reduction of postoperative pain parameters by presurgical relaxation instructions for spinal pain patients, *Spine* 10:163, 1985.
47. Lawlis GF: *The four relationship factor questionnaire,* Wichita, KS, 1974, Test Systems.
48. Levin JS: How religion influences morbidity and health: reflections on natural history, salutogenesis and host resistance, *Soc Sci Med* 43:849, 1996.
49. Levin JS: Religious research in gerontology, 1980-1994, *J Religious Gerontol,* manuscript submitted for publication, 1999.
50. Levin JS, Schiller PI: Is there a religious factor in health? *J Religion Health* 26:9, 1987.
51. Levin JS, Vanderpool HY: Is religion therapeutically significant for hypertension? *Soc Sci Med* 29:69, 1989.
52. Lindenthal JJ, Myers JK, Pepper MK, Stern MS: Mental status and religious behavior, *J Sci Study Religion* 9:143, 1970.
53. Lock BR, Hughes RH: Religion and youth substance abuse, *J Religion Health* 24(3):197, 1985.
54. Mayo CC, Puryear HB, Richeck HG: MMPI correlates of religiousness in late adolescent college students, *J Nerv Ment Dis* 149:381, 1969.
55. McClure RF, Loden M: Religious activity, denomination, membership, and life satisfaction, *Psychol Q J Hum Behav* 19:13, 1982.

56. Morris PA: The effect of pilgrimage on anxiety, depression, and religious attitude, *Psychol Med* 12:226, 1982.

57. Nash CB: Psychokinetic control of bacterial growth, *J Aican Soc Psychical Res* 51:217, 1982.

58. Nash CB: Test of psychokinetic control of bacteria mutation, *J Am Soc Psychical Res* 78(2):145, 1984.

59. O'Brien ME: Religious faith and adjustment to long-term hemodialysis, *J Religion Health* 21(1):68, 1982.

60. Oleckno WA, Blacconiere MA: Relationship of religiosity to wellness and other health related behaviors and outcomes, *Psychol Rep* 68:819, 1991.

61. O'Regan B, Hirshberg C: *Spontaneous remission,* Sausalito, CA, 1993, Institute of Noetic Sciences.

62. Oxman TE, Freeman DH, Manheimer ED: Lack of social participation or religious strength or comfort as risk factors for death after cardiac surgery in elderly, *Psychosom Med* 57:5, 1995.

63. Parker WR, St Johns S: *Prayer can change your life,* New York, 1957, Prentice Hall Press.

64. Peavey B, Lawlis GF, Govern A: Biofeedback-assisted relaxation: effect of phagocytic capacity, *Biofeedback Self Regul* 10:33, 1985.

65. Poloma MM, Pendleton BF: Religious domains and general well being, *Soc Indicators Res* 22:255, 1990.

66. Pressman P, Lyons JS, Larson DB, Strain JS: Religious belief, depression, and ambulation status in elderly women with broken hips, *Am J Psychiatry* 147:758, 1990.

67. Probst LR, Ostrom R, Watkins P, Dean T, Mashburn D: Comparative efficacy of religious and non-religious cognitive-behavioral therapy for the treatment of clinical depression in religious individuals, *J Consult Clin Psychol* 60:94, 1992.

68. Richmond N: Two series of PK tests on paramecia, *J Am Soc Psychical Res* 36:577, 1953; (b) Pleass CM, Dey ND: Using the Doppler effect to study behavioral responses of motile algae to psi stimulus, Parapsychological Association, Presented Papers 3673, 1985; (c) Metta L: Psychokinesis on lepidopterous larvae, *J Parapsychol* 36:213, 1972.

69. Salmon P: Psychological factors in surgical stress: implications for management, *Clin Psychol Rev* 12(7):45, 1992.

70. Sheehan W, Kroll J: Psychiatric patients belief in general health factors and sin as causes of illness. *Am J Psychiatry* 147:112, 1990.

71. Sicher F, Targ E, Moore D, Smith H: A randomized double-blind study of the effect of distant healing in a population with advanced AIDS, *West J Med* 169:356, 1998.

72. Solfvin GF: Psi expectancy effects in psychic healing studies with malarial mice, *Eur J Parapsychol* 4(2):160, 1982.

73. Stack S: The effect of religious commitment on suicide: a cross-national analysis, *J Health Soc Behav* 24:362, 1983.

74. Stark R: Psychopathology and religious commitment, *Rev Religious Res* 12:165, 1971.

75. Tedder W, Monty M: Exploration of long-distance PK: a conceptual replication of the influence on a biological system, *Res Parapsychol* 90, 1980.

76. Troyer, H: Review of cancer among 4 religious sects: evidence that life-styles are distinctive sets of risk factors, *Soc Sci Med* 26:1007, 1988.

77. Van Reek J, Drop MJ: Cigarette smoking in the USA. Sociocultural influences, *Revue D Epidemiol Sante Publique* (Paris) 34(3):168, 1986.

78. Watkins GK, Watkins AM: Possible PK influence on the resuscitation of anesthetized mice, *J Parapsychol* 35(4):257, 1971; (b) Watkins GK, Watkins AM, Wells RA: Further studies on the resuscitation of anesthetized mice, *Res Parapsychol* 157, 1973; (c) Wells R, Klein J: A replication of a psychic healing paradigm, *J Parapsychol* 6:144, 1972; (d) Wells R, Watkins G: Linger effects in several PK experiments, *Res Parapsychol* 143, 1974.

79. Witter RA, Stock RA, Okun MA, Haring MJ: Religion and subjective well-being in adulthood: a quantitative synthesis, *Rev Religious* Res 26:332, 1985.

80. Zuckerman DM, Kasl SV, Ostfield AM: Psychological predictors of mortality among elderly poor, *Am J Epidemiol* 119:410, 1984.

18

Therapeutic Touch: Healing with Energy

Lyn Freeman

WHY READ THIS CHAPTER?

Over the past 25 years, Dolores Krieger, the developer of therapeutic touch, has personally taught the energy technique to more than 48,000 health professionals. Estimates of the total number of persons that have learned therapeutic touch now exceed 85,000, and therapeutic touch is practiced worldwide in more than 75 countries. Therapeutic touch is used in hospital settings, private practices, hospices, and home-care settings.

Case study and clinical trials report positive outcomes with the use of therapeutic touch. Nonetheless, like many forms of energy medicine, its theory, practice, and benefits have been strongly challenged by individuals in the medical establishment. The reader is encouraged to review the history, philosophy, hypothesized mechanisms, and clinical outcomes of therapeutic touch and judge for him or herself.

CHAPTER AT A GLANCE

Therapeutic touch is defined as an intentionally directed process of energy modulation during which the practitioner uses the hands as a focus to facilitate healing.

Therapeutic touch is explained in the theoretical framework of Roger's "Theory of Unitary Man." The theory states that all persons are highly complex fields of life energy. Further, these fields of energy are coextensive with the universe and are in constant interaction and exchange with surrounding energy fields, including the human energy field. As the developer of therapeutic touch, Dr. Krieger hypothesized that by interacting with and modulating these energy fields, individuals can produce a healing effect. She further postulated that this healing capacity is a natural human potential that can be learned.

Reported physiologic effects of therapeutic touch include deep relaxation and facilitation of the healing process. Clinical trials of the effects of therapeutic touch have demonstrated reductions of anxiety and pain, increased speed of wound healing, and immune modulation.

> *Health is a state of complete physical, mental, and social well-being, and not merely the absence of disease or infirmity.*
>
> CONSTITUTION OF THE WORLD HEALTH ORGANIZATION

CHAPTER OBJECTIVES

1. Define therapeutic touch.
2. Explain the operational steps required to practice therapeutic touch.
3. Discuss the history and development of therapeutic touch.
4. Elucidate Roger's "Theory of Unitary Man."
5. Discuss the article in the Journal of the American Medical Association (JAMA) that challenged the underlying theory of therapeutic touch.
6. List the physiologic effects documented from studies on therapeutic touch.
7. Describe and evaluate the clinical trials on therapeutic touch and its effects on anxiety.
8. Describe and evaluate the clinical trials on therapeutic touch and its effects on pain.
9. Describe and evaluate the clinical trials on therapeutic touch and its effects on wound healing and immune function.

■ Therapeutic Touch Defined

Therapeutic touch (TT) is defined as an intentionally directed process of energy modulation during which the practitioner uses the hands as a focus to facilitate healing.[24] This process does not require that the patient consciously participate, nor is its effect dependent on the patient's belief in the intervention. TT may or may not involve contact with the physical body, but contact is **always** made with the energy field of the client.

In TT, a distinction is made between healing and curing. *Curing* is the process of eliminating all signs and symptoms of disease and refers to the disease model of health care. *Healing,* on the other hand, refers to the emergence of right relationship with or among body, mind, and/or spirit; it is about becoming more "whole." Healing refers to a condition of harmony, a state of unity, ordered peace, and connection. Healing may emerge as a relationship between two parts of the physical body, like cells and tissue, or it may emerge as a change in one's relationship with God, self, one's purpose, the planet, or one's relationship with others. Within the context of TT, a terminally ill patient may not be "cured," but he or she can nonetheless experience a healing. TT emphasizes that all healing and curing is ultimately self-healing and self-curing. The health practitioner can only assist in the removal of obstructions to healing and curing.[30] Practitioners of TT are often considered "midwives" of the healing process.

For the TT practitioner, the most important factor in healing is *intentionality.* The intention to heal refers to the compassionate, focused attention of the practitioner toward the patient.

■ Steps Required to Perform Therapeutic Touch

The application of TT requires performing the following operational steps:

1. *The practitioner makes the mental intention to assist the subject and centers him or herself* (i.e., becoming aware of oneself as an open system of energies in constant flux). This first step is often accomplished by the practitioner entering a meditative state of awareness, shifting the focus of attention inward, and finding within oneself an inner reference of stability. The practitioner must become *grounded.*

2. *The practitioner moves the hands over the patient's body, becoming attuned to the condition of the patient and becoming aware of changes in sensory cues via the sensations experienced through the hands.* This second step entails an assessment of the patient's energy field by moving the hands 2 to 4 inches over the patient's body from head to toe. Practitioners may feel tingling, heat, coolness, pressure, rhythm, or lack of rhythm in the field, or they may feel a sense of thickness or thinness. (Note: It is normal that a practitioner may not feel the energy field for a year or more after beginning practice.)

3. *The practitioner clears and mobilizes the energy field.* This third step is accomplished by *unruffling* the patient's energy field in areas that are perceived as nonflowing, that is, sluggish, congested, or static. The practitioner may think "relax" or "smooth" as he or she engages the energy field. The hands move in smooth sweeping motions over the body, 2 to 4 inches from the skin.

4. *The practitioner builds up a localized field between the hands and directs that excess energy through the hands to the patient, applying the energy toward wholeness.* With this fourth step, the practitioner takes the energy from the environment and visualizes it overflowing to the patient.

5. *The practitioner balances the energy field by creating the intention of wholeness and grounding.* In this final step, the practitioner pays special attention to what is happening to the patient. Has the patient had enough? Does he or she feel any discomfort? Is the patient restless?[12,21]

All of these steps are required to adequately practice TT.

■ History of Therapeutic Touch

TT is derived from the ancient practice of laying-on of hands, but it differs in that it is not performed within a religious context nor does it require a professed faith or belief in its efficacy by the practitioner or the patient. Another difference between laying-on of hands and TT is that no direct skin-to-skin contact is required between practitioner and patient. Rather, TT is believed to produce a repatterning of the environmental energy fields of both the practitioner and patient.

In an interview, Dolores Krieger described how she became involved in healing.

"I never thought I would be able to 'heal.' By chance, I was exposed to the research of a religious group called the Layman's Group. These were people from various religions in the New York area—scientists and clergy—who wanted to scientifically test certain biblical statements. They decided that laying-on of hands could be objectively tested, so they brought in many healers and studied what the healers were doing and how their patients were responding."[12]

Dr. Krieger was exposed to the laying-on of hands and to this group of scientists and clergy when she drove her friend, Dora Kunz, to one of their meetings. Dora Kunz was said to possess unusual abilities for perceiving what occurred energetically during the healing process. Dora had studied, since childhood, under the tutelage of Charles W. Leadbeater, a leader and recognized seer in the Theosophical Society.[22]

Oskar Estebany would also have a profound influence on the development of TT. During the 1960s, Bernard Grad, a psychical researcher, published studies of healing experiments with Estebany as his subject. Estebany, a gifted healer, successfully demonstrated increased rates of wound healing in mice and accelerated rates of growth in plants.[9,10]

Estebany became a healer quite by accident. His cavalry horse became ill, and he stayed up one night praying over and stroking the animal. In the morning, the horse was well. Later, the parent of a severely ill child begged Estebany to heal his child. Although Estebany was initially opposed to doing so (he believed he could only heal animals and that it might be sacrilegious to attempt to heal a person), he was persuaded to try. The child recovered completely. After his retirement from the Hungarian Cavalry, Estebany turned his full-time attention to healing with laying-on of hands.

Ms. Kunz and Dr. Krieger, board members of an establishment known as the Pumpkin Hollow Farm, eventually invited Oskar Estebany to work with patients at the Farm. Observing Estebany heal, sometimes for 16 hours a day, led Krieger to conceive a dream of nurse healers who could help the sick. However, before this dream could be realized, Krieger knew that substantive evidence demonstrating the physiologic effects of laying-on of hands was needed. Research was soon underway.

Estebany, along with Dora Kunz and Dr. Krieger, formed the core of a study group on healing. While working with Krieger and others, Estebany successfully demonstrated an elevation of serum hemoglobin in humans and an increase in activity of trypsin in vitro via the laying-on of hands.[18-20,35] It was from this original work that Krieger would later conceptualize and develop TT and postulate its effects as an interaction of energy fields between practitioner and patient.

In the 1970s, the Menninger foundation and the Association for Transpersonal Psychology held a joint conference on human consciousness at Council Grove, Kansas. Researchers on healing consciousness, including Krieger and Kunz, were invited to attend. Dr. Elmer Green of biofeedback fame ran the conference; Krieger, Kunz, and Jack Schwarz, a clairvoyant, were soon recruited for a "spontaneous" research project. They were asked to diagnose medical conditions in persons who were ill. Physicians assessed the accuracy of the diagnoses. Kunz and Schwarz diagnosed with 100% accuracy and Krieger with 80% accuracy—phenomenal rates of success. This experience "awakened" Krieger to the reality of healing.

Krieger realized that other factors, in addition to one's belief system, were significant in the healing that occurred with the laying-on of hands. It was this realization that led Krieger and Kunz to develop TT without religious emphasis.

In 1975, Dr. Krieger realized her original dream when she developed a formal curriculum for graduate level nurses called *Frontiers in Nursing* and began teaching TT at New York University. Nurses working in intensive care units and emergency rooms proved to be most interested in learning the new healing process.[12,21]

■ Philosophic Underpinnings of Therapeutic Touch

TT is based on the philosophy of holism and general systems theory.[3,17] In nursing science, holism is represented by Roger's *Theory of Unitary Man*.[32] This theory states that all persons are highly complex fields of various forms of life energy. These fields of energy are coextensive with the universe and are in constant interaction and exchange with surrounding energy fields. Thus interacting energy fields change each other because of the interaction. It is believed that the practitioner of TT channels life energy through his or her hands to the patient, resulting in a restoration of balance and an increased capacity of the patient to heal him or herself. Essentially, the practitioner serves as a conduit of this energy. The Rogerian methodology encompasses both an assessment phase and intervention phase.

Several individuals have described the philosophy supporting TT. Heidt discusses how all living systems are vibrating fields of energy, sending and receiving information from the environment surrounding them.[4,31,32,36] Through a continuous interchange of their fields, the ill person's energy field tends to become more like that of the healthy person during TT. When field repatterning occurs, the patient's own self-healing mechanisms are stimulated and the ability to regulate the mechanisms in his or her living system is enhanced.[11]

Quinn, quoting Martha Rogers, describes humans as "four-dimensional negentropic energy fields engaged in a continuous, mutual process with the four-dimensional, negentropic environmental energy field."[28] (Negentropic energy refers to that which is available for interactive exchange).

This view of humans and the environment as being inseparable and coextensive with the universe is also the foundation of many Eastern philosophies. During the last 20+ years, physicists have openly supported these age-old assumptions, even borrowing from Eastern terminology to depict a vision of energy.[5,39]

Dr. Krieger believed that the capacity to heal is a natural human potential that can be learned. There are two factors that are primary to the practice of TT: (1) focused intention to heal, and (2) transference of energy from healer to subject.[21] To date, this energy field has not been adequately identified nor has the energy hypotheses been tested directly. Quinn, a leading researcher in the field of TT, acknowledges that the energy field has not been demonstrated by standard scientific techniques. She also recognizes that empirical testing of TT as a treatment modality based in energy fields awaits the development of innovative design and measurement methods.[27]

In 1982, Janet Quinn advanced TT an additional step by taking the theoretical principle behind TT—an interaction of energy fields—and demonstrating that physical contact is not necessary for the healing effect to occur.[29] Thereafter, studies of TT were often conducted without touch and were sometimes compared with casual touch as a control treatment.

■ Response from the Traditional Medical Community

The theoretical underpinnings of TT have fueled comment from many detractors who believe that the foundation of TT is not scientific or provable. The response to the growing acceptance and use of TT in medical settings has led to serious challenges from some components of the medical community. The best-known and most publicized example of this challenge was a study by a 9-year-old girl (Emma Rosa), published in 1998 by the bulwark of the medical establishment, *JAMA*. In this reported investigation, 22 practitioners with 1 to 27 years of experience with TT were tested under blinded conditions to determine whether they could correctly identify which of their hands were closest to the investigator's hand. The flip of a coin determined the placement of the investigator's hand.[33] In this investigation, 14 practitioners were tested 10 times each, and 7 practitioners were tested 20 times each. The practitioners were asked to state whether the investigator's hand hovered around their right or left hand. The authors stated that to validate the theory of TT, the practitioners should be able to locate the investigator's hand 100% of the time. The results of the study were that TT practitioners identified the correct hand 44% of the time—no better than random chance. The authors concluded that the failure of this study to "substantiate TT's most fundamental claim (that the energy field can be felt) was unrefuted evidence that the claims of TT are groundless and that further professional use is unjustified."

To maintain scientific rigor, no one study is ever accepted as "unrefuted evidence" that the claims of any discipline are groundless. A considerable body of literature is required to draw such conclusions or refutations. When the authors of the *JAMA* article extrapolated the findings of this study to conclude "further professional use [of TT] is unjustified," their credibility and objectivity became questionable. Linda Rosa, mother of the 9-year-old Emily, represented the Questionable Nurse Practices Task Force and the National Council Against Health Fraud, Inc., a group outspoken for its opposition to TT. The 9-year-old Emily tabulated the original findings. The study itself was methodologically flawed, with small numbers of subjects, and the study tested TT intervention outside its healing context. Although this study is of interest, its greatest value may be as one of the preeminent examples of the tension existing between complementary medicine (in this case, TT) and traditional medicine.

■ Physiologic Effects of Therapeutic Touch

Although the mechanisms by which TT "works" have not been adequately assessed, physiologic effects have been attributed to the TT experience. The major effects of TT are reported to be (1) deep relaxation and a reduction in anxiety, (2) reduction of pain, and (3) facilitation of the healing process. Laboratory experimentation on TT found that it induces a state of physiologic relaxation. In one study, the TT practitioner and receivers of TT were monitored for 2 consecutive days. Electroencephalographic (EEG) and electromyographic (EMG) studies, galvanic skin response (GSR), temperature, heart rate indexes, and self-reports indicated that subjects were in a relaxed condition with a high abundance of large amplitude alpha activity in both eyes-open and eyes-closed states.[16] One TT healer (Krieger) was studied for 2 days, alone and with three patients. EEG and electrocardiogram (ECG) readings, GSRs, and temperatures were recorded. The essential finding was a preponderance of fast beta EEG activity present in the healer (Krieger).[1]

Although meditation is typically thought to produce low arousal, alpha-theta patterns, this is not always the case. The activity produced depends on the style of the meditator and the type of meditation practiced. Some authors have observed an enhancement of synchronous beta EEG patterns in advanced meditators.[2,6,26] The authors of the study using Dr. Krieger as the subject concluded that EEG findings were on a continuum, with one endpoint being alpha-theta and the other fast beta. TT, they concluded, is a form of meditation that functions on the beta end of the meditative continuum. By contrast, the three patients to whom Dr. Krieger provided TT treatments demonstrated a relaxed state with an abundance of large amplitude alpha activity, both with eyes closed and open; they also reported that the process induced a feeling of relaxation. Earlier research by Krieger also demonstrated increased hemoglobin levels in subjects after TT intervention.[18]

■ Clinical Trials of Therapeutic Touch Efficacy

The lion's share of the literature has tested the effectiveness of TT to modulate anxiety and pain. A few studies have tested TT's effects on wound healing and immune function. The following text reviews this literature and its demonstrated outcomes.

Therapeutic Touch as Treatment for Anxiety

The two landmark studies of TT for the treatment of anxiety in patients with cardiovascular disease were performed by Heidt and Quinn.[11,28] Quinn compared TT with placebo therapeutic touch (PTT), the process of mimicking the hand actions of a TT practitioner but without centering or the application of intentionality. Rather, PTT was performed while subtracting backwards by 7s from 100 to prevent accidental centering or intentionality. Quinn found that postanxiety scores were significantly reduced in patients treated by noncontact TT but not by PTT.

Heidt compared TT with a casual touch group (e.g., pulse taken at the wrists and in the feet) and with a no-touch control group (e.g., nurse seated beside patient asking questions but without touching). Heidt found that TT significantly reduced state anxiety, preintervention to postintervention, as compared with both casual touch and no-touch groups.

Other researchers have explored the effects of TT for treatment of anxiety in adult psychiatric inpatients and in persons facing stressful examinations or presentations. Olson and Sneed divided students into categories of stress (e.g., high anxiety, low-to-moderate anxiety) and compared TT with quiet time. In the high-anxiety group, but not the low-to-moderate anxiety group, TT reduced anxiety more than quiet time.[25]

Gagne and Toye compared the efficacy of TT with relaxation therapy and with PTT in a psychiatric inpatient population. Both relaxation therapy and "real" TT significantly reduced anxiety, but TT was more effective in reducing anxiety than relaxation therapy.

Two studies have been performed on the effects of TT with anxious children. Kramer compared TT with casual touch in 2-week-old to 2-year-old children hospitalized for injury, acute illness, or surgery. Outcomes were measured using biofeedback equipment.[15] TT was demonstrated more effective in reducing anxiety as assessed by pulse, skin temperature, and GSR. Kramer's findings were weakened because she failed to report random group assignment, the number of children per group, or what constituted stress behaviors.

Ireland compared TT with mimic TT (MTT) as a treatment for anxiety in a study of 20 6- to 12-year-old children with human immunodeficiency viral (HIV) infection. The TT intervention lowered mean anxiety scores, whereas MTT did not[13] (Table 18-1).

Although most of these studies were well-designed, the authors found that subject numbers ranging from 60 to 152 would be required to assess differences accurately. The use of larger subject numbers and replication of these studies would further increase scientific credibility of TT as an intervention for anxiety.

Therapeutic Touch as Pain Intervention

TT has been assessed for its capacity to reduce pain of osteoarthritis, tension headache, burns, and surgery (Table 18-2).

Gordon and others assessed the efficacy of TT to reduce pain and increase activity levels of patients with osteoarthritis of the knee. They compared (1) a combination of standard care and TT, (2) a combination of standard care and mock TT,

TABLE 18-1	Effects of Therapeutic Touch on Anxiety		
AUTHOR(S)	**TREATMENT AND CONTROL GROUPS**	**NUMBER**	**OUTCOMES**
Olson M, Sneed N: Anxiety and therapeutic touch, *Issues Ment Health Nurs* 16:97, 1995.	(1) High anxiety with TT (2) High anxiety without TT, but sitting quietly, 15 min without TT, sitting quietly (3) Low-to-moderate anxiety (4) Low-to-moderate anxiety without TT sitting quietly, 15 min	40	Subjects were caregivers and students TT administered 3 days before examination, paper, or presentation No significant difference was found among groups with TT POMS, state/trait anxiety, or visual analog scale Sample size precluded significant differences; authors concluded 152 subjects would be needed to identify differences Reduction of anxiety for high-anxiety group was greater with TT than for high-anxiety subjects not receiving TT
Quinn JF: Therapeutic touch as energy exchange: testing the theory, *Adv Nurs Sci* 6(2):42, 1984.	(1) Noncontact TT (2) PTT	60	Subjects were hospitalized cardiovascular patients Placebo TT involved mimicking the hand actions of TT but not centering and subtracting by 7s from 100 After-test anxiety scores were significantly reduced in those treated by noncontact TT, but not PTT (p<0.0005)
Gagne D, Toye RC: The effects of therapeutic touch and relaxation therapy in reducing anxiety, *Arch Psychiatr Nurs* 8(3):184, 1984.	(1) TT (2) Relaxation therapy (3) PTT	31	Patients were Veteran Administration psychiatric inpatients TT reduced state anxiety significantly (p<0.001), as did relaxation therapy (p<0.01) Movement was significantly quieted by relaxation therapy (p<0.001) Expectation did not correlate with outcome Authors concluded that both TT and relaxation therapy are beneficial for reducing anxiety in psychiatric patients
Kramer NA: Comparison of therapeutic touch and casual touch in stress reduction of hospitalized children, *Pediatr Nurs* 16(5):483, 1990.	(1) TT (2) Casual touch	30	Patients were children 2 wks to 2 yrs of age hospitalized for injury, acute illness, or surgery Stress reduction was measured by pulse, skin temperature, and GSR as measured by biofeedback instrument Casual touch meant stroking the child Results were measured at 3- and 6-min intervals Measurement demonstrated a significant difference, favoring TT (p<0.05) for 3- and 6-min intervals
Heidt P: Effect of therapeutic touch on anxiety level of hospitalized patients, *Nurs Res* 30(1):32, 1981.	(1) TT (2) Casual touch (3) No touch	90	Patients were hospitalized in a cardiovascular unit Subjects who received TT experienced a highly significant reduction in state anxiety preintervention to postintervention (p<0.001) TT subjects also had a significantly greater reduction in posttest anxiety scores as compared with casual touch or no touch
Ireland M: Therapeutic touch with HIV-infected children: a pilot study, *J Assoc Nurs AIDS Care* 9(4):68, 1998.	(1) TT (2) MTT	20	Subjects were 20 HIV-infected children, 6 to 12 yrs of age Statistically significant decrements were found in mean before and after test scores between groups, with TT producing significant reductions in anxiety (p<0.01) and MTT producing insignificant changes (p=0.20)

GSR, galvanic skin response; *HIV*, human immunodeficiency virus; *MTT*, mimic therapeutic touch; *POMS*, profile of mood state; *PTT*, placebo therapeutic touch; *TT*, therapeutic touch.

and (3) standard care alone with the TT group.[7] The group treated with a combination of standard care and TT improved significantly more than the other two groups for pain severity, improved function, and general health.

Eckes performed a study in which patients served as their own controls for 4 weeks and then received TT once a week for 6 weeks or practiced progressive muscle relaxation (PMR) once a week for 6 weeks. Study patients were older (55+

| TABLE 18-2 | Effects of Therapeutic Touch on Pain | | |

AUTHOR(S)	TREATMENT AND CONTROL GROUPS	NUMBER	OUTCOMES
Keller E, Bzdek VM: Effects of therapeutic touch on tension headache pain, *Nurs Res* 35(2):101, 1986.	(1) TT (2) PTT	60	Patients suffered from tension headaches 90% of subjects exposed to TT experienced a sustained reduction in headache pain (p<0.0001) An average of 70% pain reduction was sustained over the 4-hr period after TT that was twice the average pain reduction following the PTT (p<0.01) Authors concluded TT has benefit beyond the PTT effect in the treatment of tension headache pain
Meehan TC: Therapeutic touch and postoperative pain: a Rogerian research study, *Nurs Sci Q* 6(2):69, 1993.	(1) TT (2) MTT (3) Narcotic analgesic	108	Patients received abdominal or pelvic surgery; pain was measured 1 hr before and after intervention (TT/MTT) Subjective report of intensity of pain was greater for the TT group than for MTT group; however, this outcome did not reach statistical significance (p<0.06) MTT group experienced no reduction in pain Within the first hour and beyond after intervention, the TT group waited significantly longer before requesting analgesics than the MTT group, suggesting that TT may reduce the need for pain medication (p<0.05) Analgesic reduced pain by 42%, TT by 13%, and MTT not at all Analgesics were the superior pain treatment, followed by TT
Samarel N et al: Effects of dialogue and therapeutic touch on preoperative and postoperative experiences of breast cancer surgery: an exploratory study, *Oncol Nurs Forum* 25(8):1369, 1998.	(1) 10-min TT and 20-min dialog (2) 10-min quiet time and 20-min dialog	31	Patients with positive breast cancer biopsy received intervention 7 days before surgery and 24 hrs after hospital discharge Pain, mood, and anxiety were assessed TT and dialog group had lower preoperative state anxiety than controls (0=0.008) No differences were found for preoperative mood or any postoperative measures Because relative positive mood and low pain scores existed for both groups, authors concluded that both treatments were equally effective for the women subjects

MTT, Mimic therapeutic touch; *PMR,* progressive muscle relaxation; *POMS,* profile of mood state; *PTT,* placebo therapeutic touch; *SC,* standard care; *STT,* sham therapeutic touch; *TT,* therapeutic touch.

years) with degenerative arthritis. Pain and stress levels were significantly reduced as compared with the baseline period for both groups. The PMR group reported lower pain scores than the TT group, although the difference did not reach significance. PMR significantly reduced distress more effectively than TT.[7]

Keller and Bzdek compared TT and PTT as treatment for tension headache pain. In this study, 90% of TT subjects experienced a sustained reduction of pain (e.g., greater than 4 hours), which was twice the average length of pain reduction associated with PTT. The authors concluded that pain reduction associated with TT has benefit beyond the placebo effect.[14]

Meehan compared TT with MTT and a narcotic analgesic for pain after postoperative abdominal or pelvic surgery. Pain reduction was greater for the TT group than for the MTT group, although this difference did not reach statistical significance. TT did significantly reduce the request for analgesics as compared with those receiving MTT. Analgesics were the superior pain treatment, followed by TT.[23]

Samarel compared (1) 10 minutes of TT and 20 minutes of dialog with (2) 10 minutes of quiet time with 20 minutes dialog in a study of patients with positive breast cancer biopsies. Intervention occurred 7 days before surgery and 24 hours after hospital discharge. Pain, mood, and anxiety were assessed before and after surgery. Only anxiety differed between groups, with the TT group significantly reducing anxiety as compared with quiet time. The authors noted that the TT group displayed positive mood and low pain scores; both interventions were determined to be equally effective.[34]

TABLE 18-2	Effects of Therapeutic Touch on Pain—cont'd		
AUTHOR(S)	**TREATMENT AND CONTROL GROUPS**	**NUMBER**	**OUTCOMES**
Gordon A et al: The effects of therapeutic touch on patients with osteoarthritis of the knee, *J Fam Pract* 47(4):271, 1998.	(1) SC with TT (2) SC with MTT (3) SC alone	31	Patients with osteoarthritis of the knee received treatment once a week for 6 weeks or general care TT group improved significantly more than MTT and SC on scores for pain severity, outdoor work, activity level (general, social, away), pain severity, interference, affective distress, punishing response, and life control ($p<0.04$ to 0.0002) Medication changes did not account for these changes No improvement was noted by visual analog scales completed before or after each treatment or in the HAQ, a measure of specific functional disability Authors concluded TT decreased pain, improved function, and general health more than placebo or SC alone
Eckes-Peck SD: The effectiveness of TT for decreasing pain in elders with degenerative arthritis, *J Holistic Nurs* 15(2):176, 1997.	(1) TT (2) PMR	82	Patients were older (age 55+) with degenerative arthritis Subjects served as their own controls for 4 wks and then received 6 treatments at 1-wk intervals Pain intensity was significantly decreased from baseline after 6 treatments ($p<0.001$), as was distress ($p<0.001$) PMR group pain and distress scores were lower than the TT group ($p=0.06$ for pain and $p=0.005$ for distress)
Turner JG et al: The effect of therapeutic touch on pain and anxiety in burn patients, *J Adv Nurs* 28(1):10, 1998.	(1) TT (2) STT	99	Subjects were severe burn patients Subjects received treatment once a day for 5 days Subjects receiving TT reported significantly greater reduction in pain and anxiety than those receiving STT TT group showed a significantly decreased CD8+ lymphocyte concentration There was no significant difference between groups on medication use

Turner and others assessed pain and anxiety in burn patients receiving either TT or sham TT. Patients receiving TT reported significantly greater reduction in pain and anxiety than those receiving sham TT. The TT group also showed a significantly decreased CD8+ lymphocyte concentration and reduced medication use.[37]

It should be noted that TT seems to demonstrate an effect in moderate-to-high anxious subjects; it does not appear to reduce low levels of anxiety in healthy subjects. Essentially, TT does not seem to interfere with what could be described as a normal stress-coping response.

Therapeutic Touch and Wound Healing and Immune Function

The effect of noncontact TT on the rate of surgical wound healing was examined by Wirth in a well-designed, double-blind study.[38] A full thickness skin wound was incised from 44 healthy male subjects on the lateral deltoid region using a skin punch biopsy instrument. The instrument was used because it removed a precise, uniform, circular layer of tissue, allowing for an accurate measurement of wound perimeters. Subjects were assigned to receive TT or no treatment. Incisions were dressed with a gas-permeable dressing that permitted oxygen and carbon dioxide transmission through the material while maintaining fluid impermeability. This type of dressing was important because it maintained the naturally moist environment of the wound and helped prevent the formation of a scab; the wound was also shielded from external fluids and from contaminants. Using a direct tracing method and a digitization system, the wound surface areas were measured on day 0 (the day of incision), day 8, and day 16.

All subjects were told that the wound was being monitored for bioelectrical conductivity of the body. Every subject inserted his arm through a rubberized hole in the wall. On the other side of the wall, those randomized to receive treatment experienced 5 minutes of TT from a trained practitioner with 5 or more years of experience. The control subjects received no treatment.

Results at days 8 and 16 found that treated subjects experienced a significant acceleration in the rate of wound healing, as compared with subjects receiving no treatment. Of the 23 patients who received TT treatment, 13 healed completely by day 16, whereas 0 of the 21 patients who received no treatment were completely healed.

Placebo effects and the possible influences of suggestion and expectation of healing were eliminated by isolating the subjects from the TT practitioner, by blinding the subjects as to the nature of the therapy received, and by using an independent experimenter blinded to the nature of the therapy (Table 18-3).

Twenty-two students facing medical or board examinations who had scored one or more standard deviations above the mean on an anxiety scale were assessed. The week before examinations, the treatment group received three TT sessions; those in the control group did not. Both groups received a standard dose of *Haemophilus* vaccine so that in vivo response to a vaccination could be assessed. The differences between groups were measured on the day before the examination. When compared with the no treatment control group, there were no significant differences in production of antibody titers in response to the vaccine. However, TT subjects produced significantly higher levels of immunoglobulin A and immunoglobulin M but not immunoglobulin G or immunoglobulin subclasses. Apoptosis (i.e., programmed cell death) was found significantly different between groups, but no conclusions were drawn as to the meaning of this finding. TT subjects reported reduced stress after treatment, but not significantly so. The authors concluded that although TT seems to influence immune function, more

TABLE 18-3	**Effects of Therapeutic Touch on Wound Healing and Immune Suppression**		
AUTHOR(S)	**TREATMENT AND CONTROL GROUPS**	**NUMBER**	**OUTCOMES**
Wirth DP: The effect of non-contact therapeutic touch on the healing rate of full thickness dermal wounds, *Subtle Energies* 1(1):1, 1992.	(1) TT (2) No treatment	44	Subjects received incised, full-thickness dermal wounds in the lateral deltoid using a skin punch biopsy; wounds were dressed with gas-permeable dressings Subjects put injured arms through a hole in a door each day for 5 mins Half received TT, half received no treatment All subjects were told they were monitored by a machine TT treated wounds healed significantly faster than untreated wounds, as measured by digitized wound traces (p<0.001 on day 8, p<0.001 on day 16) Complete healing of 13 of 23 treated subjects occurred by day 16 vs 0 of 23 controls
Olson M et al: Stress-induced immunosuppression and therapeutic touch, *Alternative Ther Health* Med 3(1):68, 1997.	(1) TT (2) No treatment	22	Subjects were students facing medical or board examinations who scored one standard deviation above the mean on the anxiety measure STAI The week before examinations, subjects received 3 TT sessions Both groups received a standard dose of Haemophilus vaccine in the upper arm to compare the in-vivo response with a safe vaccine There was no significant difference between groups in titers of antibodies to Haemophilus influenzae However, subjects that received TT produced significantly different levels of IgA and IgM CD25 (mitogen stimulated T lymphocyte function) and IgG levels differed in the expected direction between groups, but not significantly so Apoptosis (programmed cell death) was significantly different between groups, but no conclusions were drawn as to the significance of this finding TT group experienced less stress after treatment, but not significantly so Authors suggested that TT may influence the immune system, but more research with larger group numbers are needed

STAI, State/Trait Anxiety Inventory; *STT*, sham therapeutic touch; *TT*, therapeutic touch.

research was needed to determine the clinical implications of TT as related to immunity and health. The authors noted that the absence of a caring person in the no-treatment control group did not control for the placebo effect from personal interaction. The small sample size may have masked benefits as well.

An Expert Speaks: Dr. Janet Quinn

Dr. Janet Quinn earned a PhD in nursing at New York University. She is Associate Professor at the University of Colorado School of Nursing and a Fellow of the American Academy of Nursing. The Federal Department of Health and Human Services and the Institute of Noetic Sciences have funded her research on TT. She has taught TT to thousands of nurses and other health care professionals around the world and has extensively published texts on TT and healing. Dr. Quinn lectures and consults internationally on mind-body-spirit medicine, TT, caring for the caregiver, healing, and caring. She is also a spiritual director and facilitates spiritual retreats, including those for caregivers and others interested in integrating spirituality with healing work.

Question. How did you become involved with therapeutic touch?

Answer. I became involved with therapeutic touch in 1974 when I was a student working on my master's degree at New York University and took a course from Delores Krieger. This was the first semester that she taught that course. I was very much a skeptic at that time until I had the direct experience of therapeutic touch with her. This was a turning point and a crisis. This meant that I really had to look at my worldview and see that the world was not how I thought it was. This was the beginning of quite a journey.

After that time, I was taking care of my mother who was dying of colon cancer, and I used a lot of therapeutic touch. That was very important in my work, because I decided afterward that it was so important to us that I would do what I could to bring it into the mainstream of nursing. After her death, I returned to graduate school to get a PhD so I could do research to make this happen; and it has happened. I would say that one of the culminating events in this process was the publication of a series of teaching videotapes produced and sponsored by the National League for Nursing. These were designed to teach nurses how to use therapeutic touch for nurses in hospitals and nursing schools. The

National League for Nursing is the national accreditation agency for nursing, so this really demonstrates how this progression of success has happened.

Question. What do you see as the present day applications of the use of therapeutic touch?

Answer. Today, you can see references to therapeutic touch in many textbooks, as this one has been envisioned. It is included in the curriculums of many nursing schools, and there is a nursing diagnosis code related to energy field disturbance that is now used by nurses to prescribe therapeutic touch. In terms of alternative or complementary therapies, it is one of the most integrated approaches, and it is being practiced by people who are already part of the mainstream helping professions. I think that it is really going strong in spite of some negative press and publicity created by people who are critical of all complementary therapies. One of the issues, of course, is that there is no evidence of measurement of a human energy field, and the point that I always want to help people remember is that the lack of a complete explanatory mechanism is a challenge that is faced by all energy medicines. It is not uniquely a therapeutic touch problem, but a problem shared by all of medical science. We give drugs all the time in which we see some evidence of efficacy but for which we have no clear understanding of the mechanisms and linkages involved.

Question. What do you see as the future implications for therapeutic touch?

Answer. We will continue to see issues of the energy field and its measurement being addressed. More studies for efficacy and mechanism will be completed. In terms of the state of the art of science, there is a body of well-controlled studies that demonstrate initial evidence of efficacy, none of which show evidence of harm, all of which need replication, and none of which show mechanism. That is what the overview of the research shows. As research continues to improve in quantity and quality, we will continue to see the easy integration of therapeutic touch into the mainstream. I think that complementary therapies are here to stay. It is no longer a question of *if* but *when* and *how* they will be integrated into our health care systems. For hospitals and clinical settings interested in using energetic medicine, therapeutic touch is a very cost-effective way to start. Because the practitioners are usually nurses salaried by the institutions, it will not cost any more to have these people use therapeutic touch. The institutions do not have to worry about credentialing additional personnel. Nurses are licensed, and therapeutic touch is already part of their practice, so this is a logical place to start. I am very optimistic about therapeutic touch—about the broader category of energy medicine—as part of the future of health care. I think that therapeutic touch has a lot to contribute to that.

■ Suggestions and Cautions When Using Therapeutic Touch

Although TT is considered safe and noninvasive, the following suggestions and cautions are offered by Krieger and others:

- Do not work with pregnant women if you are a novice.
- Do not let hands get too still over the head area. (It is believed this area is particularly sensitive to TT.)
- Do not become attached to outcomes; outcomes belong to the patient.

There are no defined contraindications for using TT. TT should be practiced within the context of the code of ethics of the practitioner's discipline; and the patient's right to refuse any treatment that is not acceptable to them, regardless of reason, must always be respected.

■ Chapter Review

TT as a group of studies has been criticized for the following reasons:

1. Lack of or inappropriate control conditions
2. Principle investigator also functions as practitioner
3. Lack of placebo control
4. Lack of testing against other forms of intervention
5. Lack of theory testing

Although these complaints are valid in many cases, the research in this field exceeds that of the research provided to support many other nursing and medical practices used in everyday medical care. More clinical research is needed to overcome these design shortcomings. Methods for documenting the existence and effect on the human energy field, if forthcoming, will do much to strengthen the theoretical underpinnings of TT. At present, scientists will have to rely on the outcomes from clinically controlled trials. These trials suggest that TT is, indeed, efficacious in the reduction of anxiety and, in some circumstances, effective in reducing pain and speeding wound healing.

CRITICAL THINKING AND CLINICAL APPLICATION EXERCISES

1. What ethical issues must be considered before performing TT on a patient?
2. TT is believed to modulate the human energy field of both the patient and healer. If this theory is correct, are there potential risks for patient or healer? If so, what are the potential risks?
3. Obtain copies of the JAMA study wherein the practitioners' ability to feel the energy field was assessed. Evaluate this study for bias, randomization, statistical analysis, hypothesis testing, conclusions, and other factors related to study integrity. What are the weaknesses of this study? What are its strengths and contributions to the literature?
4. Define Roger's Theory of Unity of Man and contrast this theory to the philosophies underpinning Chinese medicine and Ayurveda.
5. Design a study of TT that addresses (1) practitioner competence, (2) adequate subject size for statistical power, (3) effects of TT on immune function and wound healing, (4) placebo effect, and (5) psychologic effect of performing TT.

Matching Terms and Definitions

Match each numbered definition with the correct term. Place the corresponding letter in the space provided.

a. TT

b. Brain wave activity of patients receiving TT.

c. Frontiers in Nursing

d. Roger's Theory of Unity of Man

e. Dolores Krieger

f. Brain wave activity of Dolores Krieger while practicing TT

g. Postulated factors primary to the practice of TT

h. Dora Kunz

i. Oskar Estebany

j. Anxiety, pain, wound healing

_____ 1. Developer of TT

_____ 2. Intentionally directed process of energy modulation during which the practitioner uses his or her hands as a focus to facilitate healing

_____ 3. Clinical categories reported to be improved by the application of TT

_____ 4. Well-researched healer who affected plant growth and healed animals before becoming a healer for human subjects

_____ 5. Well-known clairvoyant, theosophist, and co-developer of TT

_____ 6. College course developed for nurses

_____ 7. All persons are highly complex fields of life energy that interact and exchange with surrounding energy fields

_____ 8. Focused intention and transfer of energy

_____ 9. High abundance of large amplitude alpha activity with eyes opened or closed

_____10. Preponderance of fast beta activity

References

1. Ancoli S, Porter L: The two endpoints of an EEG continuum of meditation—alpha/theta and fast beta. In Krieger D: *The therapeutic touch: how to use your hands to help or heal,* Englewood Cliff, NJ, 1979, Prentice Hall Press.

2. Banquet JP: Spectral analysis of the EEG in meditation, *Electroencephalogr Clin Neurophysiol* 35:143, 1973.

3. Battista J: The holistic paradigm and general systems theory, *Gen Sys J* 22:65, 1977.

4. Burr HS: *Blueprint for immortality: the electric patterns of life,* London, 1972, Neville Spearman.

5. Capra F: *The tao of physics,* New York, 1977, Bantam Books.

6. Das NN, Gastaut H: Variations de l'activite electrique du cerveau, du coeur et des muscles sequieletttiques au cours de la meditation et de "l'extase" yoguique, *Electroencephalogr Clin Neurophysiol Suppl* 6:211, 1955.

7. Eckes-Peck SD: The effectiveness of therapeutic touch for decreasing pain in elders with degenerative arthritis, *J Holistic Nurs* 15(2):176, 1997.

8. Gordon A, Merenstein JH et al: The effects of therapeutic touch on patients with osteoarthritis of the knee, *J Family Prac* 47(4):271, 1998.

9. Grad B: Some biological effects of the laying on of hands: review of experiments with animals and plants, *J Am Soc Psychical Res* 59:95, 1965.

10. Grad B: Telekinetic effect on plant growth, *Int J Parapsychol* 5:117, 1963.

11. Heidt P: Effect of therapeutic touch on anxiety level of hospitalized patients, *Nurs Res* 30(1):32, 1981.

12. Horrigon B, Krieger D: Healing with therapeutic touch, *Alternative Ther Health Med* 4(1):85, 1998.

13. Ireland M: Therapeutic touch with HIV-infected children: a pilot study, *J Assoc Nurs AIDS Care* 9(4):68, 1998.

14. Keller E, Bzdek VM: Effects of therapeutic touch on tension headache pain, *Nurs Res* 35(2):101, 1986.

15. Kramer NA: Comparison of therapeutic touch and casual touch in stress reduction of hospitalized children, *Pediatr Nurs* 16(5):483, 1990.

16. Krieger D: *Foundation for holistic health nursing practices: the renaissance nurse,* Philadelphia, 1981, Lippincott.

17. Krieger D et al: Therapeutic touch: searching for evidence of physiological change, *Am J Nurs* 79:660, 1979.

18. Krieger D: Healing by the laying on of hands as a facilitator of bioenergetic change: the response of in vivo hemoglobin, *Psychoenergetic Sys* 1:121, 1976.

19. Krieger D: *The relationship of touch with the intent to help or to heal, to subject in vivo hemoglobin values: a study in personalized interaction,* The proceedings of the ninth American Nurses Association Research Conference, New York, 1973, American Nurses Association.

20. Krieger D: The response if in vivo human hemoglobin to an active healing therapy by direct laying on of hands, *Hum Dimens* 1:12, 1972.

21. Krieger D: *The therapeutic touch: how to use your hands to help or to heal,* Englewood Cliffs, 1979, Prentice Hall.

22. Leadbeater CW: *The inner life,* vol II, ed 4, Wheaton, IL, 1967, The Theosophical Publishing House.

23. Meehan TC: Therapeutic touch and postoperative pain: a Rogerian research study, *Nurs Sci Q* 6(2):69, 1993.

24. Mulloney SS, Wells-Federman C: Therapeutic touch: a healing modality, *J Cardiovasc Nurs* 10(3):27, 1996.

25. Olson M, Sneed N: Anxiety and therapeutic touch, *Issues Ment Health Nurs* 16:97, 1995.

26. Peper E, Pollini SJ: *Fast beta activity: recording limitations, problems and subjective reports.* In Proceedings of the Biofeedback Research Society, Colorado Springs, 1976.

27. Quinn JF: Building a body of knowledge: research on therapeutic touch, 1974-1986, *Holistic Nurs* 6:37, 1988.

28. Quinn JF: Therapeutic touch as energy exchange: testing the theory, *Adv Nurs Sci* 6:42, 1984.

29. Quinn J: An investigation of the effects of therapeutic touch done without physical contact on state anxiety of hospitalized cardio-vascular patients, New York, 1982, New York University. (Doctor dissertation)

30. Quinn J: *Therapeutic touch: a video course for health-care professionals. Part I: theory and research,* New York, 1996, National League for Nursing.

31. Ravitz LJ: Electromagnetic field monitoring of changing state-function including hypnotic states, *J Am Soc Psychosom Dent Med* 17(4):119, 1970.

32. Rogers ME: *Introduction to the theoretical basis of nursing,* Philadelphia, 1970, FA Davis.

33. Rosa L, Rose E, Sarner L, Barrett S: A close look at therapeutic touch, *JAMA* 279(13):1005, 1998.

34. Samarel N, Fawcett J et al: Effects on dialogue and therapeutic touch on preoperative and postoperative experiences of breast cancer surgery: an exploratory study, *Oncol Nurs Forum* 28(8):1369, 1998.

35. Smith MJ: Paranormal effects on enzyme activity, *Hum Dimens* 1:12, 1973.

36. Tiller WA: New fields, new laws. In White J, Krippner S, editors: *Future science,* Garden City, NY, 1977, Doubleday.

37. Turner JG, Clark AJ, Gauthier DK, Williams M: The effect of therapeutic touch on pain and anxiety in burn patients, *J Adv Nurs* 28(1):10, 1998.

38. Wirth DP: The effect of non-contact therapeutic touch on the healing rate of full thickness dermal wounds, *Subtle Energies* 1(1):1, 1992.

39. Zukav G: *The dancing wu li masters: an overview of the new physics,* New York, 1979, William Morrow.

Appendix A: Program Research Evaluation: Methods and Statistical Overview

What methods demonstrate effectiveness (or ineffectiveness) of an alternative therapy program?

In many ways, the evaluation of an alternative therapy is one of the most interesting issues of program analysis because of the nature of the design of the program. It is interesting to begin the evaluation of a program by asking each of the principal therapy participants the actual goals of the program and by determining a consensus. Too many times, there is great variance in the program administration's perception of the outcome goals and the perceptions of the practitioners.

For example, in one evaluation in Arkansas, it was observed that the director, who wrote the grant for the program, had clear objectives for improving the quality of health in patients with cancer, specifically in the areas of reducing anxiety and depression. In contrast, the therapists collectively reported that the program outcome should improve family relations, which often revealed family dysfunction and exacerbated anxiety and depression.

Although outcome criteria (e.g., pain reduction, vocational rehabilitation) are usually clear in the design of the program, many features cannot be measured and easily assessed at exit times. Beyond the obvious, some of the most widely used outcome criteria are the following:

1. Energy and activity levels
2. Functional abilities
3. Sleep and eating behaviors
4. Disease symptoms
5. Health status
6. Satisfaction with health (or health service delivery)
7. Sex life
8. Well-being
9. Psychologic effect (i.e., increased positive features, such as self-esteem, self control and/or decreased negative features, such as anxiety, stress)
10. Life satisfaction
11. Happiness
12. Ability to work
13. Employment status
14. Economic parameters (e.g., cost-effectiveness, cost minimization)

Economic Evaluation

Since many managed care organizations and insurance companies are now considering a range of therapies with varying costs and benefits, economic analyses are becoming a common feature not only with programs but with individual practitioners as well. Even the Food and Drug Administration (FDA) is unlikely to be the agency responsible for assuring cost-effectiveness, because this responsibility could potentially confuse the FDA's mandate of safety and efficacy. Many reasons underlie the current force to conduct economic analyses.

Such studies can be conducted from the perspectives of society as a whole, the payer, the provider, and the patient. These perspectives determine the types of costs and consequences included in the evaluation.

There are four basic types of economic approaches currently used in the market: *cost minimization, cost effectiveness, cost utility,* and *cost benefit.* Although the programs are not compared directly with concurrent ones, historical data are often used as standards. For example, many programs have conducted economic analyses for patients with back pain, comparing the costs of surgery and vocational rehabilitation if patients choose the route of aggressive surgery, as compared with the clinical costs of a more conservative approach.

Cost-minimization analyses are those variables that demonstrate that a program can reduce the costs of treatment, if one assumes that the health outcomes would be the same as a more aggressive and costly approaches. In the example of pain clinics, one could assume the probabilities of health consequences (from surveys reporting frequencies of return-to-work and reduction of pain), thereby offering some assurances of reduced costs to the insurance carrier. Cost-minimization approach is most common for pain clinics.

Cost-effectiveness analyses are based on a more sophisticated methodology. Some form of unit is designed for measurement, creating a natural gradient of quantitative result. Examples of natural units may include the number of cases successfully diagnosed, years of life or work life gained, reduction of pain units (on an analogue scale), and reduction of drug use. In general, these types of analyses are the most common, because they permit cost comparisons based on common health quantifiable measures without resorting to quality of care.

Cost-utility analysis is a controversial economic measure in which a Quality Adjusted Life Year (QALY) is determined. A QALY is the time period in a given health state that is deemed equivalent to 1 year of perfect health, similar to a ratio of bad health to good health, using good health as a constant. The intention is to provide a unit of quantity combined with quality. However, from studies by the author [GFL], this method has poor interrater reliability; and when time is used as a part of judgment, validity suffers. There are instruments that provide greater accuracy to determine quality of life. The author has also discovered major cultural differences with respect to time perception, especially as a part of disease process.

In *cost-benefit analyses,* all outcomes and therapies are expressed in monetary units, such as discounted future earnings capacities or willingness to pay for improved safety or decreased health risk. In a cost-benefit analysis, the net benefit is the result when costs can be subtracted from benefits. Obviously, the major issue is to translate health factors (e.g., pleasure, pain, nausea) into dollars, because people are accustomed to this unit of measure. Cost-benefit analysis is common in safety programs and environmental studies.

Research Methodology

As a general process, the field of medical research is typically a set pattern, especially as it applies to the use of drugs that may harm. Three phases must be followed to ensure a safe research protocol. *Phase I research* tests for safety and probably uses the safest group—animals or healthy humans. Levels of toxicity and side effects are the greatest concerns in this level. *Phase II research* usually refers to the use of the therapy or drug for people with the condition for which it was designed to help. Since control groups are often not used, many program evaluations could be classified under these efforts. Efficacy of usage for a determined problem is assessed. *Phase III research* assesses efficacy, safety, and dosage, especially in comparison with standard practices. Control and comparison groups are used to determine relative effectiveness to standard care. Alternative therapies research should embrace the control model of research to achieve the objectives of professional acceptance into the literature.

In contrast to program evaluation, research methodology is more concerned with comparison with other factors, attempting to hold all conditions constant except for the experimental condition. In some ways, programs can be placed into a research methodology by establishing controls. For example, Dr. Dean Ornish's cardiovascular program was compared with a group of patients with equal severity of heart disease, and measures of artery disease were used as the *dependent variable.*

The quality of the research design depends upon the control of extraneous variances that might account for the results of the experiment. Keeping in mind that the perfect experiment has yet to be performed, the following methods have been used as the "gold standard" quality research that are most highly respected in the industry.

Control or Comparison Groups

To demonstrate that a therapy or drug has merit, a comparison is made with another treatment, preferably a traditional standard or *no-treatment* condition. Unfortunately, there are always controversies surrounding a control group, since they can never be perfectly comparable with the experimental group. Nevertheless, in most research studies the control group is treated at the same time and in the same ways, except for the experimental variable. In the most sophisticated designs, the participant does not know which group he or she is assigned (*single blind*), the researcher does not know which group the patient is assigned (*double blind*), and the person who is measuring the change (e.g., laboratory technician) does not know the group membership (*triple blind*), thereby eliminating expectations or unconscious cues.

Sometimes a placebo condition is designed to replace the "missing" experimental influence in the experimental groups, creating a closer likelihood that all participants will feel the same about the procedures. A *placebo treatment* is one in which the participants are given a treatment that has the expectation of positive response but has no ingredients that would actually produce effects. For example, some researchers have used a sugar pill that looks like the active treatment. The instructions are given with the same expectations. (In fact, in triple-blind studies, the researcher may not know at that time which is the active treatment). The results of responses to the placebo supposedly purport to measure expectation. However, it has been pointed out that placebos often simulate the bodyís responses via imagery and serve to actualize a body-mind curative reaction.

Various strategies have been used to produce equivalent groups to study, but all have problems. The major concern is for the groups to look alike, and two basic methods have been used—randomization and matching. The *randomization approach* is superior because it assumes that if a researcher randomly assigns each subject to one group, all the characteristics of error will be equally distributed, thereby meeting an implicit assumption of normalcy. This method would be preferable when the researcher wants a normal distribution and has access to enough subjects for random selection or random assignment. A thousand subjects might be safe for this method. *Matching* subjects on selected characteristics is a more plausible method, especially when there are abnormal conditions, such as disease states. The difficulties with this approach lie in the characteristics being matched (e.g., state of mind, economic levels, gender, culture), because reliance is unknown and variance may overlap.

The control group can serve as its own experimental control in some cases, such as *cross-over designs,* in which a subject will serve under one condition and then under another. *Wait-control groups* have been used in conditions in which a group of participants will be the control group initially and then be crossed over to an experimental condition. Pattern effects and time effects can be confounding.

Reliable and Valid Measures of Change

Human bodies have a tendency to change over time, regardless of what happens to them. This principle applies to attitudes and intellectual consistencies as well. Whether a person is asked the same question twice (e.g., "How do you feel?") or an independent person administers a physical measurement twice (e.g., blood pressure), chances are some change will occur. The most consistent measures are the most reliable measures, because one can be certain that the experimental condition is responsible for the outcome rather than mere

change. The outcome variables noted in program evaluation, such as the economic parameters, have been chosen in this regard to measure effectiveness of therapies and products. This stability to change is referred to as *reliability.*

A good indication of a variable's reliability can be measured by its consistency in other efforts, typically the correlation of the response from one occasion to another. For example, suppose the reliability of blood pressure was 0.80 (which it is not). The statistical prediction would be that a person would be measured at a similar magnitude relative to the norm 64% of the variance (0.80 × 0.80). One could see that even less reliable measures (e.g., number of white blood cells, subjective units of comfort) are problematic to important studies.

Validity of a variable simply means that the variable measures what it is supposed to measure. For example, does temperature rise from normalcy mean disease intensity? Does pain signify time of the pathologic condition? Does a variance in human immunodeficiency virus (HIV) relate to acquired immunodeficiency syndrome (AIDS)? Actually, very few variables have total validity, and the assumptions made about them are from past understandings of behavior and predictions. The validity of a variable is usually associated to the association it has with other understood variables. For example, if blood pressure rises as renal failure is evident, the *correlational coefficient* can label the association (e.g., 0.80).

Statistics

Since few experiments in medicine are conclusive, *probability theory* is frequently employed, which is the use of statistics. Although there are hundreds of approaches that may be applied to a project, the test of probability comes down to two approaches: (1) Are treatments different in outcome? (2) How are two (or more) measures alike? Both outcomes are compared with a randomness distribution. For example, if the experimental group outcome had an average of 50% reduction in pancreatic tumors and the control group had a 10% reduction, would we conclude that these events occurred by chance or were the result of the treatments? If one had the opportunity to run enough studies to calculate this figure using actual data, it would be an appropriate conclusion of how important this outcome was for the effectiveness of the drug or treatment. In a true empirical world, a thousand studies could be conducted that were replicates in every form and could directly assess how many times the outcomes of the studies were the same. However, a theoretical distribution chart is often relied upon for conclusions that may not have anything to do with cancer rates. For example, the *binomial distribution* is based on the probabilities of outcome based on a 50/50 outcome (i.e., flipping a coin). The *chi-square probability* table is based on equal distribution of frequencies among categories. The assumption of the selected probability table can be critical to conclusions reached in studies. In very general terminology, the lower the *probability of chance* (P<0.05), the more confident the researcher can conclude that the results are not random but consistent. The "P" in statistics refers to *probability* and the "<" or "=" is "less than" or "equal to" the number designated. In this case, "P <0.05" would be read that this event would occur in 5% of the time by chance alone; or, the expression "P=0.03" would mean that the event would occur 3% of the time by chance alone. Hopefully, the researcher has articulated the hypothesis of the design to arrive at these conclusions before the results are revealed.

Two errors in statistical conclusions are classical, referred to as *type I and II errors,* or *alpha* or *beta errors. Type I error* occurs when the researcher concludes that the findings are significant when they really are not. The use of the deviation from randomness is the fair test of this error. The deviation of 0.05 from randomness is most common, meaning that if the findings would have happened less than 5% of the time randomly, the conclusions have been tested for type I error. *Type II error* is when the results are deemed not significant when they actually are. The *power* of a statistical test is very important in this decision. Sometimes the result of the small number of subjects or the distribution of the range of measures, a statistical test simply is not sufficiently sensitive to show differences from randomness when they actually are present. The power of a statistical test should be at least 0.80 (0 to 1.00).

For example, the power of using a statistical approach, called a "chi-square," would be 0.70. This procedure is often used when the researcher has small numbers of subjects or limited sophisticated data, such as categories of outcome (e.g., "good" or "bad"). A more sophisticated statistical approach would be an *analysis of variance.* However, to be used for additional power, more numbers of subjects would be required and the higher sophistication of data, such as laboratory test scores would be necessary.

In recent years, there have been many research studies in particular areas using similar methodologies. When enough studies of quality are gathered, a *meta-analysis* can be computed to assess the magnitude of effect across studies. This means that one can statistically account for the sample size of each separate study and average the effect of a specific treatment across studies. However, in some overview of article conclusions, these methods are merely referred to as reviews in which trends are based on outcomes. For example, Christi Pattern and John Martin recently published the article, "Does Nicotine Withdrawal Affect Smoking Cessation? Clinical and Theoretical Issues" in *Annals of Behavioral Medicine* (vol. 18, no. 3, 1996). Over 100 articles were evaluated, and from those conclusions the statement was made that nicotine withdrawal was not a consistent factor in the cessation of smoking behavior.

Confounding Influences

In every study there are always *confounding variables,* those annoying but important influences that must be admitted in honest ways and discussed so that the reader is assured that the researcher was aware of these influences and controlled them as far as possible. For example, no one can control the weather, yet we know that weather conditions can influence the way a person feels on a day-to-day basis. Family crisis, automobile problems, and unknown phobias are other examples of these issues.

Ethics

Gone are the days when the scientist could make judgments solely on the value of the outcomes without regarding the risks or attitudes of the patients. It is now the practice for sponsored research to go through various boards of research behavior before final approval is given. These boards are given the task of determining the risks to the participants and researchers before proceeding. In addition, the boards usually require some type of written consent from the participants, which confirms that they thoroughly understand the risks before administration. These standards should be articulated in the professional codes of ethics for the various disciplines; however, if such a set of principles is not present and required for a professional group, research efforts will be discouraged in established hospitals and clinics.

Appendix B: Answers to Multiple Choice and Matching Questions

Chapter 1
1. p
2. h
3. k
4. e
5. n
6. d
7. r
8. g
9. m
10. s
11. i
12. b
13. v
14. a
15. f
16. q
17. c
18. j
19. t
20. l
21. o
22. u

Chapter 2
Matching
1. c
2. d
3. a
4. b

Multiple choice
1. a, d, e
2. b, c
3. a
4. e
5. a
6. d
7. c
8. g
9. e
10. e

Chapter 3
1. e
2. j
3. g
4. a

5. i
6. b
7. f
8. d
9. h
10. c

Chapter 4
Matching
1. g
2. k
3. j
4. b
5. n
6. d
7. h
8. i
9. o
10. a
11. r
12. p
13. l
14. m
15. q
16. f
17. s
18. e
19. c

Multiple choice
1. a, b, e, f
2. c
3. a, c, d
4. b, c, d

Chapter 5
1. b
2. e
3. h
4. c
5. i
6. d
7. f
8. g
9. a

Chapter 6
1. c, h
2. f
3. e
4. i
5. d
6. g
7. j
8. a
9. b

Chapter 7
No multiple choice or matching

Chapter 8
1. i
2. b
3. k
4. j
5. e
6. h
7. l
8. a
9. g
10. o
11. m
12. d
13. n
14. c
15. f

Chapter 9
1. g
2. e
3. d
4. b
5. c
6. a
7. f

Chapter 10
1. p
2. i
3. r
4. a
5. o
6. b

7. l
8. n
9. e
10. g
11. j
12. b
13. f
14. h
15. k
16. c
17. q
18. m

Chapter 11
1. 1e
2. l
3. a
4. j
5. h
6. d
7. i
8. c
9. g
10. k
11. b
12. f

Chapter 12
1. c
2. i
3. e
4. g
5. f
6. a
7. m
8. b
9. h
10. l
11. d
12. k
13. n
14. j

Chapter 13
1. j
2. a
3. i
4. g

5. c
6. k
7. d
8. e
9. b
10. h
11. f

Chapter 14
1. h
2. f
3. j
4. i
5. b
6. e
7. a
8. d
9. c
10. g

Chapter 15
No multiple choice or matching

Chapter 16
No multiple choice or matching

Chapter 17
No multiple choice or matching

Chapter 18
1. e
2. a
3. j
4. i
5. h
6. c
7. d
8. g
9. b
10. f

Appendix C: Additional Web Sites

National Institutes of Health Office of Dietary Supplements
http://odp.od.nih.gov/ods/

National Institutes of Health Center for Complementary and Alternative Medicine
http://altmed.od.nih.gov/nccam/

Food & Drug Administration (FDA) Special Nutritionals Adverse Event Monitoring System
http://vm.cfsan.fda.gov/-dms/aems.html

Appendix D: Organizations

Acupuncture

The American Academy of Medical Acupuncture (AAMA)
5820 Wilshire Boulevard., Suite 500
Los Angeles, CA 90036
(323) 937-5514
www.medicalacupuncture.org/

American Association of Acupuncture and Oriental Medicine (AAAOM)
433 Front Street
Catasauque, PA 18032
(610) 266-1433
www.aaom.org/

National Commission for the Certification of Acupuncturists (NCCA)
P.O. Box 97075
Washington, D.C. 20090
(202) 232-1404
http://acupuncture.com/tcm
Bioelectromagnetics

National Institute of Environmental Health Sciences (NIEHS)
P.O. Box 12233
Research Triangle Park, NC 27709
(919) 541-3345
www.niehs.nih.gov/

Institute for Frontier Science
6114 La Salle Avenue, P.O. Box 605
Oakland, CA 94611
(510) 531-5767
www.healthworld.com/frontierscience/

Biofeedback

Biofeedback Certification Institute of America
10200 W. 44th Avenue, Suite 310
Wheatridge, CO 80033
(303) 420-2902
www.bcia.org/

Chiropractic

American Chiropractic Association
1701 Clarendon Boulevard
Arlington, VA 22209
(703) 276-8800
www.amerchiro.org/

World Chiropractic Alliance
2950 North Dobson Road, Suite 1
Chandler, AZ 85224
(800) 347-1011
www.chiropage.com

Exercise

The Cooper Institute
600 5th Avenue South, Suite 205
Naples, FL 34102
(941) 261-3290
http://cooperinstitute.org/

Herbs

American Herbalist Guild
P.O. Box 70
Roosevelt, UT 84066
(435) 722-8434
www.healthworld/com/associations/pa/herbal
medicine/ahg/

The Herb Research Foundation
1007 Pearl Street, #200
Boulder, CO 80302
(303) 449-2265
www.healthy.com/herbalist/

American Botanical Council
P.O. Box 144345
Austin, TX 78714-4345
(512) 926-4900
www.herbalgram.org/

Homeopathy

Homeopathic educational Services
2124 Kittridge Stree
Berkeley, CA 94704
(510) 649-0294
www.homeopathic.com/

International Foundation for Homeopathy
P.O. Box 7
Edmonds, WA 98020
(425) 776-4147
www.healthy.net/pan/pa/homeopathic/ifh

National Center for Homeopathy
801 North Fairfax Street
Suite 306
Alexandria, VA 22314
(703) 548-7790
www.homeopathic.org/

Hypnosis

The American Institute of Hypnotherapy
16842 Von Karman #475
Irvine, CA 91724
(800) 634-9766
www.aih.cc/

American Society of Clinical Hypnosis
2200 East Devon Avenue, Suite 291
Des Plaines, IL 60018
(708) 297-3317
www.healthfinder/gov/text/org

International Medical and Dental Hypnotherapy Association
4110 Edgeland, Suite 800
Royal Oak, MI 48073-2285
(800)-257-5467
www.npginc.com/imdha/

Milton H. Erickson Foundation, Inc.
3606 North 24th Street
Phoenix, AZ 85016
(602) 956-6196
www.erickson-foundation.org

The National Guild of Hypnotists
P.O. Box 308
Merrimack, NH 03054-0308
(603) 429-9438
www.ngh.net/

Society for Clinical and Experimental Hypnosis
2201 Haeden Road, Suite 1
Indianap.o.lis, IN 46268
(509) 332-7555

Imagery

The Academy for Guided Imagery
P.O. Box 2070
Mill Valley, CA 94942
(800) 726-2070
www.healthy.net/agi/

Health Associates
22 Calle Alejandra
Santa Fe, NM 87505
(505) 466-1899

Massage

American Massage Therapy Association
820 Davis St., Suite 100
Evanston, IL 60201-4444
(847) 864-0123
www.amtamassage.org/contact/htm

National Certification Board for Therapeutic Massage and Bodywork
8201 Greensboro Drive, Suite 300
McLean, VA 22102
(800) 296-0664
(703)-610-9015
www.ncbtmb.com

Touch Research Institute (Tiffany Field's Organization)
Department of Pediatrics,
University of Miami School of Medicine
P.O. Box 016820
Miami, FL 33101
(305) 243-6790
www.miami.edu/touch-research

Meditation

Center for Mindfulness in Medicine, Health Care and Society
University of Massachusetts Medical Center
419 Belmond Avenue, 2nd floor
Worcester, MA 01604
www.mindfulnesstapes.com/

Transcendental Meditation Program
Maharishi Vedic School
636 Michigan Avenue
Chicago, IL 60605
(312) 431-0110
(808) 532-7686
www.maharishi.org/cgi

Psychoneuroimmunology

Psychoneuroimmunology Research Society
Attn: Virginia M Sanders,
Secretary-Treasurer, PNIRS
Dept. of Cell Biology, Neurobiology & Anatomy

Loyola University Medical Center
2160 S. First Avenue
Maywood, IL 60153
(708) 216-6728
www.PNIRS.org

Therapeutic Touch

Nurse Healers Professional Associates, Inc.
11250-8 Roger Bacon Drive, Suite 8
Reston, VA 20190
(703) 234-4149
www.therapeutic-touch.org/html/

Spiritual Medicine

Institute for Medicine and Prayer
St. Vincent Hospital
455 St. Michael's Drive
Santa Fe, NM 87505
(505) 820 5479

Index

Page number set in italic denotes illustration.
Page number with "t" denotes table.

Hypothalamus
and emotions, 9
and fever, 43
function
in autonomic nervous system, 7–8, *11*
and illustration of, 5, *7*
hormones secreted by, 9–10
illustration of in endocrine system, *374*
responding to fear, 12

I

Idiopathic sclerosis
using biofeedback to treat, 216
Iliotibial tract muscles
anatomic illustration of, *371*
Illness
definition of, 4
religion and recovery from, 473, 474–77
Illness-induced taste-aversion paradigm
conditional response technique, 69–70
Imagery
assessments and diagnoses, 273
categories of, 265–66
definition of, 260, 262
Dr. Jeanne Achterberg on, 280–81
effects on physiology and biochemistry, 266–67
future of, 281
and health, 262–81
helping depression, 270–71
history of, 262–63
and immune cell migration, 272
indications and contraindications for, 280
of mind-body interactions, 264
and music, 21
for pain treatment, 273–74
pervasiveness of, 263–64
physiology and mechanisms of, 263
and placebo effect, 264
preparation for, 279–80
summary of effects, 272–73
as therapy, 273
types of diseases treated with, 264–65, 271–77
Imhotep
using early hypnosis, 228
Immune cells
migration affected by imagery, 271–72
Immune competence
in unhappily married women and men, 113–14
Immune conditioning
Russian experiments on, 68
Immune deficiencies
types of, 35
Immune modulators
description of, 17–18
Immune responses
affected by bereavement, 120–23
of cancer patients, 130
and end-state imagery, 265
illustration of, *47*
studies on couples, 105–7
Immune suppression
loneliness and, 128
Immune suppression function
and stress, 102–3
Immune system
basics of, 39, 40t, 41
biochemical effect of social support on, 102–4
cellular makeup of, 39–54
challenges to disease treatment of, 66
description of, 34
Dr. Candace Pert on, 15–17
effects of
exercise on, 445–46
massage on, 373, *374*

Immune system—cont'd
effects of—cont'd
spiritual intervention on, 484
and electromagnetic medicine, 466
emotional repression of, 24–25
function and illustration of, 5, 8
mind-body interactions within, 5–21
nerve endings, 19–20
receptors of, 16–17
social interaction and, 95, 97–104
stimulation with echinacea, 399
strengthened with vaccines, 349
strengthening with relaxation therapy, 145–46
therapeutic touch to boost, 501–3
Immunity
Solomon and Moos on, 69
Immunocompetence
description of, 19–20
Immunodeficiency assays, 55–59
Immunodeficiency disorders
classifications of, 54–55
Immunodiffusion
radial, 62
Immunoglobulins
function of, 44
homeopathic dillution of, 351
specific immunity function of, 53t
Immunologic competence
measurements of, 54–59
Immunologic reactivity
description of, 20
Immunosuppressant agents, 36
Impotence
Gingko biloba for, 404
In vitro
definition of, 59
In vitro chemotaxis tests, 59
In vitro stimulation
of T-cells, 56–57
Inactivity
risk factor for cardiovascular diseases, 429–30
Incontinence
fecal, 205
treated with EMG biofeedback, 196, 200–201
Incubation
in early Greek hypnosis, 228
India
ancient practices of massage in, 364
Indirect thrust technique
in chiropractic, 297
Induration
following intradermal injections, 55
Industrial toxicology
early papers by Samuel Hahnemann, 347
Infants
massage therapy for, 377–79
Inflammations
feverfew for, 401–2
goldenseal to treat nasal, 408–9
Influenza
echinacea effect on, 400
homeopathic treatment of, 355
Informational substances
description of, 6
Infrared bands
classification in electromagnetic spectrum, 462
Infraspinatus muscles
anatomic illustration of, *371*
Infusion
definition of, 396
Ink blot tests
on benefits of prayer, 480
Insomnia; *See also* sleep
helped with meditation, 174

Inspiration
definition of, 437–38
illustration of mechanics, *437*
Insudation
with atherosclerosis, 429, *430, 431*
Insurance
utilization rates lowered by TM, 175–76
Integumentary system
effects of massage on, 366, *368*
Intentionality
importance of in therapeutic touch, 495
Interferon
as chemical messengers, 20
decline during academic stress, 128
effects of stress on production of, 126
Interleukins
as chemical messengers, 20
Intermittent claudication
Gingko biloba studies on, 406
Interventions
marital, 109
meditation, *177*
model, 91–92
relaxation *versus* meditation, 187–88
stress-management for Alzheimer's caregivers, 118–20
summary of relaxation therapy, 161
Intestinal lining
function and illustration of, 5, *8*
Intestines
nervous system linked to, 294
in Qi meridian system, 311, 315
Intradermal injections
for T-cell assays, 55
Ionizing
definition of, 463
Irritable bowel syndrome (IBS)
hypnosis to treat, 246, 247t
relaxation therapy for, 160
using biofeedback to treat, 216
Ischemia
A.T. Still on, 289
Ischemic reperfusion injury
bilberry for, 396
Islam
spiritual healing, 475
using early forms of hypnosis, 227

J

Jacobson, Edmund
on relaxation therapy, 140–42
Jacobson's Progressive Relaxation Therapy (JPRT)
history and philosophy of, 140–42
introduction to, 138
learning mechanics of, 141–42
Jaundice
milk thistle to treat, 412
Jewish mysticism
early meditation practices, 173–74
Jing, 314
Jobs
loss of
as mortality risk, 34, 38
studies concerning health and, 95, 97
Jogging
combining with meditation, 174
and depression, 446, 447t
Joints
chiropractic work on, 288
Juvenile rheumatoid arthritis
effects of massage on pain of, 375–76

K

Karolinska Institute, 17
"Kava dermopathy," 411